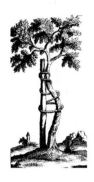

Textbook of Disorders and Injuries of the Musculoskeletal System

Third Edition

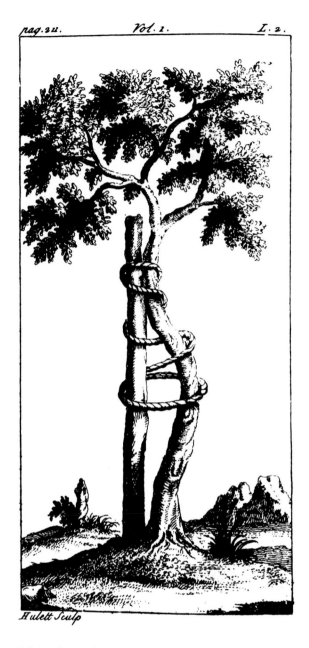

Hulett Sculp

Of Books and Patients

"To study the phenomenon of disease without books is to sail an uncharted sea, while to study books without patients is not to go to sea at all."

Sir William Osler

An Introduction to Orthopaedics, Fractures and Joint Injuries, Rheumatology, Metabolic Bone Disease and Rehabilitation

Textbook of Disorders and Injuries of the Musculoskeletal System

Third Edition

1,360 Illustrations on 860 Figures
670 New References

Robert Bruce Salter

C.C., O. Ont., F.R.S.C., M.D., M.S. (Tor.), F.R.S.C., F.A.C.S., F.H.S.C.
Hon. Dr. Med (Uppsala), Hon. D.Sc. (Memorial and Toronto)
Hon. LL.D. (Dalhousie), Hon. D. Litt.S. (Wycliffe, Toronto)
Hon. F.R.C.P.S. Glasg., Hon. F.R.C.S. Edin., Hon. F.C.S.S.A., S. Africa
Hon. F.R.C.S. Eng., Hon. F.R.A.C.S., Aust., Hon. F.R.C.S. Ire., Hon. M.C.F.P.C.

University Professor Emeritus of the University of Toronto
Professor and Chairman Emeritus of Orthopaedic Surgery, University of Toronto
Faculty, Institute of Medical Science and School of Graduate Studies
Member of the Center for Bioethics, University of Toronto
Senior Orthopaedic Surgeon Emeritus, The Hospital for Sick Children, Toronto
Honorary Consultant in Orthopaedic Surgery, The Hospital for Sick Children
Senior Scientist Emeritus, Research Institute, The Hospital for Sick Children
Consultant, The Orthopaedic and Arthritic Hospital, Toronto
Laureate of the Canadian Medical Hall of Fame

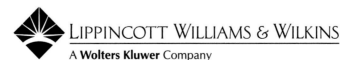

LIPPINCOTT WILLIAMS & WILKINS
A **Wolters Kluwer** Company
Philadelphia · Baltimore · New York · London
Buenos Aires · Hong Kong · Sydney · Tokyo

Editor: Eric P. Johnson
Managing Editor: Linda S. Napora
Marketing Manager: Christine Kushner
Project Editor: Kathleen Gilbert

351 West Camden Street
Baltimore, Maryland 21201-2436 USA

Rose Tree Corporate Center
1400 North Providence Road
Building II, Suite 5025
Media, Pennsylvania 19063-2043 USA

Printed in the United States of America

First Edition, 1970
Reprinted 1971, 1972, 1974, 1975, 1977, 1978, 1979, 1980, 1981, 1982
Second Edition, 1983
Reprinted 1984
Third Edition 1999

Library of Congress Cataloging-in-Publication Data

Salter, Robert Bruce.
    Textbook of disorders and injuries of the musculoskeletal system /
Robert Bruce Salter.—3rd ed.
       p.   cm.
    Includes bibliographical references and index.
    ISBN 13: 978-0-683-07499-4
    ISBN 10: 0-683-07499-7
    1. Musculoskeletal system—Diseases.   2. Musculoskeletal system—
Wounds and injuries.
    [DNLM: 1. Musculoskeletal Diseases.   2. Musculoskeletal System
injuries.   WE 140 S177t y: 1998]
    RC925.S2   1998
    616.7—dc21
    DNLM/DLC
    for Library of Congress   97-42747
                                                                 CIP

The publishers have made every effort to trace the copyright holders for borrowed material. If they have inadvertently overlooked any, they will be pleased to make the necessary arrangements at the first opportunity.

To purchase additional copies of this book, call our customer service department at **(800) 638-0672** or fax orders to **(800) 447-8438.** For other book services, including chapter reprints and large quantity sales, ask for the Special Sales department.

Canadian customers should call **(800) 665-1148,** or fax **(800) 665-0103.** For all other calls originating outside of the United States, please call **(410) 528-4223** or fax us at **(410) 528-8550.**

Visit Williams & Wilkins on the Internet: http://www.wwilkins.com or contact our customer service department at **custserv@wwilkins.com.** Williams & Wilkins customer service representatives are available from 8:30 am to 6:00 pm, EST, Monday through Friday, for telephone access.

                                                                                07
                                                                         7 8 9 10

Dedication

To You—
a student of today,
a practitioner of tomorrow,
this textbook is respectfully dedicated

Foreword

The textbook that you hold in your hands is different from other medical textbooks written by scientists, educators, and clinicians. As an inquisitive orthopaedic professional, you will ask why? Certainly the author is a scientist who has applied the scientific method to basic research and has translated his findings into improved care for patients; certainly the author is an educator who has trained many residents and has instructed students and surgeons around the world; certainly the author is a clinician who has emphasized that a complete and detailed history and physical examination followed by a rational and organized approach to the patient's problems will lead to the correct diagnosis and allow the proper treatment of each patient. The author's ability to transmit his expertise in these areas will be apparent when you read this book. What is more important, however, is that the author is also a humanitarian, and that is what I hope you, the reader, will emulate after you have read this book. Look carefully at the sections on Communication with Your Patients about the Diagnosis on page 89, General Principles of Treatment on pages 91 to 93, A Litany for Medical Practitioners on page 93, Communication with Your Patients about the Recommended Treatment on page 114, and The Doctor-Patient Relationship as Part of Treatment on page 114. These sections and similar ones in this text will serve you well.

This Third Edition of this textbook has been updated by rewriting of the text; by marked expansion of the material relating to a number of conditions; by replacement of many of the previous citations with 670 recently published references; and by addition of sections and illustrations on such topics as computerized tomographic scanning, magnetic resonance imaging, and ultrasonography. The layout has been redesigned and the text reformatted. Each of these improvements represents the author's effort to provide an up-to-date textbook that is clear, concise, and accurate, so as to provide his readers with a solid background in the diagnosis and treatment of disorders and injuries of the musculoskeletal system in both children and adults.

Even with the extensive knowledge about the musculoskeletal system that you obtain from this book, however, you will not be able to provide the best care to your patient unless you have heeded the author's message about compassion. You must realize that the extra time that you spend discussing the diagnosis and treatment with the patient and concerned family members in a way that they each can understand, is of the utmost importance in practising the art and science of medicine. In this age of technology, the book seeks to educate you to be a caring medical practitioner, one who realizes that the true practice of medicine or any of its specialties requires not only great skill and exceptional knowledge, but also concern in truly caring for your patients.

Henry R. Cowell, M.D., Ph.D.
Editor, and Chairman of the Board of Editors
The Journal of Bone and Joint Surgery
(American Volume)

Preface

An Open Letter to a Student

Dear Student:

I have written this textbook expressly for a select group, namely *you and your fellow students*. By writing this book solely for *you*, I have endeavoured to fulfill *your* specific needs as a student of today and also as a practitioner of tomorrow in relation to the exciting and fascinating subject of clinical disorders and injuries of the musculoskeletal system.

Your specific needs in relation to the musculoskeletal system are to acquire the following: first, knowledge of the normal structure and function of musculoskeletal tissues as well as their cellular reactions to disorders and injuries so that you may *understand* the natural course and clinical manifestations of the more common conditions; second, skill in eliciting, interpreting and correlating clinical information including the pertinent physical signs, radiographic features, and laboratory data so that you may recognize or *diagnose* accurately the various clinical conditions when you encounter them in your patients; third, judgment concerning the clinical application of the general principles and specific methods of musculoskeletal *treatment* to the care of patients.

An explanation of the title of this book may help to clarify its purpose and its scope. It is generally understood among teachers and publishers that a "textbook" or "text" is a book written for undergraduate students. A "textbook" as defined by Webster is "a book containing the principles of a subject, used as a basis for instruction." A textbook is, therefore, quite different from a reference book, which must be encyclopaedic in nature; it is different from a monograph, which must include virtually all available knowledge in a very limited field; it is different from an atlas of operative technique; it is even different from a synopsis, an outline, a manual, or a handbook. Thus, a textbook, as suggested by its definition, should serve as the broad base and framework upon which you may build the additional knowledge that you will gain from your own clinical teachers as well as from the patients whom you will be privileged to see in the outpatient clinics and on the wards of your own teaching hospitals.

The *purpose* of this Third Edition, like that of its two predecessors, is to introduce you to the basic sciences pertaining to the musculoskeletal tissues as well as to the clinical practice; that is, diagnosis and treatment of the wide variety of disorders and injuries from which these tissues may suffer. Accordingly, its *scope* includes the "surgical" subjects of orthopaedics and fractures as well as the "medical" subjects of rheumatology, metabolic bone disease, and rehabilitation. Woven throughout the fabric of this book, you will find the thread of emphasis on kindness and compassion which are the hallmarks of total care for the total patient as an individual person.

In the Second Edition, I had included a final chapter entitled "The Philosophy and Nature of Medical Research" in the fervent hope of stimulating, and perhaps even inspiring, you to consider the possibility of your own personal involvement, either part-time or full-time, in this essential and rewarding component of our profession's responsibilities.

In this Third Edition, I have broadened the title of this chapter, which has become "The Philosophy and Nature of Medical Research with One Example." For the one example, I have chosen the basic and applied research that a series of my Research Fellows and I have conducted over the past 28 years on the biological concept of continuous passive motion (CPM) for the healing and regeneration of articular cartilage, ligaments, and tendons. I have summarized the evolution of this concept from its origination to research to clinical applications in the heartfelt hope that this example will help you to appreciate even more fully the intellectual rewards of medical research.

While the teacher of students carries the responsibility for teaching, the responsibility for learning rests with *you*—the student. I urge you, therefore, to learn from this textbook, from your own clinical teachers, and from your observation of patients so that you may be better prepared to serve the needs of patients who will seek your advice in the years to come. As Amiel has written, "The highest function of the teacher is not so much in imparting knowledge as in stimulating the pupil in its love and pursuit."

I wish you well in your pursuit of knowledge, not only as a student of today, but also as a practitioner of tomorrow, and equally important, as a continuing student throughout your entire professional life!

Yours sincerely,

Robert B. Salter

About the Author*

Robert B. Salter, a sixth generation Canadian, is a graduate in Medicine of the University of Toronto. After serving for 2 years with the Grenfell Medical Mission in Northern Newfoundland and Labrador, he took his postgraduate orthopaedic training in Toronto and an additional year on the McLaughlin Fellowship in London, England with the late Sir Reginald Watson-Jones and Sir Henry Osmond-Clarke.

On his return to Canada in 1955, Dr. Salter was appointed to the Staff of The Hospital for Sick Children, Toronto, as well as to the Hospital's Research Institute, and 2 years later he was appointed Chief of Orthopaedic Surgery. After 9 years in this position he became Surgeon-in-Chief of the Hospital and a Professor of Surgery of the University of Toronto. Following completion of his 10-year term in this position, he was appointed Professor and Head of the Division of Orthopaedic Surgery, which includes eight Teaching Hospitals. He completed his 10-year appointment in 1986 and continues as a Professor of Orthopaedic Surgery and as a Senior Orthopaedic Surgeon of The Hospital for Sick Children, as well as a Research Project Director of the Hospital's Research Institute. In 1995 he became Professor Emeritus in the University, a Member of the Honorary Consultant Staff of The Hospital and Senior Scientist Emeritus of the Hospital's Research Institute.

A world-renowned orthopaedic surgeon, teacher, and scientist, Dr. Salter has developed numerous innovative methods of orthopaedic treatment based on his personal, clinical, and experimental investigations over a period of 40 years. These new methods include the innominate osteotomy (the "Salter operation"), which he designed in 1957 for congenital dislocation and subluxation of the hip in children and adults, and also for the severe form of Legg-Perthes' disease, a method of preventing cubitus varus as a complication of supracondylar fractures of the humerus, and a surgical operation to correct recurrent dislocation of the patella. The Salter-Harris classification of epiphyseal-plate injuries, which he created with Dr. W. Robert Harris in 1962, is still widely accepted.

As an orthopaedic teacher, he helped to develop the University of Toronto "systems-oriented" curriculum for undergraduate teaching relevant to the musculoskeletal system. He has written over 118 scientific articles in referred journals and 39 book chapters as well as three editions of his "Textbook of Disorders and Injuries of the Musculoskeletal System—An Introduction to Orthopaedics, Fractures and Joint Injuries, Rheumatology, Metabolic Bone Disease and Rehabilitation," which has also been translated into Spanish, Portuguese, Japanese, and Malaysian. He has taught as an invited Visiting Professor in 190 universities in a total of 40 countries and has delivered 69 "Named" Lectures.

As an orthopaedic statesman, Dr. Salter has served as President of the Canadian Orthopaedic Association as well as the Royal College of Physicians and Surgeons of Canada and the International Federation of Surgical Colleges (a total of 47 Colleges of Surgery worldwide).

In his capacity as an orthopaedic scientist, Dr. Salter has consistently conducted imagi-

* Updated in 1998 from "About the Author" in the Preliminary Pages of Salter's Monograph entitled, Continuous Passive Motion (CPM), a Biological Concept for the Healing and Regeneration of Articular Cartilage, Ligaments and Tendons: From Origination to Research to Clinical Applications, 1993. Published by Williams & Wilkins, Baltimore, U.S.A.

native and original basic research over a period of 43 years of continuous investigation on numerous orthopaedic problems, which include: acetabular maldirection in dysplasia of the hip, avascular necrosis of the femoral head as a complication of treatment of congenital dislocation of the hip, Legg-Perthes' Disease, the harmful effects of immobilization of joints; with and without compression and the phenomenon of hydrocortisone arthropathy. Since 1970, he has been involved with basic research concerning his exciting new biological concept of 'continuous passive motion' (CPM) for diseased and injured joints and has demonstrated the beneficial effects of CPM on the healing and regeneration of articular cartilage and peri-articular tissues in a wide variety of animal models of diseases and injuries in the rabbit. He began to apply this concept to the care of patients for specific indications in 1978, with excellent results.

For his many contributions to orthopaedic surgery through his combined clinical and experimental investigations as a clinician-scientist over a period of four decades, Dr. Salter has received numerous honors and awards. He has been elected an Honorary Fellow of six Colleges of Surgery in the English-speaking world and has received honorary degrees from four universities, including his Alma Mater, the University of Toronto. He has received the Royal College Medal in Surgery (1960), the Gairdner International Award for Medical Science (1969), the Lawrence Chute Award for Undergraduate Teaching (1971), the Nicolas Andry Award (1974), the Charles Mickle International Award for Advances in Science (1975), the Kappa Delta Award for Research (1987), the Medec Award for Medical Achievement (1989), the Robert Danis Medal of the International Society of Surgery (1989), the Arthur H. Huene International Award of the Paediatric Orthopaedic Society of North America (1992), the Ross Award of the Canadian Paediatric Society (1992), 1995 Skvere International Humanitarian Award (from Skvere Institutes of USA), and the 1996 Outstanding Contribution Award (Pioneer Award) of the Paediatric Orthopaedic Society of North America. He has been inducted into the Canadian Medical Hall of Fame (1995). In 1997, he received the F.N.G. Starr Medal, the highest award of the Canadian Medical Association.

Dr. Salter has been elected a Fellow of the Academy of Science of the Royal Society of Canada (F.R.S.C., 1979), and he has been appointed an Officer of the Order of Canada (O.C., 1977) as well as to the Order of Ontario (O. Ont., 1988). In 1981, he was appointed to the prestigious rank of "University Professor" of the University of Toronto, the University's highest honor to a member of its active faculty, "for excellence in research and teaching." This rank is held by only 15 of the 6000 faculty members at any time. In 1997, he was promoted from Officer to Companion of the Order of Canada (C.C.), his country's highest honor.

Acknowledgments

The philosophy of teaching embraces the tradition of sharing knowledge—through teaching of present and future generations of students in a given discipline—in return for what has been shared with the teacher by his or her own teachers. Accordingly, I am indebted to those persons, both living and dead, from whom I have learned and especially to those who have stimulated and encouraged me, in turn, to teach others.

The teacher who undertakes to write a textbook covering such a broad field as disorders and injuries of the musculoskeletal system in both children and adults must, of necessity, add to his own personal knowledge from that of colleagues in the same discipline as well as in related disciplines. Then, the teacher sifts and synthesizes this accumulated knowledge and offers it to students and practitioners as food for their minds in a manner that is intellectually palatable, digestible, satisfying, and nourishing.

I am particularly grateful to Dr. Henry R. Cowell, the Editor and Chairman of the Board of Editors of the American Volume of the Journal of Bone and Joint Surgery, for his typically gracious, erudite, and elegant Foreword to this Third Edition.

I have appreciated the comments and suggestions concerning the First and Second Editions offered by both students and teachers from numerous countries and I have endeavoured to respond to them in the preparation of the Third Edition. Because orthopaedic surgery is such a rapidly developing specialty, updating of a textbook such as this necessitates an extensive review of the relevant literature that has been published during the intervening years. In addition to the various journals and books of orthopaedic surgery and related fields, one particular source of new knowledge merits special mention, namely the annual Year Books of Orthopaedic Surgery from the Second Edition in 1983 to the Third Edition in 1998. These Year Books have been thoughtfully edited up to 1988 by the late Dr. Mark B. Coventry and from 1988 to 1998 by Dr. Clement B. Sledge. I am indebted to both of them for their helpful reviews of the orthopaedic literature. Another excellent source of current orthopaedic knowledge has been the series of Orthopaedic Knowledge Updates and other books published by the American Academy of Orthopaedic Surgeons.

At the University of Toronto, many friends and colleagues have read specific sections of the manuscript and have offered constructive criticisms. Accordingly, I wish to record their names (in alphabetical order) with grateful thanks.

Those whose discipline is other than orthopaedic surgery include the following: Alison Anthony (physiotherapy), Paul Babyn (diagnostic imaging), Victor Blanchette (hematology), Howard Clarke (plastic surgery), William Feldman (paediatrics), Brenda Gallie (ophthalmology and cancer), David Gilday (nuclear medicine), Duncan Gordon (rheumatology), Susan King (infectious diseases), Sang Whay Kooh (metabolic bone disease), Gideon Koren (population health sciences), Ronald Laxer (rheumatology), William Logan (neurology), Marcellina Miam (child abuse), Timothy Murray (metabolic bone disease), Brian O'Sullivan (radiation oncology), Greg Ryan (obstetrics), Louis Siminovitch (molecular genetics), Rajka Soric (rehabilitation medicine), Charles Tator (neurosurgery), Lap Chee Tsui (molecular genetics), John Wherrett (neurology), Ronald Worton (molecular genetics).

My University of Toronto colleagues who have also helped in this way include the following:
Benjamin Alman, Terrence Axelrod, Robert Bell, Earl Bogoch, John Cameron, William Cole, Timothy Daniels, Michael Ford, Allan Gross, Hamilton Hall, Douglas Hedden, John McCulloch, Michael McKee, Antonio Miniachi, Mercer Rang, Joseph Schatzker, Marvin Tile, John Wedge, James Wright.

Many of the clinical photographs from the First and Second Editions have been retained in the Third Edition because Dr. Judith Wunderly Walker (who at that time was a medical illustrator) had painstakingly prepared these illustrations in such a way as to provide uncluttered uniformity in the background of the final prints. In addition, she had done most of the line drawings. Consequently, I continue to appreciate her skill and ingenuity.

The work of providing prints and other illustrations for the Third Edition has been cheerfully accomplished by the following members of the Graphic Centre at The Hospital for Sick Children under the direction of Tiiu Kask: Diogenes Baena, Robert Teteruck, and Lisa Spodek—to them I express my sincere thanks. For the typing of the manuscript I am indebted to Harriett Davidson, Bonnie Morgan, and Anna Fazari, whose typing skills are exceeded only by their dedication to the textbook.

To the staff of Williams & Wilkins, in general, and to the Editor, Eric P. Johnson, Managing Editor, Linda Napora, and Project Editor, Kathleen Gilbert, in particular, I am most grateful for bringing my manuscript to publication.

As a science writer and a novelist, my wife, Robina, has carefully read each portion of the manuscript as it has been written and has made many valuable editorial suggestions; in addition, she has assisted with the time-consuming and exacting task of reading page proofs. More importantly, however, in her role as my wife and as the mother of our five children, Robina has been a constant source of inspiration. For her unselfish understanding and for her abiding love, I am, and always will be, most thankful.

ROBERT B. SALTER

Contents

Section II Musculoskeletal Disorders—General and Specific

9 Generalized and Disseminated Disorders of Bone, 183

10   Inflammatory Disorders of Bones and Joints, 207

14   Neoplasms of Musculoskeletal Tissues, 379

Section III Musculoskeletal Injuries

Section **IV** **Research**

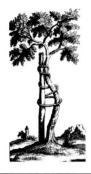

Section I

Basic Musculoskeletal Science and its Application

---

1 Introduction: The Past and the Present

"We see so far because we stand on the shoulders of giants"

—Sir Isaac Newton

BRIEF HISTORICAL BACKGROUND

As a student approaching the twenty-first century, you live in a tremendously exciting era. As you pursue your studies of the basic sciences and of modern clinical medicine or the allied professional fields, you will realize how much of what you are learning has been developed since *you* were born. This is simply an indication of the recently accelerated acquisition of scientific knowledge. However, as Cicero said: "Not to know what happened before one was born is to remain a child." The history of medicine and surgery deserves your attention not only because it is fascinating and inspiring but also because it places your present knowledge in perspective and may even stimulate original thought concerning possible developments of the future. If, after graduation, you choose to study one particular field of medicine or other health care professions in depth you would be wise to delve into the history of that particular field so that you may avoid repeating the errors of the past.

The bones of prehistoric humans provide mute testimony of disorders and injuries of the musculoskeletal system, and from the beginning caring persons sought ways to alleviate the crippling conditions of others. As early as 9000 BC, in the Paleolithic age, superstitions were being replaced by rational thinking and caregivers were beginning to use splints for weak limbs and broken bones. In the Neolithic age, around 5000 BC, crude amputations of diseased or damaged limbs were already being performed. The Egyptians had developed the concept of the crutch by 2000 BC. Greece replaced Egypt as the center of culture by the fifth century BC and Hippocrates, through his teaching and through his students, had become the "father of medicine." In the second century AD, Galen, a Greek physician who moved to Rome, became the founder of experimental investigation.

Throughout the first eighteen centuries AD, knowledge in medicine and surgery advanced slowly, culminating in the significant contributions of England's John Hunter (1728-1793), who has been revered ever since as the "father of surgical research." Understandably, however, the development and performance of major surgical operations had to await the revolutionary nineteenth century

1

discoveries of general anesthesia by Long and Morton (United States), the bacterial basis of disease by Pasteur (France), antisepsis by Lister (Scotland), and x-rays by Roentgen (Germany).

Progress in the science of medicine and surgery in the twentieth century, and more particularly in its second half, has been staggering in its rapidity. Happily, there is no end in sight for such escalating progression. Indeed this is only one of the factors that makes the study and practice of medicine in general, and orthopaedic surgery and allied professional fields in particular, so exciting and challenging.

In the twentieth century, the care of patients with disorders and injuries of the musculoskeletal system has evolved through three phases. First was the "strap and buckle" phase in which various orthopaedic splints, braces, and other types of appliances constituted the predominant form of management. Next came the phase of excessive orthopaedic operations, many of which were based more on clinical empiricism than on scientific investigation. In the third and current phase, science is rapidly replacing empiricism, as evidenced by the combination of increased *experimental laboratory investigations (basic research)*, aimed at understanding the physiology and pathology of the musculoskeletal system more completely, and both retrospective and prospective *clinical investigations* to study the natural course of disorders and critically evaluate the results of various forms of treatment in humans.

In this scientific phase, the study of clinical problems of the musculoskeletal system has become increasingly stimulating and challenging. The care of patients remains an *art*, but the art must be based on *science*.

You will gain much knowledge from those who have gone before you, both recently and in the distant past, but you may be assured that there is much more to be discovered and understood.

THE SCOPE OF ORTHOPAEDICS

Although the history of disorders and injuries of the musculoskeletal system dates back to antiquity, the specialty of orthopaedics as a branch of medicine and surgery is relatively young. In 1741, Nicolas Andry, then Profes-

sor of Medicine in Paris, published a book, the English translation of which is *Orthopaedia, or the Art of Preventing and Correcting Deformities in Children*. He coined the term "orthopaedia" from *orthos* (straight or free from deformity) and *pais* (child) and expressed the view that most deformities in adults have their origin in childhood (Fig. 1.1). Although the term "orthopaedics" is not entirely satisfac-

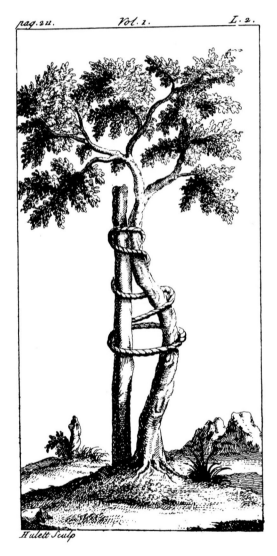

Figure 1.1. This "orthopaedic tree" from Nicolas Andry's eighteenth-century book has become the international symbol of orthopaedic surgery. It illustrates the concept that a crooked young tree—like a deformed young child—can be helped to grow straight by applying appropriate forces.

tory, it has persisted for more than two centuries and is unlikely to be replaced in your academic lifetime.

The present scope of orthopaedics has come to include all ages and is considered to consist of the art and science of prevention, investigation, diagnosis, and treatment of disorders and injuries of the musculoskeletal system by medical, surgical, and physical means—including physiotherapy—as well as the study of musculoskeletal physiology, pathology, and other related basic sciences.

Thus, the modern, sophisticated orthopaedic surgeon serves as both physician and surgeon (as implied by the American synonym "orthopedist"). To provide exemplary total care for patients with certain musculoskeletal disorders or injuries, the orthopaedic specialist must work in close collaboration with medical specialists—including rheumatologists, metabolic bone physicians, and rehabilitation physicians (physiatrists) or other surgical specialists, particularly plastic surgeons and neurosurgeons—as well as health care professionals, including physiotherapists, occupational therapists, and medical social workers.

As a group, musculoskeletal disorders and injuries are remarkably common. Indeed, it has been ascertained from numerous surveys in North America that at least 15% of the total number of patients seen by a primary care, or family physician, suffer from a disorder or injury of the musculoskeletal system either with or without some coexistent condition.

CURRENT TRENDS IN CLINICAL CONDITIONS OF THE MUSCULOSKELETAL SYSTEM

Our environment is the scene of continual change, and from decade to decade we see many changes in the nature and frequency of the musculoskeletal disorders and injuries that confront us. Although certain musculoskeletal conditions, such as congenital deformities and bone neoplasms, have remained with us, others have gradually become less common. New problems have arisen in their place and must receive increasing attention. For example, if you had been a student in the early decades of the twentieth century, you would have been taught much about bone and joint tuberculo-

sis, vitamin deficiencies of bone, and paralytic poliomyelitis. Today, these conditions have been largely brought under control by prevention, at least in developed countries. Nevertheless, in recent years there has been a resurgence of tuberculosis and the appearance of post-polio syndrome. Other conditions, such as acute bone and joint infections, have been partially controlled, but only by the application of intensive modern antibiotic treatment at the onset of disease. Thus, the current emphasis in teaching about these conditions must be on early recognition, or diagnosis, of the clinical picture and early treatment.

Severe cerebral palsy with its associated paralytic problems is even more common than before because some infants with this condition, who previously died early in life, now survive and grow up with their problem. The age span of humans has become progressively longer, and as a result the various degenerative conditions, such as degenerative arthritis, now assume greater clinical importance. Likewise, senile weakening of bone (osteoporosis), with its complication of fractures in the elderly, has become an increasingly important problem. Certain conditions, such as rheumatoid arthritis, that in previous decades were treated by medical means alone, have become partially amenable to surgical treatment. The increase in the number of automobiles, combined with their increasing speed, has been responsible in part for the great increase in the number and severity of musculoskeletal injuries—fractures and associated trauma—and in particular for the increasing number of patients who sustain multiple serious injuries involving several major systems of the body.

RECENT ADVANCES

In recent decades there has been increasing emphasis on the broad fields of medical epidemiology and statistics relevant to both basic research and clinical investigation, in particular concerning methodology and interpretation of data. Epidemiological methods have led to the development of prospective randomized, controlled double-blind investigations and clinical trials, "clinical outcome studies" (patient-derived measures of satisfaction), evidence-based medicine (including the cost-effectiveness of various forms of diagnosis and treatment), and practice guidelines. Such developments are especially important in the current era of medical cost constraints by governments and increasing demands by both governments and the public for more accountability by the medical and related professions concerning the delivery of health care.

In medical undergraduate education the method of "problem-based learning" is becoming increasingly popular as is the system of using trained "actors" or "actresses" to simulate patients. Postgraduate education has been enhanced by the establishment of technical (psychomotor) skills workshops and laboratories. An important advance in continuing medical education has been "telemedicine," which provides university-staffed audio and, more recently, audiovisual teaching for physicians, surgeons, and other health care professionals in their own communities far from the university center.

During the past three decades, the dynamism of orthopaedics has been demonstrated by many important developments that have had a significant impact on the prevention, diagnosis, and treatment of musculoskeletal disorders and injuries. *Preventive* orthopaedics has become a reality through more precise counseling as well as intrauterine detection of certain disorders by amniocentesis. The administration of folic acid to all pregnant mothers has significantly reduced the incidence of spina bifida (a neural tube defect), especially in the offspring of high-risk mothers who have already had a child with spina bifida. Earlier *diagnosis* of potentially serious orthopaedic disorders, such as congenital dislocation of the hip, has become a reality through the routine examination of all newborns, as has the early detection of scoliosis (curvature of the spine). These initiatives have been proved effective. Noninvasive diagnostic "imaging" of musculoskeletal disorders and injuries has been enhanced by radioactive isotope bone scans (scintigraphy) and ultrasound scans (ultrasonography) and especially by computed tomography (CT), both two-dimensional and three-dimensional, as well as by magnetic resonance imaging (MRI). Endoscopic examination of the interior of large joints, such as the knee, ankle, hip, wrist, elbow, and shoulder, is now possible with an arthroscope and even certain intra-articular operations, including removal of loose bodies, repair of torn menisci, or reconstruction of an anterior cruciate ligament, can be performed through the arthroscope (arthroscopic surgery).

The discovery by molecular geneticists of the gene responsible for certain diseases—for example, muscular dystrophy—raises the exciting prospect of gene therapy through genetic engineering for such diseases. In addition, some oncogenes are being found in musculoskeletal tumors.

Recent advances in orthopaedic *treatment* include the following:

- Total prosthetic joint replacements for almost every joint in the extremities and osteochondral allografts for irreversible arthritis
- More effective mechanical spinal instrumentation for scoliosis
- Back education units
- Hyperbaric oxygenation for impaired peripheral circulation
- Detection and monitoring of increased pressure in various "muscle compartment syndromes"
- More effective methods of nonoperative treatment of fractures (cast bracing), operative treatment (AO system of rigid internal fixation), stimulation of delayed fracture healing or even nonunion (electricity), and the biological resurfacing of joints through stimulation of the repair and regeneration of articular cartilage (continuous passive motion; CPM) and other methods
- More effective systemic chemotherapy for malignant diseases
- Limb salvage operations as attractive alternatives to amputations for malignant tumors of the extremities
- Steroid injection for simple bone cysts
- Resection of a bony bridge across an epiphyseal plate
- Earlier and more complete surgical correction of severe clubfeet
- More appropriate materials for splints and braces (orthoses) and for artificial limbs (prostheses)

The method of slow distraction of callus at the site of an osteotomy—the "distraction osteogenesis" technique of Ilizarov—has improved the results of surgical limb lengthening and the correction of bony deformities to a remarkable degree.

The development of surgery performed under magnification of the operating microscope (microsurgery) has made possible the replantation of completely severed digits and limbs and the transfer of free vascularized bone grafts and even vascularized and reinnervated autogenous muscle grafts.

These recent advances, which have greatly enhanced the prevention, diagnosis, and treatment of musculoskeletal disorders and injuries, are discussed in appropriate chapters of this textbook.

Thus, there have been many significant advances in orthopaedics during the past three decades. Nevertheless, there are still numerous unsolved problems that will require imaginative research to provide a solution. Indeed, much remains to be discovered and developed. As Cowper wrote, "Knowledge is proud that he knows so much; wisdom is humble that he knows no more."

SUGGESTED ADDITIONAL READING

Andry N. Orthopaedia: or the art of correcting and preventing deformities in children (facsimile reproduction of first edition in English, London, 1743). Philadelphia: JB Lippincott, 1961. Vols. 1 and 2.

Bick EM. Source book of orthopaedics. 2nd ed. Baltimore: Williams & Wilkins, 1948 (facsimile reprint of 1948 edition by Hafner Publishing, New York, 1968).

Bick EM. Classics of orthopaedics. Philadelphia: JB Lippincott, 1976.

Howorth MB. A textbook of orthopaedics. Philadelphia: WB Saunders, 1952.

Keith A. Menders of the maimed. London Froude (1919 limited editions). Philadelphia: JB Lippincott, 1951.

LeVay D. The history of orthopaedics. An account of the study and practice of orthopaedics from the earliest times to the modern era. Park Ridge, NJ: The Parthenon Publishing Group, 1990.

Lister J. On the antiseptic principle in the practice of surgery. Lancet 1867;2:253.

Lyons AS, Petrucelli RJ II. Medicine: an illustrated history. New York: Harry N Abrams Publishers, 1978.

Mayer L. Orthopaedic surgery in the United States of America. J Bone Joint Surg 1950;32B:461.

Osmond-Clarke H. Half a century of orthopaedic progress in orthopaedic surgery. J Bone Surg 1950;32B:620.

Peltier LF: Orthopedics: history and iconography. San Francisco: Norman Publishing, 1993.

Platt H. The evolution and scope of orthopaedics. In: Clarke JMP, ed. Modern trends in orthopaedics. Vol 1. London, Butterworth, 1950.

Raney RB. Andry and the orthopaedics. J Bone Joint Surg 1949;31A:675-682.

Rang M. Anthology of orthopaedics. Edinburgh and London: E & S Livingstone, 1966.

Roentgen WK. On a new kind of ray. Nature 1896; 53:274, 377.

Salter RB. Advances in paediatric orthopaedics in North America 1954 to 1987. (The American Orthopaedic Association Centennial Program). J Bone Joint Surg 1987;69A:1265-1267.

Sournia J-C. The illustrated history of medicine. London: Harold Starke Publishers, 1992.

2 Normal Structure and Function of Musculoskeletal Tissues

"Anatomy is to physiology as geography is to history; it describes the theatre of events."
—Jean Ferme (1497–1558)
On the Natural Part of Medicine (Ch. 1)

Having completed the preclinical phase of your undergraduate course, you will have learned much about the embryology, anatomy, histology, biochemistry, and physiology of the musculoskeletal tissues in humans. This is extremely important, because to understand the abnormal, you must have an understanding of the normal; indeed, your knowledge of the normal will serve as a broad base on which to build a knowledge of the abnormal. Some of the more important aspects of this broad base are reviewed to refresh your memory and to prepare you for subsequent study of the abnormal clinical conditions of the musculoskeletal system (also known as the locomotor system).

BONES AS STRUCTURES AND BONE AS AN ORGAN

The tissue bone is considered from two entirely different points of view: 1) individual bones are *anatomical structures* and 2) bone of the entire skeleton collectively is a *physiological organ* that is metabolically active.

Since the nonliving intercellular matrix of bone is calcified, or stonelike, it is one of the hard tissues. Indeed, its hardness provides the strength to individual bones as *structures* and enables them to serve three functions: 1) to provide the rigid framework for the trunk and extremities to withstand mechanical loads; 2) to serve as levers for the locomotor function of skeletal muscles; 3) to afford protection for vulnerable viscera, for example, the skull for the brain, the spine for the spinal cord, and the thoracic cage for the heart and lungs. Bone of the entire skeleton as an *organ* serves two additional functions: 4) it contains hemopoietic tissue of the myeloid type for the production of erythrocytes, granular leukocytes, and platelets and 5) it is the organ of storage or reservoir for calcium, phosphorus, magnesium, and sodium, helping to maintain the "milieu intérieur" of ionized mineral homeostasis by storing or releasing these substances as the need arises.

Thus, in addition to being bone-forming cells, osteoblasts also govern metabolism in response to a wide variety of stimuli—biochemical, mechanical, electrical, and magnetic—via specific cellular receptors.

Embryonic Development of Bones

In the initial stages of development, the tube-shaped embryo contains three primary germ cell layers: the *ectoderm* or covering layer, the *endoderm* or lining layer, and the *mesoderm* or middle layer. From the mesoderm comes the *mesenchyme,* a diffuse cellular tissue that exhibits pluripotentiality in the sense that its undifferentiated cells are capable of differentiating into any one of several types of connective tissue such as bone, cartilage, ligament, muscle, tendon and fascia. Bone and cartilage, being able to support weight through their non-living intercellular substances, may be thought of as *supporting* connective tissues.

During the fifth week of embryonic development, the limb buds, covered by ectoderm, appear. In the central axis of each limb bud, the mesenchymal cells become condensed into a short cylinder. This cylinder is segmented by less densely cellular areas at the sites of future joints and each segment represents a tiny *mesenchymal model* of the future long bone that will develop from it (Fig. 2.1). By the sixth embryonic week, the undifferen-

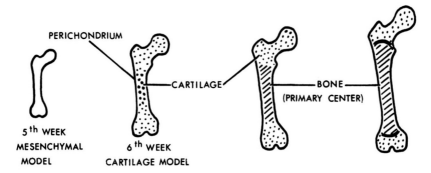

Figure 2.1. Embryonic development of a long bone during the first 6 months of embryogenesis.

tiated mesenchymal cells of each model begin to differentiate by manufacturing cartilage matrix and thereby forming a *cartilaginous model* of the future bone. The cartilaginous model grows partly from within (*interstitial growth*) and partly through the apposition of new cells on its surface (*appositional growth*) from the deeper layers of the *perichondrium* (Fig. 2.1).

After the seventh week of embryogenesis, the cartilage cells in the center of the model hypertrophy and form longitudinal rows, after which the intercellular substance, or matrix, calcifies, resulting in cell death. Vascular connective tissue then grows into the central area of dead cartilage bringing *osteoblasts* that secrete collagen and proteoglycans into the matrix; the matrix is then impregnated with calcium salts and becomes immature bone on the calcified cartilage matrix, thereby forming the *primary center of ossification*. This process of replacement of cartilage by bone is called *endochondral ossification* and it occurs only in the presence of capillaries. The endochondral ossification advances toward each end of the cartilage model, which, in turn, continues to grow in length at its cartilaginous ends by interstitial growth. The perichondrium has by this time become periosteum, and in its deeper layer, the mesenchymal cells, which have differentiated into osteoblasts, lay down bone directly by the process of *intramembranous ossification,* there being no intermediate cartilaginous phase (Fig. 2.1).

By the sixth month of embryonic development, resorption of the central part of the long bone results in the formation of a medullary cavity—the process of *tubulation*. At the time of birth, the largest epiphysis in the body (distal femoral epiphysis) has developed a *secondary center of ossification* by the process of endochondral ossification within it (Fig. 2.2). Secondary centers of ossification appear in the other cartilaginous epiphyses at varying ages after birth. Each such center, or ossific nucleus, is separated from the metaphysis by a special plate of growing cartilage—the *epiphyseal plate, or physis,* which provides growth in the length of the bone through the interstitial growth of cartilage cells.

The short bones (e.g., the carpal bones) are developed by endochondral ossification in the same manner as the epiphyses. By contrast, the clavicle and most of the skull develop bone directly in the mesenchymal model by the process of intramembranous ossification from the periosteum without going through a cartilaginous phase.

During the early weeks of intrauterine life, the developing embryo is particularly susceptible to noxious environmental factors that arrive via the placental circulation. For example, if the mother develops a rubella infection or takes a harmful drug such as thalidomide during this critical period, embryonic development is likely to be seriously affected. The extent of the resultant abnormality depends on

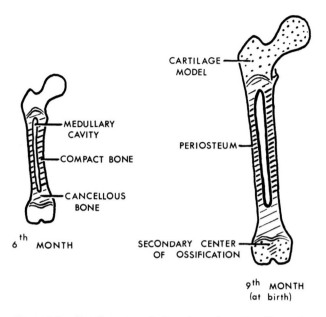

Figure 2.2.   Development of a long bone from 6 to 9 months.

the *exact* phase of embryonic development at the time; in general, the earlier the stage of development, the more extensive will be the resultant abnormality. When you consider the remarkable speed and complexity of human embryonic development, it is hardly surprising that some children are born with an obvious congenital abnormality; indeed, it is surprising that the vast majority of children are completely normal at birth.

Bone Growth and Remodeling

Bones grow in *length* by one process (involving endochondral ossification), whereas they grow in *width* by another process (involving intramembranous ossification).

Growth in Length

Since interstitial growth within *bone* is not possible, bone length can increase only by the process of interstitial growth within *cartilage* followed by endochondral ossification. Thus, there are two possible sites for cartilaginous growth in a long bone—articular cartilage and epiphyseal plate cartilage (Fig. 2.3).

Articular Cartilage

The articular cartilage in a long bone is the only growth plate for growth of its *epiphysis*. The articular cartilage in a short bone provides the only growth plate for the whole bone.

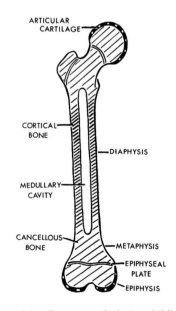

Figure 2.3.   Bone growth during childhood.

Epiphyseal Plate Cartilage

The epiphyseal plate provides growth in the length of the *metaphysis* and *diaphysis* of a long bone. In this site of growth, a constant balance is maintained between two separate processes: (1) interstitial growth of the cartilage cells of the plate, making it thicker and thereby moving the epiphysis farther away from the metaphysis and (2) calcification, death and replacement of cartilage on the metaphyseal surface by bone through endochondral ossification.

Four zones of the epiphyseal plate can be distinguished (Fig. 2.4):

1. *The zone of resting cartilage* anchors the epiphyseal plate to the epiphysis and contains immature chondrocytes, as well as delicate blood vessels that penetrate it from the epiphysis and bring nourishment to the entire plate.
2. *The zone of young proliferating cartilage* is the site of most active interstitial growth of the cartilage cells, which are arranged in vertical columns.
3. *The zone of maturing cartilage* reveals a progressive enlargement and maturation of the cartilage cells as they approach the metaphysis. These chondrocytes accumulate glycogen in their cytoplasm and produce phosphatase which may be involved in the calcification of their surrounding matrix.
4. *The zone of calcifying cartilage* is thin and its chondrocytes have died as a result of calcification of the matrix. This is structurally the weakest zone of the epiphyseal plate. Bone deposition is active on the metaphyseal side of this zone and as new bone is added to the calcified cores of cartilage matrix, the metaphysis becomes correspondingly longer.

Hormonal Control of Longitudinal Bone Growth

Throughout the world, and especially in developing countries, malnutrition remains the most common cause of retardation of longitudinal bone growth. Such malnutrition is also accompanied by disturbances of endocrine function.

Human growth hormone, which is synthesized in the anterior pituitary gland, exerts its growth-promoting effect through the production of insulin-like growth factor in the

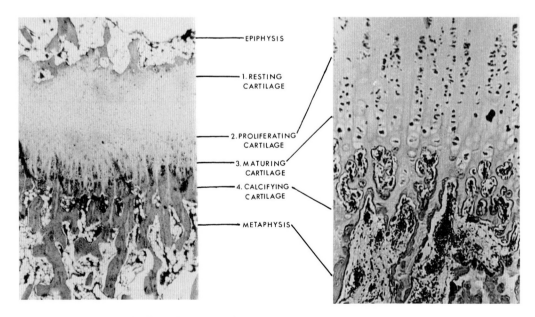

EPIPHYSIS

1. RESTING CARTILAGE

2. PROLIFERATING CARTILAGE

3. MATURING CARTILAGE

4. CALCIFYING CARTILAGE

METAPHYSIS

Figure 2.4.   Histological appearance of an epiphyseal plate (from the upper end of tibia of a child). **A.** Low power. **B.** High power.

liver. Thyroxine is also essential for normal longitudinal growth. Sex hormones are involved in the characteristic postpubertal "growth spurt" in adolescent boys and girls. Glucocorticoids (cortisones) have an inhibitory effect on growth as seen in Cushing's syndrome, whether naturally occurring or secondary to prolonged therapeutic administration of cortisone to children.

Growth in Width

Bones increase in width by means of appositional growth from the osteoblasts in the deep, or inner (cambium), layer of the *periosteum,* the process being one of intramembranous ossification. Simultaneously, the medullary cavity becomes larger through osteoclastic resorption of bone on the inner surface of the cortex, which is lined by endosteum.

Remodeling of Bone

During longitudinal growth, the flared metaphyseal regions of bone must be continually remodeled as the epiphysis moves progressively farther away from the shaft. This is accomplished by simultaneous osteoblastic deposition of bone on one surface and osteoclastic resorption on the opposite surface.

However, remodeling of bone continues throughout life, since some haversian systems, or osteons, continually erode through cell death as well as through factors that demand removal of calcium from bone; therefore, deposition of bone must also continue to maintain *bone balance.* During the growing years, bone deposition exceeds bone resorption, and the child is in a state of *positive* bone balance. By contrast, in old age, bone deposition cannot keep pace with bone resorption, and the elderly person is in a state of *negative* bone balance.

Remodeling of bone also occurs in response to physical stresses—or to the lack of them—in that bone is deposited in sites subjected to stress and is resorbed from sites where there is little stress. This phenomenon is generally referred to as *Wolff's law* and is exemplified by marked cortical thickening on the concave side of a curved bone (Fig. 2.5) as well as by the alignment of trabecular systems along the lines of weightbearing stress in the

internal architecture of the upper end of the femur (Fig. 2.6).

It is likely that the phenomenon of Wolff's law is mediated by induced electrical potentials. For example, in a bowed tubular bone—or a curved trabecula of cancellous bone—a negative electrical charge or potential exists on the concave side (compression force) and a positive charge on the convex side (tension force). Furthermore, it would seem that a negative charge induces bone deposition, whereas a positive charge induces bone resorption. (During the past decade, this concept of electrical stimulation of osteogenesis has been increasingly applied to the healing of delayed union of fractures in patients, as discussed in Chapters 6 and 15).

Anatomy and Histology of Bones as Structures

Anatomical Structure

Bones, from the viewpoint of their gross structure, are classified as 1) long bones, or tubular bones (e.g. femur), 2) short bones or cuboidal bones (e.g., carpal bones), and 3) flat bones (e.g., scapula). Furthermore, each bone consists of dense cortical bone (*compacta*) on the outside and a sponge-like arrangement of trabecular bone (*spongiosa*) on the inside (Fig. 2.7). In children, the covering periosteum is thick and loosely attached to the cortex, and it produces new bone readily. In adults, by contrast, the periosteum becomes progressively thinner and more adherent to the cortex, and it produces new bone less readily. This fundamental difference explains, in part, why fractures heal more rapidly in young children than in adults.

Blood Supply to Long Bones

Three distinct vascular systems exist in long bones: 1) an *afferent* vascular system comprising nutrient and metaphyseal arteries that together supply the inner two thirds of the cortex and periosteal arteries that supply the outer one third, 2) an *efferent* vascular system that conveys venous blood, and 3) an *intermediate* vascular system of capillaries within the cortex. The direction of blood flow through a long bone is normally centrifugal, that is,

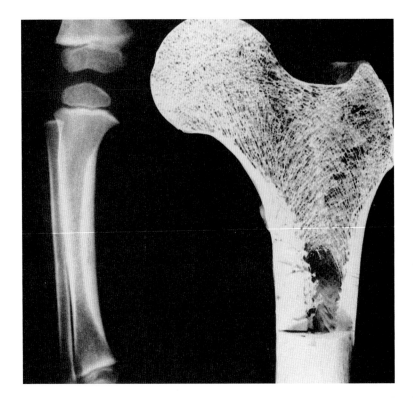

Figure 2.5.   Left. An example of Wolff's law is seen in the tibia of a 2-year-old child with a bow leg deformity. Note the significant thickening of the medial cortex, which is on the concave side of the deformity and is subjected to the most stress on weightbearing.

Figure 2.6.   Right. An example of Wolff's law is seen in the internal architecture of this dried specimen of the upper end of the femur of an adult. Note the alignment of the trabecular systems of cancellous bone along the lines of weight-bearing stresses.

from the medullary cavity to the periosteal surface.

Histological Structure

From the viewpoint of its microscopic structure, bone is classified in the following way (the commonly used synonyms are included in parentheses):

- *Immature bone* (nonlamellar bone, woven bone, fiber bone)
- *Mature bone* (lamellar bone): (1) cortical bone (dense bone, compacta); (2) cancellous bone (trabecular bone, spongiosa)

The two major histological types of bone demonstrate significant differences in their relative content of cells, collagen, and proteoglycans.

Immature Bone

The first bone that is formed by endochondral ossification during embryonic development is of the immature type; subsequently, it is replaced gradually by mature bone so that by the age of 1 year, immature bone is no longer seen under normal conditions. Nevertheless, throughout life, under any abnormal condition in which new bone is formed rapidly (such as the healing of a fracture and the reaction to an infection or a tumor), the *first* bone formed is of the immature type. Here again, the rapidly formed immature bone is subsequently replaced by mature bone. Immature bone, also called fiber bone or woven bone because of its large proportion of irregularly "woven" collagen fibers in a haphazard arrangement, is very cellular and contains more

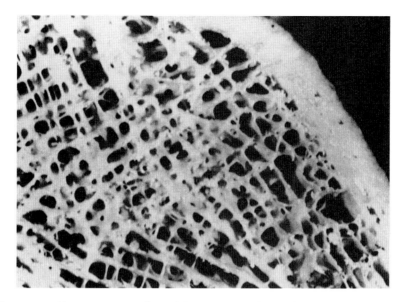

Figure 2.7.   Transverse cut surface of the innominate bone of the pelvis, exhibiting an outer shell of dense cortical bone, or compacta (at the right edge of the specimen), covering cancellous, trabecular bone, or spongiosa.

proteoglycan but less cement substance, as well as less mineral, than does mature bone (Fig. 2.8).

Mature Bone

The dense cortical (or compact) mature bone is characterized by the concentric arrangement of its microscopic layers or lamellae and also by the complex formation of *haversian systems* or *osteons,* which are well designed to permit circulation of blood within the thick mass of cortical bone (Fig. 2.9). Similar to plywood, the collagen fibrils in any given concentric layer of a haversian system course in a different direction from those of adjoining layers—an arrangement that adds strength to the cortical bone.

In cancellous (or trabecular) bone, the arrangement of the lamellae is somewhat less complex because the trabeculae are thin and can therefore be nourished by surrounding vessels in the marrow spaces (Fig. 2.10).

Cancellous bone has only one quarter of the body's mass of cortical bone, but because its surface area is eight times larger than that of cortical bone, and because bone turnover is a surface phenomenon, this turnover in can-

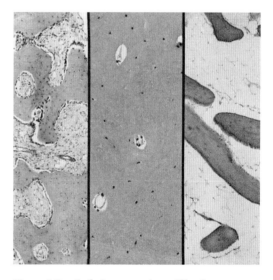

Figure 2.8.   Left. Immature bone (fiber bone, woven bone) in the human. This cellular type of bone is laid down in an irregular "woven" pattern.

Figure 2.9.   Middle. Cross-section of the dense cortex of mature bone in the human. Note the concentric arrangement of the layers, or lamellae, around a central vessel thereby forming haversian systems, or osteons.

Figure 2.10.   Right. Trabeculae of mature cancellous bone in the human. The thin trabeculae are nourished by surrounding vessels in the marrow spaces.

cellous bone is eight times greater than that in cortical bone.

Mature bone is less cellular and contains more cement substance and more mineral than does immature bone. The interstices of cancellous bone contain blood vessels, nerve fibers, fat and hemopoietic tissue. Although during childhood, hemopoietic tissue is found in cancellous bone throughout the skeleton, it is limited in adult life to the cancellous bone of the spine, shoulder, and pelvic girdle.

Bone Cells and Their Function

The *osteoblasts,* which represent one type of differentiated mesenchymal cell, are essential for *osteogenesis* or *ossification,* since they alone can produce the organic intercellular substance, or *matrix,* in which *calcification* can occur later. Because of its microscopic similarity to bone (in decalcified preparations), the uncalcified tissue is called *osteoid* (bonelike), or prebone. Once calcification occurs in the matrix, the tissue is *bone.* Thus, ossification and calcification are not synonymous. As soon as an osteoblast has surrounded itself with organic intercellular substance, it lies in a *lacuna* and is henceforth known as an *osteocyte.*

Each osteocyte, imprisoned in its own lacuna, extends cytoplasmic processes via *canaliculi* to connect with similar processes from neighboring osteocytes. It is through these tiny channels that the osteocytes receive their nutrition from tissue fluid derived from regional blood vessels (in horizontal Volkmann's canals and in longitudinal haversian canals). Unlike cartilage, bone cannot enlarge by interstitial growth because its matrix is calcified. Thus, a given bone can enlarge only by appositional growth on an existing surface.

Urist discovered a family of growth factors in the demineralized matrix of bone in 1965. These noncollagenous glycoproteins, which he has designated *bone morphogenetic proteins (BMPs),* stimulate undifferentiated perivascular mesenchymal cells to differentiate into osteogenic cells—that is, osteoblasts—and thereby induce entirely new bone formation. Some members of the family of bone morphogenetic proteins (which are related to the family of transforming growth factors, including TGF-β) have the potential to enhance the healing of bone defects and nonunions of fractures in humans.

The large, multinucleated cells that lie on the naked or uncovered bone surfaces and that are capable of resorbing or removing bone are called *osteoclasts.* It is believed that osteoclasts are derived from the fusion of many pluripotential stem cells—monocytes or macrophages—that cover or line bone surfaces. Their unique function is to resorb bone from bony surfaces. Calcium can be removed from bone only by osteoclastic activity (*osteoclasis*), which removes the organic matrix and the calcium simultaneously, a process that is more accurately described as *deossification* rather than "decalcification."

Biochemistry and Physiology of Bone as an Organ

Although the *gross appearance* of bones as structures changes slowly, particularly after the period of skeletal growth, there is much *microscopic change* taking place within the bones as a result of the active physiology of bone as an organ. The main biochemical function of bone concerns calcium and phosphorus metabolism.

Biochemistry of Bone

The biochemical composition of bone is as follows: organic substances, 30%; inorganic (mineral) substances, 60%; water, 10%.

Organic Substances

The organic component of bone includes the bone cells as well as the organic intercellular substance, or matrix. Collagen fibers and noncollagenous proteins constitute more than 95% of the organic matrix, which also contains small quantities of reticular fibrils and amorphous substances (including hyaluronic acid and chondroitin sulfate). The osteocytes constitute only 2% of the organic matrix.

Inorganic Substances

The most important inorganic substances in bone are calcium and phosphorus, but other ions include magnesium, sodium, hydroxyl, carbonate, and fluoride. Although the actual chemical composition of the bone crystal is known to vary during life, it is generally considered a hydroxyapatite crystal with the possible formula of $Ca_{10}(PO_4)_6(OH)_2$; the first deposit of mineral is probably amorphous $Ca_3(PO_4)_2$.

Enzymes. *Bone alkaline phosphatase,* which is produced by osteoblasts, may play a role in the osteoblastic production of organic matrix before calcification—that is, osteoid—and may also play a role in its subsequent calcification. The metabolism of living bone cells—and indeed of all cells—depends on multiple enzyme systems.

Calcium and Phosphorus Metabolism

The metabolisms of calcium (Ca) and phosphorus are so closely interdependent that they are best considered together. Indeed, the normal plasma levels of both calcium and inorganic phosphate (P_i) are regulated by three hormones: the active metabolites of vitamin D (now considered to be hormones rather than vitamins), parathyroid hormone (PTH), and calcitonin. The metabolically active tissues on which these three hormones act are bones, kidneys, and intestine. As a physiological organ, bone is the reservoir for 99% of the total body calcium (1000 g) and 90% of the total body phosphorus, the calcium and phosphate of bone being bound to each other as hydroxyapatite—$Ca_{10}(PO_4)_6(OH)_2$. Thus, only 1% (1000 mg) of calcium is in the extracellular fluid and only a minute, but critically important, amount (50 mg) is intracellular, mostly in mitochondria.

Maintenance of a narrow normal range of total plasma calcium is vital (9.0 to 10.4 mg/100 mL or 2.25 to 2.60 mM). Of the total plasma calcium, approximately one-half is ionized (Ca^{2+}) and the other half is protein-bound (mainly to albumin). Less critical is the maintenance of a normal plasma P_i of approximately 3 mg/100 mL or 1 mM in adults and 5 mg/mL or 1.6 mM in children. The plasma concentrations of calcium are higher in children, in whom they are inversely correlated with age.

Calcium has a large number and wide variety of functions in the body including the following:

1. It controls internal regulation of the function of all cells; calmodulin and actin have prime functions in modulating the intracellular effects of calcium
2. It regulates cell membrane permeability, nerve excitability, muscle contraction, and gland secretion.
3. Extracellular calcium ion concentration regulates synthetic and secretory functions of the parathyroid gland (for PTH) and thyroid C cells (for calcitonin).
4. It controls adhesiveness between cells.
5. It controls the hardness and rigidity of bones and teeth through hydroxyapatite [$Ca_{10}(PO_4)_6(OH)_2$].

Calcium Homeostasis

Calcium in the diet is absorbed through the small intestine into the bloodstream, and this process depends on the normal integrity of the intestinal mucosa, normal gastric acidity, the presence of the active metabolites of vitamin D, and the presence of bile salts and pancreatic enzymes (to digest fatty acids that would otherwise combine with calcium in the small bowel to form insoluble calcium soaps). Calcium is excreted both in the urine and in the feces. The calcium homeostasis in a normal adult is depicted in Figure 2.11.

Phosphate Homeostasis

Dietary P_i is also absorbed through the small intestine, both by diffusion and by active transport mechanisms stimulated in part by the active metabolites of vitamin D, especially the hormone $1,25(OH)_2D$. The precise mechanisms governing the transport of phosphate in and out of cells are not well understood. It is clear, however, that the kidney plays a pivotal role in regulating the level of plasma P_i as shown schematically in Figure 2.12.

Actions of Parathyroid Hormone

The secretion of PTH is stimulated by hypocalcemia (but not directly by hypophosphatemia). The main effect of PTH is stimulation of bone reabsorption, but it also increases

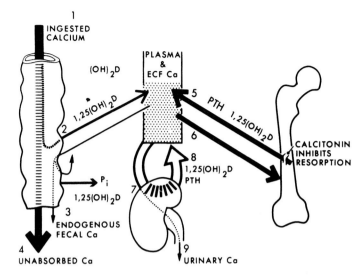

Figure 2.11. Processes that determine plasma and ECF calcium concentrations. **1.** Ingested calcium: normally 500 to 1000 mg/day (500 to 1000 mL of milk provides 1000 mg of calcium). **2.** Intestinal absorption: normally 300 mg/day; most absorption occurs in duodenum and proximal ileum. **3.** Endogenous fecal calcium; this represents an obligatory calcium loss. The calcium is excreted in bile, intestinal juices, and desquamated cells. It amounts to 150 mg/day. **4.** Unabsorbed calcium (**3 and 4**) equals total fecal calcium. **5.** Resorption from bone. **6.** Accretion into bone. In the normal adult, resorption equals accretion. The exact mechanism that couples these processes is not understood. Between 500 and 1000 mg of calcium are exchanged per day. In growth, accretion is greater than resorption. **7.** Glomerular filtration. A passive process that depends on the glomerular filtration rate and concentration of ultrafiltrable calcium, amounting to 10 g/day. **8.** Renal tubular reabsorption—an active, 99% efficient process. **9.** Urinary calcium, 50 to 300 mg/day. Net calcium balance equals intake (**1**) minus total fecal (**3 and 4**) calcium plus urine calcium (**9**). One gram of calcium is equivalent to 25 mmol. (Courtesy of Dr. Donald Fraser.)

resorption of calcium from the renal tubule. By contrast, PTH inhibits renal tubular resorption of phosphate, thereby leading to a decrease in plasma phosphate concentration. Thus, the net effects of PTH actions are elevation of plasma calcium and correction of hypocalcemia, as well as lowered plasma phosphate concentrations. In addition, PTH stimulates the synthesis of $1,25(OH)_2D$ (Figs. 2.11 and 2.12).

Actions of Calcitonin
Calcitonin, discovered by Copp in 1962, is secreted by the C cells in the thyroid. Its secretion is stimulated by hypercalcemia and inhibited by hypocalcemia. The clinical significance of calcitonin in the homeostasis of calcium and

phosphate in humans is not yet clear. It is known, however, that calcitonin decreases bone resorption by suppressing osteoclastic activity (this effect is of clinical significance in the treatment of Paget's disease and osteoporosis as discussed in Chapter 9). Calcitonin has also be found to be a powerful analgesic. Both salmon and porcine calcitonin have an effect in humans.

Actions of Vitamin D Metabolites
It is now known that vitamin D per se is metabolically inactive. Of its active metabolites, however, the most significant is 1,25-dihydroxycalciferol (1,25-dihydroxy vitamin D) $(1,25(OH)_2D)$ which acts like a steroid hormone as shown by DeLuca.

The major effect of the active normal metabolites of vitamin D (principally 1,25 (OH)$_2$D) is to increase absorption of both calcium and phosphate from the intestine; 1,25-dihydroxyvitamin D also increases the mobilization of calcium (and secondarily P$_i$) from bone. Additional actions of less apparent significance include increased renal tubular reabsorption of calcium and stimulation of synthesis of calcium-binding protein in intestinal mucosa cells. The net effect of all these phenomena is to elevate the plasma levels of calcium. Recent evidence suggests that 24,25(OH)$_2$D may participate in the deposition of mineral in the uncalcified matrix of bone—that is, in osteoid.

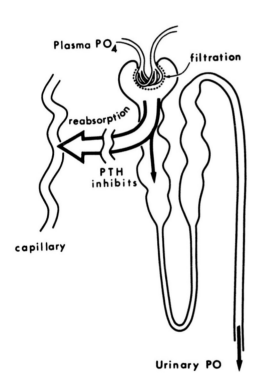

Figure 2.12. Phosphate reclamation by the kidney. Plasma P$_i$ exists in an almost completely ultrafiltrable state. Glomerular filtrate phosphate is a passive process, which is calculated from glomerular filtrate phosphate × plasma P$_i$. Renal tubular reabsorption of phosphate is normally efficient, 70 to 90% of glomerular filtrate phosphate. It is an active process, occurring mainly at the proximal convoluted tubule. Tubular reabsorption of phosphate = glomerular filtrate phosphate − urinary phosphate. (Courtesy of Dr. Donald Fraser.)

As is the case for all hormones, the synthesis of 1,25(OH)$_2$D and 24,25(OH)$_2$D is under feedback regulation. The main factors for stimulating the most active metabolite of vitamin D, namely, 1,25(OH)$_2$D, include hypocalcemia, hypophosphatemia, and PTH.

JOINTS AND ARTICULAR CARTILAGE

A joint is simply a junction between two or more bones. Joints provide segmentation of the human skeleton and allow varying degrees of motion between the segments, as well as varying amounts of segmental growth.

Classification of the Types of Joints

Five distinct types of joints exist in the body, each with its particular characteristics. They are described in the following list:

1. *Syndesmosis:* a joint in which the two bones are bound together by fibrous tissue only, as in the suture joints between the skull bones.
2. *Synchrondrosis:* a joint in which the two bones are bound together by cartilage. An epiphyseal plate is, in effect, a temporary synchrondrosis that binds the epiphysis to the metaphysis and that permits longitudinal growth. The cartilaginous joints between some of the endochrondral bones in the base of the skull are also synchondroses.
3. *Synostosis:* a joint that, at some stage, has become obliterated by bony union. Some syndesmoses and all synchrondroses eventually fuse and thereby become synostoses.
4. *Symphysis:* a joint in which the two opposing surfaces are covered by hyaline cartilage and joined by fibrocartilage and strong fibrous tissue. There may be a small central cleft (as in the symphysis pubis) but not a true joint cavity. Symphyses allow little movement but provide much stability. Intervertebral joints (usually called intervertebral discs) are a specialized form of symphysis in which the opposing cartilage-covered surface of adjacent vertebral bod-

ies are joined together by a ring of dense fibrous tissue and fibrocartilage (the annulus fibrosus). The central cleft or space is filled with a semifluid substance (the nucleus pulposus).

5. *Synovial joint:* a joint in which the two opposing surfaces are covered by hyaline articular cartilage and joined peripherally by a fibrous tissue capsule enclosing a joint cavity that contains synovial fluid. Synovial joints, which are present throughout the limbs, allow free movement, but at the expense of providing less stability than the other four types of joints.

Synovial joints provide a smooth, self-lubricating, almost frictionless gliding motion throughout an average lifetime of normal use. The resilient articular cartilage also acts as a cushion or shock absorber for the subchondral bone during impact loading. However, once cartilage is damaged, at any age, either by injury or by disease, its ability to heal or regenerate under ordinary circumstances is so limited that the inevitable result is progressive degenerative arthritis.

Embryonic Development of Synovial Joints

An articular disc of mesenchyme appears (*the primitive joint plate*) at the site of future synovial joints in the central condensation of mesenchyme of the limb bud. A dense tissue, which is the counterpart of perichondrium of the cartilaginous model, surrounds the primitive joint plate and is the forerunner of the joint capsule. By the seventh or eighth week of embryonic life, clefts or spaces, which are filled with tissue fluid, appear in the primitive joint plate (cavitation) and gradually coalesce to form a single joint cavity. The synovial fluid may be considered a mucin (hyaluronic acid) diluted by tissue fluid. The outer layer of the joint capsule differentiates into fibrous tissue, whereas the inner layer becomes specialized to form the synovial membrane.

It is known from scientific studies that from the sixth week of embryonic life, active intrauterine movement of the limbs is essential to the normal embryonic development of synovial joints (this is just one example of the critical importance of motion in maintaining healthy joints).

Anatomy and Histology of Synovial Joints

Anatomical Structure

The various anatomical structures of a typical synovial joint are best depicted diagrammatically as seen in Figure 2.13. The convex joint surface is always larger than the opposing concave joint surface—an arrangement that allows gliding motion. Articular cartilage has the consistency of firm rubber and, like rubber, it is resilient. It is also called *hyaline* cartilage (Greek *hyalos,* glass) because like "frosted" glass, articular cartilage is pearly white and partially translucent, an appearance that is due to its distinctive intercellular matrix.

Articular cartilage is a viscoelastic tissue that is a mixture of an elastic solid and a viscous liquid; as such it is admirably suited to withstand the intermittent shear and compres-

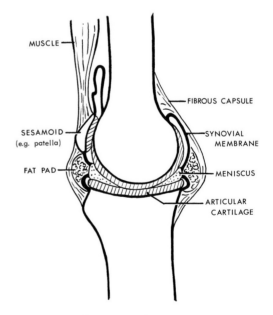

Figure 2.13. Diagrammatic representation of the various anatomical structures of a typical human synovial joint (a sagittal section of the knee viewed from the side).

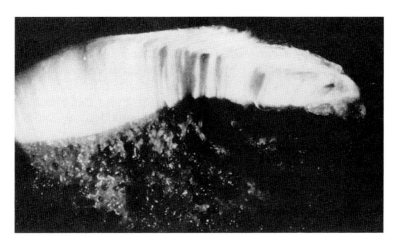

Figure 2.14.   Fracture surface of a fresh fracture involving the articular cartilage **(top)** and underlying cancellous bone of the patella in a young man. Note the vertical alignment of the bundles of collagen fibers in the deep zone of the cartilage and the horizontal alignment in the superficial zone. The bundles descend vertically from the superficial zone to the deep zone, thereby forming arcades. (Courtesy of Dr. Roby Thompson.)

sion forces of normal joint function. Through tribology (the science of friction, wear and lubrication of interacting surfaces in relative motion) we learn that the coefficient of friction between the two surfaces of a normal joint is extremely small, in fact only one-fifth that between two pieces of ice! A form of "boundary lubrication" or "weeping lubrication" is made possible by a mucin (hyaluronate) in the synovial fluid so that motion occurs between two thin layers of fluid rather than directly between two surfaces of articular cartilage.

The macroscopically smooth articular surface is provided by a tough, skinlike, limiting membrane that exhibits lines of tension (comparable to Langer's lines of the skin). Indeed, intact cartilage *in vivo* has been likened to an inflated air tent or a tire in that much water is imbibed by the hydrophilic matrix and this "inflates" the cartilage, which is therefore pressurized; the intracartilage pressure is contained by the intact surface membrane. The thickness of articular cartilage varies from one joint to another, and even from one area to another within a given joint.

Within the substance of the cartilage the bundles of collagen fibers form arcades like the curved ribs of an umbrella (Benninghoff's arcades). Thus, they rise vertically from their deep attachment to the subchondral bone,

gradually become horizontal as they reach the joint surface, and then descend in a vertical configuration again to the bone (Fig. 2.14).

The synovial membrane lines the entire joint cavity except over the surfaces of articular cartilage and menisci. It has the ability to secrete as well as absorb. Synovia-covered fat pads, which are mobile, project into peripheral spaces in the joint, thereby preventing a vacuum from developing in the cavity. The outer fibrous capsule becomes greatly thickened in some areas to form strong ligaments that help provide some degree of joint stability.

The medial and lateral menisci, which consist of fibrocartilage as opposed to hyaline articular cartilage, occupy the space between the peripheral areas of the opposing joint surfaces within the knee joint (Fig. 2.13). The extracellular matrix of the meniscus consists mainly of type I collagen fibers. Once thought to be expendable, the menisci are now known to be an integral component of the knee joint; indeed the surgical excision of a meniscus eventually leads to secondary degenerative arthritis. The menisci provide a more congruous articulating surface for the femoral condyle and the opposing tibial plateau, thereby improving joint stability and the load distribution as well as joint lubrication.

Histological Structure of Articular Cartilage

Hyaline articular cartilage is characterized by a paucity of sparsely scattered chondrocytes in a vast matrix of intercellular substance. Unlike most other tissues, such cartilage is completely devoid of blood vessels, lymphatic vessels, and nerve fibers. Indeed the chondrocytes in normal cartilage live in immunological isolation from the cells of the rest of the body, which explains the success of cartilage allografts.

The chondrocytes in their lacunae are arranged in three indistinct layers or zones (Fig. 2.15). In the superficial zone, the limiting membrane, known as the lamina splendans, is characterized by a plethora of collagen fibers that are parallel to the surface and small oval cells that are similarly aligned. Unlike bone that is clothed in periosteum, the articular surface is not covered by perichondrium. In the middle zone the chondrocytes are younger and somewhat more active than in the other two zones. Mitotic figures may be seen in this zone during childhood, but they are not normally seen in adulthood. In the deep zone, the collagen fibers are vertical and the chondrocytes are mature. During the growing years, this layer functions as the growth cartilage of the underlying epiphysis, allowing it to increase in both height and width. In adult life, however, the matrix of the deepest part of this zone becomes calcified; the border between the calcified zone and the uncalcified remainder of the articular cartilage is known as the tidemark.

The distinctive matrix, which is a resilient gel, is composed of tissue fluid (primarily water) (70 to 80%), collagen (10 to 15%) and proteoglycans (10 to 15%). Although the fluid can move in and out of the matrix, cartilage is hydrophilic, and the fluid gives this tissue its turgidity. The collagen of hyaline articular cartilage is type II (in contrast to that of the fibrocartilage of menisci, which is type I). Like

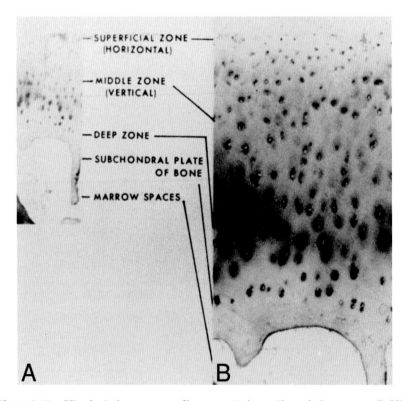

Figure 2.15.   Histological appearance of human articular cartilage. **A.** Low power. **B.** High power.

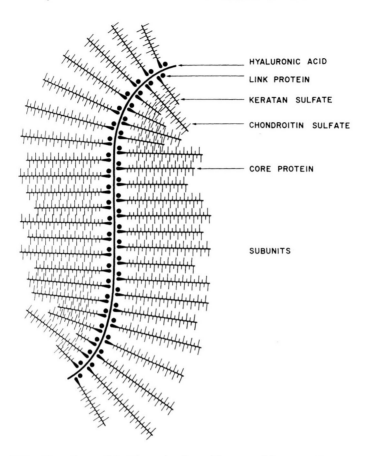

HYALURONIC ACID
LINK PROTEIN
KERATAN SULFATE
CHONDROITIN SULFATE

CORE PROTEIN

SUBUNITS

Figure 2.16. Tentative model of the molecular architecture of the proteoglycan aggregate. (Courtesy of Dr. Lawrence Rosenberg.)

the rods in reinforced concrete, the collagen fibers provide cartilage with its strength, especially in tension. It is the hydrophilic proteoglycans that bind or "glue" the collagen fibers together and provide the articular cartilage with the resilience and elasticity so necessary in resisting intermittent shear and compressive forces and in providing the rigid subchondral bone a protective shock absorber.

Rosenberg has made extensive studies of the remarkable macromolecules of proteoglycan aggregates with their central cores of hyaluronic acid, link proteins, and multiple subunits composed of a central core and bristle-like rods of three glycosaminoglycans: chondroitin-4-sulfate, chondroitin-6-sulfate and keratan sulfate (the obsolete term for glycosaminoglycans is mucopolysaccharides). These glycosaminoglycans in the subunits resemble the bristles of a test tube brush: because each "bristle" carries a negative electrical charge, they repel one another, and this is what gives articular cartilage its characteristic resilience. The complex structures of proteoglycan aggregates and their subunits are best appreciated schematically (Figs. 2.16 and 2.17).

PROTEOGLYCAN SUBUNIT

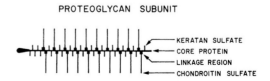

KERATAN SULFATE
CORE PROTEIN
LINKAGE REGION
CHONDROITIN SULFATE

Figure 2.17. Diagram of the proposed structure of the proteoglycan subunit. (Courtesy of Dr. Lawrence Rosenberg.)

Both the collagen and the proteoglycans are synthesized by the chondrocytes, which therefore carry the responsibility for maintaining the physical properties of the cartilage through extracellular homeostasis. Indeed these cells, once thought to be somewhat dormant, are metabolically active—more so during childhood, of course, than during adult life. Chondrocytes respond to many stimuli, including active or passive motion and substances such as growth factors, interleukins, and drugs. For example, growth hormone, androgens, insulin, and calcitonin stimulate chondrocytes to proliferate as well as to synthesize both collagen fibers and proteoglycans of the cartilage matrix. (Such synthesis is also stimulated by TGF-β.) Chondrocytes require little oxygen for metabolism, but they are dependent for their nutrition on the long-range diffusion of nutrients from the synovial fluid, which is essentially a modified type of tissue fluid. Therefore, the two most important factors in the optimal nutrition of articular cartilage are a healthy synovial membrane to produce the synovial fluid and adequate "circulation" or diffusion of this nourishing fluid through the matrix to reach the chondrocytes. Understandably, nutrition of the cartilage is enhanced by joint motion, which squeezes synovial fluid into and waste products out of the spongelike matrix. By contrast, immobilization of a synovial joint, especially if prolonged, leads to stasis of synovial fluid and disuse atrophy of the cartilage.

Bone and Cartilage: Similarities and Differences

Bone and cartilage are similar in some respects but different in others. Both these tissues are derived, or differentiated, from pluripotential mesenchymal stem cells; both consist of cells lying in lacunae that are embedded in an intercellular matrix that they have synthesized, and the matrix of both tissues is reinforced by resilient collagen fibers that are comparable to the metal rods in reinforced concrete.

By contrast, however, the matrix of bone is heavily calcified, which gives bone its stonelike quality. Furthermore, whereas the chondrocytes are nourished by long-range diffusion of synovial fluid (a modified tissue fluid) into and

out of the avascular matrix, osteocytes require more oxygen so that bone is a highly vascular tissue permeated by capillaries that course in the central haversian canals of each osteone and provide tissue fluid that reaches the embedded osteocytes via tiny canaliculi within the calcified matrix. The collagen of the matrix of bone is type I but that of the matrix of cartilage is type II.

Structure and Functions of the Synovial Membrane

The synovial membrane is composed of two distinct layers: an inner and an outer. Not a true membrane, the inner synovial lining is a thin syncytium of only a few layers of loosely connected cells supported by an outer layer of fibrous and fatty tissue that, in contrast to cartilage, has a rich supply of blood vessels, lymphatic vessels, and nerve fibers. There are two types of cells in the inner layer. The predominant type A synoviocytes, which have many features of macrophages, serve to clear the joint of waste materials, whereas the type B synoviocytes synthesize hyaluronate, which is a mucin that provides synovial fluid with its viscosity and its remarkable lubricating qualities. Because of the countless villi in the synovial membrane its functional surface area is enormous, for example, as much as 100 m² in a human knee joint.

Crystalloids, including most antibiotics, diffuse across the synovial membrane readily in both directions via the capillaries, but proteins with their large colloidal molecules leave the joint cavity via the lymphatics. Particulate matter (such as hemosiderin from a joint hemorrhage) is removed from the synovial cavity through phagocytosis by the macrophage-like type A synoviocytes, but may then remain in the synovial membrane and subsynovial tissues for many months, leading to synovial hypertrophy.

Synovial Fluid

A viscous, pale yellow, clear fluid resembling the white of an egg (from the Latin *ovum*, egg), synovial fluid is a dialysate of plasma, a type of tissue fluid to which glycoprotein and the lubricant hyaluronic acid (hyaluronate) have been added. Thus, synovial fluid serves the dual function of nourishing the articular cartilage and lubricating the joint surfaces. A normal joint contains relatively little synovial fluid; for example, the normal adult knee, which is the largest joint in the body, contains less than 5 mL. Thus, the true joint space is virtually a potential space. (The so-called joint space seen between the bony surfaces of a joint in a radiograph is more appropriately designated the cartilage space.) Synovial fluid is present not only in synovial joints but also in synovial tendon sheaths and synovial bursae.

In a normal joint, the total cell count of synovial fluid is less than 200 cells/mL; monocytic macrophages and lymphocytes predominate with only a small percentage of polymorphonuclear leukocytes. Synovial fluid contains albumin and globulin but no fibrinogen. The absence of fibrinogen may explain why normal synovial fluid does not clot. Blood, mixed with synovial fluid in a joint, likewise does not clot.

SKELETAL MUSCLES

Almost 50% of the average person's body weight is skeletal muscle, and such muscle requires almost 50% of the body's metabolism. The skeletal muscles, of which there are more than 400 in the human body, are the "living motors" that provide *active movement* of the articulated skeleton as well as *maintenance of its posture*. The basic property of skeletal muscle is *contractility* of its protoplasm (*sarcoplasm*), which enables the individual muscle to shorten, and thereby provide movement (*isotonic contraction*), to resist lengthening without allowing movement (*isometric contraction*), or allow lengthening while maintaining tension (*eccentric contraction*).

Anatomy and Histology of Skeletal Muscle

The size, shape, and gross structure of muscles vary tremendously in accordance with their particular function and workload, but the basic cellular structure is the individual *muscle cell*, which because of its long, thin, thread-like shape is called a *muscle fiber*. Skeletal muscle is designated *voluntary* muscle because it is under the individual's will, and *striated* because of its characteristic microscopic cross-

striations (Fig. 2.18). Each individual muscle cell, or fiber, is innervated by a single anterior horn cell of the spinal cord through a single axon within a peripheral nerve fiber (although a given anterior horn cell innervates more than one muscle cell in a muscle). The anterior horn cell, its axon, the myoneural junctions, and the individual muscle fibers supplied by the single anterior horn cell constitute a *single motor unit*. The connective tissue components of a skeletal muscle serve as a medium through which the rich nerve and blood supplies to the muscle fibers course; in addition, they provide a noncontractile framework or "harness" through which the contraction of muscle fibers is transmitted to bone. The connective tissue surrounding the entire muscle is termed *epimysium*, that surrounding bundles of muscle fibers is termed *perimysium*, and that surrounding each individual muscle fiber is termed *endomysium* (Fig. 2.19).

Each muscle fiber is, in fact, a thin, significantly elongated, multinucleated cell that varies tremendously in length depending on the muscle in which it is situated. Each fiber extends from its origin in a tendon or a bone to its insertion into a tendon that, in turn, is inserted into another bone. In a unipennate muscle (such as the sartorius) there is evidence to suggest that each muscle cell probably extends the full length of the muscle. The protoplasm, or *sarcoplasm*, of each muscle fiber is contained by a thin membrane, the *sarcolemma*, under which the eccentrically placed cell nuclei lie, about 40 for each millimeter length of the fiber. Of these nuclei, a small percentage represent *satellite cells* (*dormant myoblasts*), which may be important sources of muscle regeneration after injury. Each muscle fiber contains many *myofibrils*, each of which, in turn, is transversely divided into thousands of tiny cylindrical areas (*sarcomeres*) by the cross-striations (a muscle fiber 5 mm long would have about 20,000 such divisions) (Fig. 2.20). Electron microscopy reveals that each sarcomere, in turn, contains about three million thick myofilaments, consisting of molecules of the muscle protein, *myosin*, and thin myofilaments, consisting of molecules of another muscle protein, *actin* (Fig. 2.21). The

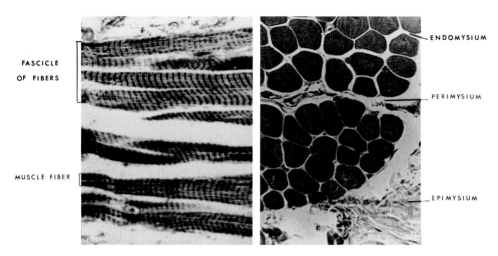

Figure 2.18.   **Left.** Longitudinal section of human skeletal muscle (voluntary, striated muscle). Note the characteristic cross-striations in each muscle fiber.

Figure 2.19.   **Right.** Cross-section of human skeletal muscle showing the connective tissue components that provide a noncontractile harness through which the contraction of the muscle fibers is transmitted to bone.

sarcomeres are, in fact, the functional units of muscle contraction.

There are two main types of muscle fibers. Type I is a slow-twitch, or slow oxidative, fiber that is most important for high-repetition, low-load endurance activities. Type II, which includes four subtypes, is a fast-twitch, or glycolytic, fiber that is better adapted for activi-

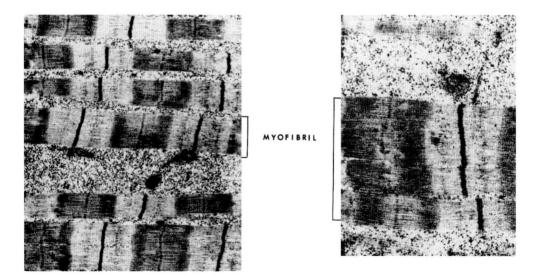

Figure 2.20.   Longitudinal section of a human skeletal muscle fiber which consists of many myofibrils each of which is divided into sarcomeres by cross-striations. Note the various "bands" in each sarcomere. Note the dark A bands alternating with the light I bands and the clearer H zone within each of the A bands. Magnification: *left*, 12,000 × ; *right*, 20,000 × .

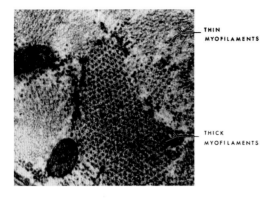

Figure 2.21. Cross-section of a sarcomere of human skeletal muscle showing thick myofilaments (myosin) and thin myofilaments (actin). Magnification 60,000 ×.

ties requiring power and speed. The functional capacity of type II muscle fibers is high-resistance training (high tension, low frequency) that results in muscle hypertrophy.

Biochemistry and Physiology of Muscle

The processes by which skeletal muscle converts stored chemical energy into mechanical energy to perform work are complex indeed. Acetylcholine is the chemical mediator of the nerve impulses at the myoneural junction, and it is believed that the energy for muscle action is derived from the breakdown of adenosine triphosphate (ATP) by adenosine triphosphatase (ATPase) with the liberation of adenosine diphosphate (ADP). Current thinking is that muscle contraction, which occurs within the individual sarcomeres, takes place as a result of the sliding of the thin myofilaments (actin) of the I bands between the thick myofilaments (myosin) of the A bands. As a result of this sliding, which may be likened to the bristles of two hair brushes that are being pushed together, the thousands of cross-striations move closer together and the entire fiber shortens (contracts). During relaxation, the thin myofilaments slide out again from between the thick myofilaments and the sarcomeres lengthen as does the entire muscle fiber.

The most important practical consideration of skeletal muscle is its ability to develop *tension,* part of which is due to its *contractile force*

and part of which is due to the *resistance of its connective tissue components to stretch.* Each muscle fiber obeys the *all-or-none law* in that it either contracts maximally or not at all. Thus, in a given muscle, the difference between a powerful contraction and a weak contraction lies in the number of individual fibers that are contracting within the muscle at that time. For each muscle there is a definite relationship between its "starting length" and the amount of tension it can develop. When the muscle is passively shortened by approximating its origin and insertion, it can develop little contractile force. The greatest contractile force is developed when the muscle is at its resting length (about halfway between its extremes of length). As the muscle is passively stretched beyond its resting length, the contractile force gradually diminishes, but the passive resistance of the connective tissue components gradually develops more tension so that the *total tension* in the muscle increases. This muscle length-tension relationship can be depicted graphically by what is known as the *Blix curve* (Fig. 2.22). You can demonstrate this phenomenon readily in your

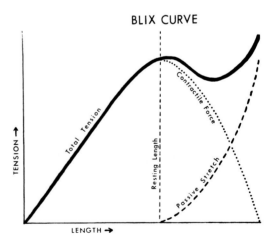

Figure 2.22. The Blix curve, depicting muscle length–tension relationship. Note that the greatest contractile force is developed when the muscle is at its resting length, about halfway between its extremes of length. As the muscle is passively stretched beyond its resting length, its contractile force gradually diminishes, but the passive resistance of the connective tissue components gradually produces more tension so that the total tension in the muscle increases.

own hand. With your fingers and wrist in the position of complete flexion, your finger flexor muscles are shortened and can develop little contractile force during an attempt to squeeze an object such as the index finger of your opposite hand; furthermore, there is no tension from passive resistance of the connective tissue components. With your wrist in the neutral position and the fingers slightly flexed, your finger flexors are at their resting length, and you can demonstrate that they have much greater contractile force. When your wrist and fingers are completely extended, there is little contractile force but much passive resistance to further stretch. Thus, the normal resting length of a given muscle is of great importance in musculoskeletal function, and any undesirable alteration in this resting length by disorders or injuries (including surgical operations) results in loss of power.

During longitudinal skeletal growth through epiphyseal plates, the muscles must also grown in length. Since the individual sarcomeres do not lengthen, the individual muscle fibers can become longer only by adding more sarcomeres, a phenomenon that occurs primarily at the musculotendinous junction.

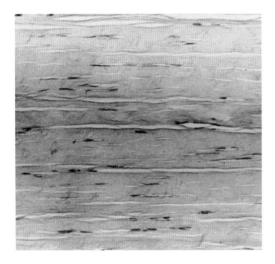

Figure 2.23.   Longitudinal section of human tendon, showing rows of flattened fibroblasts scattered between collagen fibers longitudinally aligned in the line of tension. Note that this tissue contains relatively few cells but an abundance of intercellular substance.

TENDONS AND LIGAMENTS

Tendons and ligaments, in contrast to muscles, are composed of dense connective tissue, which, because it contains an abundance of nonextensile collagen (type I) fibers, is known as fibrous connective tissue. The bundles of parallel collagen fibers are aligned in the direction of tension, which is ideal both for tendons that transmit force—that is, pull, from a muscle to a bone—and also for ligaments that resist force—that is, stretch from one bone to another across a joint. Thus, both tendons and ligaments have remarkable tensile strength.

Understandably, tendons and ligaments have a similar histological appearance—a predominance of tightly packed parallel bundles with rows of flattened *fibroblasts* scattered between them (Fig. 2.23).

In adult life, the fibroblasts become relatively dormant *fibrocytes,* and since the intercellular substance requires no nutrition, the blood supply is minimal. At sites of friction, a tendon is enveloped by a *synovial sheath,* consisting of a visceral and a parietal layer of synovial membrane and lubricated by a synovial-like fluid containing hyaluronate. The synovial sheath, in turn, is covered by a dense fibrous tissue sheath. Both tendons and ligaments gain an extremely firm attachment to bone at their sites of insertion by a continuation of their collagen fibers, which penetrate deeply into the solid substance of cortical bone and fan out within it as Sharpey's fibers. So strong is this attachment that even with severe traction injuries, neither ligaments nor tendons "pull out" of bone; instead the ligament or tendon either tears within its substance or a fragment of bone is avulsed along with the inserted tendon or ligament.

The stress deprivation that is associated with prolonged immobilization of a joint, and thereby also of its ligaments, causes progressive weakness in the ligaments and even greater weakness in their ligament-bone junctions. Indeed, it may take from 6 to 12 months after motion has been resumed before these junctions regain their normal strength.

The reactions of musculoskeletal tissues to disorders and injuries are discussed in Chapter

4, and generalized bone disorders caused by metabolic disturbances (metabolic bone diseases) are discussed in Chapter 9.

SUGGESTED ADDITIONAL READING

Andersson GB. Muscle and gait. In: Frymoyer JW, ed. Orthopaedic knowledge update 4. Rosemont, American Academy of Orthopaedic Surgeons, 1993.

Buckwalter JA. Musculoskeletal tissues and the musculoskeletal system. In: Weinstein SL, Buckwalter JA, eds. Turek's orthopaedics: principles and their application. Philadelphia: JB Lippincott, 1994.

Buckwalter JA, Rosenberg LC, Hunziker EB. Articular cartilage composition, response to injury, and methods of facilitating repair. In: Ewing JW, ed. Articular Cartilage and Knee Joint Function: basic science and arthroscopy. New York: Raven Press 1990.

Bullough PG. Bone. In: Owen R, Goodfellow J, Bullough PG, eds. Scientific foundations of orthopaedics and traumatology. London: William Heinemann Medical Books, 1980.

Bullough PG. Cartilage. In: Owen R, Goodfellow J, Bullough PG, eds. Scientific foundations of orthopaedics and traumatology. London: William Heinemann Medical Books, 1980.

Copp DH. Calcitonin: Discovery, development and clinical applications. Clin Invest Med 1994; 17:269–277.

Copp DH, Cameron EC, Cheney BA, Davidson AGF, Henze KG. Evidence for calcitonin—a new hormone from the parathyroids which lowers blood calcium. Endocrinology 1962;70:638.

Cormack DH. Ham's histology. 9th ed. Philadelphia: JB Lippincott 1987.

Cormack DH. Essential histology. Philadelphia: JB Lippincott, 1993.

Cruess RL, ed. The musculoskeletal system. Embryology, biochemistry and physiology. New York: Churchill-Livingstone, 1982.

De Haven KE. The role of the meniscus. In: Ewing JW, ed. Articular cartilage and knee joint function: basic science and arthroscopy. New York: Raven Press, 1990.

DeLuca HF. Calcium metabolism. Acta Orthop Scand 1975;46:286–314.

Einhorn TA. Bone metabolism and metabolic bone disease. In: Frymoyer JW, ed. Orthopaedic knowledge update 4. Rosemont: American Academy of Orthopaedic Surgeons, 1993.

Fraser D, Kooh SW. Disturbance of parathyroid hormone and calcitonin. In: Forfar JO, Arneil GC, eds. Textbook of Paediatrics. 3rd ed. Edinburgh: Churchill-Livingstone, 1984.

Garrett WE Jr, Best TM. Anatomy, physiology, and mechanics of skeletal muscle. In: Simon SR, ed. Orthopaedic basic science. Rosemont: American Academy of Orthopaedic Surgeons, 1994.

Hughes S, Sweetnam R. The basis and practice of orthopaedics. London: William Heinemann Medical Books, 1980.

Iannotti JP, Goldstein S, Kuhn J, et al. Growth plate and bone development. In: Simon SR, ed. Orthopaedic basic science. Rosemont: American Academy of Orthopaedic Surgeons, 1994.

Johnson EE, Urist MR, Finnerman GAM. Resistant nonunions and partial or complete segmental defects of long bones. Treatment with implants of a composite of human bone morphogenetic protein (BMP) and autolyzed antigen-extracted, allogeneic (AAA) bone. Clin Orthop 1992;277:229–237.

Kaplan FS, Hayes WC, Keaveny TM, et al. Form and function of bone. In: Simon SR, ed. Orthopaedic basic science. Rosemont: American Academy of Orthopaedic Surgeons, 1994.

Malemud CJ, Moskowitz RW. Physiology of articular cartilage. Clin Rheum Dis 1981;7:29–55.

Mankin HJ. Metabolic bone disease: an instructional course lecture. The American Academy of Orthopaedic Surgeons. J Bone Joint Surg 1994; 76-A:760–788.

Mankin HJ, Mow VC, Buckwalter JA, et al. Form and function of articular cartilage. In: Simon SR, ed. Orthopaedic basic science. Rosemont: American Academy of Orthopaedic Surgeons, 1994.

Mow VC, Fithian DC, Kelly MA. Fundamentals of articular cartilage and meniscus biomechanics. In: Ewing JW, ed. Articular cartilage and knee joint function: basic science and arthroscopy. New York: Raven Press, 1990.

Paget SA, Bullough PG. Synovium and synovial fluid. In: Owen R, Goodfellow J, Bullough PG, eds. Scientific foundations of orthopaedics and traumatology. London: William Heinemann Medical Books, 1980.

Posner AS. Bone mineral. In: Owen R, Goodfellow J, Bullough PG, eds. Scientific foundations of orthopaedics and traumatology. London: William Heinemann Medical Books, 1980.

Rodrigo JJ. Orthopaedic surgery: basic science and clinical science. Boston: Little, Brown, 1986.

Rosenberg LC. Proteoglycans. In: Owen R, Goodfellow J, Bullough PG. Scientific foundations of orthopaedics and traumatology. London: William Heinemann Medical Books, 1980.

Smith R. Calcium, phosphorus and magnesium metabolism. In: Owen R, Goodfellow J, Bullough PG, eds. Scientific foundations of orthopaedics and traumatology. London: William Heinemann Medical Books, 1980.

Thornhill TS, Schaffer JL. Arthritis. In: Frymoyer JW, ed. Orthopaedic update 4. Rosemont: American Academy of Orthopaedic Surgeons, 1993.

Uhthoff HK. The embryology of the human locomotor system. New York: Springer-Verlag, 1990.

Urist MR. Solubilized and insolubilized bone morphogenetic protein. Proc Nat Acad Sci USA 1979;76:1828–1832.

Urist MR. Bone: formation by autoinduction. Science 1965;150:893. Reprinted in J NIH Res 1997;9:43 (as a "landmark paper").

Urist MR, De Lange RJ, Finnerman GAM. Bone cell differentiation and growth factors. Science 1983;220:680.

Woo SL-Y, Kai Nan A, Arnoczky SP, et al. Anatomy, biology and biomechanics of tendon, ligament and meniscus. In: Simon SR, ed. Orthopaedic basic science. Rosemont: American Academy of Orthopaedic Surgeons, 1994.

3 Reactions of Musculoskeletal Tissues to Disorders and Injuries

"Give me facts, but above all give me understanding"

—Solomon

Having reviewed the *normal* structure and function of the various musculoskeletal tissues, you are now ready to review the *abnormal* structure and function caused by the *biological reactions* of these tissues to disorders and injuries. As a student, and later as a practitioner, you must always remember that your patient is a person—with all that this implies. Nevertheless, you will find it helpful to think about his or her tissue reactions, or pathological processes, not only in terms of the resultant *gross lesions* but also in terms of the dynamic biological activity of the *cells*, which act and react as living populations both in time and at specific sites—that is, the pathogenesis of various pathological states. Enlightened by a knowledge of these reactions, or pathological processes, you will be better prepared to understand the clinical, radiographic, and laboratory *manifestations* of the many abnormal clinical conditions of the musculoskeletal system that you will encounter in your patients. Indeed, these manifestations will enable you to make an intelligent diagnosis as, discussed in Chapter 5. In addition, you will be better able to appreciate the reason, or rationale, for the general principles and specific methods of their treatment, as outlined in Chapter 6 and described in subsequent chapters.

BONE
Reactions of Bone

Bone, which is a highly specialized type of connective tissue, is capable of only a limited number of reactions to a large number of abnormal conditions. Although the results of these reactions may be manifested by significant changes in the gross structure of a bone or bones, the basic nature of the reactions is best considered at a *microscopic, or cellular,* level because the reactions are those of living bone and the cells are the only living components.

There are just four basic ways in which bone can react to abnormal conditions: (1) *local death,* (2) *an alteration of bone deposition,* (3) *an alteration of bone resorption,* and (4) mechanical failure, that is, *fracture.*

When an area of bone is completely deprived of its blood supply, its reaction is local death (*avascular necrosis of bone*). The resultant segment of dead bone then becomes an abnormal condition in itself and incites further reactions from the surrounding living tissues, as discussed in Chapter 13. Bone that remains alive can react to abnormal conditions by either an alteration of deposition or an alteration of resorption, or both. Bone deposition, however, involves a combination of two major processes, namely, osteoblastic formation of organic matrix (osteoid) and calcification of this matrix to form bone; calcification of matrix may be less than normal (hypocalcification), but it is seldom more than normal. Thus, the reactions of living bone may be outlined as follows:

1. Altered deposition of bone
   (a) Increased deposition (increased formation of matrix with normal calcification)
   (b) Decreased deposition (either decreased formation of matrix or hypocalcification)
2. Altered resorption of bone
   (a) Increased resorption
   (b) Decreased resorption
3. Combinations of altered deposition and altered resorption

The abnormal condition may incite one or more reactions in a given bone or part of a bone (*a localized reaction of bone as a structure*) or it may incite one or more reactions in all bones (*a generalized reaction of all bone as an organ*). These reactions in bone are of more than academic interest; indeed, they are of great practical significance because they cause changes in *bone density* and therefore can be detected and studied by ordinary radiographic examination as well as by *computed tomography* (CT) and magnetic resonance imaging (MRI). Thus, either increased deposition or decreased resorption (or a combination of the two) results in *more bone* and is detected by *increased radiographic density (sclerosis)* (Fig. 3.1), whereas the opposite reactions result in *less bone* and are detected by *decreased radiographic density (rarefaction)* (Fig. 3.2).

Throughout an individual's life, bone is formed, or deposited, by osteoblasts, while at the same time bone is removed, or resorbed, by osteoclasts. Thus, to maintain a normal bone mass, it is necessary to maintain a normal balance between osteoblastic bone deposition and osteoclastic bone resorption.

Normally, an individual's bone mass increases gradually from birth to the mid-20s—that is, young adult life. It remains relatively constant throughout middle life, but in later life—that is, old age—it decreases progressively, with a consequent progressive weakening of the bone and resultant increased susceptibility to fracture.

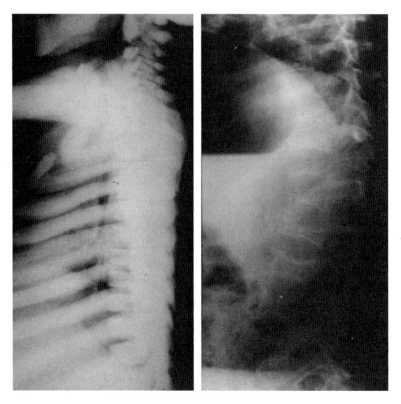

Figure 3.1.   Left. This shows an example of a generalized increase in bone. The spine of this child with osteopetrosis (marble bones) reveals increased radiographic density in all bones.

Figure 3.2.   Right. This is an example of a generalized decrease in bone osteoporosis (osteopenia). The spine of this child with osteogenesis imperfecta ("fragile bones") reveals decreased radiographic density in all bones.

Examples of Reactions of Living Bone

The various reactions of living bone may be incited by a wide variety of clinical disorders and injuries, some of which arise within the musculoskeletal system and some of which arise within other systems of the body. Examples of these abnormal clinical conditions are only mentioned here, but each is discussed in subsequent chapters. In each of these clinical conditions, there is an alteration in the normal *equilibrium*, or *balance*, between bone deposition and bone resorption.

Generalized Reactions of All Bone As an Organ
Bone Deposition Greater Than Bone Resorption (Generalized Increase in Bone)

Osteopetrosis (Marble Bones) (see Chapter 8). In osteopetrosis, bone deposition is probably normal, but bone resorption is defective, and therefore there is an increase in the total amount of bone (Fig. 3.1).

Acromegaly (See Chapter 9). Bone deposition is increased in acromegaly by excessive intramembranous ossification from the periosteum.

Bone Deposition Less Than Bone Resorption (Generalized Decrease in Bone)

Osteoporosis (Osteopenia) (See Chapter 9). Bone deposition is decreased because of decreased osteoblastic formation of matrix (osteoid) and, in addition, bone resorption is increased, with the result that there is a marked decrease in the total amount of bone. Examples of generalized osteoporosis are congenital osteogenesis imperfecta ("fragile bones") (Fig. 3.2) (see Chapter 8), disuse osteoporosis (prolonged decrease in physical activity), steroid-induced osteoporosis, and postmenopausal osteoporosis.

Rickets in Children and Osteomalacia in Adults (See Chapter 9). Although the osteoblastic formation of matrix is normal in rickets seen in children, as well as in osteomalacia in adults, there is decreased calcification (hypocalcification) of the matrix with a resultant decrease in the amount of (calcified) bone.

Localized Reactions of Bone as a Structure
Bone Deposition Greater Than Bone Resorption (Localized Increase in Bone)

Work Hypertrophy. The bone reacts to the extra stresses and strains of increased function by increased bone deposition, which is an example of Wolff's law. For example, in a rigid varus deformity of the foot in which most of the weight is borne on the foot's lateral edge, the fifth metatarsal hypertrophies (Fig. 3.3).

Degenerative Osteoarthritis (See Chapter 11). The subchondral bone underlying that portion of the joint surface taking the greatest amount of excessive intermittent pressure reacts by increased bone deposition that is seen radiographically as subchondral sclerosis.

Fractures (See Chapter 15). The periosteum and endosteum react to bony injury with a localized increase in bone deposition to form callus as part of the healing process.

Infection (See Chapter 10). The periosteum, elevated by pus, reacts to infection by deposition of new bone.

Osteosclerotic Neoplasms (See Chapter 14). The reaction of increased bone deposition to certain benign neoplasms and neoplasmlike lesions of bone (such as osteoid osteoma) is called *reactive bone*, whereas the bone produced by certain malignant bone neoplasms (such as osteosarcoma and osteoblastic metastases) is called *tumor bone*.

Bone Deposition Less Than Bone Resorption (Localized Decrease in Bone)

Disuse Atrophy (Disuse Osteoporosis). The bone reacts to the diminished stresses and strains of decreased function (disuse) by decreased bone deposition, whereas the bone resorption continues unchanged. The result is a localized decrease in bone. Thus, in a lower limb, for example, prolonged immobilization, prolonged relief of weightbearing, and severe paralysis of long duration all cause disuse atrophy of bone (Fig. 3.4).

Rheumatoid Arthritis (See Chapter 10). The bone reacts to the periarticular soft tissue inflammation of rheumatoid arthritis by decreased bone deposition and possibly increased bone resorption. Of course, disuse at-

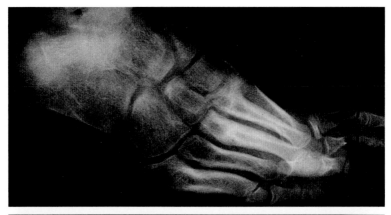

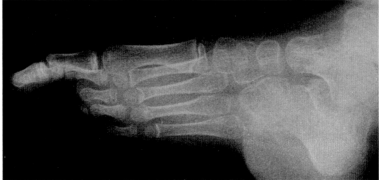

Figure 3.3.   Top. This is an example of a localized increase in bone (work hypertrophy of bone). The hypertrophy of the fifth metatarsal of this boy's foot is a reaction to the increased stresses and strains of most of the weight being borne by the lateral edge of this rigid and deformed foot.

Figure 3.4.   Bottom. This is an example of a localized decrease in bone (disuse atrophy of bone; disuse osteoporosis). The atrophy of all the metatarsals in this boy's foot is a reaction to the decreased stress and strain of no weightbearing on the forefoot because of paralysis of the calf muscles and the resultant inability of the patient to push the forefoot down against the floor or the ground while walking.

rophy may also be a factor because of the coexistent decrease in the function of the involved joint.

Infection (See Chapter 10). The inflammatory process within the bone results in destruction of existing bone by increased resorption locally (*osteolysis*), even though the periosteum reacts by new bone deposition on the outside of the bone.

Osteolytic Neoplasms (See Chapter 14). Some benign bone neoplasms and most malignant bone neoplasms (both primary and secondary) cause a localized destruction of existing bone by increased resorption (osteo-

lysis), even though the periosteum and endosteum may deposit "reactive bone."

Mechanical Failure of Bone (Fractures) (See Chapters 15 to 17)

The tough collagen fibers of the organic matrix of bone provide its strength in tension, whereas the calcified inorganic matrix of bone provides its strength in compression. Thus, an anatomical specimen of a long bone (such as the radius) that has been completely decalcified artificially, becomes in effect a soft tissue structure and can be bent—or even tied in a knot—without breaking. By contrast, an anatomical specimen of a long bone in which the organic matrix has been removed remains a hard tissue but becomes as brittle as a tube of glass and a direct blow or an angulatory force causes it to shatter.

Since the degree of mineralization of bone gradually increases during childhood, the response of a given bone to injury varies with age up to adult life. In adults, bone that is subjected to excessive force fails completely, that is, it fractures. In children, a bone that is subjected to excessive force also fractures. However, with less severe force, the child's bone may buckle or bend without an obvious fracture; this phenomenon is known as *plastic deformation of bone.*

EPIPHYSEAL PLATES
Reactions of Epiphyseal Plates

As stated previously, each epiphyseal plate is a highly specialized cartilaginous structure through which longitudinal growth of bone occurs. Like bone, it is capable of only a limited number of reactions to a large number of abnormal conditions. There are just three basic ways in which an epiphyseal plate can react: (1) *increased growth,* (2) *decreased growth,* and (3) *torsional growth.* Normal growth in each epiphyseal plate requires the plate to have an intact structure and a normal blood supply (which most commonly comes in from the epiphyseal side of the plate). Intermittent pressures associated with normal physical activity are also necessary. An injury involving the epiphyseal plate may cause part or all of it to close—that is, to ossify—and thereby stop growing. Prolonged hyperemia stimulates growth, whereas relative ischemia retards it; indeed, complete ischemia of the epiphysis results in necrosis of the attached epiphyseal plate and therefore complete cessation of growth. Excessive *continuous* pressure on an epiphyseal plate retards growth, and yet a decrease in the normal *intermittent* pressure (as occurs with decreased function of a limb) also retards growth. If either stimulation or retardation occurs in one part of an epiphyseal plate while normal growth continues in the remainder, growth becomes uneven; under these circumstances, a progressive angulatory deformity develops in the bone during subsequent growth.

Examples of Reactions of Epiphyseal Plates

As with bone, the various reactions of epiphyseal plates may be incited by a wide variety of clinical disorders and injuries, some of which arise within the musculoskeletal system and some of which arise within other systems of the body. Examples of these abnormal clinical conditions are only mentioned here, but each is discussed in subsequent chapters.

Generalized Reactions of All Epiphyseal Plates
Generalized Increase in Growth (Gigantism)

Arachnodactyly (Hyperchondroplasia) (Marfan's Syndrome) (See Chapter 8). In Marfan's syndrome, which is an inborn error of development, there is excessive cartilaginous growth (hyperchondroplasia) in all epiphyseal plates (Fig. 3.5).

Pituitary Gigantism (See Chapter 9). Excessive growth hormone from an eosinophilic adenoma of the anterior pituitary gland during childhood stimulates growth in all epiphyseal plates, resulting in pituitary gigantism.

Generalized Decrease in Growth (Dwarfism)

Achondroplasia (See Chapter 8). In achondroplasia, an inborn error of development, there is deficient cartilaginous growth in all epiphyseal plates (Fig. 3.6).

Pituitary dwarfism (Lorain type) (see Chapter 9). Deficient growth hormone from the anterior pituitary gland during childhood retards growth in all epiphyseal plates.

Rickets (See Chapter 9). The deficient calcification (hypocalcification) of the preosseous cartilage of the epiphyseal plate in the zone of calcifying cartilage results in a retardation of growth in all epiphyseal plates.

Localized Reactions of an Epiphyseal Plate
Localized Increase in Growth

Chronic Inflammation (See Chapter 10). The prolonged hyperemia associated with any chronic inflammatory condition *near* an epi-

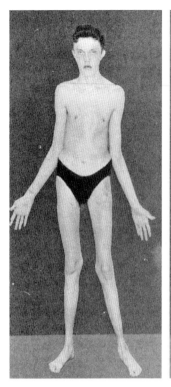
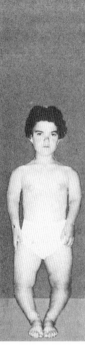

Figure 3.5.   Left. This is an example of a generalized increase in growth (arachnodactyly; hyperchondroplasia, Marfan's syndrome). This 14-year-old boy's limbs are long and thin because of excessive cartilaginous growth (hyperchondroplasia) in all epiphyseal plates.

Figure 3.6.   Right. This is an example of a generalized decrease in growth (achondroplasia; achondroplastic dwarf). This 13-year-old girl's limbs are short and deformed owing to defective growth (achondroplasia) in all epiphyseal plates.

physeal plate stimulates local growth. This phenomenon is observed in disorders such as chronic osteomyelitis and rheumatoid arthritis (Fig. 3.7).

Displaced Fracture of the Shaft of a Long Bone (See Chapter 15). When the nutrient artery to the shaft of a long bone is disrupted by a fracture, a temporary compensatory hyperemia at the epiphyseal ends of the long bone follows, and the result is a temporary stimulation of local growth.

Congenital   Arteriovenous   Malformations. The continuing hyperemia associated with the various types of arteriovenous malfor-

mations provides continuing stimulation of the epiphyseal plates in the involved limb and consequently an overgrowth of the limb.

Localized Decrease in Growth

Disuse Retardation. When a limb is not used normally over a long period, as in prolonged immobilization, prolonged relief of weightbearing, or severe paralysis of long duration, the associated decrease in the normal intermittent pressures causes a retardation of growth in the involved limb (Fig. 3.8).

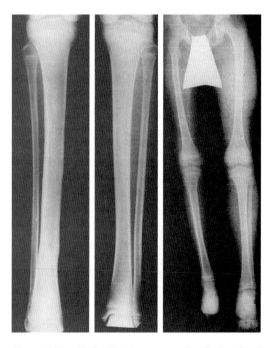

Figure 3.7.   Left. This is an example of a localized increase in longitudinal growth in the right tibia of a 14-year-old girl (chronic inflammation of a long bone). Chronic osteomyelitis of the right tibia associated with prolonged hyperemia over the preceding 7 years has stimulated local epiphyseal plate growth, thereby producing a limb length discrepancy.

Figure 3.8.   Right. This is an example of a localized decrease in longitudinal growth in the right lower limb of a 12-year-old boy (disuse retardation of bone growth). Severe residual paralysis from poliomyelitis in early childhood has resulted in a decrease in the normal intermittent pressures of muscle pull across the joints and of weightbearing on the long bones of the right lower limb, thereby leading to local disuse retardation of epiphyseal plate growth and a resultant limb length discrepancy.

Physical Injury (See Chapter 16). A fracture that either crosses the epiphyseal plate or crushes it, is frequently followed by bony union across the plate and therefore a local cessation of growth.

Thermal Injury. The cartilage of the epiphyseal plate is sometimes destroyed either by local cold (frostbite) or by local heat (burns).

Ischemia (See Chapter 13). Total avascular necrosis of an epiphysis is always associated with necrosis of the cartilage of the underlying epiphyseal plate (and cessation of growth) because the epiphyseal vessels supply both structures.

Infection (See Chapter 10). The cartilage of the epiphyseal plate is particularly susceptible to the chondrolytic action of the pus produced by some infections, especially those caused by *Staphylococcus*. The cartilage destruction usually involves only part of an epiphyseal plate, resulting in subsequent uneven growth.

Localized torsional growth

When a growing long bone and its epiphyseal plate are subjected to either continual or intermittent twisting (torsional) forces, as in certain postural habits of sitting on the floor, the bone gradually becomes twisted (develops torsion) in the same direction as the applied force. The torsional deformity in the long bone occurs through torsional growth in the involved epiphyseal plate and can usually be reversed by applying corrective torsional forces in the opposite direction. Clinical conditions caused by torsional deformities of growing long bones, and their correction, are discussed in Chapter 7.

SYNOVIAL JOINTS

In a normal synovial joint, the smooth and reciprocally shaped cartilaginous opposing surfaces permit frictionless and painless movement. By contrast, any irregularity or damage to the articular surface inevitably leads to progressive degenerative changes in the joint, with resultant limitation of movement and pain. The joint capsule is particularly sensitive to stretching and increased fluid pressure within the joint, which helps explain why abnormal conditions of joints are so painful. Indeed, disorders and injuries of joints consti-

tute the greatest single physical cause of disability in civilized humankind.

Hyaline articular cartilage, which has a rubberlike consistency, is both compressible and resilient. When loaded by normal function, it becomes somewhat flattened—that is, deformed or compressed—and when that load is removed, it returns to its resting shape. With normal cyclical loading and unloading, therefore, the matrix of the articular cartilage behaves rather like a compressible sponge in that such actions enhance diffusion of the nutrient tissue fluidlike synovial fluid into, and the waste products out of, the matrix. In addition, the cyclical pressure changes of normal joint motion are transmitted via the matrix as signals to continue synthesizing the collagen and proteoglycans of the matrix. By contrast, prolonged immobilization of a given joint significantly reduces such signals, with consequent deterioration of chondrocyte function and, hence, of the articular cartilage itself.

Reactions of Articular Cartilage

Articular cartilage, which contains no blood vessels, lymphatics, or nerves, is capable of reacting to abnormal conditions in only three ways: (1) *destruction,* (2) *degeneration,* and (3) *peripheral proliferation.*

In this section on articular cartilage, brief reference is made to four scientific investigations that we have conducted using rabbits in our laboratory in the Research Institute of The Hospital for Sick Children in Toronto. They are included here not only as research data relevant to the destruction, degeneration, and possible regeneration of articular cartilage but also as examples of the importance of the *philosophy and nature of medical research* (see Chapter 18). These four investigations include the harmful effects on articular cartilage of prolonged immobilization of a synovial joint, continuous compression of joint surfaces, and repeated intra-articular injections of hydrocortisone as well as the beneficial effects of a relatively new concept—continuous passive motion (CPM) of a synovial joint—on the healing and regeneration of articular cartilage.

The limitation of space in this textbook

precludes the possibility of recording the many excellent scientific investigations of orthopaedic surgeon–scientist colleagues in other centers.

Destruction

The powers of regeneration of articular cartilage are so limited that destruction of cartilage is a serious and irreparable lesion. Articular cartilage is destroyed by any condition that interferes with its main source of nutrition from synovial fluid as well as by the chondrolytic enzymes present in certain types of pus. Although cartilage is radiolucent, destruction of the cartilage can be detected radiographically by a decrease in the normal width, or thickness, of the *cartilage space* between the radiopaque bone ends (Fig. 3.9).

The following sections provide examples of abnormal conditions that cause destruction of articular cartilage.

Rheumatoid Arthritis (See Chapter 10). The pannus, which adheres to cartilage, interferes with nutrition of the cartilage by synovial fluid in rheumatoid arthritis.

Infections (See Chapter 10). The pus of staphylococcal septic arthritis and tuberculous arthritis is particularly chondrolytic.

Ankylosing Spondylitis (See Chapter 10). In ankylosing spondylitis, the joint gradually becomes completely obliterated by bony fusion (bony ankylosis).

Prolonged Immobilization of a Synovial joint. When a normal rabbit knee is immobilized in flexion for as little as 3 weeks, and more consistently for 10 weeks or longer, the synovial membrane becomes adherent to the articular cartilage that is not in contact with the opposing joint surface. This phenomenon obliterates the fluid space between cartilage and synovial membrane, thereby blocking the normal synovial fluid nutrition of the underlying cartilage and producing an irreparable lesion that we have called *obliterative degeneration of articular cartilage*. This lesion can also be seen in the cartilage of human patients secondary to prolonged limitation of joint motion associated with persistent joint deformity.

Continuous Compression of Articular Cartilage. When the two opposing joint surfaces of the rabbit knee are continuously compressed

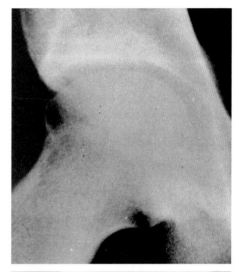
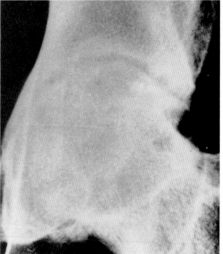

Figure 3.9. The destruction of articular cartilage caused by infection is seen in this figure. The left hip joint of this 14-year-old girl has been the site of pyogenic infection (septic arthritis). Note the decreased thickness of the cartilage space (a more accurate term than "joint space") of the left hip **(bottom)** compared with that of the normal opposite hip **(top),** indicating loss of articular cartilage.

against one another (either by means of a skeletal pin compression device or by immobilization of the joint in an extreme—i.e., a forced—position of compression) for as little as 8 days, the contact areas of the two articular surfaces are completely deprived of their synovial fluid nutrition, and the inevitable result is a "pressure sore" that we have designated *compression necrosis of articular cartilage*.

Intra-articular Injections of Hydrocortisone. After two or more weekly injections of hydrocortisone T.B.A. into the knee joint of a rabbit, the following progressive degenerative changes are seen in the articular cartilage: thinning, fissuring, fibrillation, depletion of proteoglycans, and cystic lesions containing calcium deposits within the matrix. We refer to these harmful effects as *hydrocortisone arthropathy.*

Degeneration

A slowly progressive type of degenerative change in articular cartilage is seen as part of the normal aging process—the cartilage becomes thinner and less cellular. These gradual changes of wear and tear render the cartilage less resilient and therefore more susceptible to injury; they are aggravated by excessive loads on joint surfaces (as with obesity), a decrease in viscosity of the synovial fluid, and local damage or destruction of cartilage.

Degeneration of articular cartilage is initiated by a change in the intercellular cement substance of the matrix (*chondromalacia*) and subsequent uncovering of the collagen fibrils (*fibrillation*). Finally the degenerated cartilage, which is primarily in the central or weightbearing area, becomes eroded, thereby exposing the subchondral bone, which with continued movement becomes thickened, dense (*sclerotic*), and polished (*eburnated*) (Fig. 3.10).

The following sections discuss abnormal conditions leading to degeneration of articular cartilage.

Premature Aging of Cartilage. An acceleration of the normal aging process in articular cartilage results in premature aging of the cartilage and is aggravated by excessive wear and tear.

Previous Destruction of Cartilage. All the destructive lesions mentioned previously (including obliterative degeneration, compression necrosis, and hydrocortisone arthropathy) lead to progressive degeneration in the remaining cartilage, as has been proved both experimentally and clinically.

Incongruity or Irregularity of Joint Surfaces. When, as a result of a previous disorder or injury, the two opposing joint surfaces are no longer smooth and congruous, the associated increase in localized areas of increased pressure and increased joint friction leads to excessive and uneven wearing of the articular cartilage, with resultant degeneration.

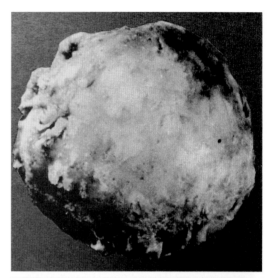

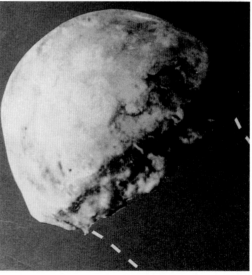

Figure 3.10. This figure shows the degeneration of articular cartilage of the femoral head of a 70-year-old man with severe degenerative joint disease (osteoarthritis) of the hip. Note the exposed, eburnated subchondral bone where the degenerated articular cartilage has almost disappeared over the weightbearing surface. Small islands of thin, degenerated cartilage have persisted over part of the femoral head. The cartilage of the nonweightbearing area is fibrillated.

Peripheral Proliferation

The peripheral articular rim of cartilage of a synovial joint, unlike the central area, is covered by a type of perichondrium that is continuous with the synovial membrane. In the presence of degeneration of the central area of cartilage and with continued movement, the peripheral perichondrium proliferates and gradually produces an almost complete peripheral ring of thickened cartilage.

Thus, the peripheral ring (which in any single view resembles a lip) is initially composed of cartilage (*chondrophyte formation*) but subsequently ossifies (*osteophyte formation*) (Fig. 3.11).

Possibility of Healing and Regeneration of Articular Cartilage. As has been demonstrated by many investigators, damaged articular cartilage is extremely limited in its ability to heal or regenerate; this accounts for the relentless progression of degenerative arthritis (osteoarthritis) as an inevitable sequel to such damage.

Despite the fact that rest and motion are the most commonly prescribed forms of treatment for musculoskeletal disorders and injuries, their relative importance, timing, and duration remain controversial. Unfortunately, the majority of involved physicians and surgeons have traditionally been "resters" rather than "movers" based more on long-established tradition and time-honored empiricism than on scientific investigations.

The aforementioned investigations on the deleterious effects of immobilization of joints, with or without compression (as well as the investigations of others), led the author to consider the exact antithesis of continuous rest, namely, continuous motion. It was obvious that because of the fatigability of skeletal muscle, continuous motion would have to be passive rather than active. Consequently, in 1970 I developed what, at that time, was the completely new concept of *continuous passive motion (CPM)* of a synovial joint in vivo based on the hypothesis that such motion would stimulate the healing and regeneration of articular cartilage through differentiation of pluripotential mesenchymal cells in the subchondral bone. Since then, a wide variety of scientific investigations in our Research Institute have proved that CPM stimulates and accelerates the healing and regeneration of articular cartilage, ligaments, and tendons much more than does either immobilization or intermittent active motion. One example of this ongoing research is an experimental model of "biological resurfacing" of a major full-thickness defect in the articular surface of the rabbit knee joint using a free autogenous periosteal graft. This experimental model and the results

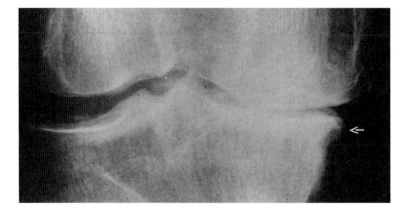

Figure 3.11.   Peripheral proliferation of articular cartilage in the right knee joint of a 60-year-old man with degenerative joint disease (osteoarthritis) is seen. Note the bony "lip" or "spur" on the medial edge of the tibial joint surface **(arrow),** indicating osteophyte formation that was preceded by chondrophyte formation.

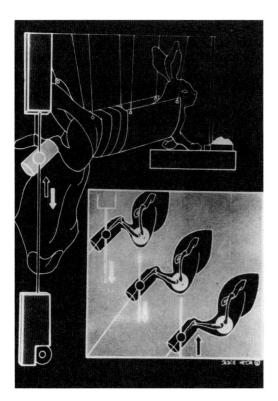

Figure 3.12. A rabbit's right hind limb is seen in the continuous passive motion apparatus, which is run by an electric motor. The range of motion used was an arc of 70° (from 40° to 110° of flexion).

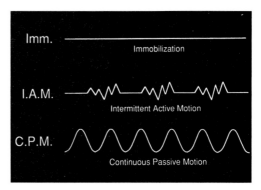

Figure 3.13. A schematic representation of the three regimens of postoperative management of the rabbits, which included knee joint immobilization, intermittent active motion (cage activity), and continuous passive motion.

of the scientific investigation are depicted in Figures 3.12 to 3.18 . This new concept has now been applied to the postoperative management of various musculoskeletal disorders and injuries in human patients, which is discussed in Chapters 6, 10, 15, 16, and 17. A summary of the author's research on CPM and its clinical applications is presented as one example of the philosophy and nature of medical research (see Chapter 18).

Reactions of Synovial Membrane

The synovial membrane, which secretes synovial fluid for nutrition and lubrication of the articular cartilage, is capable of reacting to abnormal conditions in one or more of three ways: (1) by producing an excessive amount of fluid (*an effusion*), (2) by becoming thicker (*hypertrophy*), and (3) by forming *adhesions*

between itself and the articular cartilage. A joint effusion may be *serous,* as with mild sprains; it may be an *inflammatory exudate,* as in synovitis and rheumatoid arthritis; it may be grossly *purulent,* as with septic arthritis; or it may be *hemorrhagic,* as with severe injury or hemophilia. All but the transient serous effusions are accompanied by varying degrees of synovial hypertrophy and synovial adhesion formation. Synovial adhesions can also form as a result of prolonged limitation of joint movement from any cause, including immobilization in a cast or rigid splint.

The synovial membranes of tendon sheaths and bursae are capable of the same reactions to abnormal conditions as are the synovial membranes of joints.

Reactions of Joint Capsule and Ligaments

The fibrous joint capsule and ligaments allow the desired range of movement but provide stability of the joint by preventing undesired movements. These structures react to abnormal conditions either (1) by becoming unduly stretched and elongated (*joint laxity*), thereby permitting instability of the joint, or (2) by becoming tight and shortened (*joint contracture*), thereby limiting the range of joint movement.

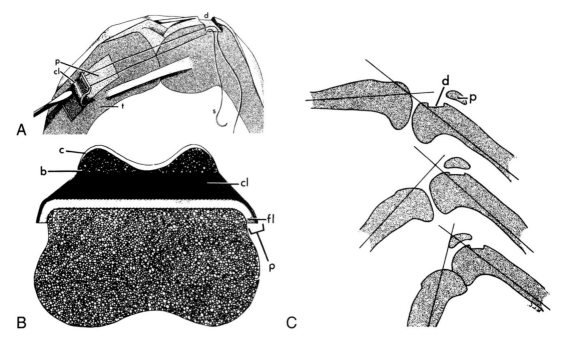

Figure 3.14.   A. Standard surgical procedure is presented in this figure. A 5-mm-wide full-thickness defect *(d)* was created across the entire width of the patellar groove. Before transplanting the graft of periosteum *(p)* from the medial side of the proximal part of the tibia into the femoral defect, a suture, or sutures, *(s)* were placed in one end of the graft and in the periosteum on one side of the femur to ensure that the deep cambium layer *(cl)* of the graft faced up into the joint in the defect. **B.** A transverse section through the periosteal graft *(p)* in the defect, with its cambium layer (cl) facing up and its fibrous layer *(fl)* facing down is seen. The base of the defect, which extended through cartilage *(c)* and bone *(b),* was flat, in contrast to the concave contour of the patellar groove. The depth of the defect ranged from 2 mm in the middle of the groove to 4 to 5 mm at the edges. **C.** The site of the defect *(d)* was selected so that the patella *(p)* would glide back and forth over it as the joint was moved passively through a range of motion from 40 to 110° of flexion.

Joint Laxity

The following abnormal conditions result in undue joint laxity.

1. Generalized congenital laxity of capsules and ligaments (see Chapter 7): This abnormality is probably determined genetically.
2. Injury (see Chapters 15 to17): Traumatic dislocation or subluxation with rupture of capsule or ligaments leads to instability of the joint.
3. Infection (see Chapter 10): In septic arthritis, the capsule may be destroyed by pus, thereby leading to a *pathological dislocation* of the joint.

Joint Contracture

The following abnormal conditions may result in a joint contracture with limitation of joint motion.

1. Congenital joint contractures: These are seen in certain congenital deformities, such as clubfeet (See Chapter 8.)
2. Infection: Fibrosis and scar formation of the capsule following infection may lead to a fibrous contracture of the joint (See Chapter 10.)
3. Chronic arthritis: Rheumatoid arthritis and degenerative joint disease both lead to progressive fibrous contracture of the joint (See Chapter 10.)
4. Muscle contracture: Ischemic contracture, (secondary to a compartment syndrome), muscle imbalance, and prolonged muscle spasm eventually result in muscle contracture, with consequent limitation of motion of the joint that is normally moved by the involved muscle (See Chapter 15.)

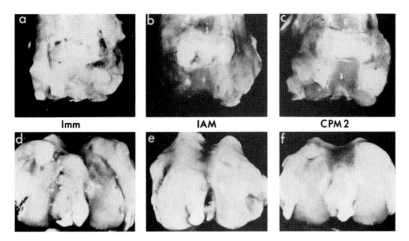

Figure 3.15. The median macroscopic results in the first three adolescent groups (immobilization *[Imm]*, intermittent active motion *[IAM]*, and 2 weeks of continuous passive motion *[CPM2]*). **a, b,** and **c** show frontal views of the defect in the patellar groove. **d, e,** and **f** are end-on views of the distal end of the femur, showing the contours of the newly formed tissues in the patellar groove defects. **a** and **d.** The immobilized knee exhibits adhesions, erosions, and only partial restoration of the patellar groove. **b** and **e.** The newly formed tissue in the knee that was subjected to intermittent active motion is irregular, and there is only partial healing of the defect. **c** and **f.** The newly formed tissue in the knee that was subjected to 2 weeks of continuous passive motion appears smooth and cartilaginous, and it has completely restored the contour of the patellar groove.

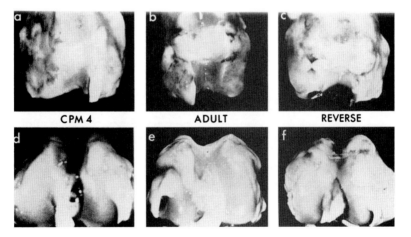

Figure 3.16. The median macroscopic results in the adolescent group that was subjected to 4 weeks of continuous passive motion *(CPM4)* and in the adult and reverse groups. **a.** The newly formed tissue in the knee of the rabbit that was subjected to 4 weeks of continuous passive motion resembles the normal adjacent cartilage, to which it is bonded. **d.** The pre-existing contour of the patellar groove has been completely restored. **b** and **e.** The defect in the adult knee has been partially healed with tissue that is smooth. **c** and **f.** The defect in the knee from the reverse group (cambian layer facing down) has been only partially repaired with irregular fibrous tissue that has not restored the contour of the patellar groove.

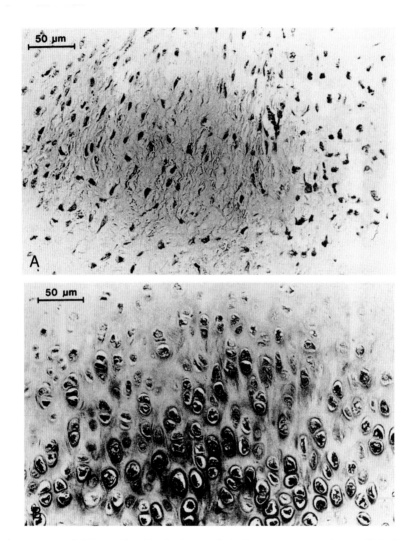

Figure 3.17.   A. The median histological result in the control group (no graft) (safranin O, 400 ×). The newly formed tissue—a mixture of poorly differentiated cartilage, mesenchyme, and fibrous tissue —does not stain well with safranin O. (Reprinted with permission from John Sevastik, Ian Goldie, eds. The young patient with degenerative hip disease. Stockholm: Almqvist and Wiksell, 1985;29.) **B.** The median histological result in the adolescent group that had 4 weeks of continuous passive motion (safranin O, 400 ×). The newly formed tissue is hyalinelike cartilage that stains well with safranin O.

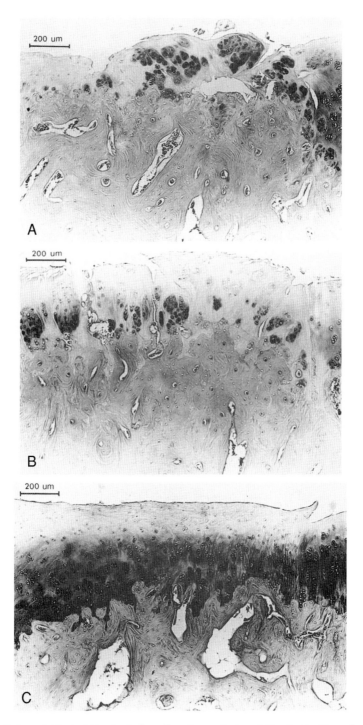

Figure 3.18. **A.** Typical histological results at 1 year in the rabbits that had been immobilized in a cast. Compared with the normal cartilage (far right), the regenerated tissue is thinner and disrupted, and it exhibits diminished uptake of safranin O (safranin O, 100 ×) and severe degenerative arthritis. **B.** Typical histological results at 1 year in the intermittent active motion group. Compared with the normal cartilage (far right), the regenerated tissue is severely fissured and exhibits diminished uptake of safranin O (safranin O, 100 ×) and severe degenerative arthritis. **C.** Typical histological results at 1 year in the continuous passive motion group. The regenerated tissue, which is smooth and intact, stains well with safranin O and closely resembles the normal articular cartilage to which it is bonded (far right) (safranin O, 100 ×). There is no arthritis.

SKELETAL MUSCLE
Reactions of Skeletal Muscle

The complex structure of skeletal muscle reacts to the many disorders and injuries of the musculoskeletal system in a limited number of ways including *atrophy, hypertrophy, necrosis, contracture,* and *regeneration.* You will recall from the discussion of muscle in Chapter 2 that a *single motor unit* of skeletal muscle consists of the anterior horn cell, its axon within a peripheral nerve fiber, the myoneural junctions, and the individual muscle fibers supplied by the single anterior horn cell. Thus, the reactions of skeletal muscle may be incited by a disorder or injury to any one of these components.

Disuse Atrophy

Skeletal muscle that is not being used normally, for whatever reason, invariably reacts by becoming weaker and smaller (*disuse atrophy*) (Fig. 3.19). Disorders of the anterior horn cell (such as poliomyelitis), the peripheral nerve fiber (such as polyneuritis), the myoneural junction (such as myasthenia gravis), and the individual muscle fiber (such as muscular dystrophy) can all incite the reaction of disuse atrophy, as can injury to any of these components. In addition, disuse atrophy is caused by prolonged immobilization of the associated joints, stiffness of the joints, and chronic joint disease. Indeed, pain arising in an abnormal joint initiates a reflex inhibition of contraction in associated muscles, a phenomenon that results in additional atrophy of muscle.

Work Hypertrophy

When a given muscle is repeatedly exercised against resistance, particularly by isometric contraction, it reacts by becoming stronger and larger (*work hypertrophy*) (Fig. 3.20). The hypertrophy is caused by an enlargement of individual muscle fibers and not by an increased number of fibers; it depends on continuation of the exercises.

Ischemic Necrosis (See Chapter 15)

Occlusion of arteries supplying muscle, whether by persistent traumatic vascular spasm, thrombosis, embolism, or a compart-

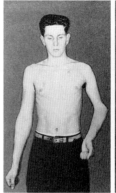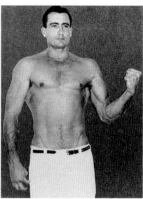

Figure 3.19.   Left. This figure shows disuse atrophy of muscle in the left arm of a 15-year-old boy resulting from prolonged stiffness of the left elbow from an old intra-articular fracture that had been treated by prolonged immobilization in a cast.

Figure 3.20.   Right. This figure shows work hypertrophy of muscle. This man vigorously exercises his muscles daily (by isometric contraction) to make them stronger and larger. The resultant hypertrophy of muscle, which results from an enlargement of individual muscle fibers, depends on continuation of the exercises.

ment syndrome, results in *ischemic necrosis* of the muscle within 6 hours, a fact that is of great practical importance, particularly when one is dealing with injuries of the limbs.

Contracture

If a muscle remains in a shortened state for a prolonged period, it develops a persistent shortening that is resistant to stretching (*muscle contracture*). Such a contracture eventually becomes irreversible. Muscle contractures also develop in certain diseases of muscle, such as polymyositis, muscular dystrophy, and cerebral palsy. In addition, the muscle fibers of a necrotic muscle are subsequently replaced by dense fibrous scar tissue, which undergoes progressive *fibrous contracture,* resulting in the production of progressive joint deformities (Fig. 3.21).

Regeneration

Injured muscle fibers may regenerate, to some degree at least, from the sarcolemma and muscle cells and possibly from the activity of the

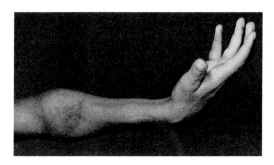

Figure 3.21.   Fibrous contracture of muscle is seen. This 10-year-old boy's forearm had been ischemic for a period of 12 hours as a result of vascular damage associated with a supracondylar fracture of the humerus. The consequential ischemic necrosis of the forearm muscles (Volkmann's ischemic necrosis) has caused replacement of muscle by dense fibrous scar tissue, resulting in fibrous contracture of the muscles.

satellite cells in each fiber. Following partial loss of innervation in a skeletal muscle, at least some of the paralyzed muscle fibers may gain a new motor nerve fiber from the remaining intact nerve fibers, in which case there is a corresponding recovery of muscle power.

MUSCULOSKELETAL DEFORMITIES

Many disorders and injuries of the musculoskeletal system are manifested by an abnormal form, or shape, of the affected limb or trunk (*musculoskeletal deformity*). Some of these deformities, such as clubfeet, are strikingly obvious on external inspection even to the casual observer, whereas others, such as a mild curvature of the spine, are more subtle and not immediately obvious. Still others, such as an abnormal shape of a joint surface, are hidden by the skin and soft tissues and are apparent only on "internal inspection" by radiographic examination. Musculoskeletal deformities may arise in bones, joints, or soft tissues, and a given deformity may involve one or more of these structures.

When confronted with a musculoskeletal deformity in one of your patients, you must consider first the *structure*, or *structures*, in which the deformity is taking place as well as the likely cause of the deformity. In addition, you must assess the *significance* of the deformity concerning not only its *appearance* but

also its present or future effect on *function*. A deformity may be *congenital* (present at the time of birth) or it may be *acquired* during postnatal life. The many musculoskeletal deformities are discussed individually in subsequent chapters. At this stage, having studied the reactions of musculoskeletal tissues to disorders and injuries, you will find it helpful to consider in a general way the types and causes of deformity in the various musculoskeletal structures. Indeed, an understanding of these aspects of deformities will help you think in terms of their diagnosis and their possible prevention as well as correction.

Types of Bony Deformity
Loss of Alignment
A long bone may be out of alignment either because it is twisted in its long axis (*torsional deformity*) or because it is crooked (*angulatory deformity*) (Fig. 3.22). If the angulatory deformity is close to a joint, the deformity may seem on external inspection to be taking place in the joint, but internal inspection by radiographic examination reveals the true site of the deformity. Angulatory deformity in a short bone, such as a vertebral body, is associated with a change in its entire shape, and since its upper and lower surface are no longer parallel, it resembles a wedge.

Abnormal Length
A long bone may be abnormally short (or even absent), or it may be abnormally long. When the deformity involves only one of a pair of limbs, the result is a *limb length discrepancy* (Fig. 3.23).

Bony Outgrowth
A lesion, such as an osteochondroma, arising from the surface of a bone may change its configuration sufficiently to produce a bony deformity that is obvious clinically (Fig. 3.24).

Causes of Bony Deformity
Congenital Abnormalities of Bony Development (See Chapter 8)
The bone may be absent because of failure to develop (*aplasia*), it may be underdeveloped (*hypoplasia*), it may be abnormally developed

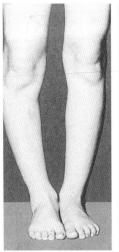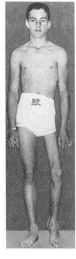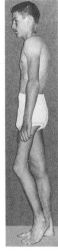

Figure 3.22.   Left. This is an angular deformity in the upper part of the right tibia in a 9-year-old girl, which resulted from retarded growth on the medial side of the proximal tibial epiphyseal plate and continuing growth on the lateral side.

Figure 3.23.   Right. Limb length discrepancy caused by retardation of growth in the epiphyseal plates of the left lower limb in a 15-year-old boy who had paralytic poliomyelitis in early childhood. Note also the marked atrophy of the limb and the knee flexion deformity.

(*dysplasia*), or it may even be doubly developed as in extra digits (*duplication*).

Fractures (See Chapters 15 to 17)
Loss of alignment may occur at the time of fracture, and if it is not corrected by adequate reduction, the bone heals with residual bony deformity (*malunion*). When a fracture fails to unite (*nonunion*), there is usually residual deformity at the site. Fractures through abnormal bone (*pathological fractures*) may be gross and produce deformities similar to those in fractures through normal bone, or they may be microscopic and repeated, in which case, they produce progressive bony deformities as in osteoporotic vertebral bodies.

Disturbances of Epiphyseal Plate Growth (See Chapters 7, 8, 13, and 16)
The deformities arising from the various reactions of epiphyseal plates to disorders and injuries have already been considered in a general way in this chapter.

Bending of Abnormally Soft Bone (See Chapter 9)
In certain generalized metabolic bone diseases, such as rickets and osteomalacia, the bone matrix (osteoid) is not normally calcified so that the bones are abnormally "soft" and will gradually bend or twist without an obvious fracture.

Overgrowth of Adult Bone (See Chapters 9 and 14)
In certain disseminated bone disorders, such as osteitis deformans (Paget's disease), the adult bone becomes thickened and crooked. Furthermore, certain bone lesions (such as osteochondroma) growing outward from the surface of bone produce a localized bony deformity which, if large and superficial, results in an obvious clinical deformity (Fig. 3.24).

Types of Joint Deformity
Displacement of the Joint
When the normal reciprocal relationship between the two joint surfaces is lost, the joint is said to be displaced. The joint may be completely displaced (*dislocated, luxated*) or only partially displaced (*subluxated*). A dislocated joint is unstable and associated with deformity (Fig. 3.25).

Excessive Mobility (Hypermobility) of the Joint
The fibrous joint capsule and ligaments normally serve as "check-reins" preventing excessive mobility (hypermobility) of the joint. If they are congenitally lax, stretched, or torn, the resultant hypermobility causes a deformity to appear when stress, such as weightbearing, is transmitted to that joint (Fig. 3.26).

Restricted Mobility of the Joint
When, for any reason, mobility of a joint is restricted, a type of joint deformity is present. For example, if a knee joint lacks the last 30° of extension, the condition is described as a 30° knee-flexion deformity (Fig. 3.27).

Causes of Joint Deformity
Congenital Abnormalities of Joint Development (See Chapter 8)
The joint may be unstable at birth and become dislocated, as in congenital dislocation of the

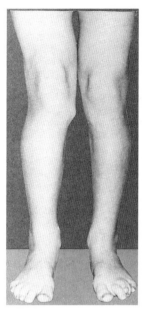
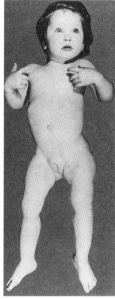

Figure 3.24. **Left.** A bony outgrowth is seen. The bony deformity on the medial side of this woman's right knee is caused by an osteochondroma (osteocartilaginous exostosis), which is a type of benign bone lesion arising from the medial surface of the upper end of the tibia.

Figure 3.25. **Right.** This figure shows displacement of a joint. This 2-year-old girl's left hip joint has been completely displaced (dislocated) since birth and is therefore unstable. Note the associated deformity of adduction and shortening of the left lower limb.

hip (also known as developmental dysplasia of the hip); it may develop with restricted mobility and contractures, as in congenital clubfoot; or it may fail to develop (*failure of segmentation*), as in congenital radioulnar synostosis. All joints of the body may be hypermobile because of congenital generalized laxity of ligaments. Any of these congenital abnormalities can produce joint deformity.

Acquired Dislocations

When a joint is dislocated, as a result of either injury (traumatic dislocation) or infection (pathological dislocation), an unstable joint deformity occurs.

Mechanical Blocks

In degenerative joint disorders, such as osteoarthritis, and displaced intra-articular frac-

tures, the opposing surfaces of the joint become irregular, and since they no longer fit well, they are said to be *incongruous.* As a result, joint mobility is restricted by a mechanical bony block. Internal derangements of a joint, such as a displaced torn meniscus and a loose body, can likewise restrict joint mobility by a mechanical block within the joint.

Joint Adhesions

In certain inflammatory joint disorders, such as rheumatoid arthritis and septic arthritis, the articular cartilage is partially or completely destroyed. The result is that adhesions may form within the joints, either between the joint surfaces or between synovial membrane and a joint surface. Likewise, following either injury or infection, muscles or their tendons may become tethered to bone by adhesions, thereby preventing normal muscle action and tendon gliding. Whether the adhesions are in the joint (intra-articular) or outside the joint (extra-articular), the associated restriction of joint motion results in joint deformity.

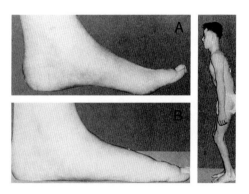

Figure 3.26. **Left.** Excessive mobility (hypermobility) of joints is seen. **A.** This 10-year-old boy's foot is hypermobile because of generalized joint laxity, but it looks normal when not bearing weight. **B.** On bearing weight, the hypermobile joints in the foot allow the foot to appear flat and therefore deformed.

Figure 3.27. **Right.** Restricted mobility of a joint is seen. This 12-year-old boy has a bilateral knee flexion deformity in that he is unable to extend his knee joints completely. The cause of this deformity is muscle imbalance caused by persistent spasticity and contracture of the hamstring muscles from cerebral palsy, an upper motor neuron lesion.

Muscle Contractures

In a given muscle, persistent shortening that is resistant to stretching (muscle contracture) may result from prolonged muscle spasm (caused by pain), prolonged immobilization, muscle diseases, and ischemic necrosis of muscle. The result of the muscle contracture is deformity in the joint, or joints, normally controlled by that muscle.

Muscle Imbalance

Persistent imbalance of power among the various muscles that control movement of a given joint may result from *flaccid* paralysis, as in poliomyelitis, or *spastic* paralysis, as in the spastic type of cerebral palsy. In either case, the continuing unequal muscle pull gradually produces a progressive joint deformity, particularly during childhood because of the added factor of skeletal growth (Fig. 3.27).

Fibrous Contractures of Fascia and Skin

Persistent shortening of fibrous scar tissue (fibrous contracture) in skin (as seen in severe burns) and of deep fascia (as seen in Dupuytren's contracture of the palmar aponeurosis) produces restriction of joint mobility with resultant deformity in the underlying and nearby joints.

External Pressures

When external pressures repeatedly force a joint into a deformed position, the ligaments on the convex side of the deformity become stretched, whereas those on the concave side become contracted. As a result, the deformity eventually becomes permanent. Common examples are the various toe deformities, for example, hallux valgus with a bunion resulting from, or aggravated by, the pressure of tight, pointed shoes in girls and women, the victims of fashion.

Joint Deformities of Unknown Cause (Idiopathic)

Certain joint deformities, such as the *idiopathic* type of lateral curvature of the spine (scoliosis), develop in otherwise healthy children for no apparent reason. Secondary bony deformities and soft tissue contractures develop eventually in idiopathic scoliosis, but the primary cause of the scoliosis has eluded detection to date and remains a challenging mystery.

SUGGESTED ADDITIONAL READING

Buckwalter JA. Musculoskeletal tissues and the musculoskeletal system. In: Weinstein SL, Buckwalter JA, eds. Turek's orthopaedics: principles and their application. Philadelphia: JB Lippincott, 1994.

Buckwalter JA, Woo Savio L-Y, Goldberg V, et al. Soft-tissue aging and musculoskeletal function. Current concepts review. J Bone Joint Surg 1993;75-A,1533–1548.

Cormack DH. Ham's histology. 9th ed. Philadelphia: JB Lippincott, 1987.

Cormack DH. Essential histology. Philadelphia: JB Lippincott, 1993.

Freeman MAR, ed. Adult articular cartilage. 2nd ed. Kent, UK: Pitman Medical, 1979.

Hughes S, Sweetnam R. The basis and practice of orthopaedics. London: William Heinemann Medical Books, 1980.

Main BJ. Effects of immobilization on the skeleton. In: Owen R, Goodfellow J, Bullough PG, eds. Scientific foundations of orthopaedics and traumatology. London: William Heinemann Medical Books, 1980.

Mankin HJ. The response of articular cartilage to mechanical injury. J Bone Joint Surg 1982;64A: 460–466.

Murphy PG, Frank CB, Hart DA. The cell biology of ligaments and ligament healing. In: Jackson DW, ed. The anterior cruciate ligament: current and future concepts. New York: Raven Press, 1993.

O'Driscoll SW, Keeley FW, Salter RB. The chondrogenic potential of free autogenous periosteal grafts for biological resurfacing of major full-thickness defects in joint surfaces under the effects of continuous passive motion. An experimental investigation in the rabbit. J Bone Joint Surg 1986;68-A:1017–1035.

O'Driscoll SW, Keeley FW, Salter RB. Durability of regenerated articular cartilage produced by free autogenous periosteal grafts in major full-thickness defects in joint surfaces under the influence of continuous passive motion. A follow-up report at one year. J Bone Joint Surg 1988;70-A: 595–606.

Salter RB, Gross A, Hall JH. Hydrocortisone arthropathy—an experimental investigation. Can Med Assoc 1967;97:374–377.

Salter RB, Field P. The effects of continuous compression on living articular cartilage. An experimental investigation. J Bone Joint Surg 1960;42A:31–49.

Salter RB, Ogilvie-Harris DJ. Healing of intra-articular fractures with continuous passive motion. American Academy of Orthopaedic Surgeons instructional course lectures. St. Louis: CV Mosby, 1979;28:102–117.

Salter RB, McNeill OR, Carbin R. The pathological changes in articular cartilage associated with persistent joint deformity. An experimental investigation. In: Studies of rheumatoid disease: proceedings of the third Canadian conference on the rheumatic disease. Toronto: University of Toronto Press, 1965.

Salter RB, Simmonds DF, Malcolm BW, Rumble EJ, Macmichael D, Clements NG. The biological effects of continuous passive motion on the healing of full thickness defects in articular cartilage: an experimental investigation in the rabbit. J Bone Joint Surg 1980;62A:1232–1251.

Salter RB. Continuous passive motion (CPM). A biological concept for the healing and regeneration of articular cartilage, ligaments, and tendons. From origination to research to clinical applications. (A monograph). Baltimore: Williams & Wilkins, 1993.

Walsh S, Frank CB, Hart DA. Immobilization alters cell metabolism in an immature ligament. Clin Orthop 1992;277:287.

Woo SLY, Kuei SC, Amiel D, Gomez MA, Hayes WC, White FC, Akeson WH. The effect of prolonged physical training on the properties of long bone: a study of Wolff's law. J Bone Joint Surg 1981;63A:780–787.

4 Some Important Pairs of Clinical Terms

Before introducing you to the various clinical conditions of the musculoskeletal system, it is important to explain the meaning of several important pairs of clinical terms in the musculoskeletal language to avoid confusion from the start. The terms of each pair have opposite meanings and, as such, are frequently confused in the minds of students (occasionally even in the minds of practitioners). All the terms describe either movements of joints or deformities in limbs; therefore, they are used frequently in discussions of clinical conditions of the musculoskeletal system. Once you have learned these terms thoroughly, they will become as much a part of your vocabulary as "right" and "left," and you will no longer have to stop and figure out which is which in any given pair.

TERMS DESCRIBING MOVEMENTS OF JOINTS
Active and Passive Movement

Movement of a joint may be either *active* or *passive*. Active movement occurs as a result of the individual's own muscular activity. Passive movement occurs as a result of an external force, such as movement of the joint by another individual (e.g., a physiotherapist), gravity, or even-—in the case of continuous passive motion (CPM)—by a motorized device (as discussed in Chapters 3, 6 and 18).

Abduction and Adduction

The movements of abduction and adduction occur at the shoulder, hip, metacarpophalangeal, and metatarsophalangeal joints.

Abduction is the movement of a part *away from* the midline of the body (Fig. 4.1).

Adduction is the movement of a part *toward* the midline of the body (Fig. 4.2).

In the hand and foot, the midline used as a reference for the digits is a line along the middle finger and middle toe, respectively.

Flexion and Extension

The movements of flexion and extension occur at the elbow, metacarpophalangeal, interphalangeal (finger), knee, and interphalangeal (toe) joints, that is, flexion from a zero position of complete extension. In these joints, extension beyond zero is called hyperextension. Flexion of the shoulder is also called forward elevation from the anatomical position (described further on).

Dorsiflexion and Plantar (or Palmar) Flexion

The movements of dorsiflexion and plantar flexion occur at the ankle and metatarsophalangeal joints. The movements of dorsiflexion and palmar flexion occur at the wrist.

Dorsiflexion is the movement of the foot or toes in the direction of the *dorsal* surface (Fig. 4.3) as well as movement of the hand in the direction of the dorsal surface (Fig. 4.4).

Plantar flexion is the movement of the foot or toes in the direction of the *plantar* surface (Fig. 4.5).

Palmar flexion is the movement of the hand or fingers in the direction of the *palmar* surface (Fig. 4.6).

Eversion and Inversion

The movements of eversion and inversion occur by simultaneous motion at the subtalar and midtarsal joints of the foot.

Eversion is the turning of the plantar surface of the foot *outward* in relation to the leg (Fig. 4.7).

Inversion is the turning of the plantar surface of foot *inward* in relation to the leg (Fig. 4.8).

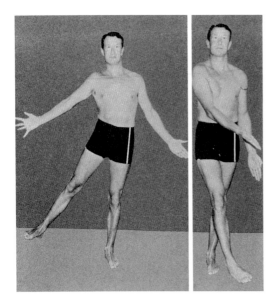

Figure 4.1.   Left. Abduction at right shoulder, right hip, and metacarpophalangeal joints of right hand.

Figure 4.2.   Right. Adduction at right shoulder, right hip, and metacarpophalangeal joints of right hand.

Internal Rotation and External Rotation

The movements of internal rotation (medial rotation) and external rotation (lateral rotation) occur at the shoulder, the hip, and to a slight degree at the knee.

Internal (medial) rotation is the turning of the anterior surface of the limb *inward or medially* (Fig. 4.9).

External (lateral) rotation is the turning of the anterior surface of the limb *outward or laterally* (Fig. 4.10).

Pronation and Supination

The movements of pronation and supination occur in the forearm through the elbow and wrist joint and in the forefoot through the midtarsal joint.

Pronation of the forearm (assessed with the elbow flexed to 90°) is the turning of the palmar surface of the hand *downward* (Fig. 4.11).

Pronation of the forefoot usually refers to a deformity in which the forefoot is maintained in a position of *eversion* (Fig. 4.7).

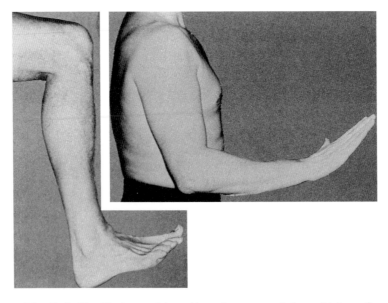

Figure 4.3.   Left. Dorsiflexion at right ankle and metatarsophalangeal joints of toes of right foot.

Figure 4.4.   Right. Dorsiflexion at right wrist.

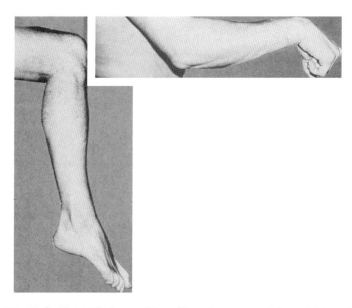

Figure 4.5. **Left.** Plantar flexion at right ankle and metatarsophalangeal joints of toes of right foot.

Figure 4.6. **Right.** Palmar flexion at right wrist, metacarpophalangeal joints, and interphalangeal joints of fingers of right hand.

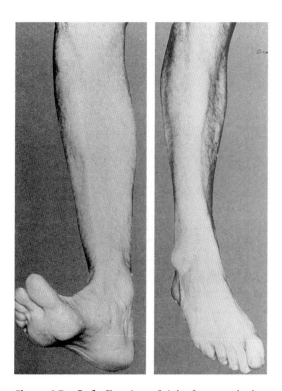

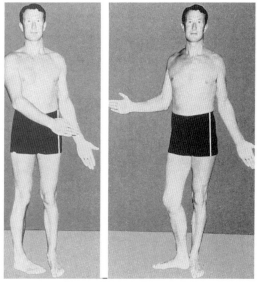

Figure 4.9. **Left.** Internal (medial) rotation at right shoulder and right hip.

Figure 4.10. **Right.** External (lateral) rotation of right shoulder and right hip.

Figure 4.7. **Left.** Eversion of right foot at subtalar and midtarsal joints.

Figure 4.8. **Right.** Inversion of right foot at subtalar and midtarsal joints.

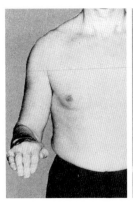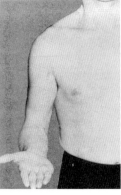

Figure 4.11.   Left. Pronation of the right forearm at proximal and distal radioulnar joints.

Figure 4.12.   Right. Supination of the right forearm at proximal and distal radioulnar joints.

Supination of the forearm is the turning of the palmar surface of the hand *upward* (Fig. 4.12).

Supination of the forefoot usually refers to a deformity in which the forefoot is maintained in a position of *inversion* (Fig. 4.8).

TERMS DESCRIBING DEFORMITIES IN LIMBS

The types and causes of musculoskeletal deformities are discussed in a general way in Chapter 3, but the descriptive terminology of such deformities merits discussion here. The following terms are used clinically in describing joint deformities.

Postural deformity is associated with, or the result of, a given posture. This type of deformity can be corrected by the patient's own muscle action.

Static deformity is one associated with the role of gravity when the body is not in motion.

Dynamic deformity occurs as a result of the patient's own muscle action. Such a deformity is usually the result of muscle imbalance and is not resistant to passive correction; it is a mobile deformity.

Fixed or structural deformity is relatively resistant to passive correction.

Calcaneus and Equinus

Calcaneus and equinus deformities occur at the ankle only (ankle calcaneus, ankle equinus).

Calcaneus is a deformity in which the foot is maintained in a position of *dorsiflexion* so that on weightbearing, only the *heel* touches the floor (Fig. 4.13).

Equinus is a deformity in which the foot is maintained in a position of *plantar flexion* so

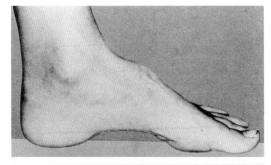

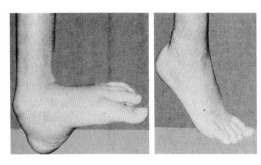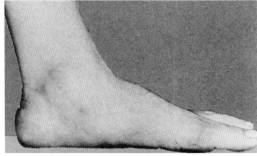

Figure 4.13.   Left. Calcaneus deformity (ankle calcaneus).

Figure 4.14.   Right. Equinus deformity (ankle equinus).

Figure 4.15.   Top. Cavus deformity of left foot (pes cavus).

Figure 4.16.   Bottom. Planus deformity of left foot (pes planus) (flat foot).

that on weightbearing, only the *forefoot* touches the floor (Fig. 4.14).

Cavus and Planus

These deformities occur only in the foot (pes cavus and pes planus).

Pes cavus is an *exaggeration* of the normal longitudinal arch of the foot, an unduly *high* arch (Fig. 4.15). The combined deformity of calcaneus of the hind foot and equinus, or plantar flexion, of the forefoot is called *calcaneocavus*.

Pes planus is a *diminution* of the normal longitudinal arch of the foot, an unduly *low* arch, or flat foot (Fig. 4.16).

Internal Torsion and External Torsion

Internal torsion and external torsion represent a twist in the longitudinal axis of a long bone, usually the tibia or femur.

In *internal torsion*, the anterior aspect of the distal end of the long bone is twisted *inward* or *medially* in relation to the anterior aspect of its proximal end, for example, internal tibial torsion (Fig. 4.17) and internal femoral torsion.

In *external torsion*, the anterior aspect of the distal end of the long bone is twisted *out-* *ward* or *laterally* in relation to the anterior aspect of its proximal end, for example, external tibial torsion (Fig. 4.18) and external femoral torsion.

Anteversion and Retroversion

Anteversion and retroversion refer to the relationship between the neck of the femur and the femoral shaft.

Femoral anteversion exists when the knee is directed anteriorly; the femoral neck is directed *anteriorly* to some degree (Fig. 4.19).

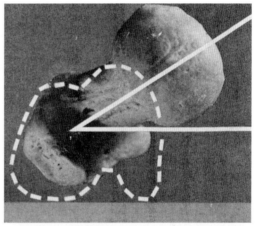

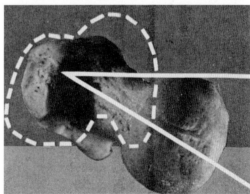

Figure 4.19.   Top. Anteversion of the femoral neck (femoral anteversion). The dotted lines outline the femoral condyles in relation to a horizontal surface. The upper solid line represents the axis of the femoral neck.

Figure 4.20.   Bottom. Retroversion of the femoral neck (femoral retroversion). The dotted lines outline the femoral condyles in relation to a horizontal surface. The lower solid line represents the axis of the femoral neck.

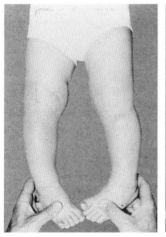
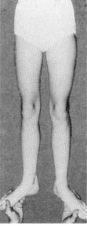

Figure 4.17.   Left. Internal torsion of the tibia (bilateral).

Figure 4.18.   Right. External torsion of the tibia (bilateral).

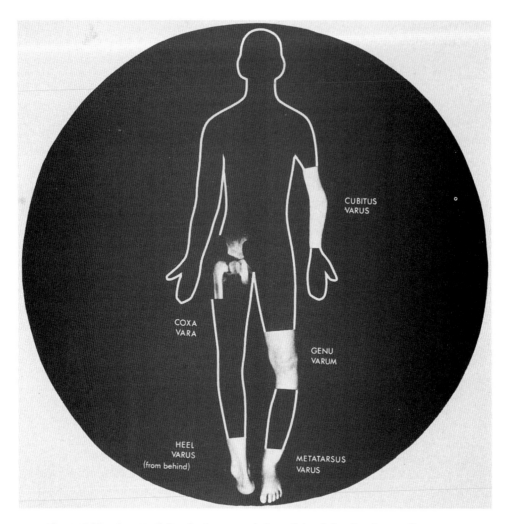

Figure 4.21.   A varus deformity is an angulation of the deformity that conforms to an imaginary circle in which the patient is placed.

Femoral retroversion exists when the knee is directed anteriorly; the femoral neck is directed *posteriorly* to some degree (Fig. 4.20.

Angulation or Bowing Deformities

An angulation deformity occurs most frequently at the site of a fracture in the shaft of a long bone but may also occur as a bowing deformity within an intact bone. Considerable confusion exists concerning the description of such angulation or bowing deformities (e.g., anterior or posterior? medial or lateral?) The adjective describing an angulation or bowing deformity refers to the direction in which the *apex of the angle* points (rather than the direction in which the distal fragment points).

Varus and Valgus

The deformities of varus and valgus refer to *abnormal angulation* within a limb. The angulation deformity is usually in a joint, or in a bone near a joint, but it may also occur through the shaft of a long bone. This particular pair of terms has probably caused more confusion than any other pair, partly because the original Latin terms had the opposite meaning to that which is now universally accepted. You will find it easy to remember which is which by thinking of the patient in the anatomical position within an imaginary circle.

Varus

Varus is an angulation that *conforms* to an imaginary circle in which the patient is placed (Fig. 4.21).

Cubitus varus is a decrease in the normal carrying angle at the elbow.

Coxa vara is a *decrease* in the femoral neck–shaft angle (less than 130°) (e.g., an angle of 90° conforms more to a circle than does the normal angle of 130°).

Genu varum is also called *bow leg* in which the knees are apart when the feet are together.

Heel varus is a decrease in the normal angle between the axis of the leg and that of the heel, as in the position of inversion.

Talipes equinovarus is an inversion deformity of the foot combined with an equinus or plantar flexion deformity of the ankle. This combination is seen in a congenital clubfoot.

Metatarsus varus is more properly called *metatarsus adductus*—an adduction deformity of the forefoot in relation to the hind foot.

Hallux varus is an adduction deformity of the great toe through the metatarsophalangeal joint.

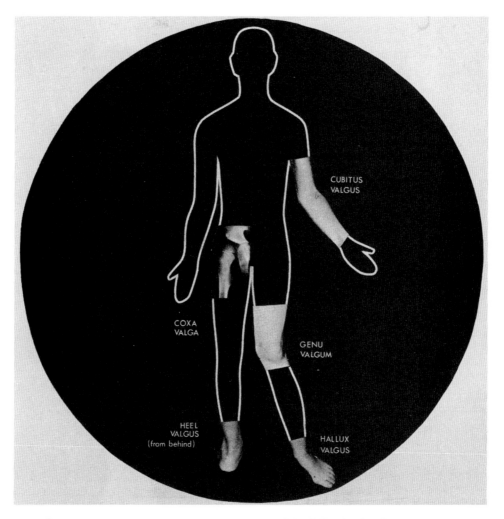

Figure 4.22. A valgus deformity is an angulation of the deformity that does not conform to an imaginary circle in which the patient is placed.

Valgus

Valgus is an angulation that does *not* conform to an imaginary circle in which the patient is placed (Fig. 4.22).

Cubitus valgus is an increase in the normal carrying angle at the elbow.

Coxa valga is an *increase* in the femoral neck–shaft angle (more than 130°), for example, an angle of 170° conforms less to a circle than does the normal angle of 130°.

Genu valgum is also called *knock-knee*. In this condition, the feet are apart when the knees are together.

Heel valgus is an *increase* in the normal angle between the axis of the leg and that of the heel, as in the position of eversion.

Talipes calcaneovalgus is an eversion defor-

mity of the foot combined with a calcaneus or dorsiflexion deformity of the ankle.

Hallux valgus is an abduction deformity of the great toe through the metatarsophalangeal joint.

CLINICAL MEASUREMENT OF JOINT MOTION AND DEFORMITY

Having learned the meaning of the pairs of clinical terms describing joint motion and de-

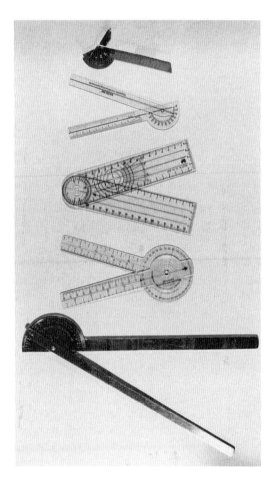

Figure 4.23.   Various types of goniometers for the accurate measurement of joint motion and deformity.

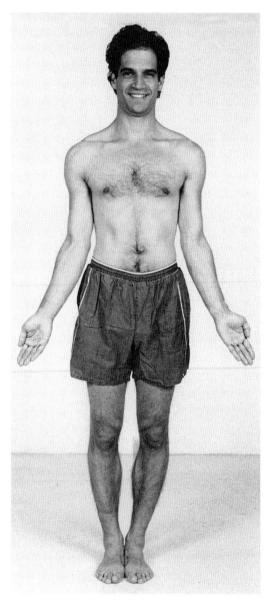

Figure 4.24.   The anatomical position.

formities, you must now learn acceptable standard methods of measuring and recording such motion and deformity in the extremities. The 1994 publication by the American Academy of Orthopaedic Surgeons entitled *The Clinical Measurement of Joint Motion* provides just such standard methods. Consequently, these methods are used throughout this textbook.

Measuring and recording joint motion and deformities are important because they provide useful data for the following activities:

1. Diagnosis of disorders and injuries of the musculoskeletal system
2. Determination of deterioration or improvement or neither in the clinical course of a disorder or injury
3. Objective assessment of the outcome of treatment, either operative or nonoperative
4. Communication about a given patient with colleagues and allied health professionals

For the sake of accuracy you should measure joint motion and deformity using some type of goniometer (Fig. 4.23).

The Anatomical Position

The starting, or zero position, for most joints in the human is the *anatomical position* in which the individual is standing erect, the head, eyes, and toes directed forward, the feet together, and the arms hanging by the sides with the palms of the hands facing forwards (Fig. 4.24).

SUGGESTED ADDITIONAL READING

Brashear HR, Crenshaw AH, Harrelson JM, Curtis PH Jr. Manual of orthopaedic surgery. 6th ed. Chicago, American Orthopaedic Association, 1985.

Blawvel CT, Nelson FRT. A manual of orthopaedic terminology. St. Louis: CV Mosby, 1977.

Green WB, Heckman WD. The clinical measurements of joint motion. Rosemont, IL: American Academy of Orthopaedic Surgeons, 1994.

Houston CS. Varus and valgus—no wonder they are confused. N Engl J Med 1980;302: 471–472.

5 Diagnosis of Musculoskeletal Disorders and Injuries

"The first step toward cure is to know what the disease is"

—Latin proverb

As a medical practitioner of the future, your first responsibility to each of your patients will be to determine what the problem or disease is (the *diagnosis*). This you must determine with great care and accuracy so that you may make the correct start toward the goal of helping your patient because, of course, he or she will have come to you as a medical practitioner primarily *to* seek help with a problem.

Problem-solving holds a certain fascination for all of us, and who among us is not stimulated by a mystery? The field of medicine affords daily opportunity to solve mysteries and other problems, not only in diagnosis and treatment but also in the many types of medical research. Solving the mystery of a diagnosis is the "detective work of medicine," and to be consistently accurate, you must emulate that greatest of all detectives, Sherlock Holmes, who constantly demanded: "Data, give me data!" (Fig. 5.1). In the investigation of a diagnostic mystery, you, like Sherlock Holmes, must be keenly interested, inquiring, attentive, alert, observant, perceptive, and skillful in correlating data, or clues, as well as in making logical deductions and conclusions from them. (It is of interest that both the literary creator of Sherlock Holmes and his "model" for the detective were members of the medical profession. Sir Arthur Conan Doyle was inspired to create the fictional figure of the master detective in 1880 as a result of his close association, as a postgraduate medical student, with Joseph Bell, a brilliant Edinburgh physician who was renowned for his remarkable powers of observation and deduction in relation to diagnosis.)

METHODS OF OBTAINING DATA (CLUES)—THE INVESTIGATION

Certain musculoskeletal conditions, such as a typical congenital clubfoot, are so obvious that their diagnosis presents little difficulty (as Holmes would say: "Elementary, my dear Watson"). However, other conditions—such as a malignant bone neoplasm in its earliest stages, or symptoms such as progressive weakness in a limb—present diagnostic problems that may require extensive investigation. Thus, not all the methods of obtaining data, or clues, are essential to making every diagnosis, but you must be prepared to use as many as necessary to solve the problem, or mystery, of diagnosis in each patient you see. The investigation to make the diagnosis of musculoskeletal disorders and injuries proceeds in the following order: 1) history taking (symptoms), 2) physical examination (signs), 3) diagnostic imaging (imaging signs), and 4) laboratory investigation (including examinations of various body fluids as well as examination of a specimen, or biopsy, of diseased tissue). Symptoms provide *subjective data,* whereas physical signs, imaging signs, and the results of laboratory tests provide *objective data.*

The Patient's Story (Clinical History)

In the current era of dramatic technological advances in a wide variety of diagnostic methods, it is more important than ever to appreciate that in most cases, a carefully and accurately obtained clinical history from the patient or the patient's relatives (or both) still contributes significantly more to a correct

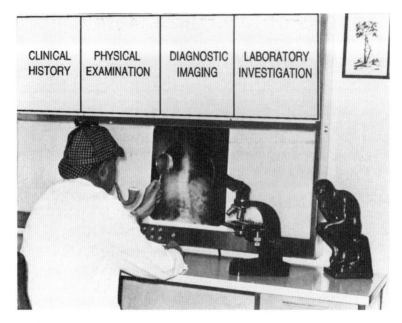

Figure 5.1.   The medical practitioner, like Sherlock Holmes, must search out and correlate all available data to solve the mystery of a diagnosis.

diagnosis than do the physical examination, diagnostic imaging, and laboratory investigation combined.

As a medical student of the present, you will have many opportunities to obtain the clinical history from patients assigned to you in the wards and outpatient clinics of your teaching hospitals. You will be wise to develop good habits of history taking during these formative years of clinical training; they will serve you well as a medical practitioner of the future.

To obtain a complete and accurate history, you must be a discerning listener and an intelligent questioner. Furthermore, you must have certain attitudes of mind toward your patient, including a sincere and kindly interest in him or her as a fellow human being, compassion, understanding, patience, and tact. Remember that for many persons, consulting a medical practitioner may be an anxious experience. Regardless of their age or level of intelligence, your patients will be quick to sense your attitude toward them, and they will either be put at ease or made to feel ill at ease by it.

Skill in history taking involves an important facet of the broad area of communication with your patients and their relatives. Goldbloom, who has described history taking as "interviewing, the most sophisticated of diagnostic technologies" offers sound advice for the interviewer, such as sitting, rather than standing, making frequent eye contact, taking sufficient time to ask relevant questions and *listen* to the patient's concerns, both spoken and, at least initially, unspoken (i.e., hidden agendas). Indeed, the public perception of the medical profession is frequently expressed by the complaint that medical practitioners are too busy to take enough time either to listen or to talk.

In recent decades, global migration has greatly increased the ethnic diversity of the population in most of the world's developed countries, especially in the larger cities. This phenomenon has created the need for interpreter services in hospitals or at least a system of obtaining a bilingual relative or volunteer to enhance the accuracy of two-way communications between the medical practitioner and a patient for whom there is a language barrier.

Under certain other circumstances (infancy, mental retardation, loss of consciousness), the patient will be unable to tell you the story himself or herself, in which case you must rely on the "hearsay" history given by a relative, a friend, or some other witness. At present, when so much medical information (and misinformation) is reported in newspapers, lay magazines, radio, and television programs, you must be discerning about your patient's interpretation of his or her symptoms or attempts at self-diagnosis—not that they should be automatically discounted (they may even be correct) but they may have misled the patient and you must not allow them to mislead *you*.

Important Data in the Patient's History
Preliminary Data

The patient's name, sex, date of birth and present age, occupation, and family responsibilities are the first items of information obtained.

The Presenting Problem or Chief Complaint

The chief complaint is the main symptom, or group of symptoms, that have prompted the patient to seek help and advice. Your opening inquiry about this should not be "What is wrong with you?" because such a question invites the obvious reaction, either silent or expressed: "That is what I have come to find out from *you*!" A preferable beginning is, "What have you *noticed* or *felt* that does not seem right to you?" Having listened to your patient describe the chief complaints in his or her own words, you need to obtain more precise information by asking further questions to determine the following: time of onset, type of onset (sudden or gradual), severity, constancy (constant or intermittent), progression, activities that aggravate it and those that relieve it, relation to any injury or other incident, and any associated symptoms.

Common Musculoskeletal Symptoms or Complaints

The following are the main reasons why a patient with a musculoskeletal condition seeks consultation with a medical practitioner:

1. **Pain.** By far the most important presenting symptom is pain, and you must inquire about it in great detail with respect to its onset, precise location, character (dull, sharp, burning), severity, duration, factors that relieve the pain as well as those that aggravate it, and its variation with day and night. There is a wide variation from person to person in relation to pain threshold and pain tolerance; the patient who "feels" more pain, or tolerates it less well than the average person, may not be exaggerating at all and requires kindly consideration. Most musculoskeletal pain is aggravated by intermittent local movement and is relieved by local rest; this suggests that during movement, such pain is caused by a sudden increase in either tension or pressure in sensitive soft tissues such as periosteum (movement at a fracture site) or joint capsule and ligaments (movement in a joint). Any such painful movement initiates muscle spasm, which in itself is painful, and this pain is superimposed on the initial pain. Pain that persists in spite of local rest suggests progressively increasing pressure in a closed space, such as occurs with an increasing amount of purulent exudate within the confines of a bone (osteomyelitis) or within a joint cavity (septic arthritis) and also with a progressively expanding bone neoplasm. Pressure on a nerve, or nerve root, produces *radiating pain* in the sensory area of that nerve or nerve root; the most common example is *sciatica*, pain radiating down the lower limb in the distribution of the sciatic nerve from pressure of a protruded intervertebral disc on a nerve root. Remember also, the phenomenon of *referred pain,* the most important example of which is pain felt in the knee (referred to the knee) but arising from a painful lesion in the hip caused by the obturator nerve pattern of hip pain. Neurological lesions may produce alterations in skin sensation, including increased or painful feeling (*hyperesthesia*), decreased feeling (*hypoesthesia*), or peculiar feeling, for example, "pins and needles" (*paresthesia*).

2. **Decrease in function.** Decreased ability to use a body part is also a common presenting complaint (chief complaint) of patients with musculoskeletal conditions. The pa-

tient may be concerned about decreased ability (disability) caused by muscle weakness or fatigue, giving way (instability) of a joint, or stiffness of a joint.

3. **Physical appearance.** The patient's chief complaint may be the physical appearance of a *deformity* such as a crooked limb or limbs (angulatory deformity), twisted limb (torsional or rotational deformity), a wasted limb (atrophy), a short leg (leg length discrepancy), or a crooked back (scoliosis). He or she may be concerned about the physical appearance of an abnormal way of walking (limp or abnormal gait). Deformities and abnormal gaits are physical signs rather than symptoms, but they may still be the patient's chief complaint or presenting problem. You must determine when the problem was first noticed, its character, clinical course (getting better, getting worse, or remaining unchanged), and the extent of any associated disability. As with tolerance to pain, patients vary widely in their tolerance, or acceptance, of deformities and abnormal gaits. A given deformity or limp may be acceptable to one patient and yet be a source of great concern (and therefore a problem) to another.

Relevant Past History

It is important to obtain a history of previous illnesses, injuries, and related treatment, including vaccinations and operations. The patient may have a tendency to ascribe his or her present symptoms or signs to a specific incident such as previous illness, an injury, or treatment, whereas you may discern that, in fact, the incident merely served to draw the patient's attention to a pre-existing and previously unrecognized condition.

Functional Inquiry

Patients with disorders of the musculoskeletal system may have coexistent disorders of some other body system, or systems, and hence the reason for inquiring into the function of all systems (*functional inquiry*). Some of the more important conditions to include are heart disease, diabetes, kidney disease, respiratory conditions, and psychogenic disturbances

with either exaggeration or falsification of symptoms. As Sir William Osler stated, "It is important to ascertain not only what kind of disease the person has, but also what kind of person has the disease." Nevertheless, you should search diligently for an organic explanation of the patient's symptoms, even though he or she may appear to be "neurotic," lest you do him or her the injustice of jumping to the wrong conclusion.

Social, Economic, and Work History

Since orthopaedic problems and their treatment frequently extend over long periods, you must obtain the relevant details of the patient's social, economic, and work history so that the proposed plan of treatment will be feasible for the particular patient.

Family History

Because some musculoskeletal conditions (both congenital and acquired) show a distinct tendency to appear in members of the same family (either in the same or in different generations), it is important to obtain such data concerning relatives by means of a *family history*.

Physical Examination

More than half the diagnoses in patients can be made on the basis of a carefully obtained, detailed clinical history, and more than three quarters of the diagnoses can be made from the combined data of the clinical history and the physical examination. Thus, these two time-honored methods are still the best combination of diagnostic tests at your disposal. Because of the importance of the clinical history and the physical examination, modern strategies—including epidemiologic and biostatistical methods—are currently being applied to test scientifically the diagnostic validity of the multitude of clinical symptoms and physical signs.

In a sense, the physical examination begins the moment the patient comes into sight. Certain striking features about the patient—body build (habitus), facial appearance (facies), way of walking (gait) as he or she approaches you, or the sitting or lying position if you are approaching him or her (body language)—may have already provided you with useful clues almost before you have had time to say "How do you do?" Your eager eyes (like those of Sherlock Holmes) will pick out every clue, and by the time the history taking part of the examination is completed, you will have detected many things about the patient (and he or she will have detected certain things about you also). Your attitude of mind toward the patient will be reflected by your methods of examination. A compassionate attitude of mind results in an awareness of the patient's feelings, as well as a respect for these feelings. Therefore, you respect the patient's modesty by ensuring that he or she is appropriately draped. Furthermore, when examining a patient of the opposite gender, you will be wise to have a nurse or other health professional in the examining room, not only as a comfort to your patient but also as a witness. You will always endeavor to be as gentle as possible in your examination so as not to produce unnecessary pain—that is, no more than is absolutely necessary to detect that a certain pressure or movement is, in fact, painful.

Apart from your own common sense and your keen senses of sight, touch, and hearing, the equipment you require for the musculoskeletal examination of the patient is simple (Fig. 5.2). The examination is conducted in systematic order: 1) *looking (inspection)*; 2) *feeling (palpation)*; 3) *moving (assessment of joint motion)*, both active and passive; 4) *listening (auscultation)* over joints and vessels; 5) *special physical tests* to elicit or exclude specific physical signs; and 6) the *neurological examination*.

Looking (Inspection)

The patient must be sufficiently exposed so that an important sign is not overlooked. Nevertheless, it is neither necessary nor appropriate to request that the patient remove his or her underclothing when examining the musculoskeletal system in older children, adolescents, and adults. Patients also appreciate the offer of an examination gown as well as the privacy to undress before and dress after the examination.

Confirm your earlier observations of the patient's habitus and facies. Observe the skin (redness, cyanosis, pigmentation) (Fig. 5.3), looking for atrophy, hypertrophy, and scars of previous injury or operation. Look for any deformity (Fig. 5.4), swelling (Fig. 5.5), or lumps (Fig. 5.6). Measure any limb shortening (Fig. 5.7) or atrophy (Fig. 5.8), always comparing the abnormal limb with the opposite limb. If the patient is able to walk, request

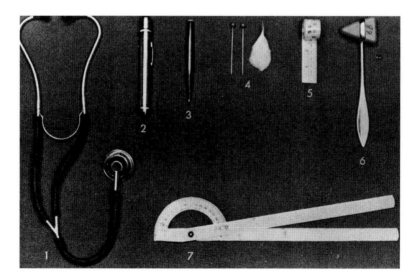

Figure 5.2. Equipment for musculoskeletal examination: stethoscope *(1)*, pocket flashlight *(2)*, skin marker *(3)*, pins and cotton wool *(4)*, tape measure *(5)*, reflex hammer *(6)*, and goniometer (to measure angles) *(7)*.

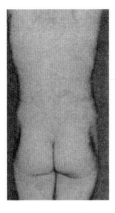

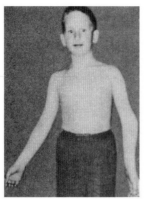

Figure 5.3. Left. The areas of light brown skin pigmentation (café au lait spots) in this boy are a clue to the diagnosis of neurofibromatosis (Von Recklinghausen's disease).

Figure 5.4. Right. The cubitus varus deformity of this boy's left arm is the result of an old supracondylar fracture of the humerus that had been allowed to heal with varus angulation.

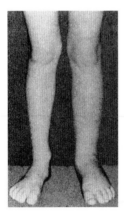

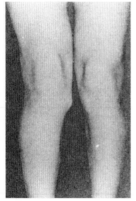

Figure 5.5. Left. The diffuse swelling of this boy's left leg results from chronic edema secondary to lymphatic vessel obstruction.

Figure 5.6. Right. The lump on the medial side of this woman's knee is a bony prominence caused by a type of benign bone lesion, an osteochondroma (osteocartilaginous exostosis), arising from the upper end of the tibia.

him or her to do so, back and forth in an unobstructed area, at least 20 feet long, because careful observation of the patient's gait may provide many important clues. Many of the

abnormal physical signs that are apparent on inspection are described and depicted in subsequent chapters.

Feeling (Palpation)
All patients appreciate a medical practitioner who has a "warm heart"; they also appreciate one who has *warm hands* and furthermore, warm hands elicit less muscle spasm than those that are cold and clammy. By palpation you will obtain data concerning skin temperature, pulse, tenderness, the nature of any swelling (indurated or edematous "pitting"), the characteristics of a lump or mass (consistency, fluctuation, size, relationship to adjacent structures), muscle bulk, and abnormal relationships of bones at their joints (dislocations). With the combination of joint movement and palpation, you will also detect joint crepitus as well as muscle tone.

Moving (Assessment of Joint Motion)
Active movement of a joint by the patient should be assessed first; it may be *limited* by pain and associated muscle spasm, muscle weakness, ruptured muscle or tendon, joint stiffness or joint contracture, or a bony block. *Passive movement* of a joint by you, the examiner, should be assessed gently; it may be *decreased* for any of the reasons already mentioned (except muscle weakness and ruptured muscle or tendon) (Fig. 5.9) or it may be *increased* as in joint instability caused by a lax capsule or torn ligaments (Fig. 5.10). Abnormal ranges of joint motion, both active and passive, should be recorded. The clinical state of the union of a healing fracture in an extremity can be assessed by detecting the presence or absence of passive motion and pain at the fracture site when a local angulatory, or torsional, force is applied to the involved extremity.

Listening (Auscultation)
Sounds arising from bones (fracture crepitus), joints (joint crepitus), or muscle action (snapping tendons) are sometimes sufficiently loud that they can be heard by both you and the patient without any effort. However, it is often informative to listen to a joint during movement through a stethoscope for more ac-

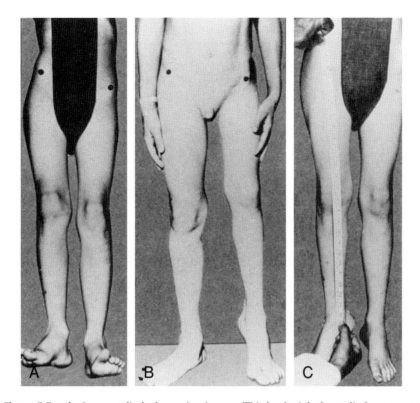

Figure 5.7. **A.** Apparent limb shortening is seen. This boy's right lower limb appears to be shorter than his left; however, they are actually the same length. The apparent shortening is caused by an adduction contracture of the right hip and resultant obliquity of the pelvis (the black dots are on the anterior superior spines). **B.** True limb shortening is seen. This boy's left lower limb is truly shorter than his right. He is almost able to compensate for this by standing on tiptoe on the shorter side. **C.** The figure shows a method of measuring true limb length from the anterior superior spine to the medial malleolus. Apparent limb length is measured from the umbilicus to the medial malleolus, with the lower limbs in line with the trunk.

curate assessment of the quality and localization of the sound (Fig. 5.11). The stethoscope is also of value in detecting the murmur of a peripheral arteriovenous fistula.

Special Physical Tests
Certain important physical signs will escape detection during the physical examination unless special tests that have been developed for the detection of these signs are carried out. The hip joint, being deeply situated and of complex structure and function, is more difficult to examine accurately than are other joints; therefore, it is not surprising that three of these special tests have been developed to demonstrate specific signs in the hip. Two of these signs are present (the test is positive) in

a variety of clinical conditions and accordingly they are considered now:

- Hip flexion deformity—the Thomas test (Fig. 5.12)
- Ineffectual hip abduction mechanism—the Trendelenburg test (Fig. 5.13)

Other specific signs are present in one condition only and are therefore more appropriately considered along with a discussion of that condition in subsequent chapters; they will be merely listed at present:

- Instability (dislocatability) of the newborn hip—the Barlow test and the Ortolani test (See Chapter 8).

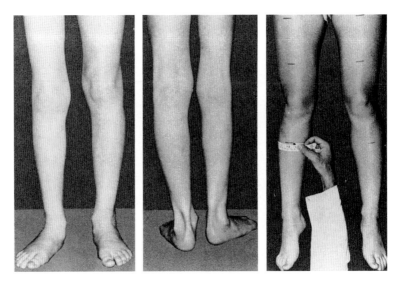

Figure 5.8.   A. The decrease in circumference of this boy's right calf and thigh results from muscle atrophy secondary to paralytic poliomyelitis. **B.** This figure shows a method of measuring limb circumference. The levels for comparable circumferential measurements should first be measured from comparable bony landmarks and marked.

- Sciatic nerve irritation Lasègue's test (See Chapter 11)
- Torn medial meniscus of the knee—the McMurray test (See Chapter 17)

Neurological Examination

Since many musculoskeletal disorders and injuries are associated with neurological deficits, it is essential to appreciate that the neurological examination is an important part of the

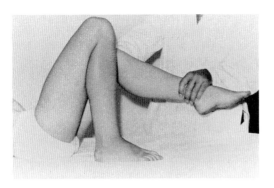

Figure 5.9.   Passive flexion of this girl's left knee was limited to 90° as a result of dense adhesions between the quadriceps muscle and the distal end of the femur after a severely displaced fracture at this site.

musculoskeletal examination. It is of particular importance when there is evidence of muscle weakness or muscle spasticity, involuntary movements of muscle, symptoms of altered skin sensation, incoordination of movement, and loss of balance. The neurological examination includes assessment of the motor system (muscle tone, power, coordination), sensory system (touch, pain, temperature, position sense, vibration), reflexes (tendon reflexes, abdominal reflexes, and plantar reflex) and rectal sphincter tone.

You will learn about the physical examination of the musculoskeletal and neurological systems most effectively from demonstrations given by your own clinical teachers as well as by practice under their supervision. These subjects justify complete textbooks; two helpful ones include two books by Hoppenfeld (one on extremities and spine, the other on orthopaedic neurology) and others referred to in the Suggested Additional Reading at the end of this chapter.

Diagnostic Imaging

Beginning in the 1970s and continuing through the 1990s, the specialty of what was

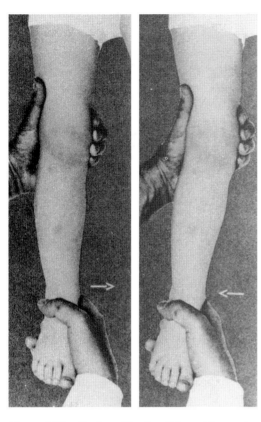

Figure 5.10. Passive adduction followed by passive abduction of this boy's right knee joint reveals an increased range of passive movement, indicating instability of the joint because of joint laxity.

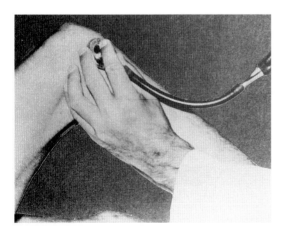

Figure 5.11. By auscultating a joint using a stethoscope, the source of joint crepitus, such as the "clunk" from an internal derangement of the joint, can usually be accurately localized during passive movement of the joint.

formerly called diagnostic radiology has been greatly expanded through a number of exciting and dramatic technological advances, including the cross-sectional imaging modalities of ultrasonography, computed tomography (CT) and, more recently, magnetic resonance imaging (MRI), only one of which (CT) involves the use of ionizing radiation. Consequently, to reflect these additional capabilities, radiography departments and departments of radiology in many hospitals are currently designated departments of diagnostic imaging. The modalities of CT and MRI, in particular, have proved to be of immense help in determining the precise location and diagnosis of many disorders and injuries of the musculoskeletal system.

Although the plain films, or radiographs, of conventional radiographic examination are still the most widely used and least expensive form of diagnostic imaging (especially for the initial examination), you will also need to become aware of the indications, merits, and indications of ultrasonography, CT, MRI, and scintigraphy (radionuclide scans of bones and soft tissues). With such a large array of imaging modalities, you will find that personal consultation with an experienced imager is helpful, not only in making the most appropriate choices but also in obtaining the most accurate interpretation of the images.

Plain (Conventional) Radiography

Prior to Roentgen's serendipitous discovery of x-rays in 1895, physicians and surgeons relied on clinical evidence to make a musculoskeletal diagnosis and follow the results of treatment. This revolutionary discovery greatly improved medical and surgical diagnosis and treatment in general, but especially in the musculoskeletal system. It is remarkable that the x-ray filament tube designed by Coolidge in 1913 has been changed little during the ensuing decades.

Examination of the musculoskeletal system by means of x-rays (radiographic examination) is, in a sense, an extension of the physical examination. It might be considered a form of "*internal inspection*" and, as such, it is of extreme value, not only in the accurate diagnosis

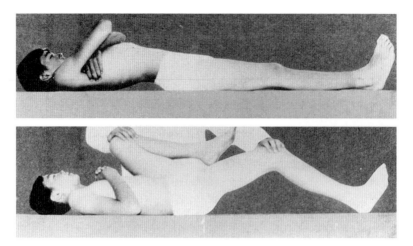

Figure 5.12. This figure describes the Thomas test for hip flexion deformity. **Top.** When the patient is lying supine, a hip flexion deformity can be masked by an increase in lumbar lordosis. **Bottom.** Passive complete flexion of the opposite hip straightens out the lumbar spine and reveals the true extent of the hip flexion deformity. This boy's hip flexion deformity was caused by the residual effects of a septic arthritis.

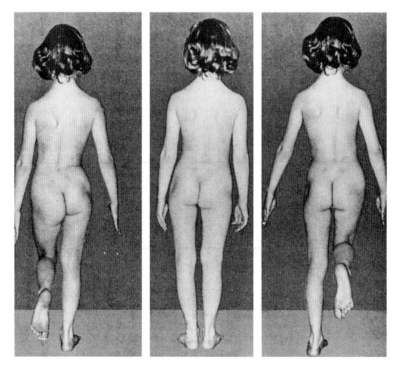

Figure 5.13. The Trendelenburg test for an ineffectual hip abduction mechanism is seen in a 4-year-old girl with congenital dislocation of the right hip. **Left.** When the child stands on her right foot (the side of the dislocated hip), the hip abductor muscles, having no fulcrum, cannot hold the pelvis level, and it drops on the opposite side. The child, in an effort to maintain balance, shifts her trunk toward the involved side. The Trendelenburg sign is also seen in the presence of coxa vara, paralyzed hip abductor muscles and painful conditions around the hip. **Middle.** The dislocation is not apparent when the child is standing with both feet on the floor (except for the slight shortening of the right lower limb). **Right.** When the child stands on her left foot (the side of the normal hip) the hip abductor muscles, having a normal function, hold the pelvis level.

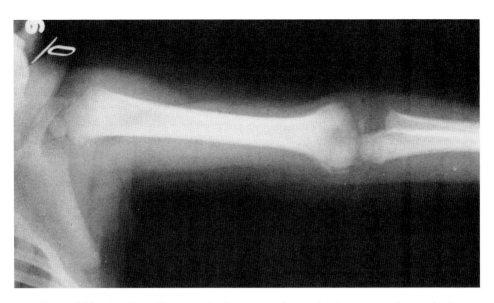

Figure 5.14.   In this radiograph, the bones, muscles, and subcutaneous fat are clearly differentiated from one another by their specific radiographic density. Note the extreme radiographic density of the metal object in the upper left corner.

of musculoskeletal disorders and injuries but also in following the subsequent course of these conditions. A brief explanation of "x-ray shadows" will make interpretation of x-ray films more interesting and more meaningful. An X-ray film (radiograph or roentgenograph) is studied against a bright light because it is a photographic "negative" rather than a "print." In radiographs, bone appears relatively white (radiopaque), whereas the soft tissues appear relatively dark (radiolucent). The radiographic density of a tissue depends on its thickness as well as its atomic weight. The thicker the tissue and the higher its atomic weight, the more radiation is absorbed and therefore the less radiation "penetrates" the tissue to expose the film, and the whiter it appears. Conversely, the thinner the tissue and the lower its atomic weight, the less radiation is absorbed and therefore the more radiation "penetrates" the tissue to expose the film, and the darker it appears. Fat has the lowest atomic weight of all the solid tissues and therefore appears darkest (most radiolucent) in the radiographic negative. Muscle, cartilage, and osteoid (not yet calcified) have approximately the same atomic weight, which is higher than

that of fat, and consequently they are more radiopaque than fat. Bone, however, because of its mineral content of calcium, phosphorus, magnesium, and other minerals, has a much higher atomic weight and is therefore much more radiopaque than the various soft tissues (Fig. 5.14). Furthermore, bone as a structure varies in its radiographic density depending on its thickness or structural density and on its calcification. Radiographically, an abnormally increased density in bone is called *sclerosis,* whereas an abnormally decreased density is called *rarefaction* (Fig. 5.15). You will recall from Chapter 3 that the radiographic density of bone clearly demonstrates the altered deposition and altered resorption of the bone as it reacts to abnormal conditions.

Air, of course, is the most radiolucent substance seen in a radiograph and, hence, it appears even darker than fat. Air is expected in the lungs, as is gas in the gastrointestinal tract. Air is also seen in the soft tissues immediately after an open surgical procedure. Air in the soft tissues at the base of the neck, however, signifies surgical emphysema, whereas widespread gas within the soft tissues of an injured part is an ominous sign of an overwhelming

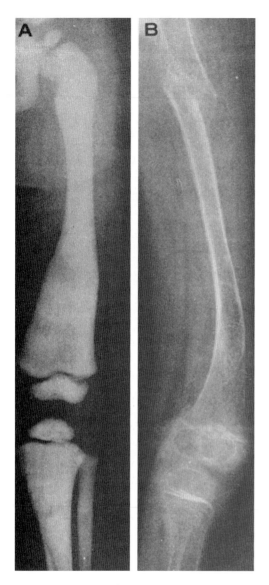

Figure 5.15. General density of bone is demonstrated in this figure. **A.** Increased density of bone (sclerosis) resulting from osteopetrosis ("marble bones"). Note also the deficit in the femoral neck and the abnormal contour of the femoral shaft. **B.** Decreased density of bone (rarefaction) due to osteogenesis imperfecta ("fragile bones"). Note also the healed fracture in the upper third of the femur.

gles to the first) is essential so that the structures can be studied from at least two projections—generally from the front (*anteroposterior projection*) and from the side (*lateral projection*) (Fig. 5.17). Sometimes additional views are required, for example, *oblique projections*. The third dimension can best be appreciated radiographically by studying two *stereoscopic projections.*

Inspection of a Radiograph
As in the inspection of your patients, you must also know what to look for when inspecting their radiographs. The following are some of the important features to look for in a radiograph:

- General density of bone—increased or decreased (Fig. 5.15)
- Local density of bone—increased or decreased (Fig. 5.18)
- Relationship between bones—dislocation and subluxation (Fig. 5.19)
- Break in bone continuity—fracture (Fig. 5.20)
- General contour of a bone—deformity (Fig. 5.21).
- Local contour of a bone—internal or external irregularity (Fig. 5.22).
- Thickness of articular cartilage—as reflected by the width of the joint space, or, more accurately, the cartilage space (Fig. 5.23).
- Changes in soft tissues—swelling, atrophy (Fig. 5.24).

You will be wise to inspect, or study, a radiograph as you would inspect, or study, a patient, initially from a distance and then from close range. In this way, your eyes move from the general to the particular and you are less likely to miss an important radiographic clue. Remember also that there may be more than one clue or sign in a given radiograph (Fig. 5.20). Comparison of a limb with the opposite limb, which has already been stressed in clinical examination, is important in radiographic examination if you are in doubt, particularly in children because of the varying appearance

and potentially fatal type of infection that causes gas gangrene (Fig. 5.16).

A radiograph, like a photograph, is only two-dimensional, and a single radiograph represents only one view, which could be misleading. Therefore, a second view (at right an-

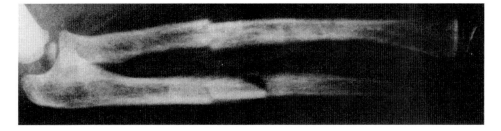

Figure 5.16. Radiograph of the forearm of a 10-year-old boy who sustained an open ("compound") fracture of the radius and ulna 3 days previously. Note the widespread gas within the soft tissues of the forearm, which is a sign of gas gangrene. So fulminating was the gas gangrene that amputation was required to save this boy's life.

of epiphyses and epiphyseal plates during the period of growth.

Because plain films do not show the soft tissues (cartilage, muscle, ligaments and tendons) well, special types of radiographic examination may be necessary to depict certain soft tissue outlines. These examinations involve the injection of a contrast medium (either a fluid that is radiopaque or air, which is radiolu-

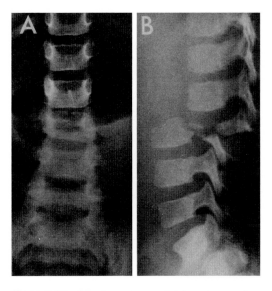

Figure 5.17. The importance of at least two projections is demonstrated in this figure. **A.** The anteroposterior projection of the lumbar spine of this severely injured boy reveals relatively little distortion of the spine. **B.** The lateral projection of the lumbar spine of the same boy reveals a severe fracture–dislocation of the spine. Two projections at right angles to each other are essential.

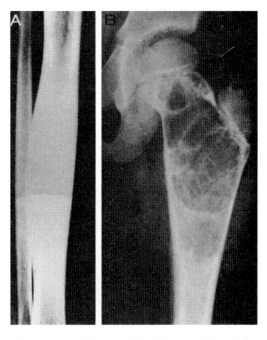

Figure 5.18. **A.** Increased local density of bone (sclerosis). The localized area of sclerosis in this boy's tibia is caused by new bone formation as a reaction to an osteosclerotic lesion (an osteoid osteoma) within the bone. In this radiograph, the osteoid osteoma itself (which is only 1 cm in diameter and is actually osteolytic) is obscured by the extensive reaction of osteosclerosis in the surrounding bone of the lateral cortex of the tibia. **B.** Decreased local density of bone (rarefaction). The localized area of rarefaction in the upper end of this girl's femur results from an osteolytic lesion (a simple bone cyst) within the bone.

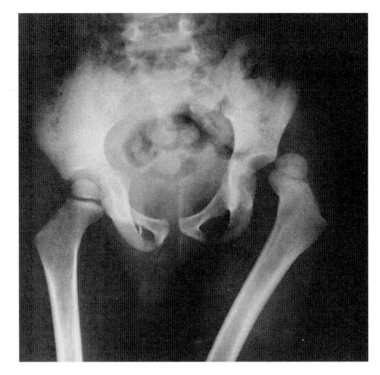

Figure 5.19.   The relationship between bones is seen in this figure. This child's left hip joint is completely dislocated as the result of a severe injury (traumatic dislocation).

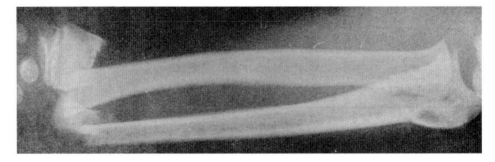

Figure 5.20.   This figure shows a break in bone continuity. The displaced fractures of the distal metaphyseal regions of the radius and ulna are obvious. However, there may be more than one clue in a given radiograph. Can you also detect the less obvious fracture? Look at the proximal end of the ulna.

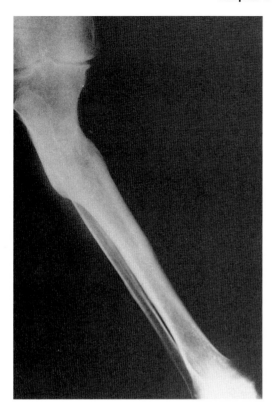

Figure 5.21. This figure demonstrates general bone contour. The varus deformity in this 60-year-old man's right tibia is the result of an old fracture that had been allowed to heal with deformity (malunion).

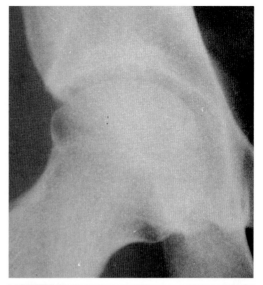

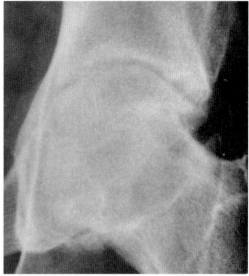

Figure 5.23. The left hip joint of this 14-year-old girl has been the site of pyogenic infection (septic arthritis). Note the decreased thickness of the cartilage space (a more accurate term than *joint space*) of the left hip compared with that of the normal opposite hip **(top)**, indicating loss of articular cartilage.

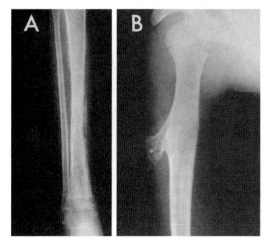

Figure 5.22. Local bone contour is seen in this figure. **A.** Internal irregularity of the distal half of the tibia in a child caused by chronic osteomyelitis. **B.** External irregularity of the humerus in a child caused by an osteochondroma (osteocartilaginous exostosis).

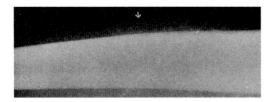

Figure 5.24. This figure demonstrates changes in soft tissues. Note the irregular density in the subcutaneous tissues overlying the tibia. This soft tissue shadow is the result of a recent hemorrhage and consequent hematoma in the subcutaneous tissues.

cent) into a body space. The following are four examples of contrast radiography.

Arthrography

Arthrography consists of the injection of a radiopaque contrast agent or air (or a combination of the two for a double-contrast examination) into the synovial cavity to detect injuries or other abnormalities of the articular cartilage, fibrocartilaginous menisci, capsule, and ligaments (Fig. 5.25).

Myelography

Injection of the contrast medium into the subarachnoid space can detect the protrusions of nucleus pulposus or soft tissue neoplasms extending into the vertebral canal (Fig. 5.26). Such protrusions are more accurately visualized by computed CT combined with myelography or by MRI imaging.

Discography

Injection of a radiopaque contrast agent into suspected abnormal intervertebral discs under local anesthesia can help in localizing the par-

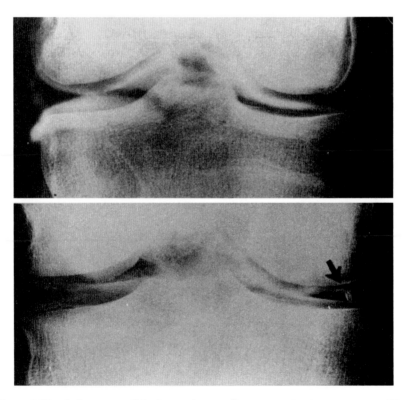

Figure 5.25. Arthrograms of the knee using a radiopaque contrast agent are seen. **Top.** Normal arthrogram of the right knee. Note the smooth wedge-shaped medial and lateral menisci clearly outlined by the dye in the joint. **Bottom.** Arthrogram of the right knee revealing penetration of the contrast agent into a vertical tear in the medial meniscus *(arrow)*. By means of several oblique projections, the location and extent of the tear can be determined. Arthrography is currently being replaced in major centers by MRI.

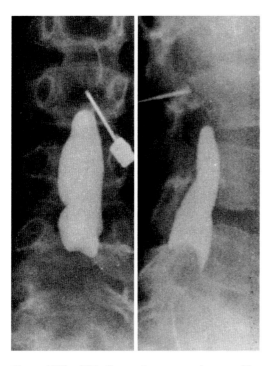

Figure 5.26. This figure shows a myelogram. The descent of the radiopaque medium (iophendylate; Pantopaque) is completely blocked at the level of the fourth lumbar vertebra by a space-occupying lesion (a neoplasm) within the vertebral canal. Nonionic contrast agents are much more satisfactory for this purpose than previously available oil-based radiopaque media.

ticular disc that is causing the patient's symptoms, not only because the injection into the responsible disc reproduces the symptoms but also because the radiographic pattern of the dye in such a disc is abnormal in that it extends beyond the normal confines of the disc. With the advent of MRI, myelography and discography are rarely performed any longer.

Sinography
Sinography consists of an injection of contrast medium into an external sinus to follow the sinus track to its source in the depths of the tissues (Fig. 5.27).

Scintigraphy
Since the 1970s, the specialty of nuclear medicine has made great strides in detecting a wide variety of lesions in bone through the use of

bone-seeking radionuclides such as technetium-99m–labeled polyphosphate; its analog, methylene disphosphate; and others. The resultant "bone scans" reflect changes in the local blood flow in bone as well as the degree of local metabolic activity.

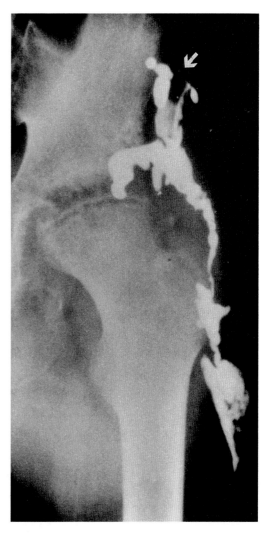

Figure 5.27. The radiopaque medium in this sinogram has been injected into a sinus on the lateral aspect of this boy's left thigh. The medium outlines the sinus tract and reveals its connection with the hip joint. The medium also outlines a radiolucent foreign body just lateral to the ilium above the hip joint *(arrow);* this was a piece of wood that had been driven into the soft tissues at the time of a penetrating injury and traumatic dislocation of the hip. Note also the evidence of destruction of the femoral head resulting from the combination of infection and avascular necrosis.

Scintigraphy has been useful in detecting and localizing a wide variety of lesions, including benign conditions (especially osteoid osteoma), primary malignant tumors, skeletal metastases, early osteomyelitis, infected endoprostheses, and even stress fractures, all of which appear on the scan as an area of *increased* radionuclide uptake (a so-called hot spot) (Figs. 5.28 and 5.29). In addition, bone scans are useful in detecting avascular necrosis of bone in its early stages, at which time there is *decreased* radionuclide uptake (a so-called cold spot).

Plain (Conventional) Tomography

Plain tomography provides images of a series of sections or slices of the tissues at varying depths from the skin surface. Such sections,

each of which is focused at a specific level, are particularly helpful in evaluating abnormalities within high-contrast tissues such as bone—for example, destructive lesions in bone, nonunions of fractures, or the completeness of bony union across an area of arthrodesis (joint fusion). Although plain, or conventional, tomography has been replaced to a large extent by CT scans and MRI scans, especially in larger centers, it still has a place in centers in which these much more expensive modalities are not available.

Computed Tomography

During the 1970s in the entire field of diagnostic radiology, CT was by far the most important and most exciting advance since 1895 when Roentgen discovered x-rays. Indeed, ra-

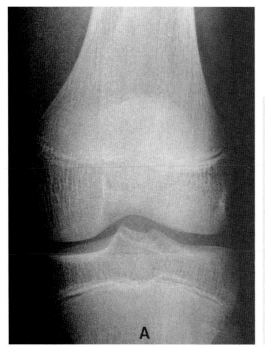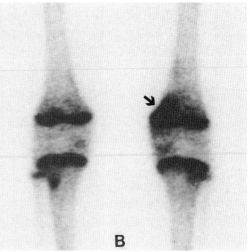

Figure 5.28.   **A.** Conventional radiograph of the distal end of the left femur in a 14-year-old boy who had sustained a direct blow to the medial side of his knee 3 days previously and who complained of increasingly severe pain at this site. Examination revealed local tenderness; he also had a fever. This is suggestive of acute hematogenous osteomyelitis (as described in Chapter 10), but it would be too early for any detectable changes in this conventional radiograph, which was interpreted to be normal. **B.** This scintogram (bone scan) of the distal ends of both femora in this patient is viewed from the front. There is focal hyperemia and increased radionuclide uptake, that is, increased bone activity (a "hot spot") in the medial part of the distal metaphysis *(arrow)* of the left femur, which is consistent with the clinical diagnosis of acute hematogenous osteomyelitis.

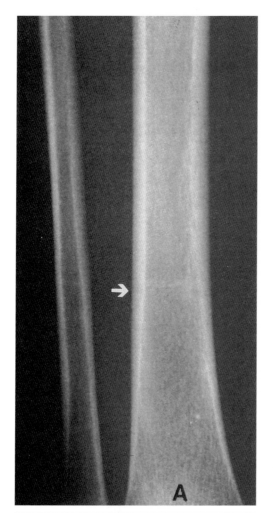

Figure 5.29. **A.** This conventional radiograph was taken of the junction of the middle and distal third of the right tibia of a 12-year-old track and field athlete who had recently started intensive spring training and who complained of local pain. There is a suggestion of a hairline stress fracture *(arrow)*, but it is too early to expect to see the fracture clearly or to see reactive new bone. **B.** The scintogram (bone scan) of this area viewed from behind reveals focal hyperemia and increased radionuclide uptake, that is, increased bone activity (a "hot spot") of the cortex of the tibia at this site *(arrow)* typical of a recent stress fracture (as described in Chapter 15).

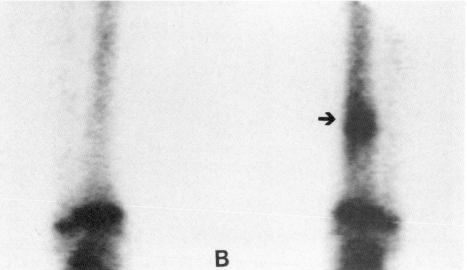

diology has entered what might be called "the era of imaginative imaging" as a result of this marvel of radiation physics, electronics, and computer science. By making extensive use of computers to reconstruct images, CT became the first cross-sectioned imaging modality.

The science and technology of CT is advancing at such a phenomenal rate that each successive generation of CT scanners soon becomes relatively obsolete.

CT, through which accurate images of "slices" of the body are generated, ingeniously overcomes many of the limitations of two-dimensional radiography and provides a degree of diagnostic accuracy not previously attainable. Originally limited to computed axial (cross-sectional) tomography and hence the term *CAT scan,* the technology has now made it possible with reformatting to look at coronal, sagittal, and even oblique slices as well. Thus, the current term, computed tomography, is more appropriate.

This sophisticated diagnostic imaging system clearly differentiates between the radiographic densities of various tissues and enables us to see lesions that are not demonstrable by standard radiography and with less radiation to the patient than conventional tomograms use.

In the musculoskeletal system, CT is of tremendous value in detecting the precise site and extent of varied disorders, such as benign and malignant tumors, pulmonary metastases, osteomyelitis, intervertebral disc herniation (CT combined with myelography), spinal stenosis, congenital abnormalities of the spine such as diastematomyelia, and meningomyelocele, as well as torsional deformities of the femur, posterior dislocation of the hip, and complex fractures of the pelvis.

More recently, some of these disorders—including benign and malignant bone and soft tissue tumors, soft tissue compression of the spinal cord by metastases, intervertebral disc herniation, and early stages of avascular necrosis of bone—can be more accurately demonstrated by magnetic resonance imaging (MRI). Nevertheless, CT is still extremely use-

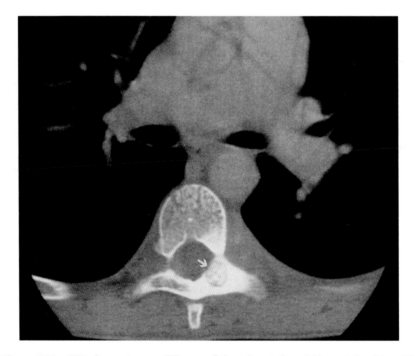

Figure 5.30.   This figure shows a CT scan of the spine at the midthoracic level in a 14-year-old boy with local pain in his back. Note the radiolucent lesion and the surrounding radiosclerotic area in the lamina *(arrow).* The diagnosis was an osteoid osteoma (as described in Chapter 14).

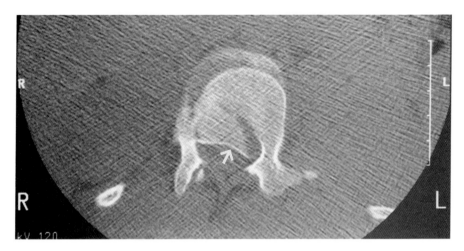

Figure 5.31.   This CT scan was taken at the level of the first lumbar vertebra in a 16-year-old boy who sustained a "burst" fracture of his spine (as described in Chapter 17). He had a neurological deficit in his lower limbs. Note the 50% decrease in the cross-sectional area of the spinal canal caused by the posterior displacement of a fracture fragment *(arrow)*.

ful in the imaging of complex fractures of the spine and the joints of the extremities as well as disc space infections and tarsal coalitions. Examples of CT scans of musculoskeletal tissues are shown in Figures 5.30 and 5.31.

Understandably, a thorough knowledge of the cross-sectional anatomy of the body is essential for the accurate interpretation of the cross-sectional slices of CT scans.

By means of highly sophisticated computer technology, three-dimensional reconstructions can be created from CT scans. Such reconstructions are especially helpful in the preoperative planning of three-dimensional reconstructive orthopaedic procedures, especially for complex problems of the pelvis and hips (Figure 5.32).

Ultrasonography (Ultrasound)
Ultrasonography, or diagnostic ultrasound, which does not involve the use of ionizing radiation, is useful in detecting joint effusions (Fig. 5.33), muscle and tendon injuries, and the precise relationship between the unossified, cartilaginous femoral head and the acetabulum in newborn infants with suspected congenital dislocation or subluxation of the hip (developmental dysplasia of the hip) (Fig. 5.34). Ultrasonography has also been used as a safe, noninvasive method to differentiate be-

tween solid soft tissue lesions and fluid-filled cystic lesions (such as a popliteal cyst).

The Doppler phenomenon using ultrasound is an accurate and noninvasive method of assessing arterial and venous blood flow in an extremity. Consequently, ultrasonography is beginning to replace invasive venography for detection of deep vein thrombosis. It is also helpful in assessing the neonatal spine and spinal cord.

Magnetic Resonance Imaging
The development of MRI in the 1980s was another major breakthrough in the field of diagnostic imaging. The most significant advantages of MRI over CT are that it uses nonionizing radiofrequency radiation rather than ionizing radiation. Using a strong magnetic field, MRI provides cross-sectional images with higher resolution than CT, and it produces better images of the brain and spinal cord. It can better differentiate the various types of soft tissue from each other and it can provide physiological as well as anatomical data (especially when used in conjunction with contrast agents and spectroscopy).

Thus, MRI is the most effective diagnostic imaging technique for the demonstration of malignant tumors of soft tissue and bone, internal derangements of joints (especially the

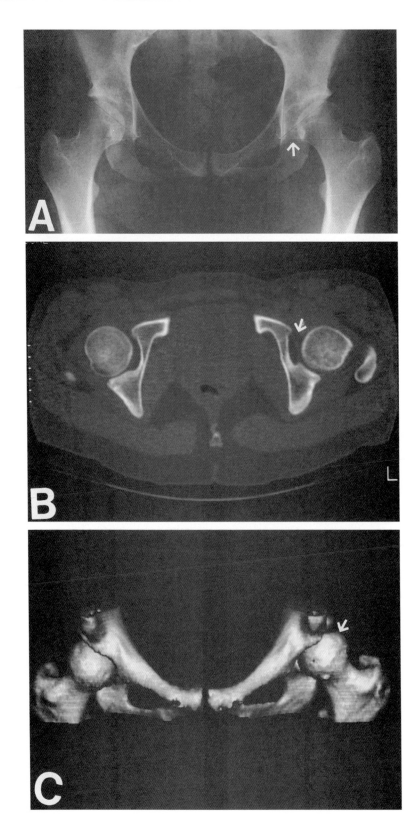

knee), rotator cuff tears in the shoulder, muscle and tendon injuries, intervertebral disc herniations, and the early stages of avascular necrosis of bone.

The various tissues of the body have two relaxation times for their specific protons; these are referred to as T1 and T2 relaxation times. The most common MRI technique is the spin echo sequence, which can be weighted to accentuate the T1 properties of tissue (T1-weighted images) or their T2 properties (T2-weighted images). In T1-weighted images, tissues with a short T1 (such as fat) have a high (bright) signal intensity, whereas fluids with a long T1 (such as cerebrospinal and synovial fluid) and tissues such as cortical bone and fibrous tissue have a low (dark) signal intensity. By contrast, in T2-weighted images, tissues with a short T2 (such as tendons and ligaments) have a low (dark) signal intensity, whereas fluids with a long T2 (such as cerebrospinal and synovial fluid) have a high (bright) signal intensity.

A recognized risk of MRI is the forceful attraction, and hence movement, of ferromagnetic objects within the patient's body—objects such as shrapnel, metallic foreign bodies in the eye, cardiac pacemakers, and intracranial aneurysm clips. Metallic prosthetic joint replacements (artificial joints) are not generally made of ferromagnetic materials. It is recommended that MRI not be used during the first trimester of pregnancy. Consequently, all patients being considered for MRI need to be screened carefully in regard to these contraindications.

Examples of MRI scans of musculoskeletal tissues are shown in Figures 5.35 and 5.36.

Laboratory Investigation

The fourth source of data that may be required, at least in some cases, to solve the problem of diagnosis is the laboratory examination of specimens of body fluids and tissues. These examinations, or tests, involve hematology, biochemistry, immunology, bacteriology, and pathology. Of the multitude of laboratory examinations available, those of most value in the diagnosis of musculoskeletal disorders are the following:

- *Blood:* Hemoglobin determination, a red blood cell count, a white blood cell count, a stained smear or film of blood, sedimentation rate, blood coagulation studies, uric acid values, and blood culture are performed.
- *Serum:* Serum calcium, inorganic phosphate, alkaline phosphatase, acid phosphatase, and protein values are obtained. Immunological or serological tests include the VDRL (Venereal Disease Research Laboratory) test for suspected syphilis, the human immunodeficiency virus (HIV) test for acquired immunodeficiency syndrome (AIDS) (only with the patient's written consent), the Mantoux test for tuberculosis, and the Rose test for rheumatoid disease.
- *Urine:* The urine's gross appearance is assessed. Determinations of albumin, glucose, cells, casts, calcium, and phosphorus are obtained, and a urine culture is performed.
- *Cerebrospinal fluid:* The gross appearance is assessed as are cerebrospinal fluid pressure and cells. Protein levels are determined and a culture is performed.
- *Synovial fluid:* The gross appearance and cells are assessed. Protein and glucose levels

Figure 5.32.   **A.** This figure shows a conventional radiograph of the hip joints of a 30-year-old woman with residual congenital subluxation of her left hip despite treatment for a congenital dislocation in early childhood. Note the increased distance between the left femoral head and the medial wall of the acetabulum *(arrow)* compared with that of the right hip. **B.** This is a CT scan of the hips of the same patient as seen in **A.** Note the increased space between the left femoral head and the medial wall of the acetabulum *(arrow).* **C.** Three-dimensional reconstruction of the hip joints of the same patient seen in **A and B.** Note the poor coverage of the lateral margin of the left femoral head by the acetabulum *(arrow).*

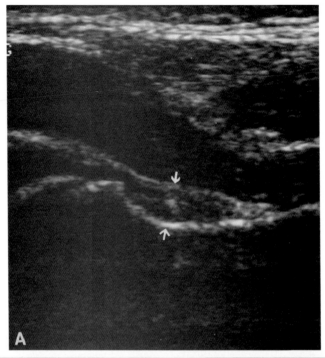

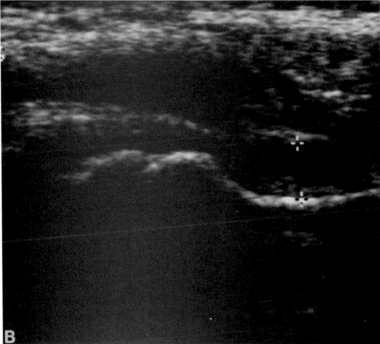

Figure 5.33. **A.** This figure shows a normal parasagittal sonogram of the left hip joint in a 6-year old-boy. The upper arrow indicates the anterior capsule of the hip joint, and the lower arrow indicates the anterior cortical surface of the neck of the femur. The space between the two arrows contains the normal amount of synovial effusion. **B.** This figure shows an abnormal parasagittal sonogram of the same boy's opposite hip, which was painful. The widened space between the two asterisks is explained by an increase in fluid within the hip joint—a synovial effusion (synovial fluid), a hemarthrosis (blood) or a pyoarthrosis (pus). Needle aspiration of the joint is required to differentiate among these three types of fluid.

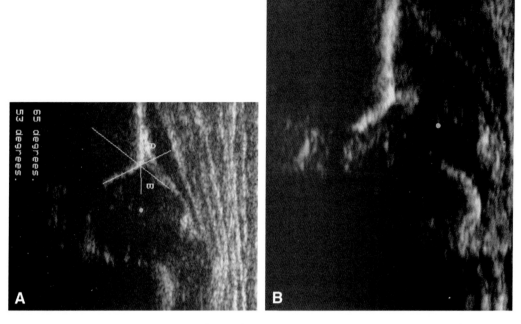

65 degrees.
53 degrees.

A

B

Figure 5.34.   A. This is a normal coronal sonogram of the left hip joint in a neonate. The white dot is over the center of the femoral head. The alpha (A) angle of 65° and the beta (B) angle of 53° are normal and the femoral head is in normal relationship within the acetabulum (i.e., it is in the socket). **B.** An abnormal sonogram of the left hip joint in a neonate is seen. The white dot is over the center of the femoral head. Note that the head of the femur is dislocated laterally and proximally from the acetabulum (i.e., it is out of the socket).

are obtained, and culture is performed. The analysis of synovial fluid obtained by joint aspiration (arthrocentesis) is of considerable value in the laboratory diagnosis of joint disorders such as septic arthritis; normal synovial fluid contains a total protein content of approximately 1.8 mg/100 mL, with relatively more albumin than globulin, and is relatively acellular (10 to 200 cells/mL, predominantly mononuclear). Synovial fluid from noninflammatory joints is usually clear, has few cells (with a normal distribution), and a low protein content, whereas the synovial fluid from inflammatory joints is usually turbid (from white blood cells or crystals, or both), has many more cells (predominantly polymorphonuclear leukocytes), and a high protein count. In septic arthritis, bacteria may be found, as may a low level of joint fluid glucose. The presence of crystals in "chemical" arthritis can be diagnostic. Monosodium urate crystals are diagnostic for gout and calcium pyrophosphate crystals are diagnostic for pseudogout.

- *Abnormal fluids (effusions, exudates):* The gross appearance is assessed as are cells. A direct smear and culture are performed. When an organism is grown in culture, further examinations are required to assess its sensitivity as well as its resistance to various antibiotics.
- *Body tissues (specimen obtained by biopsy):* Bone marrow is usually obtained by either sternal or iliac crest puncture (*aspiration biopsy*). Bone and soft tissue specimens are obtained either by open operation (*open biopsy*) or by withdrawing a small piece of tissue through a hollow cannula (*punch biopsy*). The microscopic examination of these tissues is of particular value in the diagnosis of musculoskeletal neoplasms.

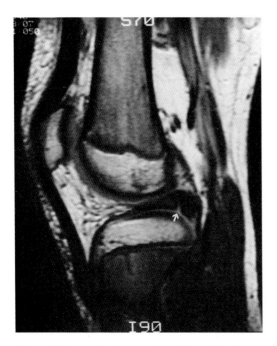

Figure 5.35. This shows a sagittal T_1-weighted MRI image of the knee joint in a 10-year-old boy with an internal derangement of his knee. Note the dark, thick discoid meniscus that is "buckled" and displaced posteriorly *(arrow)*.

Examples of the role of these various laboratory examinations in the diagnosis of specific musculoskeletal disorders are provided in subsequent chapters.

Diagnostic Arthroscopy

Following the lead of urologists, who for decades have been able to visualize the interior of the bladder by means of the cystoscope, in the mid-1960s orthopaedic surgeons developed sophisticated fiber-optic arthroscopes (especially for the knee joint) that can allow more complete visualization of most large joints than can be obtained by an open operation (arthroscopy) of the joint. Indeed, diagnostic arthroscopy has increased the accuracy of diagnosis of internal derangements and other disorders to more than 95%. Although arthroscopy is currently the most frequently performed orthopaedic procedure in North America, it should not be considered a substitute for the clinical history, physical examination, diagnostic imaging, or laboratory investigation.

During the early years of arthroscopy, the orthopaedic surgeon looked inside the joint through the optical system of the arthroscope. Currently, through the use of miniaturized color television cameras, it is possible for the surgeon, as well as everyone else in the operating room, to see the same moving picture of the interior of the joint in color on a television screen (Fig. 5.37).

It is now even possible to perform certain surgical procedures using the arthroscope plus specially designed instruments that are inserted either through the scope or into the knee through a separate portal (arthroscopic surgery). Procedures such as removal of a loose body, partial or total meniscectomy, drilling defects in the articular surface, abrading areas of chondromalacia, and even reconstruction of cruciate ligaments can be performed.

Arthroscopy of the knee and even arthroscopic surgery can be performed under either local or general anesthesia, usually on an outpatient or "day-care" basis, with considerably less morbidity than is associated with open arthrotomy. Because of the inaccessibility of some areas of the knee joint, arthroscopy may have to be combined with double-contrast (air and dye) arthrography in the diagnosis of "problem knees." Arthroscopy has also been developed for other joints, including the shoulder, elbow, wrist, ankle, and even the hip.

Arthroscopy identifies patients for whom arthrotomy can be obviated; for those patients requiring arthrotomy, arthroscopy makes the planning for such open surgery more accurate.

Understandably, diagnostic arthroscopy and arthroscopic surgery are more readily accepted by patients than are open operations, and this accounts, at least in part, for their popularity. As with other such procedures, however, there is a risk of abuse, such as overuse and questionable indications—a risk that has been well stated in the literature by international leaders in the field.

Antenatal Diagnosis

Since the mid-1970s, the field of antenatal, or prenatal, diagnosis of congenital abnormalities has expanded dramatically because of the combination of a safe method of amniocente-

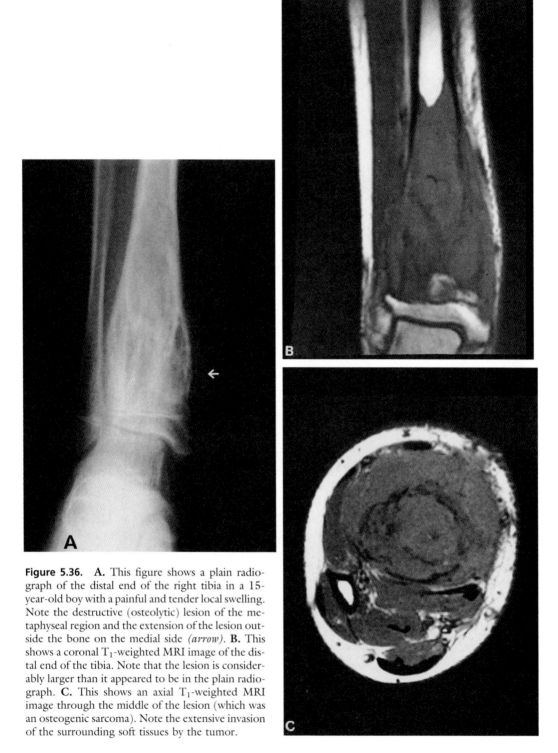

Figure 5.36. **A.** This figure shows a plain radiograph of the distal end of the right tibia in a 15-year-old boy with a painful and tender local swelling. Note the destructive (osteolytic) lesion of the metaphyseal region and the extension of the lesion outside the bone on the medial side *(arrow)*. **B.** This shows a coronal T_1-weighted MRI image of the distal end of the tibia. Note that the lesion is considerably larger than it appeared to be in the plain radiograph. **C.** This shows an axial T_1-weighted MRI image through the middle of the lesion (which was an osteogenic sarcoma). Note the extensive invasion of the surrounding soft tissues by the tumor.

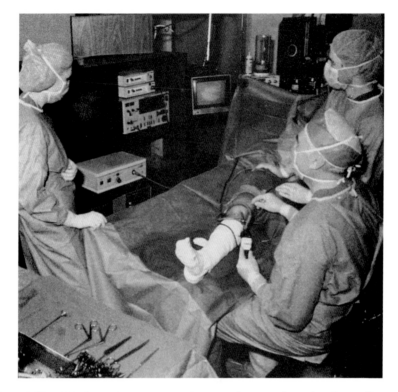

Figure 5.37. This figure demonstrates arthroscopy being performed under sterile conditions in an operating room. The surgeon's left hand is holding the arthroscope with its miniaturized camera, which displays the interior of the joint on a color television screen (Courtesy of Dr. RW Jackson).

sis (whereby the aspirated amniotic fluid is studied both biochemically and genetically) and highly specialized ultrasonography (ultrasound). The once popular technique of direct endoscopic visualization of the fetus through a fetoscope, which was associated with complications for the fetus, has been largely replaced by the safe, noninvasive, and yet effective diagnostic imaging technique of ultrasonography.

The diagnostic capabilities of these sophisticated techniques with respect to the antenatal diagnosis of congenital abnormalities of the musculoskeletal system are discussed in Chapter 8 (Congenital Abnormalities).

CORRELATION OF ALL DATA (CLUES)

As you proceed with the investigation of the patient's problem, possible diagnoses come to mind and you direct the investigation along appropriate lines. Having collected the pertinent data or clues, you, like Sherlock Holmes, are then ready to review the overall picture and to correlate the data––that is, relate the clues to each other. By means of logic, deduction, and previous experience, you then endeavor to arrive at a probable solution (*provisional diagnosis*) of the problem. When there is insufficient proof, or evidence, for a single solution, the possibilities can at least be narrowed to a few "suspects" (*differential diagnosis*), following which the investigation continues with the collection of more data.

From a study of 50 clinicopathological conferences published in the *New England Journal of Medicine*, Eddy and Clanton concluded that the following six steps are taken to arrive at a diagnosis:

1. aggregation of groups of findings into patterns
2. selection of a "pivot" or key finding

3. generation of a cause list
4. pruning of the cause list
5. selection of a diagnosis
6. validation of the diagnosis

If your personal experience is limited, you would naturally wish, in the interests of your patient, to seek consultation with a more experienced colleague.

COMMUNICATION WITH YOUR PATIENTS ABOUT THE DIAGNOSIS

Solving the problem of diagnosis for your patients is just the first of many steps toward the goal of helping them with their problem. Having made a diagnosis of the present situation, you must then consider the future outlook *(prognosis)* for your patients and be prepared to communicate with them at their level of understanding. They and their close relatives have the right to know (if they wish) just what your diagnosis means in relation to them and their future. How often one hears patients say of their medical practitioner: "He *said* quite a bit, and used some big words that I could not understand, but he really didn't *tell* me anything, and I am confused and concerned." No matter how brilliant you have been in the scientific aspect of your investigation, it is of little comfort to your patient unless you have developed the art of communication. It is, of course, not only unnecessary, but also unwise, to explain the minutiae of your patients' diagnosis and treatment to them as though they were medical students or medical doctors. Nevertheless, it is essential that you give them an understanding of their condition and also that you be *aware* of their particular needs and fears.

Your patients may either fear death from a progressive disease such as cancer, or fear life with a painful, crippling, or disabling condition. They will want and need to know the answers to questions such as "What is wrong with me? How serious is it? Can it be treated? How successfully? What is the treatment? How long will I be away from my home or from my work? What would happen if it is not treated?"

Wilson has written that the medical doctor communicates best when he or she is honest, compassionate, caring, calm, readily available, sensitive and trustworthy.

The practice of medicine is becoming progressively more scientific and this is as it should be because science must always be the basis of medical knowledge. At the same time, however, you must develop the art of communicating with your patients, which, in effect, requires that you acquire a keen and sympathetic awareness of their needs as well as their concerns, for as Sir William Osler stated so clearly "The practice of medicine is an art based on science."

SUGGESTED ADDITIONAL READING

AbuRahma AF, Dietrich EB, Reiling M. Doppler testing in peripheral vascular disease. Surg Gynecol Obstet 1980;150:26–28.

Apley AG, Solomon L. Apley's system of orthopaedics and fractures. 7th ed. Oxford: United Kingdom: Butterworth-Heinemann, 1993.

Brower AC. Arthritis in black and white. Philadelphia. WB Saunders, 1988.

Conway WF. Imaging. Editorial overview. Curr Opin Orthop 1992; 3:135–136.

Eddy DM, Clanton CH. The art of diagnosis. Solving the clinicopathological conference. N Engl J Med 1982;306:1263–1268.

Einhorn TA: Bone metabolism and metabolic bone disease. In: Frymoyer JW, ed. Orthopaedic knowledge update 4. Rosemont, IL: American Academy of Orthopaedic Surgeons, 1993.

El-Khoury GY, Resai K, Moore TE. Imaging of the musculoskeletal system. In: Weinstein SL, Buckwalter JA, eds. Turek's orthopaedics: principles and their applications. Philadelphia: JB Lippincott, 1994.

Feldman W. On ordering tests (editorial). Ann R Coll Phys Surg Can 1993;26:269–270.

Goldbloom RB. Interviewing: the most sophisticated of diagnostic technologies. Ann Roy Coll Phys Surg Can 1993;26:224–228.

Hayes CW, Conway WF. Magnetic resonance of imaging of articular cartilage. Curr Opin Orthop 1992;3:152–157.

Hoppenfeld S. Physical examination of the spine and extremities. New York: Appleton-Century-Crofts, 1976.

Hoppenfeld S. Orthopaedic neurology: a diagnostic guide to neurologic levels. Philadelphia: JB Lippincott, 1977.

Hughes SPF. Radionuclides in orthopaedics surgery. J Bone Joint Surg 1980;62B:141–150.

Jackson RW, Dandy DJ. Arthroscopy of the knee. New York: Grune & Stratton, 1976.

Keller MS, Harbhajan SC, Weiss A. Real-time sonography of infant hip dislocation. Radiographics 1986;6:447–456.

Kessel L. Color atlas of clinical orthopaedics. Chicago: Year Book Medical, 1980.

Kim HKW, Babyn PS, Harasiewicz KA, Gahunia HK, Pritzker DPH, Foster FS. Imaging of immature articular cartilage using ultrasound backscatter microscopy at 50 MHz: J Orthopaedic Research 1995;13:963–970.

Mankin HJ: Metabolic bone disease: an instructional course lecture. American Academy of Orthopaedic Surgeons. J Bone Joint Surg 1994; 76-A:780–788.

Marshall KW, Mikulis DJ, Guthric BM. Quantitation of articular cartilage using magnetic resonance imaging and three-dimensional reconstruction. J Orthop Res 1995;13:814–823.

McGinty J, Caspari RB, Jackson RW, Poehling GG. Operative Arthroscopy. New York: Raven Press, 1991.

McGinty JB, Johnson LL, Jackson RW, McBryde AM, Goodfellow JW. Uses and abuses of arthroscopy: a symposium. Current Concepts Review. J Bone Joint Surg 1992;74-A:1563–1577.

McRae R. Clinical orthopaedic examination. 3rd ed. Edinburgh: Churchill Livingstone, 1990.

Nyberg D, Mahony BS, Pretorius D. Diagnostic ultrasound of fetal anomalies. St. Louis: CV Mosby, 1990.

O Keefe D, Mamtora H. Ultrasound in clinical orthopaedics. J Bone Joint Surg 1992;74-B: 488–494.

Ozonoff MB. Pediatric orthopedic radiology. 2nd ed. Philadelphia: WB Saunders, 1992.

Paul DJ, Gilday DL. Polyphosphate bone scanning of non-malignant bone disease in children. J Can Assoc Radiol 1975;26:285–290.

Post M. Physical examination of the musculoskeletal system. Chicago: Year Book Medical, 1987.

Resnick DJ, Sartoris DJ. Imaging of the musculoskeletal system. In: Orthopaedic knowledge update 3. Rosemont, IL:American Academy of Orthopaedic Surgeons, 1990.

Romero R, Pilu G, Jeantry P, Ghidini A, Hobbins JC. Prenatal diagnosis of congenital abnormalities. Norwalk, CT: Appleton & Lange, 1988.

Sackett DL, Rennie D. The science of the art of the clinical examination. JAMA 1992; 267:2650–2652.

Sissons HA, Murray RO, Kemp HBS. Orthopaedic diagnosis: clinical, radiological and pathological coordinates. Berlin: Springer-Verlag, 1984.

Smith FW, Gilday DL. Scintigraphic appearances of osteoid osteoma. Radiology 1980; 137:191–195.

Springfield DS. Radiolucent lesions of the extremities. J Am Acad Orthop Surg 1994;2:306–316.

Stoller DW. Magnetic resonance imaging in orthopaedics and sports medicine. Philadelphia: JB Lippincott, 1993.

Watt I. Magnetic resonance imaging in orthopaedics (invited article). J Bone Joint Surg 1991; 73B:539–550.

Wilson D. Communication and the family physician. Can Fam Phys 1980;26:1710–1716.

6   General Principles and Specific Methods of Musculoskeletal Treatment

You can appreciate from the first five chapters of this textbook, as well as from your own preclinical and clinical experience to date, that humans are subject to a large number and wide variety of disorders and injuries of the musculoskeletal system. In addition, a given disorder or injury may present different problems for different kinds of individuals. It is not surprising, therefore, that the specific methods of treatment for patients with musculoskeletal conditions are both numerous and varied. Before discussing the many disorders and injuries of the musculoskeletal system and their treatment in subsequent chapters, it seems wise at this time to consider the *general principles* as well as the *specific methods* of treatment of musculoskeletal conditions so that you may become aware of the therapeutic methods and also so that the subsequent discussions may be more meaningful for you.

GENERAL PRINCIPLES OF TREATMENT

Principles are those fundamental truths that provide both a basis for reasoning and a guide for conduct. In the practice of medicine, general principles are formulated from natural laws ("laws of nature")—laws of the behavior of body tissues under various conditions as well as laws of human behavior—laws that you must constantly respect. As Leonardo da Vinci stated, "Nature never breaks her own laws." Thus, the general principles of treatment must be the basis for your reasoning in selecting the specific method of treatment for your patients as well as the guide for your conduct during their total care. It is important not only to know *what* you are doing or planning to do but also to know the reason *why*.

The following general principles are expressed in the form of advice to you as a practitioner of the future. These principles of treatment, like your own professional conscience, ought to be obeyed always.

1. First do no harm (primum non nocere)

As a result of the many important scientific advances in recent years, you will have powerful and effective methods of treatment to help your patients. Remember, however, that although these methods have a potential for great benefit, they also have a potential for great harm. Treatment can be a double-edged sword. The expression *iatrogenic disease* means a harmful condition in a patient produced unwittingly and inadvertently by the practitioner. You must be constantly aware of this danger and on guard against it. In planning a method of treatment for your patients, its potential benefit must be weighed against its potential harm. Not to be made better by treatment is discouraging, but to be made worse is devastating for your patients! Understandably, iatrogenic disease is the main reason for litigation (i.e., a lawsuit brought against the practitioner by the patient or the relatives).

2. Base treatment on an accurate diagnosis and prognosis

It is obvious that you cannot help your patients if you treat them on the basis of a wrong diagnosis—for example, if you treat them for rheumatic fever when, in fact, they have acute osteomyelitis or if you treat them for osteomyelitis when, in fact, they have a sarcoma of bone. Moreover, you will not be helping your patients as much as you should if you treat only a secondary manifestation of their disease (a symptom or a sign) without making an accurate diagnosis of the underlying or primary disease—for example, if you merely treat their pain without diagnosing its cause or if you treat their paralytic foot deformity without recognizing that the primary cause, or condition, is an enlarging spinal cord neoplasm. Furthermore, you will do your patients a disservice if you treat them (other than by reassurance) for a condition with such a good prognosis that it would improve spontaneously without treatment or if you fail to treat them, thinking their prognosis is good when, in fact, it is not. You may think that all such errors of omission and commission are surely uncommon, but regrettably, they are not!

3. Select treatment with specific aims

Although the general aim of treatment must always be to help the patient, the treatment must have specific aims to deal with the specific problem. You will recall from Chapter 5 that the common presenting problems, or chief complaints, of patients with musculoskeletal disorders and injuries are 1) pain, 2) a decrease in function, and 3) the physical appearance of either a deformity or an abnormal gait. Therefore, having made an accurate diagnosis of the underlying, or primary, condition responsible for the presenting problem or complaint and having planned treatment of the primary condition, you must also select a treatment with the specific aim of dealing with the complaint itself. Thus, the musculoskeletal treatment will have as its specific aim one or more of the following: 1) the relief of pain, 2) the improvement of function, 3) the prevention or correction of deformity, and 4) the improvement of gait.

4. Cooperate with the laws of nature

The natural restorative powers of humans are truly remarkable and constitute your strongest ally in treating a patient's disorders and injuries. Work *with* these powers and you will accomplish much for your patients; work *against* them and you will accomplish little. You must appreciate the *natural laws of the behavior of body tissues* under various circum-

stances in order to work *with* them through the appropriate choice of a general type of treatment as well as the specific method and particular technique of treatment. Furthermore, with a knowledge of the *natural laws of human behavior,* you will be much more aware of the patient's need for your understanding, compassion, kindness, and reassurance, as well as his or her need to have confidence in you—the practitioner. As you treat patients in cooperation with the laws of nature, you will come to realize how much you depend on these natural powers of restoration, just as Ambroise Paré, a famous 16th century French surgeon, realized when he said, "Je le pansay, Dieu le guarit" (Old French, meaning "I dressed his wounds, God healed him").

5. Be realistic and practical in your treatment

Certain methods of treatment that may seem attractive in theory may be neither realistic nor practical for your particular patient. Common sense and sound judgment will lead you to ask yourself three important questions concerning any proposed treatment:

"Precisely what am I aiming to accomplish by this method of treatment—what is its specific aim or goal?"

"Am I, in fact, likely to accomplish this aim or goal by this method of treatment?" If the answer to this question is "no," obviously you must make another choice. If the answer is "yes," you must ask yourself a third question.

"Will the anticipated end result justify the means or method. Will it be worth it for your patient in terms of what he or she will have to go through—the risks, the discomfort, the period away from home, work, or school? If the carefully considered answer to this third question is "yes," you will have selected a realistic and practical method of treatment for your patient. If, however, the answer is "no," you must select another method of treatment and ask the three questions again.

6. Select treatment for your patient as an individual

The treatment of many nontraumatic disorders of the musculoskeletal system is elective rather than emergency in nature. This means that there will be ample time to elect, or select, the particular method of treatment most suitable for your particular patient and his or her particular disorder in relation to his or her particular needs. In this way, you will avoid merely selecting a method of treatment for a "case" or for a diagnosis as though it existed in isolation rather than in a human individual with individual needs. A given disorder may present a different problem for one individual than it does for another, not only in relation to age, sex, occupation and any coexistent disease but also in relation to his or her personality and his or her resultant psychological reaction to the problem. Therefore, your choice of treatment will be influenced by all these factors so that it may be tailored to fit the particular needs of the particular patient. You are, in fact, hoping through your treatment to do something *for* your patients rather than just *to* them.

We must forever remember that our function as practitioners is "to cure sometimes, to relieve often and to comfort always" (anonymous folk-saying of the 15th century).

A LITANY FOR MEDICAL PRACTITIONERS

Some of these important general principles are epitomized by Sir Robert Hutchinson, of The London Hospital, England, in the following litany which he wrote for medical doctors (1953):

"From inability to let well alone;

From too much zeal for the new and contempt for what is old;

From putting knowledge before wisdom, science before art, and cleverness before common sense;

From treating patients as cases, and from making the cure of the disease more grievous than endurance of the same,

Good Lord, deliver us."

GENERAL FORMS AND SPECIFIC METHODS OF TREATMENT
Forms of Treatment

Patients with musculoskeletal conditions are cared for by various general forms, or types, of treatment, each of which includes a number of specific methods; furthermore, each specific method may be achieved by a variety of specialized techniques. It will be apparent to you that at this stage of your training, it is more important for you to learn about the general principles, the general forms or types, and the specific methods of treatment than it is to learn the details of specialized techniques.

The *seven general forms* or *types of treatment* include the following: 1) psychological considerations, 2) therapeutic drugs, 3) orthopaedic apparatus and appliances, 4) physical and occupational therapy, 5) surgical manipulation, 6) surgical repair and reconstruction, 7) electrical stimulation, 8) continuous passive motion, and 9) radiation therapy. Treatment is sometimes described as either *conservative* (when no surgical operation is involved) or *radical* (when the treatment consists of operation). However, under many circumstances, these terms lose their significance and meaning and therefore, the terms *nonoperative* and *operative* are more appropriate.

The importance of rehabilitation is given special emphasis in a later section of this chapter.

Specific Methods of Treatment

In subsequent chapters, reference is made to the various forms and specific methods of treatment relating to specific musculoskeletal disorders and injuries. In this chapter, however, all the forms and their specific methods are discussed as a group so that you may consider them in perspective and so that references to treatment in subsequent chapters may be more meaningful for you.

For each specific method of treatment, there are favorable circumstances in which the method should be used (*indications*) as well as unfavorable circumstances in which it should not be used (*contraindications*). Knowledge of the indications and contraindications is of great importance in selecting a specific method, or methods, of treatment for a particular patient with a particular problem. There is not always unanimity of opinion, even among experts, about indications and contraindications in relation to the treatment of many disorders and injuries because these opinions are based not only on general principles but also on individual experience and the present state of knowledge. With continuing advances in knowledge as well as improvements in both methods and techniques, indications and contraindications become modified. There may be more than one therapeutic pathway by which to reach a desired goal, but some pathways are smoother, easier, and safer than others for your patient.

1) Psychological Considerations

Socrates, in about 400 BC, admonished that we "ought not treat the body without the mind." Every one of your patients requires and deserves some psychological consideration in the form of compassion and sympathetic understanding as well as the assurance that everything possible will be done to help him or her. For patients with minor disorders or musculoskeletal variations of normal, the only type of treatment needed may be reassurance. However, this important form of treatment requires both time and skill; your patient's concern, or anxiety, is usually greater than you realize. He or she may not be reassured if you merely state that there is nothing seriously wrong and that there will be no treatment. Some of your patients may interpret the statement "there will be no treatment" as meaning that nothing *can* be done rather than that nothing *needs* to be done. Your thoughtful reassurance will do much to allay their fears and restore their peace of mind.

2) Therapeutic Drugs

Many of the disorders and injuries of the musculoskeletal system are *physical* conditions for which there is no specific drug therapy. For example, there is no specific therapeutic drug available (as yet) that will accelerate the *normal* healing of injured musculoskeletal tissues or that will make a weak muscle stronger, a lax ligament tighter, a stiff joint mobile, or a deformed bone straight. Nevertheless, certain types of drugs do have an important place in musculoskeletal treatment. Since specific drug preparations are continually changing as a result of pharmaceutical advances, it is prefera-

ble in a textbook such as this to discuss types of drugs rather than specific preparations or "trade names."

Analgesics

The relief of pain, which is of such immediate importance to the patient, can and should be provided by appropriate analgesics. However, the underlying *cause* of the pain must be determined lest you make the error of treating only a symptom of an underlying condition that, in itself, requires specific treatment. Salicylates and other mild analgesics are effective in relieving mild musculoskeletal pain. Narcotics must be used with great caution, particularly for chronic pain because of the danger of *iatrogenic* drug addiction.

Nonsteroidal Anti-inflammatory Drugs

During the past two decades, nonsteroidal anti-inflammatory drugs (NSAIDs), of which there are many varieties, have become among the most frequently prescribed drugs, especially for disorders of the musculoskeletal system. They decrease inflammation by inhibiting the synthesis of prostaglandins. However, this mechanism can also cause toxic complications, such as gastrointestinal ulceration and bleeding as well as renal failure and aggravation of any pre-existing heart failure. In noninflammatory musculoskeletal disorders, nonsteroidal anti-inflammatory drugs are no more effective than simple analgesics such as acetaminophen.

Chemotherapeutic Agents

Antibiotics and other chemotherapeutic agents can be of great value in the treatment of specific musculoskeletal infections, particularly osteomyelitis and septic arthritis. However, they must be administered intelligently by determining, insofar as is possible, the specific causative organism as well as its sensitivity, or its resistance, to the various agents. Antibiotic therapy is discussed in Chapter 10.

During the past two decades, the use of powerful cytotoxic agents in the chemotherapy of cancer has done much to increase the survival rate and prolong life, although not necessarily improve its quality. These anticancerous agents are discussed in Chapter 14.

Corticosteroids

The anti-inflammatory action of corticosteroids has been of some value in decreasing certain of the manifestations of nonspecific inflammations associated with conditions such as bursitis and rheumatoid arthritis, but these drugs do not cure the underlying disease. Furthermore, the prolonged systemic administration of corticosteroids can produce many harmful effects. Therefore, these drugs should be used with caution in the systemic treatment of chronic musculoskeletal conditions. The infrequent injection of corticosteroids can be helpful. However, the author has demonstrated through basic research in the rabbit that repeated intra-articular injections of hydrocortisone can be deleterious to the articular cartilage.

Vitamins

Vitamin C is the specific therapeutic agent for scurvy, and vitamin D is specific for the classic type of vitamin D–deficiency rickets. Other types of rickets are refractory to ordinary doses of vitamin D; the treatment of the various generalized disorders of bone is presented in Chapter 9.

Specific Drugs

Colchicine is one of the few examples of a specific therapeutic drug that provides dramatic relief for one specific condition—acute gouty arthritis, as discussed in Chapter 10.

3) Orthopaedic Apparatus and Appliances

Before the advent of anesthesia in the nineteenth century, much of the treatment of musculoskeletal disorders and injuries involved the use of various types of orthopaedic apparatus and appliances designed to provide local rest, support, and corrective forces. These methods, which are still important and will continue to be important in the future, are best considered in relation to their specific aims in musculoskeletal treatment.

Rest

For centuries, it was thought, on the basis of empiricism, that total body rest (bed rest) was necessary for certain severe disorders and injuries of the musculoskeletal system. However, prolonged and continuous bed rest is associated with many harmful effects, including 1) disuse atrophy of muscles with resultant generalized weakness, 2) disuse atrophy of bone (generalized osteoporosis), 3) increased calcium excretion, 4) deep vein thrombosis with the threat of pulmonary embolism, and 5) pressure sores (decubitus ulcers) that can be prevented only by excellent nursing care. Therefore, a bedridden patient should be encouraged to exercise uninvolved limbs and, whenever feasible, should be helped from the bed to a chair, or wheelchair, or even a "walker" or crutches for at least part of each day. It is remarkable that the concept of early ambulation of patients after major operations was not accepted until the middle of the twentieth century!

For centuries, it was also thought, on the basis of the same empiricism, that *local rest*—that is, *immobilization* of varying degree—aids the healing of inflamed and injured musculoskeletal tissues and also helps to relieve pain that is related to movement.

On the basis of the author's scientific investigations of continuous passive motion (as mentioned in a subsequent section of this chapter), however, it has become apparent that enforced local rest, or rigid immobilization, are *not* essential either for the healing of inflamed and injured musculoskeletal tissues or for the relief of pain.

Relative rest for a limb may be provided by simply preventing its usual function with a sling for an upper limb or crutches for the relief of weightbearing in a lower limb. For relief of weightbearing, a sling for the lower limb may be used with crutches (Fig. 6.1). Another form of relative rest for a limb is provided by *continuous traction*, which can be achieved by many techniques. Continuous traction is used for the following purposes: 1) to stretch gradually soft tissues that have become shortened secondary to a long-standing joint deformity or dislocation (e.g., continuous traction prior to reduction of a congenital dislocation of the hip) (Fig. 6.2A), 2) to relieve painful muscle spasm associated with joint inflammation or injury, and 3) to maintain length of the limb and alignment of fracture fragments in unstable fractures of the shafts of long bones (Fig. 6.2**B**).

A useful method of supporting a painful, or irritable, hip or knee that enables the patient to move the affected joint freely is the combination of *slings and springs*. The padded slings that support the limb above and below the knee are suspended by springs that are attached to an overhead beam (Fig. 6.2**C**).

Fairly rigid and continuous local rest (*immobilization*) is used to maintain or stabilize

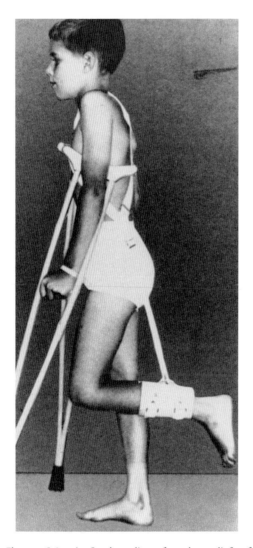

Figure 6.1. A Snyder sling for the relief of weightbearing in a lower limb. This form of management is acceptable for short-term treatment, but for long-term treatment the problem, understandably, is lack of patient compliance.

the position of a fracture or a dislocation after its reduction as well as to maintain the desired position of a part following injury, surgical manipulation, or surgical operation. This type of immobilization is most commonly obtained by the application of plaster of Paris casts of varying design (Fig. 6.3).

You must realize, however, that prolonged immobilization of a limb, and its synovial joints, is associated with many harmful effects, including 1) disuse atrophy of local muscles and resultant muscle weakness, 2) disuse atrophy of local bone (localized osteoporosis), 3) local venous thrombosis with resultant edema, and 4) the complication of pressure sores (cast sores) and most importantly, muscle contractures, joint capsule contractures, and intra-articular adhesions, all of which lead to persistent joint stiffness. These iatrogenic effects of immobilization may require many months for reversal, with or without physiotherapy. If the involved limb has been immobilized for a long time (more than 1 or 2 months), especially after an intra-articular injury or operation, the joint may never recover completely and consequently may develop secondary post-traumatic arthritis.

Support for Muscle Weakness and Joint Instability

A patient with extensive muscle weakness in the upper limb can be helped by the use of *functional braces* which are designed to transmit movement to the weak part of the limb from some other muscle group (Fig. 6.4). A weak or unstable and painful spine can be given some degree of support by a *spinal brace* (Fig. 6.5). In the lower limb, when either muscle weakness or joint instability interfere with weightbearing and walking, the involved limb can be supported by means of an appropriate *brace*, which prevents unwanted motion while permitting desired motion (Fig. 6.6, **top row**). Hypermobile joints in the feet occasionally require temporary support by appropriate shoe corrections such as arch supports and sole wedges. Mild soft tissue injuries of joints may be given temporary support with carefully applied *adhesive tape strapping*.

In recent years, the time-honored terms *braces* and *splints* have been replaced by the

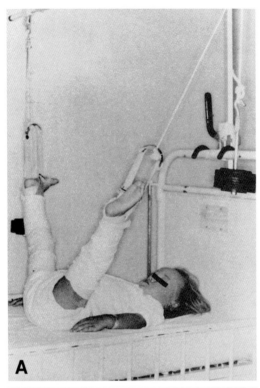

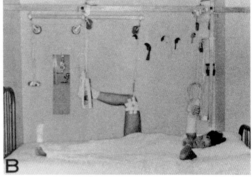

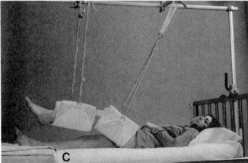

Figure 6.2. **A.** Skin traction through special adhesive tape has been applied to the lower limbs of this child to stretch the shortened muscles secondary to bilateral congenital dislocation of the hips prior to reduction of the dislocations. **B.** Skin traction through special adhesive tape for an unstable fracture of the humerus and skeletal traction through a metal pin in the distal end of the femur for an unstable fracture of the upper third of the femoral shaft. **C.** Slings and springs that support the lower limb while enabling the patient to move the hip and knee actively and easily.

more sophisticated collective term *orthoses,* and the individuals who produce such devices are no longer *brace makers* or *splint makers* but *orthotists.* By the same token, artificial limbs have become *prostheses* and are produced not by *limb makers* but by *prosthetists.* Light plastic materials such as polypropylene have made present-day orthoses not only lighter but also cosmetically more acceptable (Fig. 6.6, **lower row**).

Prevention and Correction of Deformity
When the development of a joint deformity is anticipated, as with muscle imbalance in either

spastic or flaccid paralysis or with muscle spasm in chronic arthritis, it is frequently possible to prevent the deformity by means of *intermittent immobilization* in a removable splint made of plaster of Paris or light plastic materials (Fig. 6.7A). Following correction of a joint deformity and the subsequent period of continuous immobilization, it may be necessary to use a removable splint for intermittent immobilization to prevent recurrence of the deformity. The gradual correction of certain torsional deformities in growing long bones is possible over a period of months with removable night splints specially designed to

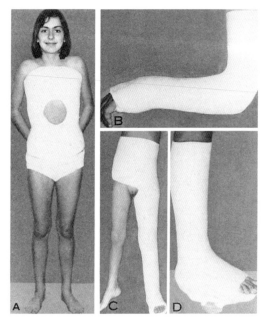

Figure 6.3. Plaster of Paris casts of varying design to provide immobilization: body cast (**A**); above-elbow cast (**B**); hip spica cast (**C**); and below-knee walking cast (**D**).

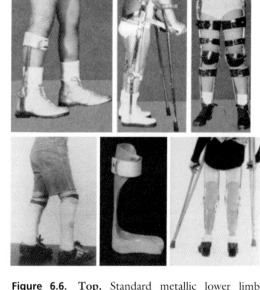

Figure 6.6. Top. Standard metallic lower limb braces, which prevent unwanted motion while permitting desired motion in weak or unstable limbs. **Bottom.** Present-day orthoses constructed of light plastic materials such as polypropylene.

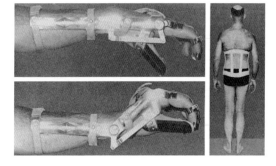

Figure 6.4.   Left. This functional brace is used to compensate for loss of power in the finger flexors. It is designed so that active dorsiflexion of the wrist causes the paralyzed fingers to flex and the thumb to oppose them.

Figure 6.5.   Right. A spinal brace is seen in this figure. This type of lumbosacral brace is designed to limit the extremes of motion of the spine and is used to relieve certain types of low back pain. It is not possible to immobilize the spine completely with any type of brace.

transmit corrective forces to the epiphyseal plates (Fig. 6.7*B*).

4) Physical and Occupational Therapy (Fig. 6.8)

The *aims* of the closely related forms of physical and occupational therapy are to regain and maintain joint motion, to increase muscle strength and to improve musculoskeletal function. Although there is considerable overlap, physical therapy (physiotherapy) tends to focus primarily on gross motor function, whereas occupational therapy is more likely to address fine motor skills. The specific methods of physical and occupational therapy are carried out by trained therapists at the request, and on the prescription of, the patient's own practitioner who, of course, is the coordinator of all the forms of treatment required for the patient. Following are some of the specific methods of such therapy in relation to their specific aims.

Joint Motion

The safest method of regaining motion in a painful stiff joint is *active movement* (by the patient's own muscle action) through the available range of motion. This is encouraged and directed by the therapist. The pain that arises at each end of the range of motion produces a reflex inhibition of muscle action that "protects" the joint from being forced. *Intermittent passive movement* (by the therapist) of such a joint is potentially dangerous, especially if it is forceful, because it may produce further irritation and injury to the abnormal synovial membrane and joint capsule and thereby result in more stiffness. Intermittent passive movement is of greatest value in *maintaining joint motion* and thereby *preventing deformity* in a joint that the patient cannot move actively because of paralysis. Passive movement is also

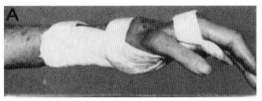

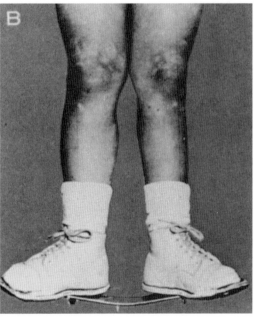

Figure 6.7. This figure shows some removable splints. **A.** This splint is worn at night and during part of the day to help prevent deformity in the patient's hand, which is affected by rheumatoid arthritis. **B.** This Denis-Browne splint is being worn at night by a child with internal tibial torsion. It is designed to exert a torsional force on the epiphyseal plates of the tibiae.

of some help in the gradual stretching of existing muscle contractures.

Muscle Strength

A muscle is strengthened only by *active exercise*. Even when a limb is immobilized, as in a cast, muscles can be strengthened by *isometric* exercises (muscle action without joint motion). *Isotonic* exercises (producing joint motion) serve the dual purpose of increasing muscle strength and helping to regain motion. Muscle exercises performed against progressively increasing resistance are particularly effective for increasing strength. When a muscle has an intact nerve supply but is "inhibited" following injury or operation, it can be electrically stimulated to contract by means of a *faradic* current applied to its motor nerve, thereby teaching the patient volitional control. A muscle that has lost its nerve supply gradually atrophies and undergoes fibrosis, but if there is hope of nerve recovery, these changes can be minimized pending nerve recovery by means of a *galvanic* current that stimulates muscle fibers directly.

Improvement of Musculoskeletal Function

Functional training involves more than joint motion and muscle strength; it involves coordination of muscles in skillful and purposeful activity by the patient. The therapist helps the patient to help himself or herself by training him or her in musculoskeletal activities required for daily life, such as walking, going up and down stairs, dressing, and eating. Adaptation to the patient's environment is addressed by both the physical therapist and the occupational therapist to optimize that patient's potential function.

5) Surgical Manipulation

The aims of surgical manipulation are to *correct deformity* either in a bone that is fractured or in a joint that is dislocated and to a lesser extent, to *regain motion* in a stiff joint. Such manipulations, which are usually performed under anesthesia, involve passive movement of the parts by a surgeon. The great majority of fractures and dislocations can be treated by manipulation of the parts

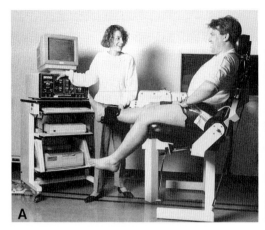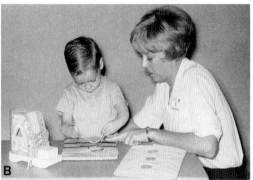

Figure 6.8. **A.** The physiotherapist is instructing the patient about a strengthening program on an isokinetic computerized dynamometer for the quadriceps and hamstring muscles. This device provides resistance throughout the range of knee joint motion. **B.** The occupational therapist is training the child to develop skill in his weak and deformed hands.

into a satisfactory position (*closed reduction*). Likewise, many congenital dislocations of the hip can be treated by closed reduction, at least in young children. The gradual correction of joint deformities caused by contracture of muscle and capsule can often be obtained by repeated gentle stretching of the tight structures at intervals; immobilization of the joint in a position of correction not only helps to maintain correction but also allows the contractures to soften somewhat so that further correction may be obtained at the time of the next stretching. This gentle type of manipulative treatment can be performed without anesthesia and is of particular value in the gradual correction of congenital deformities such as clubfeet. Forceful manipulation of stiff joints under anesthesia carries the risk of either producing further joint damage or causing a fracture through osteoporotic bone. Nevertheless, manipulation of a large joint, under anesthesia and without undue force, is of value in regaining motion when the stiffness is caused by simple joint adhesions rather than severe contractures of the muscle or joint capsule. Such manipulation, of course, must be followed either by active exercises or by a continuous passive motion device to maintain the increased motion that has been gained. The anatomical

effects of manipulation of the cervical or lumbar spine are not well understood as yet, but some surgeons believe that such manipulations frequently relieve pain arising from the musculoskeletal tissues in these areas. Manual fracture of a bone (*osteoclasis*) under anesthesia was commonly used in the past to correct deformities but is seldom used now except with abnormally weakened bone.

6) Surgical Operations
As a result of advancing clinical and experimental knowledge, improved surgical techniques, and improved anesthesia, open surgical operations have come to play an increasingly important role in the treatment of musculoskeletal disorders and injuries. Nevertheless, the operative form of treatment is indicated only for certain specific musculoskeletal problems. Many patients can be treated successfully without an operation and therefore do not need one, whereas others cannot be helped by an operation and therefore should not be subjected to one. Surgical operations have a potential for providing great benefit to the patient, but they also have a potential for producing great harm to that patient. Thus, the general principles of treatment discussed at the beginning of this chapter, as well as the indications and con-

traindications of the various surgical operations, must be thoughtfully considered by the orthopaedic surgeon, who is primarily a *musculoskeletal physician* who has also been trained and taught *how* to operate, *when* to operate, and most important, *when not* to operate. Indeed, the *decision* is more important than the *incision*.

The aims of surgical operations for musculoskeletal conditions include relief of pain, improvement of function and ability, and the prevention or correction of deformity. The general methods of operative treatment by which these aims are achieved involve various combinations of *repair, release, resection, reconstruction,* and *replacement* of involved tissues. For each general method, there are several specific methods, and for each specific method there are a variety of surgical techniques. As a student of the present, and as a practitioner of the future, you should know about the available surgical methods, but you do *not* need to know the details of surgical techniques. The numerous surgical methods are discussed briefly in relation to the *tissue* involved and the *aim* of the operation.

Operations on Muscles, Tendons, and Ligaments

Increased pressure from bleeding or edema within a closed muscle compartment (compartment syndrome) can be relieved by surgical division of the fascia (*fasciotomy*). A cut tendon is repaired by suture (*tenorrhaphy*) (Fig. 6.9). If a segment of the tendon has been irreparably damaged, that segment may be replaced by a *free tendon graft* using an autogenous, but unimportant, tendon (such as the

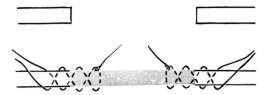

Figure 6.10. The autogenous free tendon graft replaces an irreparably damaged segment of tendon.

tendon of the plantaris muscle) (Fig. 6.10). When a tendon is tethered by adhesions, it may be freed (*tenolysis*), or if its range of excursion is limited by a constricting fibrous tunnel, it may be *released* by either *incision* or *excision* of the tunnel. A shortened muscle may be dealt with by simple division of its tendon (*tenotomy*), subcutaneously or at open operation, or by formal *tendon lengthening* (Fig. 6.11). The action of a paralyzed or damaged muscle may be replaced by transferring the tendinous insertion (or origin) of a nearby normal muscle to improve muscle balance (*muscle transfer* or *tendon transfer*) (Fig. 6.12). In order to check, or limit, an undesired joint motion, the tendon of a muscle (usually a paralyzed muscle) may be separated from its muscle and implanted into bone to serve as a check rein or ligament (*tenodesis*) (Fig. 6.13). A major ligament that has been completely torn may be sutured (*ligamentous repair*), but if it is irreparably damaged, it may have to be replaced by a tendon, or by a free graft of fascia lata (*ligamentous reconstruction*).

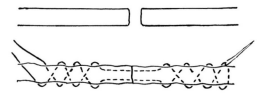

Figure 6.9. For tenorrhaphy (tendon suture) to be successful, the external surface of the repaired tendon must be smooth so that it may glide within its sheath.

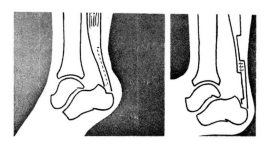

Figure 6.11. Tendon lengthening. Following the long step-cut in this Achilles' tendon, the ends are allowed to shift in relation to each other and are then sutured in the elongated position.

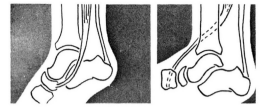

Figure 6.12. The tendon of the tibialis posterior muscle has been rerouted through the interosseous membrane and transferred to the lateral cuneiform bone on the dorsum of the foot. In its new position, it will serve as a dorsiflexor of the ankle and an evertor of the foot.

Operations on Nerves

A cut nerve is repaired by *nerve suture,* but if the gap is too large a *nerve graft* may be required. An abnormally thickened perineural sheath, or other constricting soft tissues, may compress the nerve, which must then be released (*neurolysis*) or *decompressed.* When a spinal nerve root is subjected to continued pressure from a protruded intervertebral disc (nucleus pulposus), decompression of the nerve root is performed after it has been exposed by removing part of the overlying lamina (*laminectomy*). If a peripheral nerve is being stretched and irritated at the level of a deformed joint (such as the ulnar nerve with a cubitus valgus deformity), the course of the nerve can be changed by transposing it to the flexor aspect of the joint (*transposition of a nerve*).

Operations on Joints

A joint may be opened (*arthrotomy*) and *explored* to remove a loose body; to excise part or, if necessary, all of a damaged fibrocartilaginous meniscus; to reduce a difficult dislocation (either congenital or acquired); or to provide adequate drainage of pus in septic arthritis. For recurrent dislocations or for congenital dislocations, the lax, elongated fibrous capsule of the joint is tightened and repaired (*capsulorrhaphy*). In severe joint contractures, it is usually necessary to divide or *release* the shortened fibrous capsule (*capsulotomy*) or even to *resect* it (*capsulectomy*). In serious conditions of synovial joints, such as rheumatoid arthritis and villonodular synovitis, it may be necessary to resect the diseased synovial membrane (*synovectomy*).

A reconstructive operation designed to regain or maintain motion in a chronically painful joint (such as in degenerative joint disease) by means of altering or replacing one or both joint surfaces is called an *arthroplasty;* removal of one joint surface is a *resection or excision arthroplasty* (Fig. 6.14); replacement of one joint surface, or both, is a *replacement arthroplasty* or *prosthetic joint replacement* (Fig. 6.15) (this important development is discussed in the next paragraph); and removal of cartilage surfaces and interpositioning of tissue (such as fascia or dermis) or of a metal

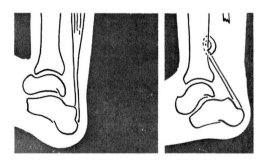

Figure 6.13. The Achilles' tendon of the paralyzed calf muscle is separated from the muscle and transplanted into the tibia so that it will serve as a check rein, or ligament, and thereby limit passive dorsiflexion (tenodesis).

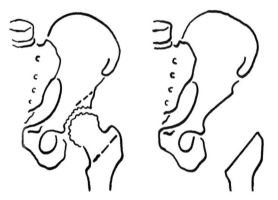

Figure 6.14. Resection (excision) arthroplasty is seen in this figure. The head and neck of the femur are excised, thereby removing one of the hip joint surfaces. The operation produces a false joint (pseudarthrosis), which allows passive movement and relieves pain but at the expense of losing stability.

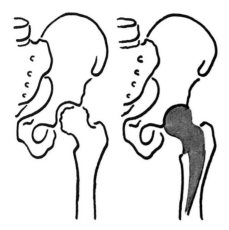

Figure 6.15. Replacement arthroplasty is seen in this figure. The head and neck of the femur are excised and replaced by a metallic internal prosthesis (endoprosthesis) to allow movement.

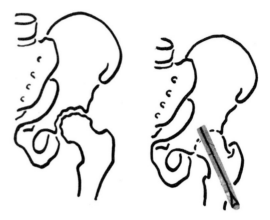

Figure 6.17. In arthrodesis, the cartilaginous joint surfaces are excised from each joint surface and the raw bony surfaces are encouraged to unite to each other (fuse). Internal fixation and bone grafts may be required. The completely fused joint is immobile but is stable and painless.

mold is an *interposition arthroplasty* (Fig. 6.16). When a single joint is severely damaged and painful, or completely unstable and disabling, and when loss of its motion would not interfere significantly with the patient's function, it can be *fused* by producing bony union across it (*arthrodesis*) in the optimal position (Fig. 6.17).

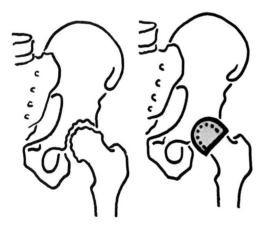

Figure 6.16. In interposition arthroplasty, the cartilaginous surfaces of both joint surfaces are removed and shaped so that an interposition substance, such as a metallic cup-shaped mold, can be inserted. Movement occurs on both the internal and external surfaces of the mold, and eventually new fibrocartilaginous tissue forms on the newly shaped bony surfaces.

Prosthetic Joint Replacement ("Total Artificial Joint")

Without question, the most dramatic and significant technological advance in orthopaedics in the twentieth century has been the concept of *prosthetic joint replacement* or total artificial joint—that is, complete excision of an arthritic joint and replacement by an "endoprosthesis" composed of artificial materials. Acknowledged as the pioneer in the science and practice of modern-day prosthetic joint replacement was the late Sir John Charnley of England who, in 1962 after much research, developed his "low friction arthroplasty" of the hip joint (even though McKee had begun to use his own total joint replacement in England somewhat earlier).

Although there are now scores of modifications of prosthetic hip joint replacements, most include a metallic femoral component and a plastic (high-density polyethylene) component, both of which are usually held firmly in place within the reamed-out femoral shaft and acetabulum by means of bone "cement" (methyl methacrylate) (Fig. 6.18).

Prosthetic hip joint replacement is indicated primarily for severe arthritis in patients who are greater than 60 years of age and who, therefore, have an average life expectancy of only one or two decades and who are unlikely

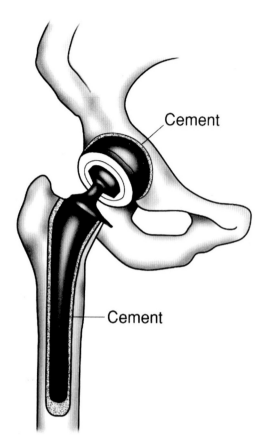

a prosthetic joint replacement, Charnley and others designed "clean-air surgical enclosures" to minimize this risk. More recently, porous, coated prostheses have been developed to allow living bone to grow into the interstices and thereby eliminate the need for bone cement. These noncemented prosthetic joints are more appropriate than the conventional cemented prosthetic joints for somewhat younger patients (Fig. 6.19).

The early clinical results of prosthetic hip joint replacements or "total hips" are dramatic, and even published results after 10 years reveal a high rate of success in older patients.

Figure 6.18.   This figure shows a cemented type of prosthetic hip joint replacement (total artificial hip). Note the metallic femoral component (head, neck, and intramedullary stem) and the metallic acetabular component (lined by high-density polyethylene). The metallic components are held firmly in place within the reamed-out femoral shaft and acetabulum by means of bone "cement" (methyl methacrylate).

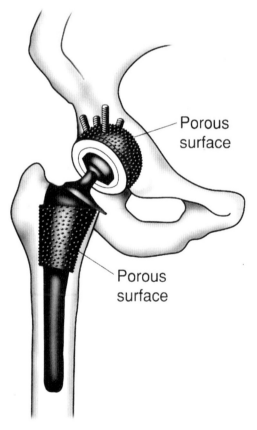

to place excessive demands on the artificial joint. These procedures are also indicated for younger patients with disabling arthritis and serious generalized disease with a limited life expectancy; they are contraindicated, of course, for children as well as for healthy, vigorous young and middle-aged adults. The complications of prosthetic hip joint replacements include loosening of one or both components of the prosthesis, "fatigue fracture" of the metallic stem, dislocation, wear of the plastic acetabulum, and infection, all of which may necessitate reoperation ("revision"). Because of the devastating effects of infection on

Figure 6.19.   The noncemented type of prosthetic hip joint replacement (total artificial hip) is seen in this figure. In this type of joint replacement, attachment of the metallic components depends on ingrowth of bone at the sites of a porous, coated surface. In this particular design, attachment of the acetabular component is augmented by metallic screws.

Although the concept of prosthetic joint replacement began with the hip, it has now been applied to virtually every joint in the upper and lower extremities—finger, thumb, wrist, elbow, shoulder, ankle, and knee. Multiple prosthetic knee joint replacements have been developed, including the hemi-arthroplasty of MacIntosh in 1957 and the hinged prosthesis of Waldius; the first non-hinged prosthetic knee joint replacement was designed by Gunston in 1968 while working with Charnley. The relatively high failure rate with the fully constrained, or hinged, prostheses has been reduced by the use of semiconstrained prostheses (Fig. 6.20). Nevertheless, the arthritic knee has been found to be a more challenging problem to solve through prosthetic joint replacement than the hip, and the early good results of "total knees" do not seem to stand up as long as those of "total hips."

Prosthetic finger joint replacements, especially of the Swanson type, have proved successful. Early designs of prosthetic elbow replacements were rather unsatisfactory, but newer designs are more promising, as are those for the shoulder joint.

After an external amputation of an extremity, the external prosthesis, or artificial limb, can be revised or replaced without reoperation. By contrast, however, total joint excision is an "internal amputation" with an "internal prosthesis" or artificial joint—a prosthesis that cannot be revised or replaced without reoperation. Furthermore, the results of such revision operations are rather discouraging.

In the current phase of phenomenal, widespread enthusiasm for total joint excision and prosthetic joint replacements, it is important to appreciate that they are neither biological nor physiological and hence may not be the final answer to the problem of arthritis. In the meantime, however, prosthetic joint replacements represent a tremendous advance in surgical technology. Nevertheless, it is essential to adhere strictly to their indications and contraindications lest surgical technology be allowed to triumph over surgical judgment.

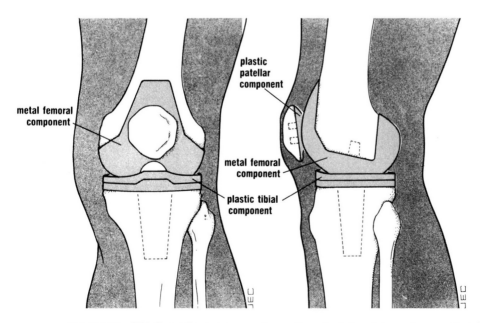

Figure 6.20.   This figure shows a cemented type of prosthetic knee joint replacement (total artificial knee). Note the metallic femoral component and the plastic (polyethylene)–covered metallic tibial components. The metallic components are held firmly in place within the host bone by means of bone cement (methyl methacrylate).

Osteocartilaginous Allografts

As an alternative to prosthetic knee joint replacement in young and middle-aged adults in whom only one side of the joint is arthritic (unicompartmental arthritis), Gross and Langer have used small osteocartilaginous allografts (from fresh cadavers) since 1971 with encouraging results without clinical or radiographic evidence of graft rejection despite the fact that no immunosuppressive therapy was given. In addition, they, as well as Mankin, have used massive osteocartilaginous allografts or transplants to replace defects from extensive local resection of malignant bone tumors.

Arthroscopic Surgery

As mentioned in Chapter 5, certain surgical procedures on the knee joint can now be performed without an open arthrotomy by using an arthroscope and specially designed surgical instruments that are inserted into the knee joint through a separate portal (Fig. 6.21). The current scope of arthroscopic surgery includes removal of a loose body, partial or total meniscectomy, repair of peripheral tears in menisci, drilling defects in the articular surface and abrading areas of chondromalacia, synovectomy, and even reconstruction of a torn anterior cruciate ligament. Understandably, the postoperative morbidity is less than that with open arthrotomy.

Operations on Bones

Draining pus from within the metaphysis of a bone may become necessary in acute hematogenous osteomyelitis and is accomplished by *bone drilling*. In chronic osteomyelitis, a sequestrum, which is a separated piece of infected dead bone, is removed (*sequestrectomy*). Occasionally, in severe and extensive chronic osteomyelitis, it is necessary to lay a bone open for drainage by removing the cortex on one side (*saucerization*). Removal of a part or all of a bone (*bone resection*)) is frequently necessary in the treatment of certain localized neoplasms.

Division of a bone with a sharp instrument (*osteotomy*) is a particularly effective type of reconstructive operation. Osteotomy is used to correct either an angular or rotational deformity in a bone (Fig. 6.22); to deal with a

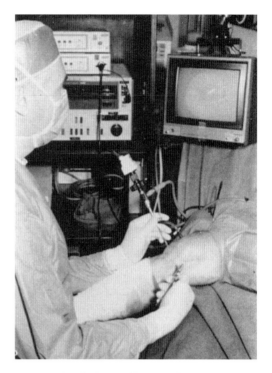

Figure 6.21.   Arthroscopic surgery is portrayed in this figure. The surgeon is holding the arthroscope in his left hand after inserting the tip of it into the patient's knee joint through one portal. Note the miniature camera attached to the opposite end of the arthroscope. The color image of the interior of the joint is displayed on the television screen. In his right hand, the surgeon is holding a specially designed surgical instrument that has been inserted into the patient's knee joint through a separate portal. Many different instruments have been designed to perform the various operations of arthroscopic surgery (Courtesy of Dr. Robert W. Jackson).

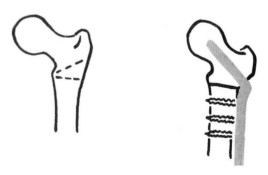

Figure 6.22.   Osteotomy to correct angular deformity in a long bone is seen in this figure. Following removal of a suitably shaped wedge of bone, the fragments are placed in the desired position, held by internal fixation, and allowed to unite like a fracture (closed-wedge osteotomy).

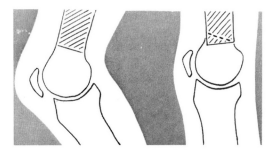

Figure 6.23. Osteotomy is used to deal with a joint deformity by producing a compensatory bony deformity near the joint. The knee flexion deformity persists, but the limb is made straight by the compensatory osteotomy in the supracondylar region of the femur.

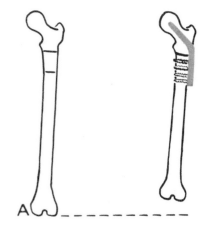

joint deformity by producing a compensatory bony deformity near the joint (Fig. 6.23); to redirect a joint surface and thereby improve the line of weightbearing forces or decrease pressure between the joint surfaces (Fig. 6.24); to permit either surgical shortening of a bone (by resection of a segment or overlapping the fragments) (Fig. 6.25**A**) or surgical lengthening of a bone in children (by gradual distraction of the osteotomy site in the presence of an intact periosteum) (Fig. 6.25**B**). Surgical lengthening of a bone by the Ilizarov technique, which involves delayed and slow distraction of callus (*callotasis*) (Fig. 6.26) and also the Debastiani modification of this technique, is capable of producing dramatic and impressive results (Fig. 6.27). In

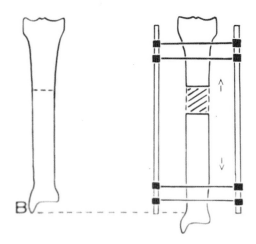

Figure 6.25. **A.** Osteotomy is carried out to shorten a bone. Following resection of a segment of bone, the fragments are brought together, held by internal fixation, and allowed to unite like a fracture. **B.** Osteotomy is used to lengthen a bone. Following simple division of the bone (usually by drilling and osteoclasis), the fragments are slowly distracted over a period of weeks to gain length. New bone from the surrounding periosteum eventually fills the gap.

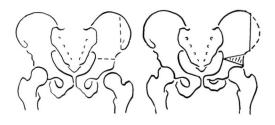

Figure 6.24. Osteotomy is used to redirect a joint surface. The innominate bone is divided, the distal fragment is redirected, and a bone graft is placed in the opening to maintain the position (open-wedge osteotomy). The redirected acetabulum provides better coverage of the femoral head and a larger weightbearing surface of articular cartilage.

the treatment of certain difficult and unstable fractures, it is sometimes necessary to expose the fracture site to replace the fragments under direct vision (*open reduction of a fracture*) and also to fix the fragments rigidly together by means of metallic devices such as screws, staples, plates, or intramedullary nails (*internal skeletal fixation*). The various methods of internal fixation and external fixation of fractures are discussed in Chapter 15.

In leg length discrepancy, an epiphyseal plate in the shorter limb can be stimulated to grow a little faster by increasing its circulation (*epiphyseal plate stimulation*), or an epiphyseal plate in the longer limb can be prevented from further growth (*epiphyseal plate arrest*) either by bone grafts (*epiphyseodesis*) or metal staples (*epiphyseal plate stapling*).

Transplantation of bone from one location (donor site) to another (host site), or *bone*

grafting, may involve the use of multiple small fragments, or strips, of cancellous bone, or solid pieces of dense cortical bone. The transplanted (donor) bone graft (the cells of which are, for the most part, dead) is slowly united or fused to the host bone by inducing deposition of new bone at the host site; eventually, the dead graft, which acts as a skeletal framework, is gradually replaced by new living bone through the simultaneous process of donor

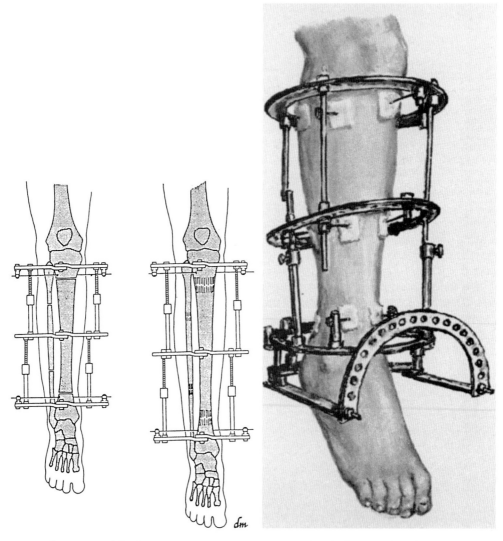

Figure 6.26.   This figure shows the Ilizarov technique of surgical lengthening of the tibia, which involves slow distraction of callus (*callotasis*) in the osteotomy site. Note that in this illustration the surgical lengthening of the tibia is taking place at two sites—one proximal and one distal. Multiple pins that traverse the bone are attached to the Ilizarov rings (external appearance seen here).

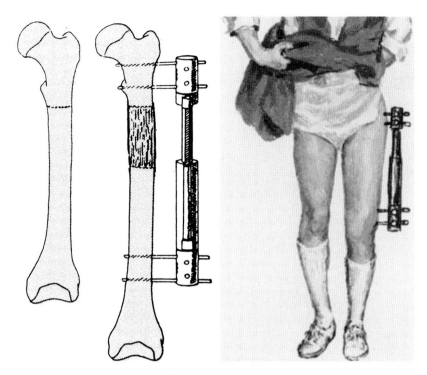

Figure 6.27. The Debastiani modification of the Ilizarov technique for surgical lengthening of the femur is seen in this figure. After the osteotomy, the callotasis is obtained by the distractible external skeletal fixation device. With both the Ilizarov method and the Debastiani modification, the patient may be allowed to bear weight throughout the prolonged period of surgical lengthening. This figure shows the external appearance of the distraction device.

bone resorption and host bone deposition. The ideal bone graft is from the patient (*autograft*) because there is no immunological graft rejection phenomenon. Less satisfactory, but sometimes practical, is stored or "banked" bone from another individual (*homograft, allograft*). Least satisfactory and seldom indicated is bone from another species (*heterograft, xenograft*). Bone grafting is used to promote bony union in a fracture that has failed to unite (nonunion) or that is unduly slow in uniting (delayed union) (Fig. 6.28); to promote fusion of a joint (arthrodesis) (Fig. 6.29) or of an epiphyseal plate (epiphyseodesis); to maintain the angulation of an "open wedge" osteotomy (Fig. 6.24); and to fill and thereby strengthen a bony defect following local bone resection or curettage of a cystic lesion or a benign intramedullary neoplasm (Fig. 6.30).

For certain serious limb conditions—such as an extensive radioresistant malignant neoplasm, irreparable injury, gangrene, or a severe congenital deformity that cannot be corrected by reconstructive operations—it may be necessary to remove part (or all) of the limb through bone (*amputation*) or through a joint (*disarticulation*) and to provide the patient with an artificial limb (*prosthesis*).

In recent decades, amputation for malignant neoplasms of the extremities has been replaced to a large extent by operations that achieve wide resection of the neoplasm and immediate reconstruction of the resultant defect, thereby sparing the remainder of the extremity (*limb sparing or limb salvage operations*).

Microsurgery

Surgery performed under the magnification of an operating microscope using microinstruments and microsutures (*microsurgery*) has

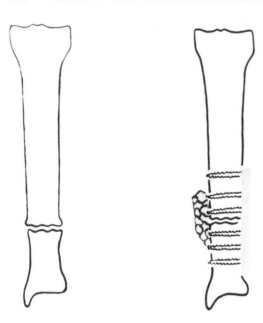

Figure 6.28. The bone graft for transplantation of bone to promote bony union for the nonunion or delayed union of a fracture may be cortical and held with screws or it may consist of multiple small chips of cancellous bone.

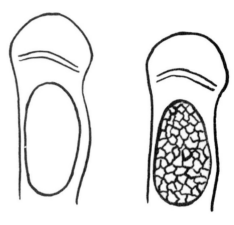

Figure 6.30. This figure shows transplantation of bone (bone grafting) to fill a bony defect following curettement of the lining of a cystic lesion in bone.

developed extremely rapidly since 1960 (Fig. 6.31). This exciting advance in surgical technology has had a significant impact on surgical disorders and injuries of the musculoskeletal system in that it is now possible to replant completely severed digits and limbs (*surgical replantation*), to repair with great accuracy divided peripheral nerves, to transfer free vascularized autogenous bone grafts with or without skin and other soft tissues, to transfer a toe

to replace a lost thumb, and even to transfer vascularized and reinnervated autogenous muscle grafts that will function as soon as the motor nerve regenerates down the transplanted motor nerve.

7) Electrical Stimulation of Fracture Healing

During the last three decades, electricity has been used both in experimental animals and in humans as an alternative to bone grafting to stimulate osteogenesis in the treatment of established nonunion of fractures. To date, the following three electrical systems have

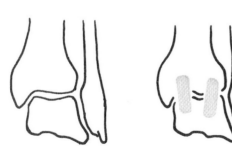

Figure 6.29. This figure shows transplantation of bone (bone grafting) to promote fusion of a joint (arthrodesis). In this example, two bone grafts are shown crossing the ankle joint.

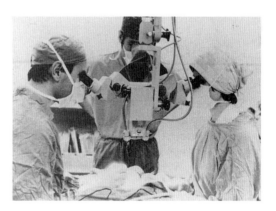

Figure 6.31. A surgeon (**left**) and an assistant are performing microsurgery through an operating microscope. A third surgeon is observing the operation through a "teaching arm" of the microscope.

been developed: constant direct current through percutaneous wire cathodes (semi-invasive) (Brighton); constant direct current through implanted electrodes and power pack (invasive) (Dwyer and also Paterson); and inductive coupling through electromagnetic coils (noninvasive) (Bassett and also de Haas). Each method has its advantages as well as its disadvantages, but all three provide the same reported overall success rate of approximately 80%. Continuing investigations, both experimental and clinical, are required to provide more data on this development.

8) Continuous Passive Motion

You will recall from Chapter 3 that since 1970 the author's concept of continuous passive motion (CPM) has been studied and continues to be studied by him in his laboratory at the Research Institute of The Hospital for Sick Children in Toronto, using experimental models of a wide variety of joint disorders and injuries in rabbits. Encouraged by the results of the first 8 years of these scientific investigations and convinced of the comfort and efficacy of CPM, we have now applied the concept to the postoperative management of carefully selected patients.

The *indications* for postoperative CPM in our preliminary clinical trials have been the following types of surgical procedures in adolescent and adult patients: 1) arthrotomy, capsulotomy, débridement, and arthrolysis of joints with painful restriction of motion secondary to post-traumatic arthritis; 2) open reduction of intra-articular fractures as well as metaphyseal and diaphyseal fractures; 3) patellectomy; 4) repair of ligamentous injuries; 5) synovectomy for rheumatoid arthritis and hemophilic arthropathy; 6) arthrotomy and drainage (combined with appropriate antibiotics) for acute septic arthritis; 7) biological resurfacing (with a periosteal graft) for a major defect in a joint surface; 8) surgical repair of a complete laceration of a tendon; 9) rigid internal fixation of a metaphyseal osteotomy; and 10) total prosthetic joint replacement.

The results of the preliminary clinical trials in the University of Toronto Teaching Hospitals have been gratifying. As with the rabbits, the CPM devices have been applied to the in-volved limb in patients at the completion of the operation while they are still under general anesthesia. The device moves the joint continuously day and night at a rate of approximately one cycle per minute for at least 1 week during which the patients are remarkably comfortable and after which they can usually maintain an excellent range of motion by their own active exercises.

We have collaborated with John Saringer, a mechanical engineer at the University of Toronto, in the design of these electric motor-driven devices to provide CPM for the ankle–knee–hip, the wrist, the elbow, and the finger (Fig. 6.32).

The experience with these clinical applications is summarized in the second part of Chapter 18.

9) Radiation Therapy (Radiotherapy)

Radiation therapy or radiotherapy, is a highly scientific and technical form of treatment involving the administration of ionizing radiation that is prescribed by physicians in the specialty that has come to be known as *radiation oncology.*

The value of ionizing radiation as a form of treatment lies in its relatively selective destruction of the more rapidly multiplying cells in malignant neoplasms and certain other conditions. Immature cells and undifferentiated cells are particularly vulnerable, or sensitive, to the effects of ionizing radiation (*radiosensitive*). Thus, it is possible by means of highly developed techniques to deliver a *lethal tumor dose* of radiation to a malignant lesion and yet produce relatively little radiation effect in the surrounding normal tissues. Radiation at therapeutic levels produces profound chromosomal changes in cells, but the effects of these changes are not apparent until the time of the next cell division (*mitosis*), when the cell will either fail to divide or will do so in an abnormal way. Thus, the radiation effect is related to the turnover rate of the cell population of the various types of irradiated tissue cells. The cells of the neoplasm, having a rapid turnover rate, show the radiation effect early, whereas those in the bed of the neoplasm (fibrous tissue and blood vessels), having a slow turnover rate, show the radiation effect later. The most

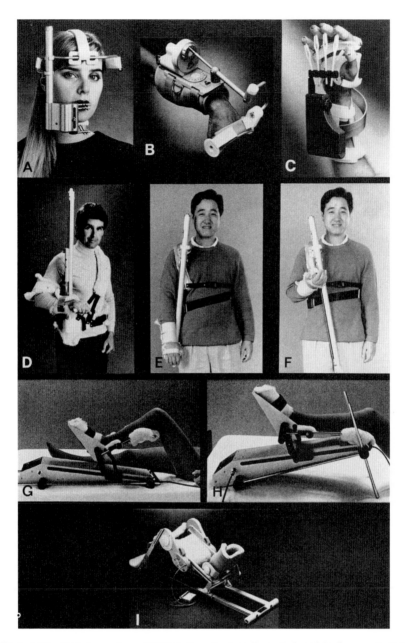

Figure 6.32.   This figure shows CPM devices that have been designed for humans by John H. Saringer, P.Eng. in collaboration with the author: for the temporomandibular joints opening and closing of the mouth (**A**); for the wrist circumduction (**B**); for the fingers and thumb flexion and extension (**C**); for the shoulder abduction and adduction (it can be modified to provide flexion and extension) (**D**); for the elbow flexion and extension combined with supination and pronation (**E and F**); for the ankle–knee–hip flexion and extension (**G**); same device as seen in **G** but set up to provide motion for the ankle only plantar flexion and dorsiflexion (**H**); and 1990 model for the ankle–knee–hip flexion and extension (**I**).

significant changes in the bed of the neoplasm are slowly progressive fibrosis and ischemia. The *total* effect of radiation therapy, therefore, is delayed rather than immediate.

The source of therapeutic ionizing radiation is usually either a high-voltage x-ray machine or a radioactive isotope such as cobalt ("the cobalt bomb"). Of the three types of energy released during the disintegration of radium (alpha rays, beta rays and gamma rays), the gamma rays have by far the greatest ability to penetrate tissues and are therefore the most effective in radiation therapy. The quantitative physical unit of *absorbed* radiation which used to be *rad*, is now termed a Gray (Gy) and is equal to 100 rad. Compared with neoplasms arising in other tissues, those arising in bone are relatively *radioresistant* and require high dosages of radiation (70 Gy or more fractionated over a period of several weeks). However, certain skeletal neoplasms, such as Ewing's sarcoma and malignant lymphoma of bone, may be at least locally destroyed by appropriate radiation techniques even though they may recur subsequently, either locally or elsewhere. For such neoplasms, radiation therapy may be the treatment of choice, whereas neoplasms that are more radioresistant, such as osteogenic sarcoma and, to a lesser extent chondrosarcoma, usually require radical surgical resection or amputation either with or without radiation.

Radiation therapy has been used empirically in the treatment of poorly understood conditions such as Langerhan's cell histiocytosis and ankylosing spondylitis as well as villonodular synovitis, but it is employed with great caution. In general, any nonmalignant condition that can be treated satisfactorily by some other form of treatment should not be treated by radiation. The most serious radiation effects on normal skeletal tissues are the following: epiphyseal plate damage with resultant growth disturbance; radiation necrosis of bone with subsequent pathological fracture; and rarely, at a much later date, radiation-induced malignancy.

REHABILITATION—A PHILOSOPHY IN ACTION

As a medical practitioner of the future, regardless of whether you are a family physician or a specialist, you will be involved in the *rehabilitation* of patients who suffer from either chronic or permanent disabling problems. Rehabilitation is not a specialized technique of treatment, not a method of treatment, not even a principle of treatment; rehabilitation is a *philosophy in action*—the philosophy of total care *of* your patients as well as continuing care *for* them. The broad aim, or goal, of rehabilitation is to correct, insofar as is possible, your patient's problem (whether it be physical, mental, or social) and *in addition* to continue to help him or her by treatment, training, education, and encouragement to cope with the residual uncorrectable portion of the problem and his or her attitude toward it, in order that his or her life may be changed from one of dependency to one of independence, from one that is empty to one that is full. In a sense, rehabilitation is "*going the second mile*" and often farther with your patient, and it is applicable to the disabling problems of all fields of medicine and surgery.

Those patients with disabling disorders and injuries of the musculoskeletal system require, and deserve, rehabilitation in its broad sense. Some examples of such disabling musculoskeletal conditions are extensive paralysis from spina bifida with meningomyelocele, poliomyelitis, spinal cord injury (paraplegia), head injury, cerebral palsy, and cerebral vascular accidents ("strokes"); extensive congenital deformities and deficiencies of limbs and acquired amputations; severe and multiple musculoskeletal injuries; generalized muscle diseases such as muscular dystrophy; neurological disorders such as disseminated sclerosis and amyotrophic lateral sclerosis (Lou Gehrig's disease); and chronic generalized rheumatoid arthritis. The rehabilitation of such patients, the total care *of* them as well as a continuing care *for* them, cannot be accomplished by one person; indeed the philosophy of rehabilitation requires the coordinated efforts of a large group, or team of professional persons, including the rehabilitation physician, the orthopaedic surgeon, the nurse, the physical therapist and the occupational therapist, the brace maker (orthotist), the limb maker (prosthetist), the psychologist, the medical social worker, the teacher, and the vocational adviser. Through continuing advances in all these fields, rehabilitation is becoming progressively more realistic and effective, and it will be of even greater importance in the future than it has been in the past.

COMMUNICATION WITH YOUR PATIENTS ABOUT THE RECOMMENDED TREATMENT

Gone are the days when it was customary and even acceptable for the physician to exhibit a paternalistic or maternalistic attitude toward the patient that conveyed the message, "I am the doctor, I know what is best for you, so don't question my decisions."

In the current era, patients and their relatives are better informed about medical matters and have higher expectations from their physician or surgeon than ever before. Their main sources of information–namely, television programs, books, and newspaper and magazine stories—may not have been completely understood or the information may not be entirely relevant to their particular disorder or injury. Nevertheless, many of your patients will, rightly, expect to learn from you the details of your recommended treatment; the implications of that treatment for them, including the benefits and the risks; and also the natural course of their condition without treatment, as well as the pros and cons of other treatment options, so that when they sign a consent form it is truly an *informed* consent. In essence, you will be wise to allow your patients to express their views in the decision-making process concerning your recommended treatment.

The Doctor–Patient Relationship as Part of Treatment

The motivating philosophy of caring for your patients is not only to treat the specific disorder or injury effectively but also to treat him or her as a fellow human being in the manner in which you would want one of your loved ones, or even yourself, to be treated, namely, in keeping with *the golden rule* "Do unto others as you would have them do unto you," a widely accepted religious and philosophical concept.

The philosophy underlying the ideal doctor–patient relationship requires that you:

1. Exhibit the following qualities toward your patients as part of their treatment: warmth, kindness, compassion, courtesy, respect, sensitivity, awareness of anxieties, empathy, professionalism and patience.
2. Take time to listen as well as to inform.
3. Make frequent eye contact.
4. Use lay terms as much as necessary in conversation with your patients in order to be understood.
5. Make your patients feel that you are willing to consider their wishes with respect to all relevant decision-making processes.
6. Encourage your patients to ask questions, not only during each appointment but also, if necessary, between appointments by telephone or letter.

As a medical student of today, and a medical practitioner of tomorrow, you will do well to develop the habit of establishing good doctor–patient relationships right from the beginning of your professional life. By so doing, you will have happier, more appreciative, more contented, and more cooperative patients as well as better clinical outcomes for them. As a consequence, you, the medical practitioner, will derive more pleasure and satisfaction from your care of patients.

SUGGESTED ADDITIONAL READING

Aichroth PM, Cannon WG Jr. Knee surgery, current practice. New York: Raven Press, 1992.

Ballard WT, Lowry DA, Brand RA. Resection arthroplasty of the hip. J Arthroplasty 1995;10:772–779.

Bassett CAL, Mitchell SN, Gaston SR. Treatment of ununited tibial diaphyseal fractures with pulsing electromagnetic fields. J Bone Joint Surg Am 1981;63A:511–523.

Berger RG. Nonsteroidal anti-inflammatory drugs: making the right choices. J Am Acad Orthop Surg 1994;2:255–260.

Brien FW, Terek RM, Healy JH, Lane JM. Allograft reconstruction after proximal tibial resection for bone tumors: an analysis of function and outcome comparing allograft and prosthetic reconstruction. Clin Orthop 1994;303:116–127.

Brighton CT. The treatment of non-unions with electricity. Current concepts review. J Bone Joint Surg Am 1981;63A:847–851.

Brotzman SB. Handbook of orthopaedic rehabilitation. St Louis: Mosby–Year Book, 1996.

Brown KLB, Cruess RL. Bone and cartilage transplantation in orthopaedic surgery. A review. J Bone Joint Surg 1982;64A:270–280.

Charland LC, Dick PT. Should compassion be included in codes of ethics for physicians? Ann Roy Coll Phys Surg Can 1995;28:415–418.

Charnley J. Low friction arthroplasty of the hip theory and practice. Berlin: Springer-Verlag, 1979.

Charnley J. Trends in arthroplasty of the hip. In: Straub LR, Wilson PD Jr, eds. Clinical trends in orthopaedics. New York: Thieme-Stratton, 1982.

Cox JP, ed. Moss' radiation oncology. 7th ed. St Louis: Mosby–Year Book, 1994.

Crenshaw AH, ed. Campbell's operative orthopaedics. 8th ed. St. Louis: Mosby–Year Book, 1992.

de Haas WG, Watson J, Morrison DM. Noninvasive treatment of united fractures of the tibia using electrical stimulation. J Bone Joint Surg 1980;62B:465–470.

Detsky AS, Naglie IG, Krahn MD. Clinical decision analysis. Review article. Ann Roy Coll Phys Surg Can 1994;27:157–159.

De Vita VT, Hillman S, Rosenberg SA. Cancer: principles and practice of oncology. 4th ed. Philadelphia: JB Lippincott, 1993.

Dwyer AF, Wickham GG. Direct current stimulation in spine fusion. Med J Aust 1974;1:73.

Gross AE, Silverstein EA, Falk J, Falk R, Langer F. The allotransplantation of partial joints in the treatment of osteoarthritis of the knee. Clin Orthop 1975;108:7–14.

Hall EJ. Radiology for the radiologist. 4th ed. Philadelphia: JB Lippincott, 1994.

Harris WH, Sledge CB. Total hip and total knee replacement. (First of two parts). N Engl J Med 1990;323:725–731.

Harris WH, Sledge CB. Total hip and knee replacement. (Second of two parts). N Engl J Med 1990;323:801–807.

Ilizarov GA. The tension-stress effect on the genesis and growth of tissues. Part II. The influence of the rate and frequency of distraction. Clin Orthop 1989;239:263–285.

Johnson LL. Arthroscopic surgery, principles and practice. Vol. 1 and Vol. 2. 3rd ed. St Louis: CV Mosby, 1986.

Kocher MS. History of replantation: from miracle to microsurgery. World J Surg 1995;19: 452–467.

Kostuik JP, Gillespie R. Amputation surgery and rehabilitation: the Toronto experience. New York: Churchill Livingstone, 1981.

Mankin HJ, Fogelson FS, Thrasher AZ, Jaffer F. Massive resection and allograft transplantation in the treatment of malignant bone tumors. N Engl J Med 1976;294:1247–1255.

McGinty J, Caspari RB, Jackson RW, Pochling GG. Operative arthrosurgery. 2nd ed. New York: Raven Press, 1995.

Morrissy RT, Weinstein SH. Lovell and Winter's pediatric orthopaedics. 4th ed. Philadelphia: Lippincott-Raven, 1996.

Nickel VL, Bottle MJ. Orthopaedic rehabilitation. 2nd ed. New York: Churchill Livingstone, 1992.

Novack D, Till J. Doctor/patient communication: the Toronto Consensus. Ontario Med Rev 1992;11–14.

Paley D. Problems, obstacles and complications of limb lengthening by the Ilizarov technique. Clin Orthop 1990;250:81–104.

Paterson DC, Lewis GN, Cass CA. Treatment of delayed union and nonunion with an implanted direct current stimulator. Clin Orthop 1980; 148:117–128.

Pendleton D, Hasler J, eds. Doctor–patient communication. New York: Academic Press, 1983.

Richards J, McDonald P. Doctor–patient communication in surgery. J Roy Soc Med 1995;78: 922–924.

Roter DL, Hall JA. Doctors talking with patients/ patients talking with doctors: improving communication in medical visits. Westport, CT: Greenwood Publishing Group, 1992.

Rougraff BT, Simon MA, Kneisl JS, Greenberg DB, Mankin HJ. Limb salvage compared with amputation for osteosarcoma of the distal end of the femur: A long-term oncological, functional and quality-of-life study. J Bone Joint Surg 1994;76-A:649–656.

Salter RB. Continuous passive motion—CPM—a biological concept for the healing and regeneration of articular cartilage, ligaments and tendons: from origination to research to clinical applications. Baltimore: Williams & Wilkins, 1993.

Salter RB, Gross AE, Hall JH. Hydrocortisone arthropathy—an experimental investigation. Can Med Assoc J 1967;97:374–377.

Schatzker J, Tile M. The rationale of operative fracture care. 2nd ed. Berlin: Springer-Verlag, 1996.

Scott G, King JB. A prospective double-blind trial of electrical capacitive coupling in the treatment of non-union of long bones. J Bone Joint Surg 1994;76-A:820–826.

Simpson M, Buckman R, Stewart M, Maquire P, Lipkin M, Novak D, Till J. Doctor/patient communication: the Toronto consensus. Br Med J 1991;303:1385–1387.

Stewart MA. Effective physician–patient communication and health outcomes: a review. Can Med Assoc J 1995;152:1423–1433.

Stockley I, McAuley JP, Gross AE. Allograft reconstruction in total knee arthroplasty. J Bone Joint Surg Br 1992;74-B:393–397.

Zatsepin ST, Burdygin VN. Replacement of the distal femur and proximal tibia with frozen allografts. Clin Orthop 1994;303:95–102.

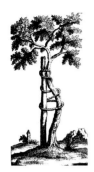

Section II

Musculoskeletal Disorders—General and Specific

7 Common Normal Variations

When you consider the astronomical number of permutations and combinations of genes and chromosomes that determine the form and function of each human being, as well as the influence of innumerable environmental factors, it is not surprising that, apart from identical (uniovular) twins, each person in this world is different from every other person. While one speaks of an *average* infant, an *average* child, and an *average* adult, it is important to appreciate that there exists *an extremely wide range of normal* in body form and function. However, the normal variations change with age so that a normal variation that is present at birth and normally changes spontaneously with age may no longer be considered normal if it persists into adult life.

It is obvious that it is necessary to know the wide range of normal variations in humans so that when you see patients, it will be possible to distinguish the normal (physiological) from the abnormal (pathological), and you will not make the error of treating a condition that neither requires nor merits treatment.

During the past two decades, several clinical investigators—including Staheli as well as Wenger and Rang—have conducted scientifically sound studies of the efficacy of various forms of treatment of normal variations of the musculoskeletal system and have concluded

that treatment such as corrective shoes, braces, splints, and exercises have little or no significant effect on the natural course or prognosis of such variations.

Thus, it is inappropriate to "treat" anxious parents by subjecting their child with a normal variation to a form of treatment that is neither necessary nor of scientifically proven value. Nevertheless, the borderline between the *extremes* of normal variation and the beginning of abnormal variation is not always clearly defined, particularly in the musculoskeletal system. Therefore, if the normal variation is extreme and may not correct itself spontaneously, it may be a source of major concern to your patient and to his or her relatives. Only under these circumstances may simple, safe, and empirically effective methods of treatment be justifiable to prevent the need for operative treatment, such as femoral or tibial osteotomies, near the end of the child's skeletal growth.

The underlying *cause;* the *natural course,* or *prognosis,* without treatment; and whether or not any *treatment* is indicated must be understood for each of these common normal variations.

Management of the various normal, or physiological, variations of the musculoskeletal system includes excluding an abnormal or pathological variation and then spending as much time as necessary with the concerned parents to enlighten them, and thereby reassure them, of the good prognosis for their child. They need, and deserve, just as much kindness and compassion as do the parents of a child with a more serious problem.

COMMON NORMAL VARIATIONS IN CHILDREN

As a medical practitioner, you will see many children with normal variations of musculoskeletal form and function, particularly in the lower limbs. The most common group of such conditions in childhood are (in lay terms) flat feet, knock knees, bow legs, toeing out, and toeing in. These conditions are extremely common in young children but become progressively less common toward adolescence, indicating that they tend to improve spontaneously. Nevertheless, these normal variations in perfectly healthy children cause much concern in the minds of the child's parents, grandparents, neighbors, well-meaning friends, and shoe salesmen. An appreciation of the underlying cause and the natural course (prognosis) of these variations will enable you to deal with them intelligently. They are best considered in two main groups based on their underlying cause: those caused by looseness, or hypermobility, of joints (joint laxity) and those caused by twisting, or torsional, deformities of the growing long bones of the lower limbs.

Variations Caused by Hypermobility of Joints (Joint Laxity)

The degree of mobility of joints varies widely in normal children. Hypermobile joints throughout the body result from lax ligaments and are extremely common in infancy, less common in childhood, and relatively uncommon in adult life. The lax ligaments, which are probably an inherited variation, seem to become less lax as the child gets older, with the result that the hypermobility of the joints tends to improve spontaneously; only the most severe degrees of the condition persist into adult life. Two common clinical variations that are secondary to hypermobility or joint laxity are *flat feet* (hypermobile pes planus) and *knock knees* (genu valgum). Understandably, both these variations are aggravated by obesity, which should be dealt with by a dietitian.

Flexible Flat Feet (Hypermobile Pes Planus)

At the age of 1 year, when most children have begun to stand, all the joints are normally hypermobile. As a result, the feet, being flexible, look flat, but only with weightbearing (Fig. 7.1). Indeed, if these children walked on their hands, they would have "flat hands" because the hypermobility of the joints is generalized rather than localized (Fig. 7.2). When the child is asked to stand on tiptoe, the longitudinal arch reappears. As the ligamentous laxity

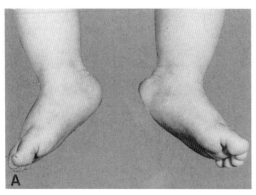
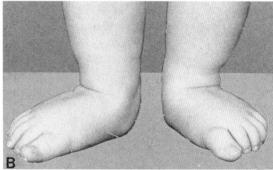

Figure 7.1.   Flexible flat feet (hypermobile pes planus) in a 1½-year-old child. **A.** The feet look normal when the child is not standing. **B.** They look flat only when weightbearing.

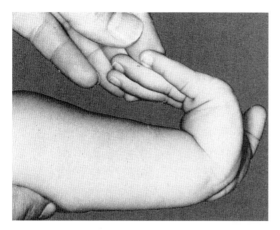

Figure 7.2. Hypermobility of the joints in the upper limb of the child in Figure 7.1, indicating generalized joint laxity. If these children walked on their hands they would have "flat hands," and no one, not even the parents, would be worried about that!

school age child, the same type of corrections added to low shoes have relatively less effect on the natural course of severe flexible feet but do serve to make the shoes last longer. Excessive corrections in low shoes, however, force the child's foot to slide to the lateral side

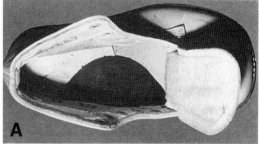

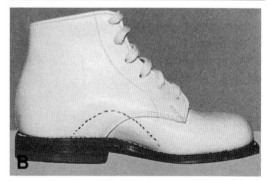

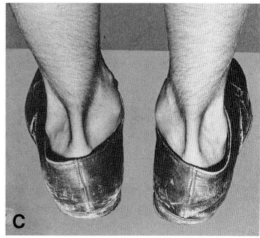

and associated hypermobility of the joints improve spontaneously, the flat appearance of the child's feet becomes less marked, which explains why flexible flat feet are so common in young children and yet relatively uncommon in adults. The term *flexible flat feet* avoids the stigma of the term *congenital flat feet,* whereas the frequently used expressions of *fallen arches* and *weak arches* are not only inaccurate but also sound unnecessarily ominous to the already anxious parents.

Once the underlying cause, as well as the natural course, of flexible flat feet are appreciated, it becomes obvious that the mild and moderate degrees of this condition require no treatment apart from reassuring the parents. It is also important to assure the parents that flexible flat feet in young children are not painful and are unlikely to become so. For severe degrees of flexible flat feet, the aim of treatment is simply to prevent further stretching of the already lax ligaments of the feet until such time as the generalized ligamentous laxity improves spontaneously. This is readily accomplished in preschool children by means of boots to which a sponge rubber arch support ("scaphoid pad") has been added (Fig. 7.3A and B). However, the child need not be denied the joy of running barefoot, or in soft running shoes, at least part of the time. For the

Figure 7.3. **A** and **B.** This boot is to be used only for preschool children with severe flexible flat feet. A sponge rubber arch support ("scaphoid pad") has been added simply to prevent further stretching of the lax joints of the feet. **C.** Excessive correction in the shoes of a 6-year-old boy with flexible flat feet. The feet slide to the lateral side of the shoe; the shoes are pushed out of shape and cause the boy discomfort.

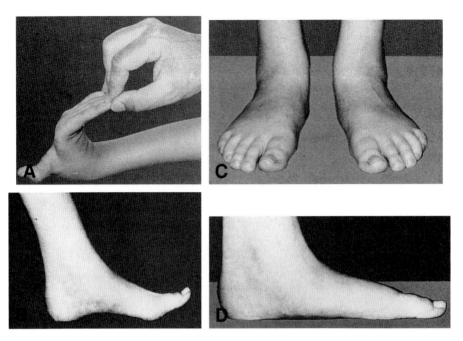

Figure 7.4. Flexible flat feet and flexible hands (**A and B**) in a 10-year-old boy with persistent generalized joint laxity. The feet appear flat only when bearing weight (**C and D**). This boy was active and did not have any pain in his feet.

of the shoe and cause unnecessary discomfort (Fig. 7.3C). Plastic longitudinal arch supports and heel cups may also be uncomfortable. Exercises designed to strengthen supposedly weak muscles are, understandably, of no value in the management of flexible flat feet because, of course, the muscles are not weak.

In adolescence, only individuals with more severe joint laxity still exhibit flexible flat feet (Fig. 7.4). Of these individuals, the majority are completely comfortable, even with ordinary footwear, in spite of being active. A small percentage of adolescents and adults with flexible flat feet complain of either discomfort or tiredness in their feet and limit their activities as a result. Carefully molded arch supports usually relieve these symptoms, but in the rare circumstances in which they do not—and only under these circumstances—some form of operative treatment such as fusion (arthrodesis) of the subtalar joint is justifiable at or near the end of skeletal growth.

Flexible flat feet associated with a tight Achilles tendon should make you think of the possibility of either mild cerebral palsy or early muscular dystrophy. Flexible flat feet must also be differentiated from the less common, but more serious, conditions of rigid valgus feet and accessory tarsal scaphoid, which are described in Chapter 8.

Knock Knees (Genu Valgum)
By far the most common cause of knock knees in young children is hypermobility of the knee joints which, in turn, is simply another manifestation of generalized joint laxity. Thus, knock knees, like flexible flat feet, are much more common in young children than in adolescents, and for the same reason. Consequently this type of knock knee corrects itself spontaneously in more than 90% of children. Since the valgus deformity is secondary to the lax medial collateral ligaments of the knee, it is most noticeable when the child is standing and also when the ligamentous laxity is tested (Fig. 7.5). The aim of treatment should be simply to prevent further stretching of the already lax medial collateral ligaments. The habitual position of sitting on the floor with the

knees in front and the feet out to the side (which has become known as the *W, or television position*) should be avoided because it stretches these ligaments further (Fig. 7.6). Boots with inside heel wedges are frequently prescribed with the idea of altering the line of weightbearing and thereby decreasing the strain on the medial collateral ligaments of the knees, but their efficacy is completely unproved.

In the few older children with persistent joint laxity and associated marked knock knees, secondary bony deformity may gradually develop because of uneven epiphyseal plate growth in the region of the knee (Fig 7.7). Under these circumstances, a specially designed night splint may be used to overcome the bony component of the deformity by influencing subsequent growth (Fig. 7.8). Day braces are both cumbersome and ineffectual, and operative treatments such as epiphyseal stapling or osteotomy are almost never necessary.

This common type of knock knees, or genu valgum, must be differentiated from the much less common but more serious type of genu valgum that occurs through bone secondary to an epiphyseal plate disturbance from con-

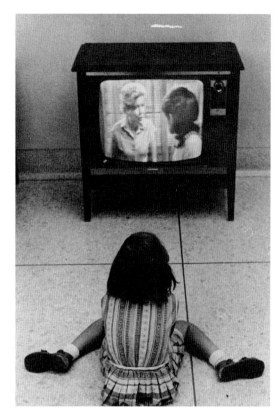

Figure 7.6. The W, or television position, of sitting. This habitual position of sitting should be avoided because it not only applies a torsional force to the femora but also stretches the medial collateral ligaments of the knees.

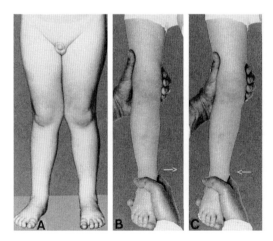

Figure 7.5. Knock knees (genu valgum) in a 4-year-old boy with generalized joint laxity. **A.** The deformity is most noticeable on weightbearing because it occurs through the lax knee joints. **B and C.** The hypermobility of the knee is demonstrated by passive adduction, which corrects the deformity, and passive abduction, which aggravates it.

genital abnormalities (Chapter 8), metabolic conditions (Chapter 9), or injury (Chapters 15 and 16).

Variations Caused by Torsional Deformities of Bones

The growing long bones of children respond to repeated twisting, or torsional, forces by an alteration of the normal growth pattern in the epiphyseal plates. The affected long bone becomes twisted in its long axis—that is, it develops either an internal or an external torsional deformity. Prenatal intrauterine positions and certain postnatal habitual sleeping and sitting positions place torsional forces on the growing long bones and are responsible for the torsional deformities that cause either toeing out or toeing in.

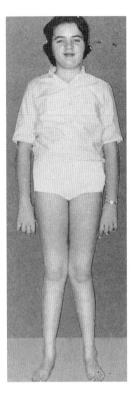

Figure 7.7.   Knock knees (genu valgum) in a 12-year-old girl with persistent generalized joint laxity. A secondary bony deformity has developed and, consequently, spontaneous correction is no longer likely.

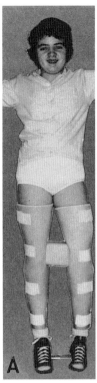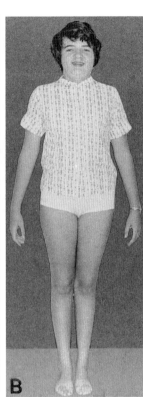

Figure 7.8.   A. This specially designed corrective splint was worn at night for 9 months to influence epiphyseal plate growth at the knees. **B.** The bony deformity was gradually corrected by the use of the night splint. Such a splint is justified only for older children whose genu valgum has failed to correct itself spontaneously.

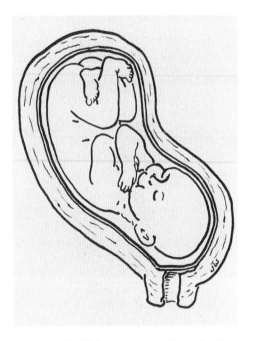

Figure 7.9.   In this intrauterine position, the hips are always flexed and externally rotated, whereas the knees are usually flexed and the feet turned inward.

Before birth, the hips are always flexed (there being no "standing room" in utero) and externally rotated, whereas the knees are usually flexed and the feet turned inward (Fig. 7.9). As a result of the torsional forces associated with this position, almost all newborn infants exhibit some degree of external femoral torsion and internal tibial torsion, both of which normally correct themselves spontaneously with subsequent growth. However, certain common habitual positions of sleeping and sitting during childhood exert torsional forces on the growing lower limbs and either prevent the spontaneous correction of the deformities present at birth or create new torsional deformities. An appreciation of this basic concept is pivotal in understanding the causes and the natural course (prognosis) of the common clinical variations of toeing out and toeing in.

Toeing Out
External Femoral Torsion (Lateral Femoral Torsion)

Toeing out, which is common in young children, is nearly always caused by external femoral torsion (Fig. 7.10). Examination reveals that when the extended lower limbs are rotated outward (externally), the knees turn out to about 90°, whereas when they are rotated inward (internally), the knees can be brought only to the neutral position (Fig. 7.11). If the child habitually sleeps face down with the femora externally rotated (Fig. 7.12), the external femoral torsion persists and, in addition, external tibial torsion may develop as a result of the associated outward torsional force on the tibia. This sleeping position, however, is seldom assumed after the age of 2 years. Thus, the prognosis for external femoral torsion is good. Rarely, in the older child, it may be necessary to use a simple night splint in which the feet are turned inward to correct the residual external femoral torsion.

External Tibial Torsion (Lateral Tibial Torsion)

Toeing out caused by external tibial torsion alone is rare, although external tibial torsion may aggravate the toeing out caused by external femoral torsion, as already mentioned; it may also compensate to some extent for internal femoral torsion, as will be mentioned later. In addition, external tibial torsion may develop secondary to the muscle imbalance of paralytic conditions such as spina bifida, cerebral palsy, and poliomyelitis (Chapter 12).

External rotation of the entire lower limb at the hip, without any torsional deformity, can result from congenital dislocation of the hip in the younger child (Chapter 8) and from a slipped upper femoral epiphysis in the older child (Chapter 13).

Toeing In
Internal Femoral Torsion (Medial Femoral Torsion)

Since the femora are never internally rotated in utero, internal femoral torsion is never seen in the newborn or even during infancy. However, if the child subsequently acquires the habit of sitting on the floor with the knees in front, the femora internally rotated, and the feet out to the side (the W, or television position) (Fig. 7.13), the associated torsional force on the growing femur gradually produces an internal femoral torsion by the time the child is about 5 years of age. Examination reveals

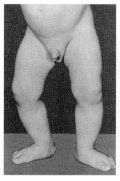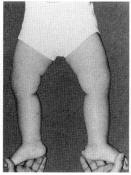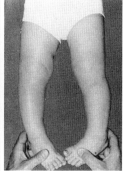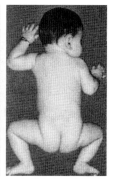

Figure 7.10.   Left. External femoral torsion with resultant toeing out in a 1-year-old boy.

Figure 7.11.   Middle. This figure shows external femoral torsion. When the extended lower limbs are rotated outward, the knees turn out to 90°, whereas when they are rotated inward, the knees can be brought only to the neutral position, indicating that the torsional deformity is in the femora.

Figure 7.12.   Right. This sleeping position with the femora and tibiae externally rotated prevents spontaneous correction of the external femoral torsion and may even produce external tibial torsion.

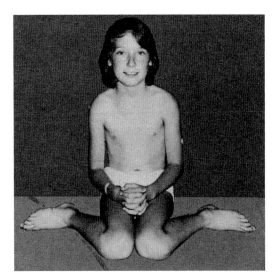

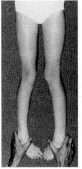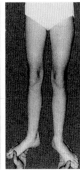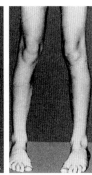

Figure 7.14.   Left. Internal femoral torsion is seen in this figure. When the extended lower limbs are rotated inward, the knees turn in to about 90°. When they are rotated outward, the knees can be brought only slightly beyond the neutral position, indicating that the torsional deformity is in the femora.

Figure 7.13.   The W, or television position of sitting has gradually produced an acquired internal femoral torsion and external tibial torsion in this 9-year-old girl.

Figure 7.15.   Right. Internal femoral torsion is seen in a 9-year-old girl. Note that both the knees and the feet are turned inward.

that when the extended lower limbs are rotated inward (internally), the knees turn in to about 90°, whereas when they are rotated outward (externally), the knees can be brought only slightly beyond the neutral position (Fig. 7.14). As a result, the child walks with both the feet and the knees turned inward (Fig. 7.15). If the child continues to assume this sitting position, the associated external force on the tibia gradually produces an external tibial torsion, in which case the child begins to walk with the knees turned in but the feet pointing straight ahead. Internal femoral torsion, being a gradually acquired torsional deformity in older children, exhibits much less tendency to correct spontaneously than do the other torsional variations.

The aim of treatment is simply to prevent further internal torsional forces from being exerted on the femora by training the child to stop sitting in the position that has caused the deformity; in addition, corrective external torsional forces can be applied to the femora by training the child to sit in the *tailor* or cross-legged position (Fig. 7.16). For more severe and persistent internal femoral torsion in children older than 8 years of age, it may be necessary to use a specially designed night splint

in which the lower limbs are kept externally rotated (Fig. 7.17). Straight last shoes may minimize the appearance of the toeing in, but wedges in the soles and twister cables are of

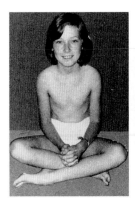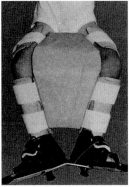

Figure 7.16.   Left. The tailor or cross-legged position, in which an external torsional force is applied to the femur, helps to correct the internal femoral torsion.

Figure 7.17.   Right. This specially designed corrective splint is used at night to apply a mild external torsional force to the growing femur and thereby correct internal femoral torsion. Both feet are turned outward 90° on the bent bar of the Denis-Browne component of the splint.

no value. Rotation osteotomy of the femur is not necessary for simple internal femoral torsion in the growing child. Wedge and colleagues have shown that internal femoral torsion is not a cause of osteoarthritis of the hip in adults.

Toeing in caused by internal rotation contracture of the hip joint secondary to the muscle imbalance of paralytic conditions such as spina bifida, cerebral palsy, and poliomyelitis should present little difficulty in the differential diagnosis (Chapter 12).

Internal Tibial Torsion (Medial Tibial Torsion)

In young children, the most common cause of toeing in is internal tibial torsion. Examination reveals that when the knee is facing forward, the foot is turned inward (Fig. 7.18). Some degree of this deformity is present in almost all infants because of the common intrauterine position (Fig. 7.9). Normally, the internal tibial torsion corrects itself spontaneously with subsequent growth. However, if the infant adopts the habitual position of sleeping on the knees with the feet turned in (Fig. 7.19), or of sitting on top of inturned feet (Fig. 7.20), the internal tibial torsion not only fails to correct itself spontaneously but also may increase over the years.

The aim of treatment is to prevent internal torsional forces from being applied to the tibiae by training the child to avoid the aforementioned harmful positions of sleeping and sitting. When this is accomplished, the internal tibial torsion gradually corrects itself spontaneously over a period of several years. However, if the internal tibial torsion is sufficiently severe in a child older than 2 years that the child is repeatedly tripping over his or her own feet, treatment is justifiable, since it consists of simply holding the feet in external rotation in a night splint (Fig. 7.21). The mild external torsional force exerted by this splint each night gradually corrects the internal tibial torsion by influencing epiphyseal plate growth over a period of 4 to 8 months, depending on how rapidly the child is growing at the time. Straight last shoes may minimize the appearance of the toeing in, but wedges in the soles of the shoes and twister cables are of no value. Rotation osteotomy of the tibia for simple internal tibial torsion in young children is not necessary and could even be considered risky because of the associated complications.

Toeing in that results from foot deformities such as metatarsus varus (forefoot adduction) and clubfeet should be obvious, although it should be remembered that in both these conditions, there is usually an element of internal tibial torsion as well (Chapter 8).

Bow Legs (Genu Varum)

The most common cause of bow legs in children is internal torsion and varus of the tibia along with external torsion of the femur (Fig. 7.22). Thus, the common type of bow leg deformity is not simply the opposite deformity of knock knees. These combined deformities are frequently present at birth because of the intrauterine position but usually improve spontaneously. However, they may even be increased by the aforementioned habitual positions of sleeping and sitting (Figs. 7.19 and 7.20).

In more severe degrees of persistent genu varum in children older than 2 years of age, it may be necessary to use a specially designed night splint to correct the varus element in the tibia, while the opposing torsional deformities in the femora are allowed to correct them-

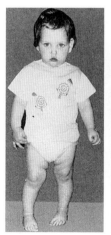
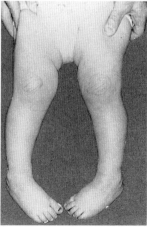

Figure 7.18.   This figure shows internal tibial torsion. When the knee is facing forward, the foot is turned inward.

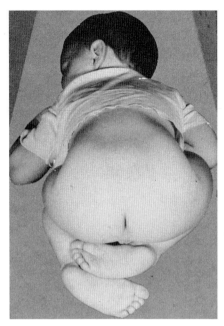
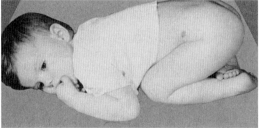

Figure 7.19.   This sleeping position with the feet turned in and underneath the infant applies further torsional force to the tibiae and not only prevents spontaneous correction of the internal tibial torsion but also aggravates it.

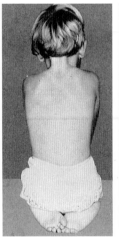
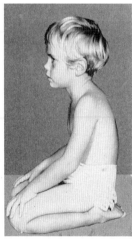
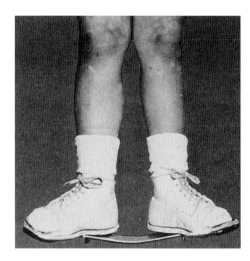

Figure 7.20.   This sitting position with the feet turned in and underneath the girl applies further torsional force to the tibiae, preventing spontaneous correction of the internal tibial torsion and perhaps actually aggravating it.

Figure 7.21.   A Denis-Browne night splint with the feet externally rotated applies a mild external torsional force to the growing tibiae and gradually corrects internal tibial torsion over a period of 4 to 8 months.

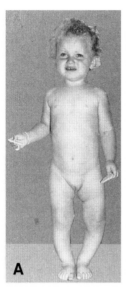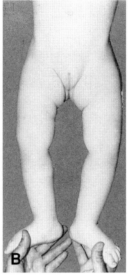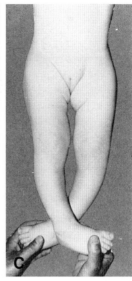

Figure 7.22. **A.** Bow legs (genu varum) caused by a combination of internal torsion and varus of the tibia along with external torsion of the femur in a 2-year-old girl. **B and C.** Passive rotation of the extended limbs outward and inward reveals the combination of torsional deformities responsible for the appearance of bow legs.

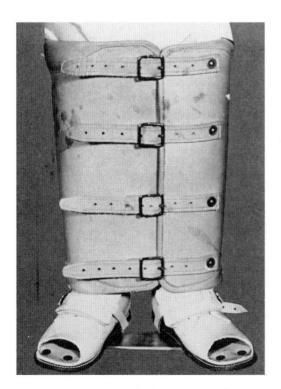

Figure 7.23. This specially designed corrective splint for children older than 2 years of age is used at night to influence epiphyseal plate growth and thereby correct the genu varum.

selves spontaneously (Fig. 7.23). Day braces for bow legs are ineffectual, and osteotomy of the tibia is not necessary for this physiological type of bow legs in young children.

The marked bow leg deformities associated with the various types of rickets (Chapter 9), tibia vara (Chapter 13), and epiphyseal plate injuries (Chapter 16) are readily differentiated from the common type of bow legs by radiographic examination.

NORMAL VARIATIONS IN ADULTS

The normal variations of joint laxity and torsional deformities just described in children may, if severe and untreated, persist into adult life, in which case they can no longer be considered within the normal range for adults. Indeed, the more severe degrees of residual flat feet, knock knees, and bow legs, although relatively rare in adults, may produce symptoms because of premature degenerative changes in the associated joints.

Normal Aging Process in the Musculoskeletal System

As individuals grow older, many changes gradually take place in their tissues as part of the aging process, changes that are as normal

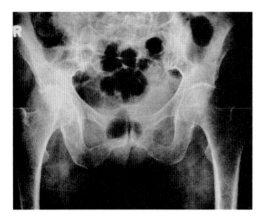

Figure 7.24. Generalized osteoporosis seen in the pelvis and femora of a 76-year-old woman. In this condition, the femoral necks are weak and particularly susceptible to fracture with minimal trauma.

as graying of the hair and wrinkling of the skin. Changes of normal aging in the musculoskeletal system include a gradual decrease in muscle strength and a gradual decrease in joint mo-

tion. Synovial joints normally "last a lifetime" in spite of gradual thinning of articular cartilage. Chondromalacia (softening of cartilage), however, is seen to some extent in the patella of almost all adults older than 30 years of age. In addition, there is a gradual decrease in the water content of the intervertebral discs, with resultant narrowing of the disc spaces and, in turn, a gradual decrease in body height during the later decades of adult life.

In the senior years, particularly in women, there is always some degree of generalized osteoporosis, with resultant weakening of bone (Fig. 7.24). This type of "senile" osteoporosis renders certain areas of the skeleton, such as the spine, the femoral neck, and the distal radius especially susceptible to fracture from minor injury. Osteoporotic cancellous bone in the vertebral bodies may gradually become deformed over the years even without an obvious fracture, thereby producing the familiar "round back" or dorsal kyphosis of the elderly (Fig. 7.25).

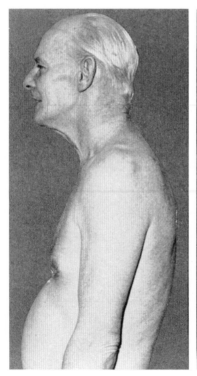
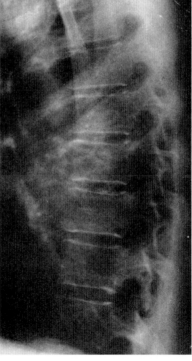

Figure 7.25. Dorsal kyphosis (round back) associated with osteoporosis of the spine in a 61-year-old man. Note the generalized rarefaction of the vertebral bodies.

It is important that you learn to distinguish the normal (physiological) from the abnormal (pathological) for each age of human development so that you may deal with them intelligently. The pathological degrees of osteoporosis are considered in Chapter 9.

SUGGESTED ADDITIONAL READING

Benson MKD, Fixen JA, Macnichol MF. Children's orthopaedics and fractures. Edinburgh: Churchill Livingstone, 1994.

Lloyd-Roberts GC, Fixen JA. Orthopaedics in infancy and childhood. 2nd ed. London: Butterworth-Heinemann, 1990.

Morrissy RT, Weinstein SL. Lovell and Winter's pediatric orthopaedics. 4th ed. Philadelphia: Lippincott-Raven, 1996.

Staheli LT. Fundamentals of pediatric orthopedics. New York: Raven Press, 1992.

Wedge JH, Munkaski I, Lobak D. Anteversion of the femur and idiopathic osteoarthritis of the hip. J Bone Joint Surg 1989;71A:1040.

Wenger DR, Rang M. The art and practice of children's orthopaedics. New York: Raven Press, 1993.

Williams PF, Cole WG. Orthopaedic management in childhood. 2nd ed. London: Chapman and Hall, 1991.

8 Congenital Abnormalities

"When I look upon a child I am filled with admiration—not so much for what that child is today as for what it may become"
—Louis Pasteur

GENERAL FEATURES
Definition and Variety

Congenital abnormalities may be defined as defects in the development of body form or function that are present *at the time of birth.* When you consider the remarkable speed and complexity of the embryonic development of the human, as discussed in Chapter 2, it is hardly surprising that some children are born with a congenital abnormality; indeed, what is surprising is that the vast majority of children are perfectly normal at birth.

The congenital musculoskeletal abnormalities vary greatly, both in extent and severity. They may be *localized,* as in a single clubfoot, or *generalized,* as in osteogenesis imperfecta (fragile bones). Furthermore, a clubfoot, for example, may be a mild and readily correctable deformity, or it may be a severe deformity that is resistant to simple methods of treatment; in either case, the deformity is easily detected at birth. Osteogenesis imperfecta may be mild and not clinically detectable at birth—indeed it may not be detected until several years after birth when the affected child sustains the first pathological fracture—or it may be so severe that pathological fractures have occurred even before birth.

Incidence

The exact incidence of congenital abnormalities is understandably difficult to determine, not only because some of the abnormalities are not detectable at birth, and therefore not reported at that time, but also because of the indefinite borderline between minor abnormalities and normal variations. Even large surveys differ, but the incidence of abnormalities detectable at birth (including stillbirths) is approximately 3%, whereas the incidence of ab-

normalities detectable at 1 year of age is approximately 6%. Significant congenital abnormalities of the musculoskeletal system are common, being exceeded in frequency only by those of the central nervous system and cardiovascular system. Furthermore, the presence of one congenital abnormality should always make you search diligently for others because it is not unusual for two, or even more, abnormalities to coexist in a given child.

Etiological Factors

Congenital abnormalities may be caused by a variety of factors, including genetic defects or environmental influences, or a combination of the two. A brief review of these factors should prove helpful to you at this stage.

Genetic Defects

In the nucleus of human cells, there are 23 pairs of *chromosomes,* and of these, 22 pairs (44 chromosomes) are called *autosomes* in which the two members of each pair are alike. The 23rd pair of chromosomes, unlike the rest, differ in males and females and, accordingly, are called *sex chromosomes.* In this pair of chromosomes, the female has two similar X chromosomes (XX), whereas the male has one X chromosome and a smaller Y chromosome (XY). The estimated 100,000 genes of each cell nucleus are located on the various pairs of chromosomes and are also paired. In these gene pairs, (*alleles* or *allelomorphs*), one gene is inherited from the *father* and one gene is inherited from the *mother.* If the two genes of a pair are alike, the individual is *homozygous;* if they are different, he or she is *heterozygous.*

Genetic defects may be inherited from either parent, or from a more remote ancestor, or they may appear for the first time in a given family as the result of a fresh *mutation,* either in a chromosome or in one of its genes. The *pattern of inheritance* of abnormalities depends on whether the abnormal gene is *dominant* (dominates the normal gene of the pair and is therefore expressed in heterozygotes) or *recessive* (is dominated by the normal gene of the pair and is therefore expressed only in homozygotes) and also on whether the gene locus concerned is *autosomal* or *sex-linked (X-linked)*.

An individual who carries one abnormal *autosomal dominant gene* and a normal gene as the allele (other member of the pair) will exhibit the abnormality; although this gene pair is *heterozygous,* the abnormal gene dominates the normal gene. When the individual mates with a normal individual, the chances of their children exhibiting the abnormality are one in two; thus, half the children (on average) will be affected. Osteogenesis imperfecta is an example of a congenital abnormality that is transmitted by an autosomal dominant gene.

In the case of an *autosomal recessive gene,* the abnormality is exhibited only in individuals in whom *both* genes of the pair have the same abnormality and are therefore homozygous (there being no normal gene by which the recessive gene can be dominated). When these gene pairs in each parent are heterozygous and the parents therefore are each *carriers* of the recessive gene but do not exhibit the abnormality, a child must inherit the abnormal recessive gene from *both* parents and so have a *homozygous* gene pair to exhibit the abnormality. The chances of the abnormality appearing in the children are one in four; thus, a quarter of the children (on average) will be affected. Sprengel's deformity of the shoulder (undescended scapula) is an example of a congenital abnormality that is transmitted by an autosomal recessive gene.

Most sex-linked (X-linked) congenital abnormalities are caused by recessive genes carried on the X chromosome. A male (XY) who carries the abnormal *recessive* gene on the X chromosome exhibits the abnormality even though the gene is recessive because it is not counterbalanced (dominated) by a normal al-

lele (there being only one X chromosome). A female (XX) who carries the abnormal recessive gene on the X chromosome, however, is normal because the expression of the abnormal recessive gene is counterbalanced (dominated) by a normal allele on the other X chromosome of the pair. Nevertheless, such a female is a carrier. The abnormal gene is transmitted by a carrier mother to half of her sons (who will exhibit the abnormality) and to half of her daughters (who will be normal but will also be carriers). An affected father who carries the abnormal gene on the X chromosome will produce normal sons because he contributes only the Y chromosome (of the XY pair) to his sons. However, his daughters, to whom he has contributed the X chromosome, will all be carriers and therefore capable of transmitting the abnormality to their sons. Hemophilia, one of the bleeding diseases, is an example of a congenital abnormality that is transmitted by a sex-linked (X-linked) recessive gene; hypophosphatasia exemplifies an abnormality that is transmitted by a sex-linked (X-linked) dominant gene.

The Genetic Revolution

The era of genetic medicine is well established; furthermore, it is expanding extremely rapidly to produce a genetic revolution. As a result, it is now well known that many diseases (such as cancer, heart disease, and Alzheimer's disease) that were previously not thought to have a genetic origin are, in fact, caused entirely or partly by defective genes that have been either inherited from a parent or have been irreversibly changed by a mutation in the somatic cells. Coming to understand the genes and their encoded proteins in a specific disease will elucidate, in molecular detail, the underlying biological processes of that disease. In due course this type of new knowledge could lead to the prevention, prediction, diagnosis, treatment and, possibly, even the cure of many genetically determined diseases.

This era of genetic medicine has stimulated the origination of the International Human Genome Project, the genome being defined as the complete genetic material of an individual. This project, which has been described as biology's equivalent of the "moonshot," is a

$3 billion attempt by scientists in many research laboratories around the world to sequence the entire human genome. It has also been referred to as the most important organized scientific endeavour ever undertaken by the human race! This stunningly exciting collaborative project will identify and characterize each of the estimated 100,000 genes (consisting of 7 billion base pairs of DNA) that constitute the complete genome of a human being and will determine the amino acid sequence and eventually the structure and function of the 50,000 to 100,000 proteins that are encoded in the genes.

As you can imagine, the current and future discoveries of genetics, gene therapy (delivering normal genes into target cells), and genetic engineering will definitely have a major impact on the practice of medicine. At the same time, these discoveries will raise many relevant ethical, social, and legal issues, including the confidentiality of an individual's genetic information as opposed to the potential availability of such information to insurance companies and possible employers.

Environmental Influences

Harmful environmental influences may alter the germ cells of either parent before fertilization takes place, or they may alter the normal development of the child during intrauterine life. Many experimental investigations in animals have shown that the effects of various harmful environmental influences are nonspecific in that several such influences are capable of producing the same congenital abnormality. Furthermore, the *type* of abnormality produced, as well as its *severity,* depends on the *timing* of the environmental influence in relation to the *precise stage of embryonic development.* Although experiments have shown that many environmental factors can produce congenital abnormalities in animals (*experimental teratogenesis*), the teratogenic effect of relatively few such factors has been proved in the human. Two definitely teratogenic factors in the human are maternal infection with the *rubella* virus (German measles) and maternal ingestion of the drug *thalidomide* (a tranquilizer), both of which exert their devastating effects during the critical first 3 months of preg-

nancy. The *severity* of the resultant abnormality is related to the precise stage of embryonic development at the time of the harmful influence. For example, during the very early development of the limb buds, thalidomide may arrest the entire process, with the result that all four limbs are grossly deficient at birth. If the drug is taken at a later stage when the limbs are more completely formed, the resultant defect may be limited to only part of a limb, such as an absence of the radius. The tragic experience with thalidomide in many countries during the late 1950s has served to emphasize the importance of drugs as potential teratogenic agents; this group of congenital abnormalities, at least, should be preventable.

Combination of Genetic Defects and Environmental Influences

Experimental teratogenesis in animals, as well as clinical observations in identical (monozygous) human twins, suggests that some congenital abnormalities occur because of a genetically determined susceptibility to a harmful environmental influence. For example, in congenital dislocation (developmental displacement, or dysplasia) of the hip, it is felt that a genetically determined abnormal degree of hip joint laxity may render such a hip joint particularly susceptible to the harmful environmental influence of the sudden change from the intrauterine position of hyperflexion to the position of extension (by passive movement) at the time of birth; thus, a hip joint that genetically was only lax and prone to dislocation may, in fact, become dislocated.

Types of Congenital Musculoskeletal Abnormalities

Localized Abnormalities

All localized congenital abnormalities of the skeleton are manifestations of one or more various types of disturbances in its normal growth and development. Thus, a bone may fail to form entirely (*aplasia*); it may fail to grow to a normal size (*hypoplasia*); its growth may be abnormal (*dysplasia*); or it may overgrow (*hypertrophy or local gigantism*). Extra, or supernumerary, parts of the skeleton may form (*duplication*), as in extra digits (*polydactyly*). Skeletal development may be *arrested* at any stage during intrauterine life; for example, when the normal descent of the scapula is arrested (Sprengel's deformity) or when the normal bony closure of the posterior part of the spinal canal is arrested, as in the various degrees of spina bifida (neural tube defect).

Localized congenital abnormalities of joints include those in which a joint is either merely *unstable* or actually *dislocated,* as in congenital dislocation (developmental displacement, or dysplasia) of the hip; those in which a joint has failed to form (*failure of segmentation*), as in congenital radioulnar synostosis; and those in which a resistant contracture of one or more joints is present at birth, as in a congenital clubfoot.

Generalized Abnormalities

Generalized congenital abnormalities can involve many parts of the musculoskeletal system and include developmental defects of epiphyseal plate growth, as in achondroplasia; congenital imbalance between bone deposition and bone resorption, as in osteogenesis imperfecta; and inborn errors of metabolism, as in certain types of refractory rickets. In addition, all joints of the body may be unduly *hypermobile* (congenital generalized joint laxity), or they may be unduly *rigid,* as in amyoplasia congenita (arthrogryposis).

Diagnosis of Congenital Abnormalities

Antenatal Diagnosis

The rapidly developing field of fetal medicine deals with the antenatal diagnosis, selective treatment, and perinatal management of an increasing number of fetal abnormalities. Its greatest impetus has come from the introduction and widespread availability of high-resolution real-time ultrasound. In expert hands under ultrasonographic guidance, most fetal tissues can now be sampled safely and used for a host of cytogenetic, biochemical, hematologic, and DNA studies. Thus, it is now possible to diagnose a wide range of conditions from chromosomal abnormalities (e.g., Down's syndrome) to structural anomalies

(e.g., spina bifida or neural tube defects [NTDs]) to inborn errors of metabolism (e.g., the mucopolysaccharidoses). Consequently, a completely new dimension has been added to genetic counseling.

NTDs, such as meningomyelocele or myelocele, are good examples of congenital abnormalities that are amenable to antenatal diagnosis. When a fetus has an open NTD, the maternal serum alpha fetoprotein (MSAFP) level is elevated, and this is used as a screening test. A raised MSAFP level should prompt a meticulous, detailed ultrasonographic evaluation of the fetal anatomy; such an evaluation can identify 95% of NTDs as well as most other fetal causes for an elevated MSAFP level. Rarely, it may be necessary to resort to amniocentesis to confirm this diagnosis, and both α-fetoprotein and acetylcholinesterase can be measured in the amniotic fluid. A woman considered at high risk of carrying a fetus with an NTD might be taking anticonvulsants or may have an affected close relative—a parent, sibling, or previous child—in which case the risk of recurrence is 2 to 5%.

Other musculoskeletal abnormalities that are amenable to antenatal diagnosis include achondroplasia, osteogenesis imperfecta, and amyoplasia congenita (arthrogryposis), all of which are discussed in subsequent sections of this chapter.

Once the diagnosis of a serious congenital abnormality has been established, the parents must be counseled as to the findings, their implications, and the full range of options and services available to them, including those of additional pregnancy support, termination, (i.e., abortion), and, when appropriate, fetal therapy. The ongoing development of new techniques for antenatal diagnosis and treatment understandably will continue to raise a number of controversial moral and ethical issues.

Postnatal Diagnosis

The responsibility for the early postnatal diagnosis of congenital abnormalities is shared by the family physician, obstetrician, and pediatrician who first see the child. Some abnormalities, such as clubfeet, are so obvious at birth that their recognition presents no difficulty.

Others, however, such as congenital dislocation (developmental displacement, or dysplasia) of the hip are not at all obvious at birth and are detected only by careful and specific methods of examination. You may be surprised to learn that this serious and potentially crippling condition is one of the most frequently undetected congenital abnormalities in the newborn period simply because of the failure on the part of the attending physician to examine the infant specifically for it. Still other congenital abnormalities are not detectable at birth but can and should be diagnosed at the time of their first clinical manifestation. Failure to recognize a congenital abnormality at the earliest possible time is an injustice, not only to the unfortunate child but also to his or her devoted parents.

Principles and Methods of Treatment

Most of the localized congenital musculoskeletal abnormalities are compatible with longevity and, therefore, their total care demands farsighted planning, skillful orthopaedic treatment, and prolonged supervision because the results must last a lifetime. At this time, you may wish to review the general principles and specific methods of musculoskeletal treatment discussed in Chapter 6, because they are as applicable to congenital abnormalities as they are to acquired disorders and injuries.

A knowledge of the *significance* and *prognosis* of a given congenital musculoskeletal abnormality is essential in relation to its treatment. Many localized abnormalities involving joints, such as congenital clubfoot and congenital dislocation (developmental displacement, or dysplasia) of the hip, become progressively more difficult to treat as time goes on because of progressive secondary changes in the involved joints and surrounding muscles. For these conditions, early recognition and early treatment are mandatory to obtain the most satisfactory results. Other abnormalities, such as single hemivertebra, have a reasonably good prognosis in that significant curvature of the spine (scoliosis) is unlikely to develop with subsequent spinal growth. By contrast, asymmetrical fusion (failure of segmentation) on one side of the spine always leads to progressive scoliosis with growth and therefore requires early treatment.

The parents of a child who is afflicted with a congenital abnormality need kindly and considerate counseling so that needless and harmful feelings of *guilt* and *negative self-pity* may be replaced by the more *positive* and helpful attitudes of *acceptance* of the problem and *cooperation* with its treatment. These parents are anxious and, indeed, entitled to know something of the prognosis, particularly with respect to the anticipated future appearance and function of the involved part as their child grows and reaches adult life. In addition, a geneticist can be of considerable help to parents who are concerned about the likelihood of a similar abnormality occurring in their subsequent children as well as in their children's children.

LOCALIZED CONGENITAL ABNORMALITIES OF THE LOWER LIMB
The Foot
Toe Deformities

Congenital overriding of the fifth toe, which results from a dorsal subluxation of the metatarsophalangeal joint, is associated with a shortened extensor tendon and tightness of the overlying skin (Fig. 8.1A). Irritation of the dorsally displaced toe (by shoes) justifies operative correction of the deformity by Z-plasty of the skin, tenotomy of the extensor tendon, and dorsal capsulotomy of the joint.

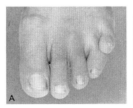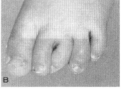

Figure 8.1.   A. This figure shows congenital overriding of the fifth toe. Surgical repositioning relieved the discomfort of pressure from shoes. **B.** Congenital varus deformity of the third toe is seen in this figure. The child had no symptoms and did not require treatment of the deformity.

Congenital varus of the small toes (curly toes) is common, particularly in the third toe (Fig. 8.1**B**). The end of the curved toe tends to lie under its medial neighbor but almost never causes discomfort. Strapping is ineffectual, and operative treatment is seldom necessary because the deformity usually corrects itself spontaneously.

Metatarsus Primus Varus

A varus, or adduction, deformity of the first (prime) metatarsal in relation to the other four metatarsals is designated *metatarsus primus varus*. The medial border of the forefoot is curved inward, and there is a wide space between the first and second toes (Fig. 8.2). If treated early by the application of a series of corrective plaster casts, the deformity is readily overcome. Unfortunately, this relatively mild

deformity is frequently overlooked for several years during which time the pressure of shoes gradually pushes the first toe (hallux) laterally, thereby, producing the secondary deformity of *adolescent hallux valgus* (Fig. 8.3). When hallux valgus develops during adolescence, it is usually progressive; because the prognosis is poor, the deformity should be corrected by a soft tissue procedure around the metatarsophalangeal joint combined with corrective osteotomy at the base of the medially deviated first metatarsal.

Metatarsus Adductus (Metatarsus Varus)

An adduction, or varus, deviation of all five metatarsals in relation to the hindfoot causes the foot to have a concave inner border and a convex outer border, especially when it is held in a weightbearing position (Fig. 8.4). This congenital abnormality, which is relatively common (2 in 1000 live births), is referred to as either *metatarsus adductus* or *metatarsus varus*, although the former is more accurate. In addition to the adduction of the forefoot, there may be supination of the fore-

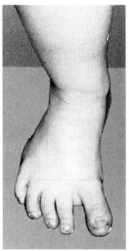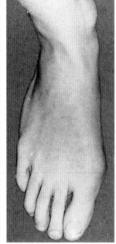

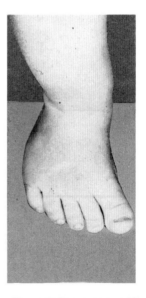

Figure 8.2. Left. Congenital metatarsus primus varus in a 3-year-old girl is seen. Note the inward curve of the medial border of the foot and the increased space between the first and second toes because of medial deviation of the first metatarsal. This deformity should be corrected early in life to prevent the development of adolescent hallux valgus.

Figure 8.3. Right. This figure demonstrates adolescent hallux valgus in a 13-year-old girl. In the presence of an underlying metatarsus primus varus, pressure from footwear has gradually produced a valgus deformity at the metatarsophalangeal joint (hallux valgus). When this deformity develops during adolescence, it tends to be progressive and should be corrected surgically.

Figure 8.4. Congenital metatarsus adductus (metatarsus varus) in a 3-month-old child is seen. The whole forefoot is deviated medially (adducted) and supinated, but the hindfoot is normal. There is frequently an associated internal tibial torsion. This child's deformity was corrected by a series of plaster casts over a period of 3 months, and the correction was maintained by the use of a Denis Browne night splint.

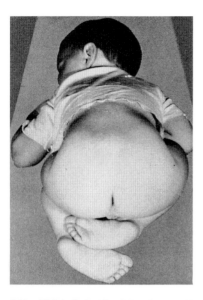

Figure 8.5. This is the habitual sleeping position with the feet curled in. This position tends to aggravate metatarsus adductus and the associated internal tibial torsion.

foot as well as internal tibial torsion. The neutral position of the heel, and hence the subtalar joint, and the normal range of motion in the ankle joint distinguish metatarsus adductus from the much more serious congenital abnormality clubfoot (which is described in the next section). Three grades of severity of metatarsus adductus (mild, moderate, and severe) are determined by the degree of flexibility of the deformity and, conversely, its resistance to correction during the initial assessment. The prognosis depends on the grade of severity.

The hip joints of these infants should be examined carefully because of an associated 2% incidence of congenital dislocation (developmental displacement, or dysplasia) of the hip.

In most children, the forefoot deformity is both mild, (i.e., flexible) and not resistant, in which case the prognosis is good with or without simple stretching by the parent and the avoidance of sleeping face down with the feet curled in (Fig. 8.5). When the deformity is more marked and rigid or resistant (as it is in approximately 20% of affected infants), the prognosis is not as good, and treatment should be started at least within the first few weeks of life. It is regrettable that metatarsus adductus of the resistant type frequently escapes detection for several months, or even longer, because the deformity becomes progressively resistant with each passing month. *Treatment* involves the careful application of a series of plaster casts in which the heel is maintained in the neutral position and the forefoot is molded into abduction and pronation. The casts are changed every 2 weeks, and the duration of cast treatment varies from 6 to 12 weeks, depending on the resistance to correction. A Denis Browne type of boot splint is then applied nightly for a few months, not only to maintain correction but also to overcome the associated internal tibial torsion (Fig. 8.6). An alternative device to maintain correction is a specially designed plastic ankle-foot orthosis known as a Wheaton brace.

Untreated congenital metatarsus adductus in a child older than 2 years of age may require a soft tissue releasing operation and, if the child has reached the age of 4 years without correction, it may be necessary to perform an osteotomy at the base of each metatarsal.

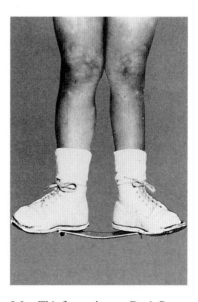

Figure 8.6. This figure shows a Denis Browne night splint, which is used following plaster cast correction of metatarsus adductus to maintain the correction and also to overcome the internal tibial torsion.

Clubfoot (Talipes Equinovarus)

The most important congenital abnormality of the foot is *clubfoot* or *talipes equinovarus,* a deformity that is easy to diagnose but difficult to correct completely, even in the hands of an experienced orthopaedic surgeon. A congenital clubfoot consists of a combination of deformities, including forefoot adduction and supination through the midtarsal joint, heel varus through the subtalar joint, equinus through the ankle joint, and medial deviation of the whole foot in relation to the knee (Fig. 8.7). The medial deviation of the foot results partly from an angulation in the neck of the talus and partly from internal tibial torsion. The degree of severity of the deformity, which may be mild, moderate, or severe, is better assessed by its feel of flexibility or, conversely, of rigidity or resistance to correction than by its appearance.

Incidence. Congenital clubfoot is common (incidence of 2 in 1000 live births), is bilateral in half of the afflicted children, and affects boys twice as often as girls. A genetic factor would seem to be responsible in about 10% of the children, but in the remainder the abnormality appears to be caused by an initial mutation in the family tree. However, if one parent and one child have clubfeet, the chances of a subsequent child being so afflicted is one in four.

Etiology and Pathology. The cause of congenital clubfoot remains one of the many unsolved puzzles of the musculoskeletal system, although the ultrastructural and histochemical studies of Handelsman suggest a neuromuscular cause. The deformity is known to exist from the early stages of embryonic development when the foot first begins to form. The muscles on the posterior and medial aspect of the leg (particularly the calf muscle and the tibialis posterior) are unduly short and, in addition, the fibrous capsules of all the deformed joints are thick and contracted on the concave side of the deformity. These soft tissue contractures become progressively resistant to correction as the weeks go by—both before and after birth—and lead to *secondary* changes, not only in the shape of the actively growing bones but also in the involved joints. An appreciation of this observation should serve to emphasize the tremendous importance of early treatment. The pathological anatomy of clubfoot (as well as its surgical correction) is well described by Carroll.

Diagnosis. Although the typical clubfoot of moderate severity is easily diagnosed, the *mild* clubfoot must be distinguished from *positional equinovarus,* which results simply from intrauterine position and can therefore be readily corrected to a normal position. The *severe true* clubfoot must be differentiated from the less common, but more troublesome, teratologic type of severe clubfoot deformity associated with either *spina bifida* or *arthrogryposis* (amyoplasia congenita).

Treatment. One of your responsibilities is to reassure the anxious parents at the outset that with early and expert treatment, their child will not be "crippled"—rather that he or she will be able to enjoy a normal life, including sports, both as a child and as an adult. The general principles of treatment, which should be applied early—at least within the

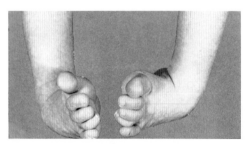
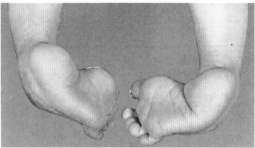

Figure 8.7. Congenital clubfeet (talipes equinovarus) in a newborn infant is seen in this figure. Note the forefoot adduction and supination, the heel varus, the ankle equinus, and the internal tibial torsion. The deformities of this infant's feet were assessed as moderately severe on the basis of the feel of resistance to passive correction.

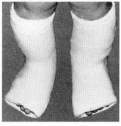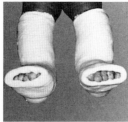

Figure 8.8. Carefully molded plaster casts are used for the initial correction of clubfeet. The skin has been painted with tincture of benzoin (Friar's balsam) and covered by a bandage before the cast is applied to prevent the child from kicking the cast off. These casts are changed at weekly intervals, and at the time of each change, further correction is obtained.

first few days of life—include gentle passive correction of the deformities, maintenance of correction for a long period, and supervision of the child until the end of growth. Even after full correction of a clubfoot, the apparent failure of the contracted soft tissues to grow adequately in length tends to produce some degree of limited motion in about half of the children; furthermore, possible recurrence of deformity should be watched for and treated, particularly during periods of rapid skeletal growth. Consequently, these children should be seen at regular intervals until they have reached skeletal maturity.

The specific methods of treatment of clubfoot vary considerably, but the following general plan of treatment, which has proved extremely satisfactory, is suggested for the average clubfoot seen within the first month of life. Nevertheless, it must be remembered that the treatment of an individual clubfoot must be tailored to fit the needs of that particular foot.

1. Plaster casts are applied weekly (following gentle and progressive correction of the deformities in the aforementioned order). This phase of treatment requires about 6 weeks (Fig. 8.8).
2. Cast treatment may then be continued or the feet may be strapped to a Denis Browne type of clubfoot splint by adhesive tape. The affected foot is progressively turned outward and into valgus (Fig. 8.9).

The adhesive is changed weekly for about 8 weeks and, during this phase of treatment, correction of the deformity is maintained while some movement is allowed in the involved joints.

3. Either a Denis Browne type of boot splint or an articulated ankle-foot orthosis (AFO) is to be worn day and night (and removed only for bathing) during the ensuing 3 months, following which it is left off for longer and longer periods until the child is walking (Fig. 8.10). It is most important that the splint be used at night for at least another year or longer to decrease the chances of recurrence.
4. Straight last or outflare boots are used for day wear until the child is 3 years of age; occasionally an outside sole wedge is added. Approximately 40% of congenital clubfeet treated early by these nonoperative methods will have responded satisfactorily within the first 3 to 4 months of treatment. Assessment of the completeness of correction of all components of the clubfoot deformity requires specific radiographic examinations.

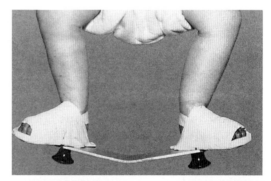

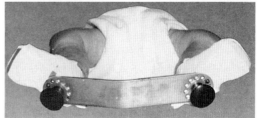

Figure 8.9. A Denis Browne clubfoot adhesive splint is shown. This exercise splint maintains correction of the deformity while allowing movement in the involved joints.

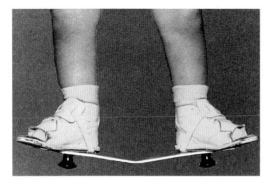

Figure 8.10.   This is a Denis Browne clubfoot boot splint. This removable splint is worn at night for at least 1 year, and usually longer, after correction of the clubfoot. It is the best type of prevention of recurrence of the deformity.

The remaining 60% of congenital clubfeet are *resistant* to these methods and consequently, under these circumstances, continuation of nonoperative treatment leads to eventual failure, either because of persistent incomplete correction or recurrence of the deformity. Immobilization of an incompletely corrected clubfoot in a forced position in a cast can even cause the iatrogenic lesion of *pressure necrosis* of joint cartilage as described in Chapter 3. In such resistant clubfeet, it is better judgment to perform a meticulous soft tissue correction of all tendon and joint contractures at 4 to 6 months for *resistance* rather than to delay surgical treatment and be forced to perform a major operation at a later date for *recurrence,* at which time the results are less satisfactory. Following this type of early surgery, the aforementioned nonoperative plan is resumed to maintain the correction. Even with excellent correction of the foot deformity, the child's calf will always be smaller than normal but not significantly weaker. Neglected clubfeet and recurrent clubfeet always require operative treatment, the extent of which depends on the severity of the various components of the residual deformity.

In general, soft tissue operations (such as capsulotomies, tendon lengthening, and tendon transfer) are effective in the first 5 years of life but become less effective in older children because of the increasingly abnormal shape of the bones. Thus, in the older child, bony oper-

ations (such as arthrodesis of the subtalar and midtarsal joints) are usually necessary to correct any residual deformity but are best deferred until the age of about 10 years.

The relatively recent emphasis on early complete surgical correction for *resistant* clubfeet at 3 to 4 months of age has greatly decreased the number of recurrences and has been an important factor in improving the overall results of treatment for this serious congenital abnormality.

Talipes Calcaneovalgus

At the time of birth, some children are found to have one or both feet maintained in a dorsiflexed and everted position, a condition commonly referred to as *congenital talipes calcaneovalgus* (Fig. 8.11). This mild and transient deformity of an otherwise normal foot is the result of intrauterine position rather than a true congenital abnormality of development; thus, it is comparable to positional equinovarus rather than to congenital talipes equinovarus. Daily passive stretching of the soft tissues by a parent usually produces excellent and permanent correction of the deformity; indeed, many of these feet improve spontaneously. Only the more resistant deformities require the application of one or two plaster casts.

Congenital Plantar Flexed (Vertical) Talus

Congenital plantar flexed talus is an uncommon, but serious congenital abnormality of

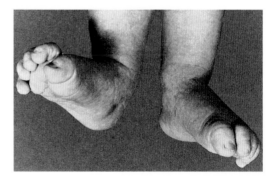

Figure 8.11.   Congenital talipes calcaneovalgus in a newborn infant is seen in this figure. Note the everted and dorsiflexed position of the foot, which is probably related to intrauterine position. This infant's foot was normal 3 months later, the only treatment having been daily stretching of the foot by the mother.

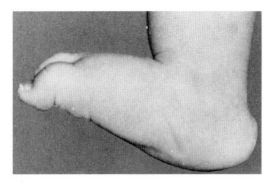

Figure 8.12. This figure demonstrates congenital plantar flexed (vertical) talus. The convex, rockerlike appearance of the sole of the foot is caused by a combination of plantar flexion of the hindfoot and dorsiflexion of the forefoot. This deformity is rigid and difficult to correct completely, even with extensive surgical operations.

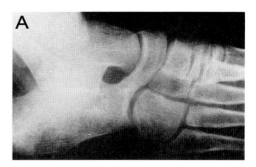

Figure 8.14. This is an oblique radiograph of a congenital calcaneonavicular bar (coalition) in the right foot of a 15-year-old boy. The abnormal bony bar joining the calcaneous to the navicular is cartilaginous in early childhood but ossifies during adolescence and blocks normal midtarsal movement.

the foot in which the talus is rigidly fixed in a position of extreme equinus, whereas the front of the foot, which is equally rigid, is dorsiflexed and everted, resulting in a sole of the foot being convex—a complete reversal of the normal longitudinal arch (Fig. 8.12). The diagnosis is confirmed by a lateral radiograph of the foot (Fig. 8.13). The condition is sometimes associated with either spina bifida or arthrogryposis. Nonoperative measures of treatment are seldom adequate, and a soft tissue releasing operation is indicated. At the first stage, the front of the foot is brought into

alignment with the plantar flexed talus by capsulotomies, and at the second stage the tight posterior tendons and joint capsules are released so that the whole foot, including the talus, can be dorsiflexed as a unit. More recently, there has been a trend toward correcting all components of the deformity in a single-stage procedure. Partial recurrence of the deformity is common and may necessitate subtalar arthrodesis in the growing child or combined subtalar and midtarsal (triple) arthrodesis in the older child.

Tarsal Coalition (Rigid Valgus Foot)

Any two of the tarsal bones in the hindfoot may be congenitally joined together by a bridge or bar (*coalition*), which at birth and in early childhood is still cartilaginous (a synchondrosis) but which in adolescence becomes ossified (a synostosis). As a result of coalitions such as *talocalcaneal bridge* and *calcaneonavicular bar*, movement in the involved tarsal joints is restricted (Fig. 8.14). The foot, which almost always goes into a position of valgus, looks flat, but unlike the hypermobile, or flexible type of flatfoot, this type of flatfoot gradually becomes both rigid and painful and is associated with secondary spasm and contracture of the peroneal muscles (it is also called *peroneal spastic flatfoot*) (Fig. 8.15). These congenital abnormalities usually pass undetected during the first 10 years of life, after which time secondary degenerative arthritis in the talonavicu-

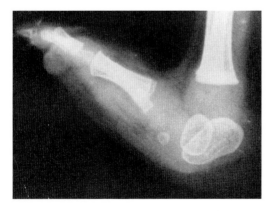

Figure 8.13. This is a lateral radiograph of the congenital plantar flexed (vertical) talus. Note the almost vertical position of the plantar flexed talus and the dorsiflexed position of the metatarsals.

lar joint produces a painful foot that causes the child to walk with a shuffling gait. Computerized tomography (CT) of the area of a suspected talocalcaneal bridge is particularly helpful in revealing this type of coalition. Nonoperative measures of treatment, such as a period of cast immobilization, are of only temporary value. Excision of the area of coalition is usually satisfactory in children who have several years of skeletal growth remaining, but for older children it is often inadequate (especially if secondary degenerative changes are present in the talonavicular joint). The most certain form of treatment for this latter group of children is combined subtalar and midtarsal (triple) arthrodesis.

Accessory Tarsal Navicular

The tarsal navicular, which is cartilaginous at birth, is sometimes congenitally larger than normal, and over the years a separate center of ossification appears within it on the medial side. This accessory bone (sometimes referred to as an os tibiale externum), into which part of the tibialis posterior tendon is inserted, is not rigidly joined to the body of the navicular and produces on the medial side of the foot a bony prominence that may become painful

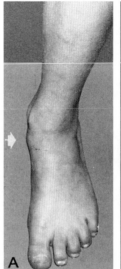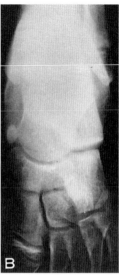

Figure 8.16. **A.** This figures demonstrates congenital accessory tarsal navicular in a 13-year-old girl's left foot. Note the bony prominence on the medial side of the foot in the region of the navicular, which was associated with local tenderness *(arrow)*. **B.** This is a congenital accessory tarsal navicular demonstrating the separate center of ossification in the abnormally large navicular to which one portion of the tibialis posterior muscle is attached. A false joint develops between the two bony parts of the navicular, and this is the site of pain. Relief of symptoms followed surgical excision of the separate center (accessory bone) along with the prominent medial portion of the navicular.

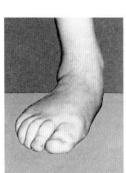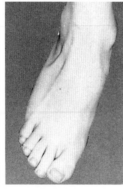

Figure 8.15. This figure shows the rigid valgus right foot (peroneal spastic flat foot) resulting from congenital calcaneonavicular bar in the 15-year-old boy whose radiograph is shown in Figure 8.14. Note that the foot is flat and in valgus even when not bearing weight. This boy's foot was extremely painful and required surgical treatment consisting of arthrodesis of the subtalar, talonavicular, and calcaneocuboid joints ("triple arthrodesis").

and tender in early adolescence (Fig. 8.16). If symptoms persist, it is necessary to excise the accessory bone along with the prominent portion of the navicular, preserving the deep insertion of the tibialis posterior tendon.

The Long Bones

Pseudarthrosis of the Tibia

In this rare but very serious abnormality, the tibia, which has failed to grow normally in width, becomes angulated in its lower third, resulting in an anterior bowing of the leg before birth. Thus, the infant is born with congenital prepseudarthrosis. The abnormality is often associated with neurofibromatosis. Wright and colleagues have suggested from their experimental model in the rat tibia that the underlying pathogenesis may be a constricting band of soft tissue encircling the tibia at this level. The thin, sclerotic bone at the site of angulation is

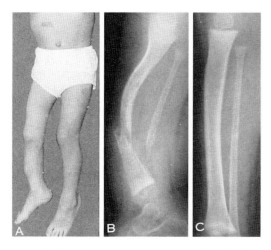

Figure 8.17. **A.** congenital pseudarthrosis of the tibia in a 2-year-old child is seen. Note the anterior angulation of the right tibia and also the area of pigmentation—a café au lait spot—on the child's abdomen and left thigh suggestive of a relationship with neurofibromatosis. **B** and **C.** Congenital pseudarthrosis of the tibia in the same child, demonstrating the pathological fracture that has failed to unite and has produced a pseudarthrosis (false joint). Note also the thin diameter of the tibia in this area compared with the normal tibia.

brittle and consequently a prepseudarthrosis should be splinted for many months, and even years, to prevent an otherwise inevitable pathological fracture from occurring in early childhood. Since the abnormal bone is avascular at this site, the fracture fails to unite and a *pseudarthrosis* (false joint) develops, with a resultant increase in the angular deformity (Fig. 8.17). Congenital pseudarthrosis of the tibia is certainly the most difficult type of nonunion confronting the orthopaedic surgeon and requires special techniques of bone grafting for its correction. Good results have been obtained from free vascularized autogenous bone grafts using the opposite fibula (performed using microsurgery) as well as from electrical stimulation. Recently, Paley and colleagues also reported good early results from the Ilizarov method of resection of the pseudarthrosis followed by distal transport of a proximal vascular segment of the involved tibia. Even a united tibia may refracture, necessitating a second operation to avoid an amputation, which, until relatively recently, was often the final method of treatment.

Hypoplasia of the Long Bones

Hypoplasia of the long bones is a rare, but very deforming congenital abnormality, which may involve the fibula, tibia, or femur. They are commonly called *congenital absence* of the particular bone. However, since some portion of the long bone, or at least of its cartilage model, is normally present at each end, the term *hypoplasia* would seem to be more appropriate. The severity of hypoplasia varies considerably.

Congenital hypoplasia of the fibula is accompanied by anterior bowing of an abnormally short tibia and a fixed equinovalgus deformity of a hypoplastic foot, the lateral portion of which is usually deficient (Fig. 8.18). Soft tissue operations are helpful in partially correcting the resistant foot deformity, but a large, ugly, built-up foot and brace are usually required because of the shape of the foot and the progressive leg length discrepancy. When the foot deformity and the shortening of the limb are severe, removal of the hypoplastic foot at the ankle (a Syme's amputation) will permit the use of a prosthesis that improves both function and appearance.

Congenital hypoplasia of the tibia is a rare, but serious, defect (Fig. 8.19). Reconstructive operations seldom provide satisfactory functional or cosmetic results, and hence amputation through the knee (disarticulation) is usually indicated, following which the child is provided with a suitable prosthetic limb.

Congenital hypoplasia of the femur varies greatly in degree but is usually severe, with resultant extreme shortening of the lower limb (Fig. 8.20). When the leg length discrepancy is marked, a built-up boot is inadequate and should be replaced by a prosthesis that may or may not have to be preceded by reconstructive bony operations.

The Knee

Dislocation of the Knee

Dislocation of the knee is an uncommon congenital abnormality and is often a manifestation of arthrogryposis. It consists of an anterior dislocation of the knee joint (Fig. 8.21). The dislocated knee, which is hyperextended and abducted, frequently requires operative reduction and lengthening of the contracted

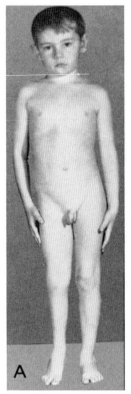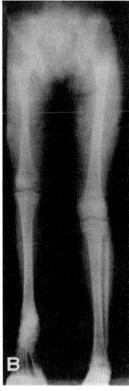

Figure 8.18.   A. This is congenital hypoplasia of the fibula in an 8-year-old boy showing the short leg (resulting from associated angulation and shortening of the tibia) and the equinovalgus deformity of the foot. This boy is attempting to compensate for the shortening by standing on tiptoe and lowering the pelvis on the short side. **B.** Congenital hypoplasia of the fibula is seen. Note the absence of ossification in the fibula and the shortening of the tibia as well as of the femur.

capsule and muscles on the anterior aspect of the knee. More commonly, congenital hyperextension of the knee (genu recurvatum) without dislocation is seen in otherwise normal infants; this less serious abnormality is usually amenable to nonoperative methods of treatment involving a series of plaster casts.

Dislocation of the Patella

The dislocation of a patella, which itself is hypoplastic, is lateral and can occur either with or without congenital dislocation of the knee. An early reconstructive soft tissue operation involving the quadriceps mechanism is indicated.

Discoid Lateral Meniscus

In this isolated abnormality, the lateral meniscus (semilunar cartilage) is thicker than normal, somewhat disc-shaped, and lacks adequate peripheral attachment posteriorly. As the child's knee extends, the thick meniscus is suddenly pushed forward and the femoral condyle rides over it, pushing it suddenly backward and accounting for the loud "clunk" that occurs during extension of the knee and that can be heard across a room. The diagnosis can be confirmed either by arthrography or magnetic resonance imaging (MRI). The discoid meniscus usually produces pain in early childhood, in which case it should be surgically "sculpted" to a more normal shape. Only if its inadequate peripheral attachment is irreparable should a discoid meniscus be totally excised because such an excision inevitably leads to degenerative arthritis of the lateral compartment of the knee in adult life.

The Hip

Developmental Coxa Vara

In developmental coxa vara, a localized congenital defect of ossification in the femoral neck results in the gradual development of a progressive varus deformity in the upper end of the femur (*coxa vara*) over the years (Fig. 8.22). For this reason, the coxa vara is usually referred to as *developmental* rather than congenital. The clinical examination reveals mild shortening of the lower limb and limitation of passive abduction of the hip. A positive Trendelenburg sign develops because the distance from the greater trochanter to the iliac crest is less than normal and the efficiency of the hip abductor muscles is consequently decreased. (The Trendelenburg sign is described in the next section.) Accordingly, the child walks with a painless Trendelenburg, or lurching, type of limp. There would seem to be some relationship between developmental coxa vara and congenital hypoplasia of the femur because in the former, the femoral shaft is frequently short, and in the latter, there is always a coexistent and severe coxa vara. The most effective treatment for developmental coxa vara is an abduction (valgus) subtrochanteric osteotomy of the femur, which not only corrects the adduction, or varus deformity, but

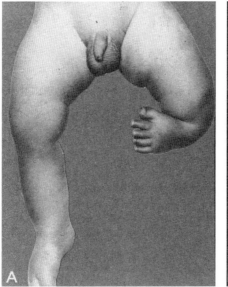
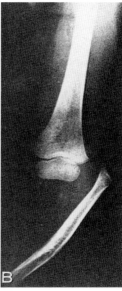

Figure 8.19. **A.** Congenital hypoplasia of the tibia in an infant is seen. The tibia is absent and the fibula is short. Thus there is neither a knee joint nor an ankle joint. This rare but serious anomaly is usually best treated by amputation through the site of the knee joint (disarticulation) and provision of a prosthesis. **B.** Congenital hypoplasia of the tibia is seen. Note the absence of the tibia and the marked shortening of the fibula.

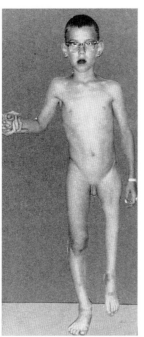
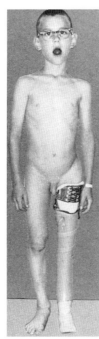
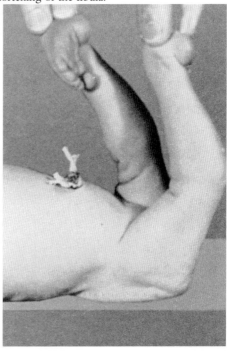

Figure 8.20. Congenital hypoplasia of the left femur in a 9-year-old boy is seen. Note the marked shortening of the lower limb, which is best managed by a suitable prosthesis preceded, when necessary, by a reconstructive bony operation. In this boy, amputation of the foot was not necessary.

Figure 8.21. This figure shows congenital dislocation of the knees in a newborn infant, demonstrating the severe hyperextension deformity. In this infant, surgical lengthening of the quadriceps muscles was required to reduce the dislocation. Note also the bilateral clubfeet.

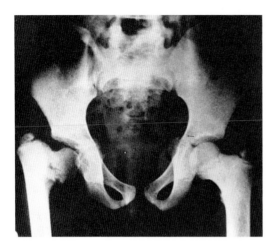

Figure 8.22.   Congenital (developmental) coxa vara of the right hip in a 10-year-old boy is seen. Note the defect of ossification in the right femoral neck, which has allowed a progressive varus deformity. The boy walked with a Trendelenburg type of limp on the right side. Following abduction subtrochanteric osteotomy of the right femur, the femoral neck defect ossified and the boy's gait became normal.

also encourages ossification of the defect in the femoral neck. The operation is most effective if performed before a marked varus deformity has developed.

Dislocation and Subluxation of the Hip (Developmental Displacement of the Hip; Developmental Dysplasia of the Hip)

One of the most important and challenging congenital abnormalities of the musculoskeletal system is *congenital dislocation of the hip,* including the related abnormalities of *congenital subluxation of the hip* and *congenital dysplasia (abnormal growth) of the hip.* Although the term *congenital dislocation of the hip* and the abbreviation CDH have been widely used for centuries, the more acceptable term at present is *developmental displacement of the hip (DDH).* Klisic, in 1989, recommended this term because "it realistically indicates a dynamic disorder, potentially capable, as the baby develops, of getting better or getting worse." Furthermore, this new term reflects the documented fact that at least a small percentage of hips that by all criteria seem normal at birth may actually

become dislocated or subluxated as late as 6 to 10 months of age when the infant's hips extend to stand erect. Under these circumstances, of course, the dislocation or subluxation is not truly congenital (i.e., present at birth), and this has important medicolegal implications. Subsequently, some authors (especially in North America) have interpreted the abbreviation DDH to mean "developmental dysplasia of the hip" or even "developmental dislocation of the hip."

Developmental displacement of the hip is meant to include not only dislocation and subluxation but also the related secondary dysplasia (failure of adequate bony development of the acetabulum and the proximal femur). In this chapter, the new term *developmental displacement of the hip* (DDH) is used rather than the traditional term *congenital dislocation of the hip* (CDH), although you should appreciate that the latter term is still preferred by some.

Developmental displacement of the hip is an abnormality that is almost as common as clubfoot and yet is not so obvious at birth; it is an abnormality that demands a specific method of examination for its detection in the newborn and yet, regrettably, is still not being recognized sufficiently early (and may even escape detection until after the child has started to walk); and finally, it is an abnormality that, unless treated early and well, inevitably leads to painful crippling degenerative arthritis of the hip in adult life. Indeed, at least one third of all degenerative joint disease, or arthritis, of the hip in adults is caused by the sequelae of developmental displacement of the hip (Fig. 8.23). In no other congenital abnormality of the musculoskeletal system is the effort to make an early diagnosis so rewarding—and the failure to make this effort so tragic! You can meet this challenge by *resolving* that throughout your professional lifetime you will *always* examine the hip joints of *every* infant entrusted to your care.

Developmental displacement of the hip is best considered in a temporal sense as a process or chain of events that, in the beginning at least, can be arrested and even reversed. A description of certain terms is helpful at this time. *Dislocation (luxation)* of the hip refers

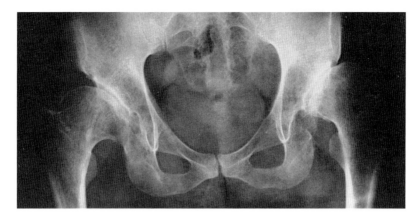

Figure 8.23.   This figure shows degenerative joint disease of both hips in a 38-year-old woman secondary to residual subluxation following inadequate treatment of congenital dislocation (developmental displacement, or dysplasia) of the hips in childhood. The patient walked with a marked limp and had pain in both hips. The serious and disabling condition could have been prevented by diagnosis and adequate treatment at birth.

to the femoral head being completely outside the socket, or acetabulum, but still within the stretched and elongated capsule (intracapsular). *Subluxation* of the hip refers to the femoral head riding laterally and proximally but still in contact with at least part of the acetabulum; such a hip is usually reduced and stable when the hip is flexed and abducted, but is subluxated (less than dislocated) when the hip is extended and adducted. If the hip remains dislocated or subluxated, the bony development of the acetabulum and proximal femur (which was normal at birth) becomes progressively abnormal (*acetabular and femoral dysplasia*). Thus, the dysplasia is secondary to the displacement and, therefore, developmental rather than congenital. The present discussion concerns only the common and typical type of developmental displacement in otherwise normal children, as opposed to the less common prenatal (teratologic) type of truly *congenital* dislocation associated with spina bifida and arthrogryposis.

Incidence
Developmental displacement of the hip is common (incidence of 1.5 in 1,000 live births). The abnormality is bilateral in more than half of the afflicted children (dislocation of both hips, subluxation of both hips, or one

of each) and affects girls eight times as often as boys. It is also more common when there is a positive family history or a breech presentation of the infant. A study of the geographic incidence, which varies tremendously throughout the world, suggests that a higher incidence is related, in part, to the custom of maintaining the hips of newborn infants in extension and adduction by various means of swaddling, including cradleboards in North American Indians and tightly wrapped blankets in all cultures (Fig. 8.24). Infants with either congenital muscular torticollis or metatarsus adductus have a higher incidence of congenital dislocation than do otherwise normal infants.

Etiology and Pathology
Unlike most of the congenital musculoskeletal abnormalities, developmental displacement of the hip is the end result of combined genetic and environmental factors. Although this complex subject is still controversial because of the lack of adequate data, the following explanation seems most reasonable and is presented briefly at this time without discussing the available evidence. The hip joint develops well *in utero*, where it is constantly maintained in acute *flexion* (Fig. 8.25A). At birth, 1 child in 80 exhibits an undue degree of congenital

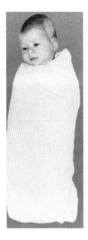

Figure 8.24. This newborn infant is tightly wrapped in a blanket that maintains the newborn hips in the harmful position of extension and adduction. This custom is one factor in the cause of the initial dislocation of a congenitally unstable hip and therefore should be avoided.

hip joint laxity, and this is probably genetically determined. If at the moment of birth, or even within the first few weeks, the previously flexed hips are passively *extended* in the presence of such marked hip joint laxity, the femoral head may dislocate and subsequently either reduce (relocate) or remain dislocated. Con-

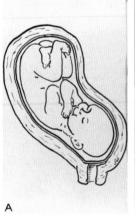
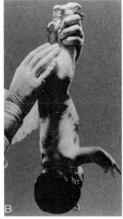

A   B

Figure 8.25. **A.** This is the fetal position in utero. The hip joints are always constantly maintained in complete flexion. **B.** Sudden passive extension of the previously flexed hips immediately after birth should be avoided because it is one factor in the initial dislocation of a congenitally unstable hip.

sequently, the age-old practice of suspending a newborn infant by the ankles is no longer acceptable (Fig. 8.25**B**). Thus, at birth, the abnormal hip can be dislocated but is not permanently dislocated, that is, it is *dislocatable.* Indeed, the majority of such hips become stable spontaneously within the first 2 months. However, if a vulnerable hip is *maintained* in extension, it tends to *remain* either dislocated or subluxated (Fig. 8.24). Persistent dislocation and subluxation cause progressive *secondary* changes in all the structures in and around the hip joint. These important secondary changes include abnormal development (*dysplasia*) of the acetabulum, which becomes *maldirected;* an increase in the normal *femoral neck anteversion;* hypertrophy of the elongated capsule; and contracture and shortening of the muscles that cross the hip joint, especially the adductor and the iliopsoas muscles.

It will be obvious to you, even from this brief description, that each and every one of the progressive secondary changes increases the difficulty of not only reducing the hip but also maintaining its reduction. Furthermore, as time goes on, these changes become not only progressively more marked but also progressively *less reversible.* All these facts should serve to emphasize the extreme importance of *early diagnosis,* the responsibility for which rests with the family physician, obstetrician, and pediatrician who are the first to see and examine infants. Indeed, it is possible that if a newborn infant's hips were *never* passively extended and *never* maintained in extension during the first few months of life, the great majority of genetically vulnerable hips could be *prevented* from dislocating or subluxating and would therefore go on to develop *normally.* Thus, the possible *prevention* of at least *most* developmental displacements of the hip and all their tragic sequelae becomes an exciting challenge!

Diagnosis and Treatment

The clinical and radiographic diagnosis, as well as the orthopaedic treatment, of developmental displacement and subluxation of the hip vary so greatly with the child's age that they are best considered in relation to several specific age groups. Nevertheless, the importance of *very early diagnosis* and *very early treatment* merits repeated emphasis. The general principles of treatment include gentle reduction of the hip followed by maintenance of the reduction with the hip in a stable position until the various components of the hip are well developed and the hip has become stable even in the position of weightbearing.

Birth to Three Months. Birth to 3 months of age is the most important period of greatest opportunity, during which the abnormality is *never obvious,* which means that *you must seek it out* by careful examination of *every* infant you see. The instability of the dislocatable hip can be detected at birth by the Barlow "provocation test," in which the flexed hips are alternately adducted while pressing the femur downward, and abducted while lifting the femur upward (Fig. 8.26). In the presence of instability you will feel—and see—the hip dislocate posteriorly as it is adducted and reduce as it is abducted. A positive Barlow test indicates that the hip is dislocatable but is not dislocated.

If the hip is already *dislocated,* the femoral head lies posterior to the acetabulum when the hip is in the flexed position, and it can be reduced by abduction while lifting the femur forward (i.e., it is reducible); this is the Ortolani sign. Extra skin creases on the inner side of the thigh and external rotation of the lower limb should make you at least suspicious of developmental displacement of the hip, even though both of these signs may also be seen in normal infants.

Tredwell and Bell have demonstrated the impressive efficacy of routine neonatal examination in all infants as a method of diagnostic screening in their area. In most other centers, however, neonatal screening by various methods have been somewhat less successful. All infants should be re-examined physically and radiographically at 4 months of age as a special precaution. Limitation of passive abduction of the flexed hip (caused by contracture of the adductor muscles) is an important sign, particularly after the first month (Fig. 8.27). Limitation of abduction does not necessarily indicate a complete dislocation, but it does indicate an abnormal hip and should always be investi-

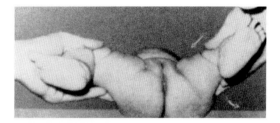

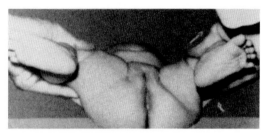

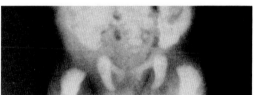

Figure 8.26. **Top.** A Barlow test is performed to demonstrate instability of the hip in the newborn period. When the flexed hip is adducted slightly while pressing downward along the long axis of the femur, the femoral head slides posteriorly out of the acetabulum. **Middle.** When the flexed hip is then abducted slightly while lifting the femur upward and pressing forward on the greater trochanter, the femoral head is suddenly reduced into the acetabulum with a "jerk." The instability can be both felt and seen. You must perform this test in every newborn infant you see to avoid the serious error of overlooking the diagnosis of developmental displacement of the hip in the newborn period. **Bottom.** This is a radiograph of the infant shown at top. The left hip is dislocated in the extended position as evidenced by the slight upward and lateral displacement of the adducted femur. Note that the acetabulum in this newborn infant has not yet become dysplastic.

gated further by radiographic examination (Fig. 8.28).

During the first 3 to 6 months of an infant's life, much of the acetabular roof and all of the femoral head is still cartilaginous, that is, it is composed of preosseous cartilage that is radiolucent. Consequently, the accurate interpretation of plain radiographs in such young infants is difficult and *ultrasonography* of the hip

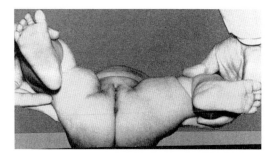

Figure 8.27. This figure shows limitation of passive abduction of the right hip in a 2-month-old infant with a developmental displacement, or dysplasia (congenital dislocation), of the right hip. This sign is more apparent after the first month of life. Note also the asymmetry of the skin folds on the medial aspect of the thighs.

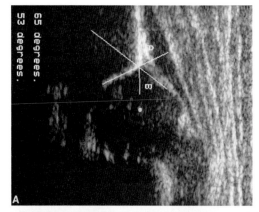

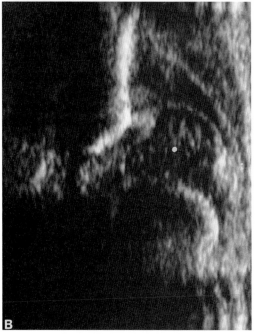

as developed by Graf and also by Harcke and Kumar is preferable (Fig. 8.29). Although routine ultrasonography of all newborn infants is not recommended for the purpose of diagnostic screening, it is definitely indicated for all infants younger than 6 months of age who have positive clinical findings and also those who are at high risk of having developmental displacement of the hips—that is, those with a positive family history, breech presentation, and generalized ligamentous laxity. Dynamic ultrasonography, which provides the examiner with a "moving image" of

Figure 8.29. **A.** A normal coronal sonogram of the left hip joint of a neonate is seen in this figure. The white dot is over the center of the femoral head. The alpha (A) angle of 65° and the beta (B) angle of 53° are normal and the femoral head is in normal relationship within the acetabulum (i.e., it is in the socket). **B.** An abnormal sonogram of the left hip joint of a neonate is shown in this figure. The white dot is over the center of the femoral head. Note that the head of the femur is dislocated laterally and proximally from the acetabulum (i.e., it is out of the socket).

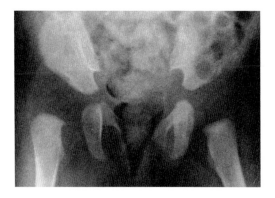

Figure 8.28. This figure shows the developmental displacement, or dysplasia (congenital dislocation), of the right hip in the 2-month-old infant seen in Figure 8.27. Note the upward and lateral displacement of the right femur and the delayed development (dysplasia) of the bony part of the right acetabulum.

the hip, is more reliable than static ultrasonography in detecting either dislocatability or subluxatability of the hip. After the age of 6 months, by which time the ossific nucleus of the femoral head has usually appeared and the ossification of the acetabular roof is more advanced, plain radiographs are preferable to ultrasonograms.

Treatment during this most favorable first 3-month period involves gentle *reduction* of the hip, which usually is not difficult at this stage, followed by *maintenance* of the hip in the stable position of flexion and abduction in some type of device such as the Frejka pillow splint (Fig. 8.30). An alternate form of management during the first 3 to 4 months is the Pavlik harness, which maintains the hips in flexion while permitting motion in other directions; when properly used, this harness produces excellent results, even for a frankly dislocated hip, and with relatively few complications (Fig. 8.31). Inappropriate use of the Pavlik harness, however, can cause avascular necrosis of the femoral head. Occasionally, after 3 weeks of treatment, the hip is still too unstable to be reduced by either type of splint, in which case a gentle closed reduction of the

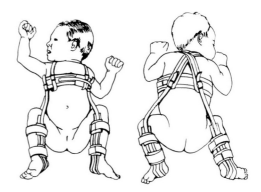

Figure 8.31. The Pavlik harness prevents both active and passive extension of the hips but permits all other movements and thereby helps to stimulate the development of the reduced hip.

hip followed by the application of a plaster hip spica cast is indicated in the "human position" (described in a subsequent paragraph). A period of about 4 months' protection is usually necessary for the capsule to become tighter and for the reduced femoral head to stimulate development of the hip and thereby reverse the secondary changes. The effects of treatment must be regularly assessed both clinically and ultrasonographically.

Three Months to Eighteen Months. In the 3- to 18-month period, the adduction contracture is more marked, and physical signs resulting from this contracture, such as limitation of passive abduction, apparent and real shortening of the involved lower limb, and prominence of the hip, become progressively more obvious (Fig. 8.32). With unilateral dislocation, shortening of the thigh is most apparent when the hips are flexed and the level of the knees is compared (Galeazzi's sign) (Fig. 8.33). The presence of a dislocation is confirmed by feeling the hip go in and out of the joint during the previously mentioned Ortolani test, but this phenomenon becomes progressively more difficult to elicit the longer the hip has remained out of joint, and it cannot be elicited with a subluxation. In the presence of a complete dislocation, a push-pull maneuver on the femur will demonstrate the phenomenon of *telescoping* as the femur moves to and fro within the thigh (Fig. 8.34). Radiographs reveal an excessive slope of the *ossified* portion of the acetabulum (an indication of

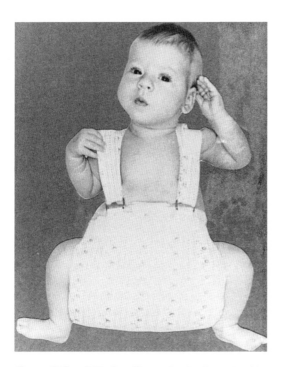

Figure 8.30. A Frejka pillow splint is shown in this figure. This 2-month-old girl had a congenitally unstable left hip joint with a positive Ortolani test. The pillow splint keeps the hips in the stable position of flexion and abduction while allowing some active movement of the hips.

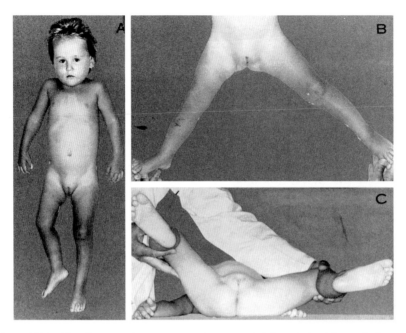

Figure 8.32. Developmental displacement (congenital dislocation) of the right hip in a 14-month-old girl. **A.** Note the adduction contracture of the right hip, resulting in apparent shortening of the right lower limb (added to the true shortening from the dislocation), the prominence of the right hip, and the external rotation of the lower limb. **B** and **C.** Note also the limitation of passive abduction of the right hip in both extension and flexion.

acetabular dysplasia and maldirection), delayed ossification of the femoral head, and varying degrees of upward and lateral displacement of the head of the femur (Fig. 8.35).

Treatment in this age group involves preliminary lengthening of the tight adductor and hamstring muscles by continuous tape traction for a few weeks (at home whenever feasible) (Fig. 8.36), and always a subcutaneous adductor tenotomy, followed by gentle *closed reduction* of the hip under general anesthesia. After the hip has been reduced and the perfection of the reduction has been confirmed radiographically, the reduced hip is *maintained* in a hip spica cast in a stable position of marked flexion and only moderate abduction (which the author originated and called the "human position," as opposed to the traditional "frog" position) (Fig. 8.37). Retention of the hip in an extreme or forced frog position of abduction or internal rotation must be avoided because it is probably the most important cause of *avascular necrosis* of the femoral head, which is a serious complication of treatment.

Postreduction radiographs obtained through the cast may be difficult to interpret, in which case computed tomography will provide a more accurate image of the relationship of the femoral head to the acetabulum. The hip spica cast is changed every 2 months until radiographs reveal satisfactory development of both the acetabulum and femoral head. The period of immobilization of the reduced hip required to bring about reversal of the secondary changes varies directly with the number of months the hip had been dislocated before treatment, but is usually between 5 and 8 months. During the last part of this period of retention, adequate *protection* of the reduction can usually be maintained by a large Frejka pillow splint or, alternatively, by the use of two long leg casts separated by an abduction bar; this type of cast allows some movement of the hip within a safe range and thereby provides further stimulation for development of the acetabulum and femoral head.

The results of gentle and careful closed treatment instituted between 3 and 18 months of age are good in approximately 80%

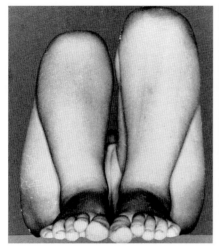
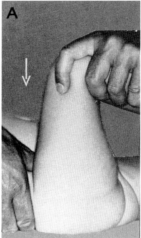
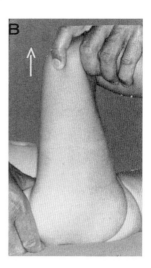

Figure 8.33.   Left. This figure shows Galeazzi's sign (also called Allis' sign) of developmental displacement (congenital dislocation) of the right hip in a 14-month-old girl. This sign, which is of value only with a unilateral dislocation, demonstrates that when the hips are flexed to 90°, the femoral head lies posterior to the acetabulum, and as a result the thigh on the dislocated side is shortened as evidenced by the lower level of the knee.

Figure 8.34.   A and B. Telescoping of the thigh in developmental displacement (congenital dislocation) of the hip in a 14-month-old girl is seen. With the involved hip flexed, a push-pull maneuver demonstrates that the femur, being dislocated at the hip, moves to and fro within the thigh.

of patients. However, it must be remembered that the percentage of good results is much higher when treatment is started at 3 months than at 18 months.

If attempted closed reduction of a dislocated hip fails to obtain a perfectly reduced hip, or if the immobilization fails to maintain

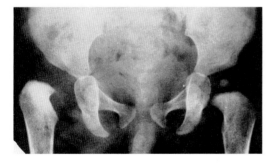

Figure 8.35. This figure shows developmental displacement of the right hip in a 14-month-old girl. Note upward and lateral displacement of the right femur, delayed ossification of the right femoral head, and delayed ossification of the right acetabulum (acetabular dysplasia).

an obtained reduction, open reduction, iliopsoas muscle release, and capsular repair should be performed through an anterior approach. For children younger than one year of age, open reduction through a medial approach is a reasonable alternative. Although this approach does not allow a capsular repair, such repair is considered by some to be less necessary in this young age group.

Eighteen Months to Five Years. In children 18 months to 5 years of age, the secondary changes are not only more severe but also less reversible. By this time, the child is walking, and a typical limp is added to the aforementioned clinical signs, all of which are more marked. When the child is asked to stand on one foot (on the side of the dislocated hip), the hip abductor muscles, having no fulcrum, cannot hold the pelvis level and it drops on the opposite side; the child, in an effort to maintain balance, shifts his or her trunk toward the involved side. These observations indicate a positive *Trendelenburg sign* (Fig. 8.38). The limp is another manifestation of this phenomenon. When the dislocation is unilateral, the child walks as though the lower limb on that side is too short and shifts the trunk toward the involved side when weight is borne on that hip. When the dislocation is bilateral, the child shifts the trunk from one side to the other while walking and gives the impression of waddling like a duck. With a subluxation, the Trendelenburg sign and the limp are not nearly as apparent as in a dislocation, but they are more readily detected when the muscles are fatigued, for example, after a long period of walking.

Treatment in this age group is associated with difficulties, dangers, and disappointments even in the most experienced hands. The muscle contractures, which by this time have become very resistant, must be overcome by a longer period of tape traction as well as by subcutaneous adductor tenotomy. For children older than 3 years of age with a high dislocation, femoral shortening is a reasonable alternative to preoperative traction. In children older than 18 months, the likelihood of obtaining a perfect closed reduction becomes progressively less and, consequently, open reduction, (i.e. *operative reduction*) is indicated. At the time of open reduction, the secondary soft tissue abnormalities, particularly the tight iliopsoas muscle and the elongated joint capsule, must be dealt with. The main problem in this age group is not the reduction but rather *maintaining the reduction;* this is a manifestation of the significant instability of the reduced, but poorly developed, hip joint, the most important component of which is the abnormal direction in which the acetabulum faces. Many bony operations involving either the femur or the acetabulum have been designed to overcome this problem of instability, but the most reliable in our experience has been innominate osteotomy, which the author designed in 1957 and first reported in 1961 to provide stability of the reduced hip by redirecting the entire maldirected acetabulum (Fig. 8.39).

The long-term results of closed reduction in this age group are depressing because only

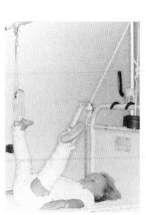
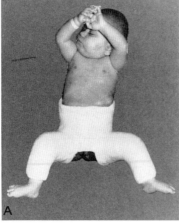
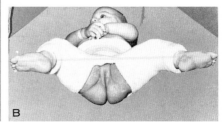

Figure 8.36.   Left. Continuous skin traction with adhesive tape is used on the lower limb for developmental displacement (congenital dislocation) of the hip in this 1-year-old girl. The traction, which is maintained for a few weeks, gradually stretches the shortened muscles around the hip in preparation for a safe and gentle closed reduction.

Figure 8.37.   A and B. A bilateral hip spica plaster cast for congenital dislocation of the hip in a 1-year-old girl. This type of cast is applied following adductor tenotomy and gentle closed reduction and maintains the reduced hip in the stable position of marked flexion and moderate abduction (the "human position"). This child required a total period of 8 months in a cast, during which time the hip responded well. Earlier diagnosis and treatment would have shortened the period of immobilization.

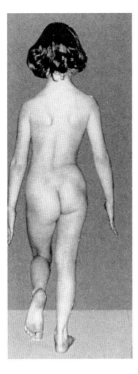
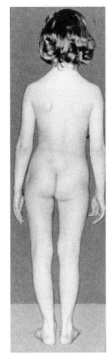
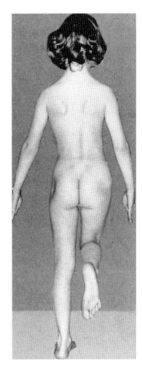

Figure 8.38.   The Trendelenburg sign is seen in a developmental displacement (congenital dislocation) of the hip in a 4-year-old girl. **Left.** When the child stands on the right foot (the side of the dislocated hip), the hip abductor muscles, having no fulcrum, cannot hold the pelvis level and it drops on the opposite side; the child, in an effort to maintain balance, shifts her trunk toward the involved side. **Middle.** The dislocation is not apparent when the child is standing with both feet on the floor (apart from the slight shortening of the lower limb). **Right.** When the child stands on the left foot (the side of the normal hip), the hip abductors, having a normal fulcrum, hold the pelvis level. The Trendelenburg sign is also seen in the presence of coxa vara, paralyzed hip abductors, and painful conditions around the hip.

30% are excellent or good. Following careful open reduction and the improvement of stability by innominate osteotomy, the long-term results are much better (87% excellent or good up to 33 years after operation) but still not as good as the results of successful closed treatment instituted in the first 3 months of life, all of which provides mute testimony to the extreme importance of early diagnosis and treatment.

After the Age of Five Years. Fortunately, few children now reach the age of 5 years with previously untreated congenital dislocation of the hip, although the same cannot be said for congenital subluxation. By this time, the secondary changes in a complete dislocation are so marked and their reversibility so limited that even extensive operative procedures (in-cluding femoral shortening) cannot be expected to meet with success, particularly in children with bilateral dislocations who are older than 6 or 7 years of age; beyond this age, it is unwise even to attempt reduction (Fig. 8.40). Residual subluxation is less difficult to treat in this age group than is dislocation and can be improved considerably by innominate osteotomy up to the end of the growing period and beyond. For unfortunate older children with irreducible congenital dislocation of the hip, palliative and salvage types of operative procedures are frequently required for the relief of pain in early adult life.

Early diagnosis and gentle treatment are still the most important aspects of developmental displacement of the hip. Neonatal screening for congenital dislocation of the hip

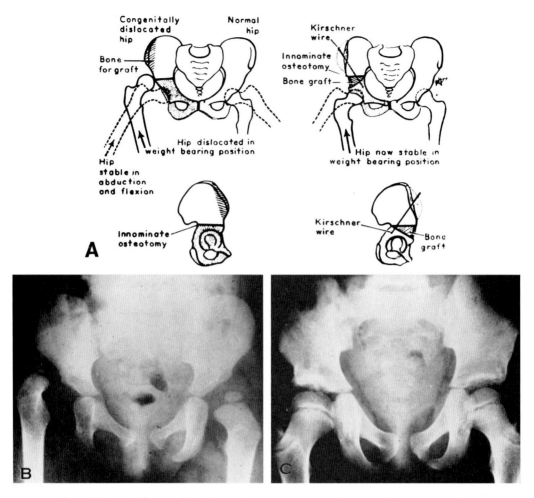

Figure 8.39.   A. The principle of innominate osteotomy is redirection of the entire acetabulum in such a way that the reduced hip, which previously was stable only in a position of flexion and abduction, is rendered stable with the limb in the normal position of weightbearing. **B.** Developmental displacement (congenital dislocation) of the right hip and congenital subluxation in the left hip in a 3-year-old girl. Note the severity of the secondary dysplasia of each acetabulum and each femoral head, which is greater in the dislocated hip than in the subluxated hip. **C.** The same girl 4 years after open reduction and innominate osteotomy of the right hip and innominate osteotomy alone of the left hip. The girl walked normally. Early diagnosis and treatment would have rendered such surgical treatment unnecessary.

in *all* infants during the first few days of life has been effective in reducing the incidence of "missed" dislocations and, hence, in reducing the number of children requiring extensive surgical treatment. Subluxations are more difficult to detect at birth, but routine physical and radiographic re-examination at 4 months of age would be useful in their detection as well.

It is to be hoped that during your professional lifetime, you will *never* allow developmental displacement, or dysplasia of the hip to go unrecognized in a newborn infant!

Amputations in the Lower Limb

Absence of the distal part of a limb at birth is, in effect, a *congenital amputation;* it is less common in the lower limb than in the upper limb. The defect may be as minor as absence of a single toe or as major as complete absence of both lower limbs. Congenital amputations

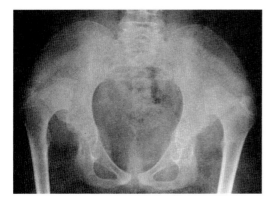

Figure 8.40. This figure shows bilateral developmental displacement (congenital dislocation) of the hip in a 9-year-old girl. The secondary changes in the acetabulum and femur, as well as in the soft tissues, are so severe and so irreversible at this age that it is not possible to obtain a good result with any form of treatment. Therefore, this girl is doomed to a disability for the rest of her life, a disability that could have been prevented by early diagnosis and early treatment.

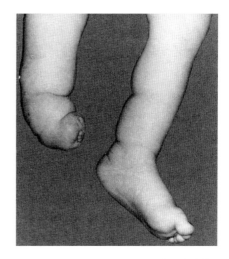

Figure 8.41.   Annular constricting band of the right lower limb with hypoplasia and edema of the limb distally.

are often associated with congenital *annular constricting bands,* which probably represent a failure of circumferential growth of the skin and soft tissues at that level during intrauterine development. Shallow constrictions may be seen without any abnormality distally; deeper constrictions are associated with hypoplasia and distal enlargement caused by chronic edema (Fig. 8.41); the deepest constrictions result in distal loss of the limb at some time during intrauterine life. When the amputation has occurred early, the stump is well healed at birth, but occasionally the intrauterine amputation is so recent that the child is born with an incompletely healed stump (Fig. 8.42A).

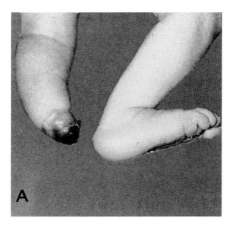
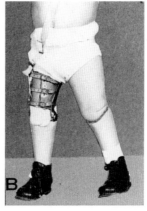

Figure 8.42.   A. This figure demonstrates intrauterine amputation. The infant was born with an incompletely healed stump, indicating that the final separation of the distal part of the limb (secondary to an annular constricting band) was recent. B. Bilateral artificial limbs (prostheses) for a 2-year old-boy with congenital amputations. This boy quickly learned to walk with almost no limp.

Treatment of children with significant congenital amputations of the lower limb involves early fitting with artificial limbs (*prostheses*) of special design to meet the specific needs of the child (Fig. 8.42B). The fact that frequent changes will be necessary during the child's growing years is no excuse for makeshift prostheses. In recent years, major improvements in prosthetic design and function have been developed as a result of the establishment of juvenile amputee clinics in which surgeons, engineers, and limb makers (prosthetists) combine their knowledge and skill.

Hemihypertrophy

Congenital enlargement of a lower limb and an upper limb on the same side as well as that of half the trunk and face (relative to the opposite side) is known as *congenital hemihypertrophy* (Fig. 8.43). The structures of each half of the body are perfectly normal, but the two halves are asymmetrical. Function of the limbs is normal, and the only clinical problem that occasionally arises is significant overgrowth of the larger lower limb in length. The resultant leg length discrepancy may be dealt with either by surgical epiphyseal arrest at the appropriate age or by surgical shortening of the femur at the end of growth.

A malignant neoplasm of the kidney, Wilms' tumor, develops in 2% of children with congenital hemihypertrophy. This association should be looked for by physical examination and ultrasonography at the time of diagnosis of the hemihypertrophy and at least once or twice a year during the first 5 to 6 years of life.

LOCALIZED CONGENITAL ABNORMALITIES OF THE UPPER LIMB
The Hand
Trigger Thumb

A constantly flexed interphalangeal joint of the thumb in children is usually caused by a congenital constriction (*stenosis*) of the fibrous sheath of the flexor pollicis longus tendon and a *secondary* nodular enlargement in the tendon at the proximal edge of the constriction. This combination always prevents

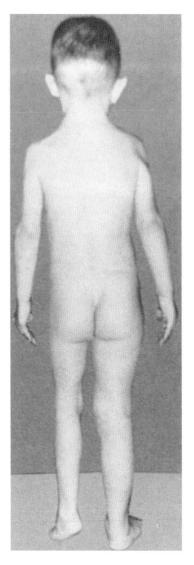

Figure 8.43.   Congenital hemihypertrophy is seen in this figure. Note that the right half of this boy's body is considerably larger than the left half. The disparity between the two sides of the body involves the face, ears, and trunk as well as the extremities.

active extension of the interphalangeal joint and frequently prevents even passive extension so that the "trigger phenomenon" of sudden, snapping flexion is seldom seen in the congenital type, even though the abnormality is commonly referred to as trigger thumb. Under the proximal skin crease, the enlargement in the tendon is readily felt as a nodule that moves with the tendon during passive movement of the interphalangeal joint (Fig. 8.44). Surgical

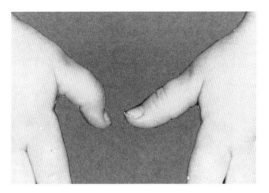

Figure 8.44.   Congenital right trigger thumb caused by congenital constriction (stenosis) of the fibrous sheath of the flexor pollicis longus tendon is seen. This 1-year-old child could not actively extend the interphalangeal joint of the right thumb; a nodule was palpable on the flexor tendon just proximal to the fibrous sheath (under the proximal skin crease). This anomaly responded well to simple division of the fibrous sheath.

treatment, which consists of longitudinal division of the constricted fibrous sheath through a transverse skin incision, allows free gliding of the tendon, after which the secondary enlargement in the tendon gradually disappears.

Webbing of the Fingers (Syndactyly)

Webbing of the fingers of varying degree is probably the most common congenital abnor-

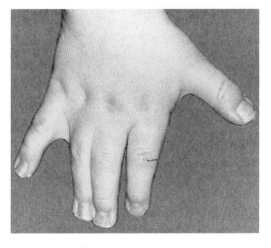

Figure 8.45.   This figure shows congenital webbing of the middle and ring fingers. Improvement in appearance and function followed surgical separation of the otherwise normal fingers at the age of 4 years.

mality of the hand. When two adjacent and otherwise normal fingers are joined by a skin web proximally, or throughout their length, satisfactory appearance and function may be expected from a reconstructive operation that includes the judicious use of skin grafts (Fig. 8.45). Although incomplete webbing may be corrected during infancy, the optimal age for reconstruction of the complete web is about 4 years.

The Forearm

Hypoplasia of the Radius (Clubhand)

Hypoplasia of the radius is a relatively uncommon, but serious, abnormality, which consists of varying degrees of hypoplasia, or even aplasia, of the radial ray of the upper limb, including the radius, scaphoid, trapezium, first metacarpal, and thumb as well as the associated muscles, nerves, and blood vessels. When the abnormality is severe, radial deviation of the hand is invariably present, the ulna is short as well as curved, and even the proximal part of the upper limb may be hypoplastic (Fig. 8.46).

The principles of treatment of this difficult problem include early correction of the radial deviation of the hand, maintenance of this correction during growth and, finally, improvement of hand function. Passive stretching of the contracted soft tissues on the concave side of the deformity is of limited and temporary value. Much more effective is an early soft tissue operation consisting of Z-plasty of the skin, division of the fibrous band (anlage) in the location of the defective radius, and maintenance of correction for several months in casts followed by appropriate removable splints. Permanent correction of the radial deviation may necessitate bony operations, such as implantation of the distal end of the ulna into a slot fashioned in the carpus. If the condition is bilateral and both thumbs are absent, the index finger of at least one hand can be surgically repositioned to function as a thumb (*pollicization*) to improve pinch and grasp functions (Fig. 8.47). It should be remembered, however, that resourceful individuals with congenital absence even of both thumbs may develop surprisingly good function of the hands without operation.

The Elbow

Dislocation of the Head of the Radius

This rare congenital abnormality is not usually detected early because there is relatively little deformity and little disability. The radial head is dislocated laterally and as a result, the radius overgrows in length (Fig. 8.48). A prominence is seen on the lateral aspect of the elbow, and there is some limitation of supination. The condition may be brought to attention for the first time following an injury during childhood, but it is readily differentiated radiographically from a traumatic dislocation by the overgrowth in length as well as changes

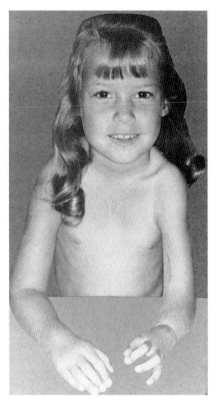

Figure 8.47. Congenital hypoplasia of the radius (clubhand) seen in the same patient seen in Figure 8.46 6 years after surgical correction of the radial deviation of each hand and pollicization of the left index finger.

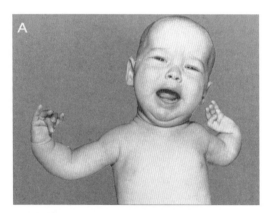

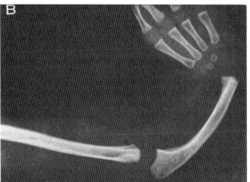

Figure 8.46. Congenital hypoplasia of the radius (clubhand) is seen in this figure. **A.** In this little girl, the anomaly is bilateral but much more severe in the left upper limb than in the right. Note the absence of a thumb, the radial deviation of the hand, and the short, curved forearm. This child also had congenital heart disease requiring operative correction. **B.** This radiograph of the left arm of the same patient reveals absence of the radius, curvature of the hypoplastic ulna, radial deviation of the hand, and absence of the thumb and first metacarpal.

secondary to any longstanding dislocation. Reconstructive procedures seldom improve function. Excision of the prominent radial head is unwise during childhood because of a subsequent growth disturbance in the radius and resultant radial deviation deformity at the wrist. Thus, such surgery should be deferred until the child has reached skeletal maturity.

Radioulnar Synostosis

Congenital bony continuity (synostosis) between the radius and the ulna at the proximal radioulnar joint is a rare abnormality that may be bilateral (Fig. 8.49). The forearm is rigidly fixed, usually in slight pronation, but because the afflicted child unwittingly compensates for the lack of supination by movements through the shoulder (adduction and external rota-

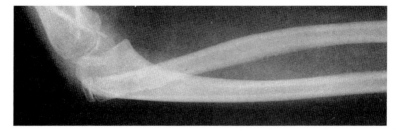

Figure 8.48. Congenital dislocation of the head of the radius is seen in a 9-year-old girl. The radiograph demonstrates complete dislocation of the radial head. The radius is already overgrown in relation to the ulna, and this indicates that the dislocation is congenital rather than acquired. This congenital anomaly is better left untreated.

tion), the abnormality is seldom detected during the first few years of life.

Operative treatment designed to provide movement is doomed to failure because of the associated soft tissue abnormalities, but fortunately the disability is so minimal that surgical treatment is unwarranted.

When the synostosis is bilateral, however, it may be necessary to reposition one forearm by means of a proximal osteotomy so that the patient may put the hands together in a more normal manner, that is, palm to palm.

Hypoplasia of the Clavicles

Hypoplasia of the clavicles is an uncommon congenital abnormality that is manifested by drooping and excessive mobility of the shoulders. It is usually bilateral and may be associated with delayed ossification of the skull (both the clavicle and the skull are "membrane bones" because they are formed by intramembranous ossification). The combination is referred to as *cleidocranial dysostosis* (Fig. 8.50). No treatment is required. When the hypoplasia involves only the middle portion of one clavicle, it should be differentiated from the extremely rare conditions of nonunion and congenital pseudarthrosis of the clavicle.

High Scapula (Sprengel's Deformity)

Since the scapula normally descends during embryonic development, a congenitally high scapula is more accurately considered *undescended* rather than elevated (Fig. 8.51). This arrested scapular development is sometimes associated with abnormalities of the cervical spine, and there is usually a ligamentous connection (*omovertebral ligament*) between the medial border of the scapula and the lower cervical spinous processes (Fig. 8.52). Subsequently, the ligament ossifies and is then the *omovertebral bone*. The scapula is not only high

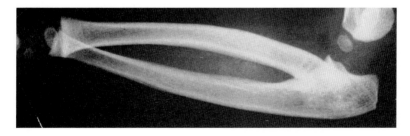

Figure 8.49. This figures shows congenital radioulnar synostosis in a 6-year-old boy. The radiograph reveals congenital bony continuity (synostosis) between the radius and ulna proximally. This anomaly was an incidental finding during examination of the boy for a finger injury. Neither the boy nor his parents were previously aware of his complete lack of supination or pronation. There was no significant disability and no treatment was necessary.

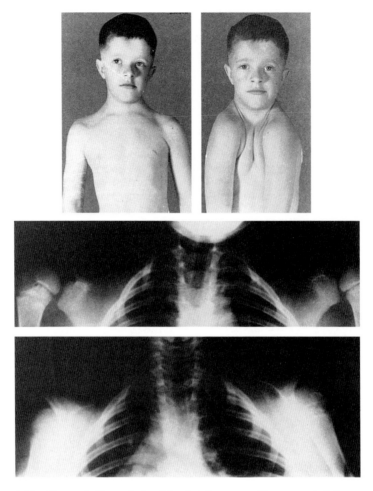

Figure 8.50.   Congenital hypoplasia of the clavicles is seen. The congenital absence of this 8-year-old boy's clavicles allowed excessive mobility of the shoulders, which could almost be brought to the midline anteriorly. The radiographs reveal an absence of clavicles and also demonstrate the excessive mobility of the scapulae. There was no significant disability, however, and no treatment was necessary.

and small but is also rotated downward (adducted), with resultant limitation of shoulder abduction. Function is seldom improved by operative treatment, but the clinical deformity can be improved cosmetically by resection of the upper third of the scapula and omovertebral bone or by surgically lowering the scapula.

AMPUTATIONS IN THE UPPER LIMB

The general discussion in a previous section of this chapter dealing with congenital amputations in the lower limb is equally applicable to those in the upper limb. Indeed, a given child may be born with a congenital amputation in both a lower limb and an upper limb, or even in all four limbs. Normal function in the upper limb is so precise and so highly specialized that the development of a truly functional upper limb prosthesis is exceedingly difficult. Nevertheless, the infant with a congenital amputation in the upper limb should be fitted with a prosthesis of simple design even before beginning to crawl (Fig. 8.53). By school age, the child should be wearing a prosthesis with full adult controls (Fig. 8.54). Much care and supervision are required to ensure that the upper limb pros-

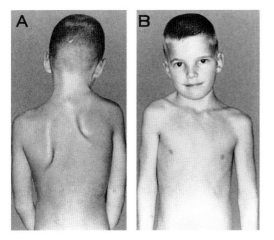

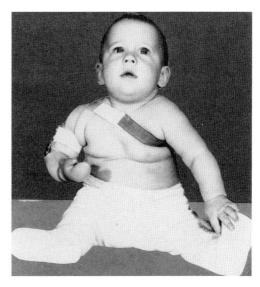

Figure 8.51. Congenital high scapula (Sprengel's shoulder) is seen in this 6-year-old boy. Note that the right scapula is not only smaller and higher than the left but also that it is adducted; consequently, abduction of the shoulder is correspondingly limited. This boy participated actively in sports. His appearance was improved by surgical resection of the upper third of the scapula.

Figure 8.53. This figure shows a prosthesis of a simple mitten design for an infant with a congenital amputation through the forearm. Such a prosthesis is fitted very early to help the child become bimanual.

thesis is both comfortable and practical so that the child will accept it as an extension of his or her deficient limb and will come to enjoy the privilege of bimanual activities. The school age child should also be given a cosmetic prosthesis (Fig. 8.55). Important technical advances in recent years have provided external power for upper limb prostheses by various

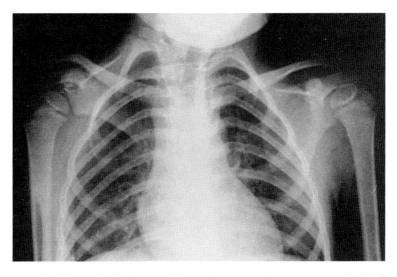

Figure 8.52. Congenital high scapula (Sprengel's shoulder) is demonstrated in this figure. The radiograph reveals the high and adducted position of the small right scapula and a bony attachment (the omovertebral bone) between the superomedial corner of the scapula and the lower cervical spinous processes.

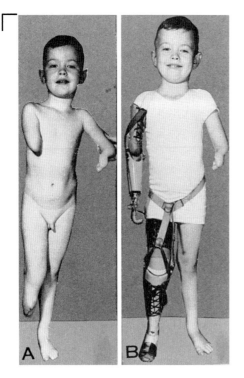

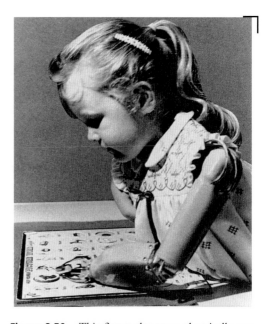

Figure 8.54. This 4-year-old boy has triple congenital amputations and has been fitted early with prostheses that have full adult controls. He is wearing two of his three prostheses and is relatively independent.

Figure 8.56. This figure shows an electrically controlled and battery driven prosthesis for a 4-year-old girl with a congenital defect of the upper limb and a small hand attached to the shoulder. She has learned to press on separate switches within the prosthesis with her fingers and thereby control opening of the terminal device, rotation of the forearm, and flexion of the elbow.

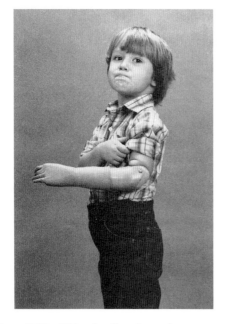

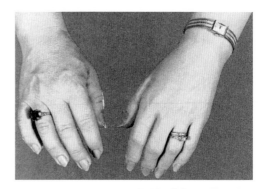

Figure 8.57. This is a cosmetic hand prosthesis for a young married woman with an amputation though the midforearm. The appearance of the plastic left hand is made to match that of the normal hand as closely as possible.

Figure 8.55. This schoolboy is wearing a cosmetic prosthesis while at school as an alternative to his functional prosthesis. You can tell from the marvelous expression on his face that he is determined to overcome the disability of his amputation.

means, including the incorporation of compressed gases as well as complex electrical and electronic devices (Fig. 8.56). The perfection of cosmetic hands represents a significant improvement in prostheses (Fig. 8.57). The previously mentioned establishment of juvenile amputee centers has resulted in a tremendous improvement in the care of these unfortunate children.

LOCALIZED CONGENITAL ABNORMALITIES OF THE SPINE
Spina Bifida

The most common congenital abnormality of the spine, by far, is *spina bifida,* which includes varying degrees of incomplete bony closure of one or more neural arches. The defect, which is also known as a neural tube defect, may occur at any level, but the most frequent site is the lumbosacral region, which is normally the last part of the vertebral column to close. Although minor defects are very common indeed, spina bifida of sufficient degree to be obvious at birth has an incidence of 2 in 1000 births.

Etiological Factors
It is well established that most mothers who give birth to a baby with an open type of spina bifida (neural tube defect) have an elevated serum α-fetoprotein level early in the pregnancy. In addition, many have a detectable inadequate dietary intake of the vitamin folic acid (folate) even before and at the time of conception. More recently, Irish scientists have discovered the first gene responsible for spina bifida as well as the fact that both parents must carry the gene for the defect to develop.

The Possible Prevention of Spina Bifida
At the beginning of this chapter, reference was made to the antenatal diagnosis of the more severe open types of spina bifida (meningomyelocele and myelocele) through an elevated maternal serum α-fetoprotein level. Indeed, this test can be used as a screening tool during early pregnancy; a positive test is an indication for a meticulous, detailed ultrasonographic evaluation of the fetal anatomy, which can detect 95% of cases of spina bifida. Rarely, it may be necessary to resort to amniocentesis to con-

firm this diagnosis, and both α-fetoprotein and acetylcholinesterase levels can be measured in the amniotic fluid. In the past two decades, prenatal diagnosis and abortion of affected fetuses have reduced the number of babies born with the open type of spina bifida, thereby reducing the prevalence (at birth) but not the initial incidence of the defect.

Following the original research by Wald and by Czeizel and Dundal, who demonstrated the role of folic acid (folate) in preventing the open types of spina bifida, Koren, the Director of the Motherisk Program in Toronto, and his colleagues have emphasized the need for government-approved fortification of food staples such as bread and cereals with folic acid for all women of childbearing age to prevent up to 75% of open spina bifida cases before conception.

Pathology of Spina Bifida
The most significant aspect of this abnormality is not the bony defect itself but rather the frequently associated neurological deficit that results from the defective development of the spinal cord (*myelodysplasia*). When present, the neurological deficit may vary from mild muscle imbalance and sensory loss in the lower limbs to complete paraplegia. Thus, spina bifida must always be considered as a possible cause of neurogenic deformities and trophic ulcers in the lower limbs as well as of bladder and bowel incontinence. Some severe teratologic types of congenital clubfeet and congenital dislocation of the hip are secondary to the prenatal paralysis and failure of muscle development associated with spina bifida. Furthermore, during childhood, various neurogenic deformities of the lower limbs may appear and increase in severity with growth as a result of residual muscle imbalance secondary to spina bifida. The varying degrees of spina bifida are best classified morphologically and are discussed on this basis.

Spina Bifida Occulta
The mildest degree of spina bifida occurs without any external manifestation and is truly hidden (occult), being detectable only by radiographic examination (Fig. 8.58). This extremely common form of spina bifida occurs in about 10% of the population and is least

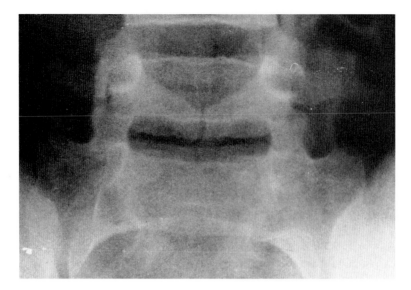

Figure 8.58.   This radiograph reveals incomplete closure of the neural arch of the fifth lumbar vertebra in the midline, the most common site of spina bifida occulta. The defect was an incidental finding in this 12-year-old boy and was not associated with any symptoms or any neurological deficit.

serious because it is rarely associated with a neurological deficit. When there is some external manifestation of the abnormality, such as a dimple, hairy patch, pigmented area, or hemangioma (Fig. 8.59), the underlying spina bifida is more likely to be complicated by a midline spur that splits the spinal cord (*diastematomyelia*) or by a *congenital benign neo-*

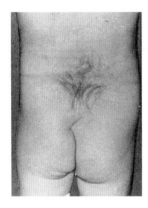

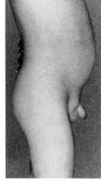

Figure 8.59.   Spina bifida of the fifth lumbar neural arch associated with an overlying hairy patch in a 2-year-old child who had a neurogenic deformity in one foot because of muscle imbalance.

plasm such as a lipoma, hemangioma, or dermoid cyst, either inside or outside the spinal canal. Under these circumstances, a neurological deficit may be present at birth, or it may develop gradually during the subsequent years of spinal growth.

Spina Bifida with Meningocele
The meninges may extrude through a larger defect in the neural arches, thereby forming a *meningocele* covered by normal skin and containing cerebrospinal fluid and some nerve roots (Fig. 8.60). The spinal cord remains confined to the spinal canal, and there is usually little or no neurological deficit clinically detectable at birth. However, as in the type of spina bifida occulta with some external skin manifestation, a neurological deficit may develop gradually during the subsequent years of spinal growth.

Spina Bifida with Meningomyelocele
When the abnormality is more severe, the spinal cord as well as the nerve roots are involved and may either lie free within the sac or constitute part of its wall. The overlying muscles and subcutaneous fat are usually defi-

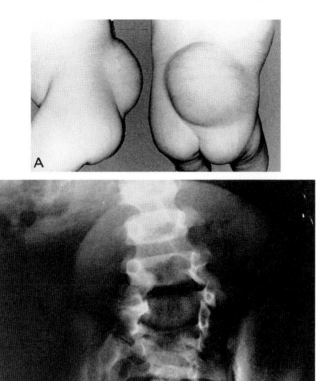

Figure 8.60. **A.** This figure shows spina bifida with meningocele. The prominent meningocele is well covered by normal skin and subcutaneous tissue. **B.** A radiograph of the same patient seen in **A.** Note the wide defect in the neural arch of the fourth and fifth lumbar vertebrae. The curved line of density proximal to the bony defect represents the outline of the proximal edge of the meningocele.

cient, and under these circumstances the covering skin is thin and translucent. In severe meningomyeloceles, the skin may be absent, in which case the cord is covered by the arachnoid and dura and sometimes by the arachnoid alone (Fig. 8.61). As might be expected, a meningomyelocele is always associated with a serious neurological deficit, which often includes bladder and bowel incontinence as well as sensory and motor loss in the lower limbs with typical deformities. When only nerve roots are involved in the meningomyelocele, the resultant paralysis is flaccid, whereas spinal cord involvement results in a spastic type of paralysis; thus, in a given child there may be a *mixed* flaccid and spastic paralysis. In almost half of these children, hydrocephalus coexists as either a potential or an actual complication. The hydrocephalus is secondary to either downward prolongation of the brainstem and part of the cerebellum through the foramen magnum (*Arnold-Chiari malformation*) or other developmental defects of the brain, such as *aqueduct stenosis.*

Spina Bifida with Myelocele (Rachischisis)

In spina bifida with myelocele, the most severe degree of spina bifida, even the skin and dura have failed to close over the neural tube so that the spinal cord and nerve roots lie completely exposed (Fig. 8.62). Inevitable infection usually results in death during early infancy.

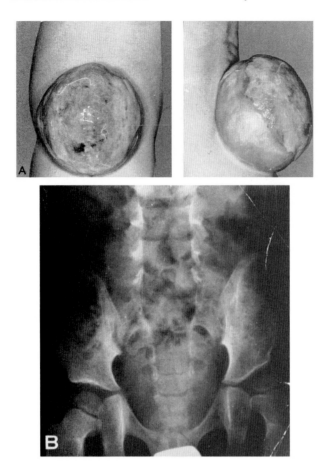

Figure 8.61.   A. This figure demonstrates spina bifida with meningomyelocele. The meningomyelocele is partly covered by thin skin, but in the central area the dura is exposed. This infant had extensive paralysis in the lower limbs. **B.** This figure shows a child with a meningomyelocele. Note the extremely large defect in the neural arch of the last three lumbar vertebrae and of the sacrum. Note also the paralytic subluxation of this child's left hip joint and secondary dysplasia of the acetabulum.

Clinical Course of the Neurological Deficit

Although the neurological deficit is usually present from the beginning and tends to remain static, it may actually increase during the first few days or weeks of life as a result of increasing nerve root tension and infection. Even when the deficit remains static, the resultant muscle imbalance in the lower limbs produces deformities that are accentuated by longitudinal growth of the limbs (Fig. 8.63). Furthermore, abnormal fixation of the neural elements to the defective area of the spine—that is, a "tethered cord"—may interfere with the normal ascent of the distal end of the spinal cord by the tethering effect and thereby produce an increasing traction lesion of the cord and a resultant increasing neurological deficit, particularly during periods of rapid vertebral growth.

Treatment of Spina Bifida with Neurological Deficit

In no other congenital abnormality of the musculoskeletal system is the *team* approach of greater importance than in the management of children afflicted by spina bifida with neurological involvement. *Neurosurgical treatment* includes careful removal of the sac whenever feasible and as early as possible, fol-

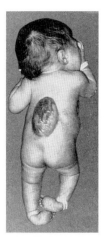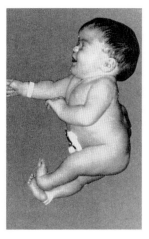

Figure 8.62. This figure demonstrates spina bifida with myelocele (rachischisis). In this newborn infant, the spinal cord and nerve roots lie completely exposed on the surface. Note also the poorly developed lower limbs and the neurogenic clubfeet.

lowed by the provision of good skin coverage; in addition, any associated hydrocephalus is decompressed by appropriate shunting operations with plastic tubes (ventriculoperitoneal

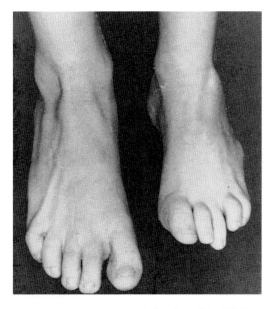

Figure 8.63. Neurogenic deformity of the left foot (cavus and varus) resulting from muscle imbalance that was secondary to spina bifida with a meningocele is seen.

shunt, ventriculocardiac shunt) to prevent irreversible brain damage. In addition, it may become necessary to release a tethered cord.

During the past two decades, the indications for immediate surgical "closure" of the open type of spina bifida in newborn infants have been controversial.

In the 1960s, surgeons in some major centers recommended emergency operations to excise the sac and provide skin coverage for *all* newborn infants with the open type of spina bifida within the first few hours of life. It was hoped that such operations might prevent the otherwise inevitable progression of the neurological deficit and thereby decrease the residual paralysis and sensory loss. The early enthusiasm for such "routine" surgery has waned as it became apparent that those infants with extremely *severe* forms of spina bifida (thoracolumbar lesions with complete paralysis of the lower limbs, severe spinal deformities, and hydrocephalus) were not really helped by such an approach. Such infants (who without surgical treatment are destined to die from the complications of their abnormality within the first 6 months of life) could be kept alive, but the end results of multiple operations—neurosurgical, urological, orthopaedic, and plastic—were so dismal that most neurosurgeons feel that for these extremely affected infants, surgical treatment on the first day of life is not justifiable. Nevertheless, excision of the sac and provision of skin coverage in the first few weeks may be justified even in this severely involved group of infants to facilitate their nursing care. For newborn infants with all lesser degrees of involvement, most neurosurgeons would recommend surgical closure in the first hours of life. Thus, the initial decision to operate or not at birth is made on the basis of sound surgical judgment tempered by the wishes of the distressed parents; understandably, such a decision, which raises philosophical and ethical issues, can be exceedingly difficult for everyone concerned.

The principles of *orthopaedic treatment* for flaccid paralysis are similar to those to be discussed for poliomyelitis in Chapter 12. When the paralysis is of the spastic type, the principles are comparable to those to be discussed for cerebral palsy in Chapter 12. Particular care is required, however, to prevent pressure sores in areas of skin deprived of normal sensation. *Urological treatment* is of great importance, not only in overcoming the distressing problem of urinary incontinence but also in preserving renal function by preventing or controlling recurrent urinary infection. Thus, the neurosurgeon, the orthopaedic surgeon, and the urological surgeon all have a significant contribution to make and all three must be cognizant of the importance of the overall *rehabilitation* of afflicted children in relation to their social development, special education, and vocational guidance so that they may reach their full potential in life.

Scoliosis

Lateral curvature of the spine (*scoliosis*) resulting from congenital abnormalities of the vertebral column and associated tissues varies widely both in severity and prognosis. Failure of one half of a vertebral body to form (*hemivertebra*) results in a short, relatively mild curvature that is usually well compensated above and below by the normal spine (Fig. 8.64). The clinical deformity is usually inconspicuous, and the diagnosis is frequently made when a radiograph is taken for some other purpose. Progression of such a curvature is unlikely, but the child should be seen at least at yearly intervals for clinical and radiographic reassessment.

Multiple congenital abnormalities of the spinal column and ribs, including multiple hemivertebrae, asymmetrical fusion of vertebral bodies, and absent ribs or fused ribs, are seldom balanced in their distribution and result in a severe congenital scoliosis that is unrelentingly progressive with subsequent growth (Fig. 8.65). Severe and progressive congenital scoliosis necessitates early operative treatment that includes spinal fusion, even in growing children, to prevent extreme deformity. The prognosis of congenital scoliosis in any given child, however, may be difficult to predict and, therefore, repeated clinical and radiographic examinations at regular intervals are required to choose the most appropriate form of treatment.

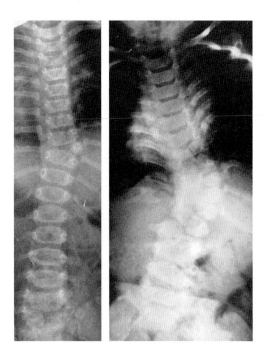

Figure 8.64.   Left. This figure shows congenital scoliosis caused by a hemivertebra at the level of the ninth thoracic vertebra in a 1-year-old child. The scoliosis involves a short segment of the thoracic spine, is well compensated above and below, and is clinically inconspicuous. The prognosis for this type of congenital scoliosis is good.

Figure 8.65.   Right. This figure demonstrates congenital scoliosis resulting from multiple congenital anomalies of the spine, including multiple hemivertebrae, fused ribs, and a congenital synostosis of pedicles on the concave side of the curve. The prognosis for this 2-year-old child's scoliosis is poor in that the curvature will definitely increase with growth. Early correction and spinal fusion are indicated.

Congenital scoliosis may be accompanied by congenital abnormalities of the kidneys, heart, or spinal cord.

Synostosis of the Cervical Spine (Klippel-Feil Syndrome)

Failure of vertebral segmentation in the cervical spine results in congenital fusion (*synostosis*) between varying numbers of cervical vertebrae. Clinically, the child's neck is not only unduly short but also relatively stiff, and the posterior hairline is low and transverse (Fig. 8.66A and **B**). The head is usually straight but is occasionally tilted to one side,

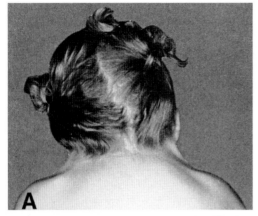

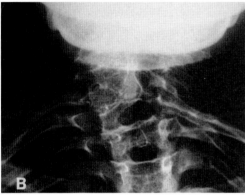

Figure 8.66.   A. Congenital synostosis of the cervical spine (Klippel-Feil syndrome) in a 5-year-old girl is seen. This girl's neck is not only short and stiff but also webbed. The posterior hairline is low and transverse. The appearance of this girl's neck was improved by a Z-plasty operation on the skin and subcutaneous tissue of each side of the neck to remove the skin webbing. **B.** The radiograph reveals multiple fusions (synostoses) of cervical vertebrae with resultant shortness of the neck.

least 40% of the infants have experienced a difficult delivery. The deformity is minimal at birth, but within the first few weeks of life a large, firm swelling develops in one sternocleidomastoid muscle. This swelling, called a *sternocleidomastoid tumor*, which is probably the result of hypertrophy of the fibrous tissue elements within the muscle, gradually disappears but leaves a *contracture* (shortening) of the involved muscle. As a result, the head becomes tilted, or laterally flexed, toward the affected side and rotated toward the opposite side (Fig. 8.67). The contracture of the muscle prevents its normal growth in length and, therefore, as the cervical spine grows, the muscle fails to keep pace and becomes relatively shorter. This relative shortness of the muscle on one side not only causes an increase in the tilting and rotation of the head but also results in progressive facial asymmetry during the growing years (Fig. 8.68). Radiographic examination is helpful in differentiating congenital muscular torticollis from the uncorrectable bony type of torticollis seen in cervical synostosis (Klippel-Feil syndrome).

It is important to remember that 20% of all infants with congenital muscular torticollis also have developmental displacement, or dys-

resembling muscular torticollis from which it must be differentiated. A congenital high scapula may coexist, and in some children a bilateral soft tissue web extends from the mastoid process of the skull toward the shoulder. Surgical treatment is limited to improving the child's appearance by operative procedures such as partial excision of a high scapula and Z-plasty of soft tissue webbing.

Muscular Torticollis (Wry Neck)

The exact cause of this congenital muscular abnormality remains a mystery, although at

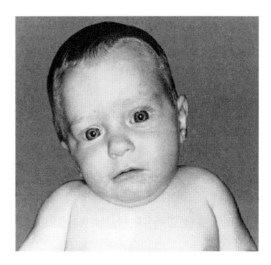

Figure 8.67.   Congenital muscular torticollis in a 1-year-old girl is seen. The girl's head is tilted to the right and slightly turned to the left, indicating that the involved sternocleidomastoid muscle is on the right side (as it is in 85% of afflicted children).

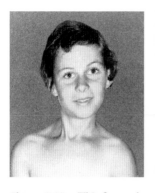 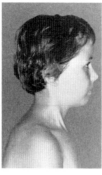

Figure 8.68.   This figure shows congenital muscular torticollis in a 10-year-old girl. Note the prominent, shortened right sternocleidomastoid muscle and also the facial asymmetry that is caused by delayed development of the right side of the face. This girl's face became more symmetrical over a 5-year period of growth following surgical division of the tight sternocleidomastoid muscle.

plasia of one or both hips. Early recognition and treatment of the torticollis are important because during the first few months of life, at least, the shortened muscle seems to respond well to daily stretching. Initially, the *treatment* is best carried out by an experienced physiotherapist who subsequently trains the parents in the exact method of stretching required. Such treatment, if instituted within the first month and continued for at least a year, results in complete and permanent correction of the torticollis in 90% of the children. In children untreated during the early months, the torticollis may become progressively resistant to stretching. Resistant and recurrent muscular torticollis require operative division of the contracted sternomastoid muscle and, in older children, secondary contractures of surrounding soft tissue must also be released.

GENERALIZED CONGENITAL ABNORMALITIES
Generalized Abnormalities of Bone

Of the multitude of generalized congenital abnormalities of bone formation and growth, only the five most significant are discussed here. Lest you be confused by their terminology, the various synonyms for these abnor-

malities are included in parentheses. Some of the generalized bone disorders that reflect inborn errors of metabolism are discussed in Chapter 9.

Osteogenesis Imperfecta (Fragilitas Ossium; Brittle Bones)

The salient feature of osteogenesis imperfecta, a relatively common form of skeletal dysplasia, is a genetically determined congenital osteoporosis characterized by weakness and fragility of all bones of the body, with resultant frequent pathological fractures.

The broad term *osteogenesis imperfecta* embraces a heterogeneous disorder with a wide variety of degrees of severity, most if not all of which are caused by mutations (either inherited or spontaneous) of type I collagen genes. The basic biochemical abnormality is an alteration of the structure and function of type I collagen which is the main type of collagen in bone, dentin, sclera, and ligaments (the tissues most involved in osteogenesis imperfecta and dentinogenesis imperfecta). Consequently, affected children exhibit varying degrees of failure of periosteal and endosteal osteogenesis with or without failure of dentinogenesis, blue sclerae, and lax ligaments.

The following four types of osteogenesis imperfecta have been classified on the basis of their clinical and radiographic features:

Type I: This is the most common and also the mildest form of osteogenesis imperfecta in which the pathological fractures begin to occur only after the child has started to walk. The sclerae are blue because they are abnormally translucent like thin skin and, consequently, they filter the red color of the underlying choroid plexus of blood vessels, just as a bruise or a subcutaneous hematoma appears blue through thin translucent skin. The child's head appears large in relation to the body but not in relation to his or her age, and the limbs are deformed. Radiographic examination reveals the slender, deformed, and osteoporotic bones. In osteogenesis imperfecta type I, the bones seem to become stronger after puberty and hence fractures occur less frequently in afflicted adults (although it is possible that the adults have learned to be more cautious). Deafness may occur at an early age. In subtype

I-A the teeth are normal, whereas in subtype I-B there is associated dentinogenesis imperfecta.

Type II: This type of osteogenesis imperfecta, which is the most severe, is both fetal and lethal with multiple intrauterine fractures. The sclerae are blue. This type is usually fatal in the perinatal period.

Type III: This type is also severe, with a number of birth fractures and multiple fractures occurring even before walking age. The limbs become progressively bowed even without gross fractures, in which case the progressive deformities result from multiple microfractures (Figs. 8.69 and 8.70). The epiphyseal plates (physes) of the limb bones become disrupted, with resultant premature closure and dwarfing. Kyphosis and scoliosis are also common, and most children with untreated osteogenesis imperfecta type III are unable to continue walking. The sclerae, which are pale blue initially, later become white.

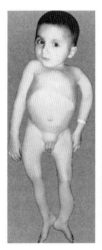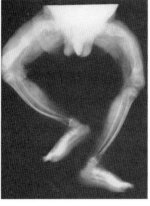

Figure 8.69. Left. Osteogenesis imperfecta type III (fragile bones) in a 4-year-old boy is seen in this figure. Note the multiple deformities in the poorly developed limbs from a long series of pathological fractures. Note also the short trunk relative to the head size. This boy's sclerae are pale blue but may become white when he is older.

Figure 8.70. Right. Osteogenesis imperfecta (fragile bones) in the same boy shown in Figure 8.69. Note the multiple healed fractures of both femora. Note also the slender, bent tibiae with extremely thin cortices and the generalized osteoporosis.

Type IV: This type is similar to type I-B in that it is usually associated with dentinogenesis imperfecta, but the sclerae are normal.

No effective medical treatment is as yet available for the underlying defect of osteogenesis imperfecta. The prevention of fractures is virtually impossible, but reasonable precautions should be taken by the child and by the parents; frequently, protective long leg braces or inflatable splints and crutches are necessary. The pathological fractures are usually treated by ordinary means, but prolonged immobilization must be avoided because it adds the problem of disuse atrophy (disuse osteoporosis) to the pre-existent osteoporosis. In the moderately severe type III osteogenesis imperfecta, the operative procedure of multiple segmental osteotomies of long bones and intramedullary metal rod fixation, developed by Sofield and Millar, serves the dual purpose of correcting severe bony deformities and providing internal support to prevent further fractures and recurrence of deformity. This method of treatment has certainly saved many severely afflicted children from a wheelchair existence.

Bailey has designed an extensible intramedullary rod, or nail, that is like a telescope and elongates as the child's bone grows in length; it offers an advantage over the conventional type of intramedullary rod.

Achondroplasia (Chondrodystrophia Fetalis)

The most striking feature of *achondroplasia*, and one that can be detected even in infancy, is dwarfism of the short limb type, the limbs being disproportionately shorter than the trunk (Fig. 8.71). It is an autosomal dominant anomaly, the majority of cases resulting from new spontaneous mutations.

The underlying defect is a failure of longitudinal growth in the cartilage of the epiphyseal plate (achondroplasia). Thus, all bones that form by endochrondral ossification, including the long bones and facial bones, are affected, whereas the membrane bones, such as those in the cranium, grow normally. This accounts for the extremely short limbs (about half of normal length) and the typical facial appearance caused by the disproportion between the size of the hypoplastic midface and that of the jaw and the rest of the head (Fig. 8.72). The total height seldom exceeds 4 feet. Radiographically, the bones are thick (because the periosteal intramembranous ossification is normal) but are frequently deformed as indicated by cubitus varus, genu varum, coxa vara, and lumbar lordosis. Spinal stenosis may develop in adult life, with the resultant neurological impairment. Operative correction of bony deformities in the lower limbs is sometimes indicated to improve both function and appearance.

The surgical lengthening of the short upper and lower limbs by the Ilizarov method has somewhat improved the appearance of a few

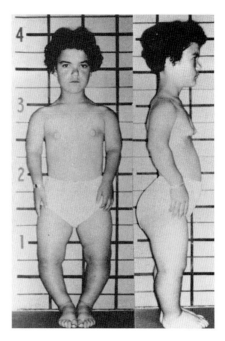

Figure 8.72.   Achondroplasia (chondrodystrophia fetalis) in a 15-year-old girl is seen. Note the dwarfism of the short limb type, the limbs being disproportionately shorter than the trunk. The limbs are bowed and there is an increase in the lumbar lordosis. The face is small relative to the head.

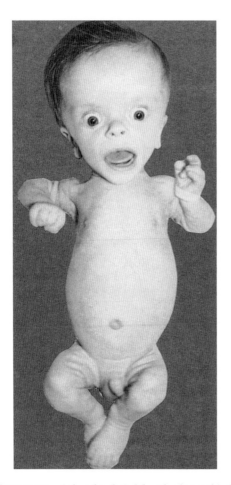

Figure 8.71.   Achondroplasia (chondrodystrophia fetalis) in a 3-month-old infant. Note the short limbs relative to the trunk and the small face relative to the large head.

achondroplastic dwarfs in recent years, but the benefits may not outweigh the associated complications and morbidity. Consequently, this particular use of the Ilizarov method remains controversial.

Achondroplastic dwarfs have a normal mentality and a normal life expectancy. Therefore, an important aspect of their total care concerns helping them to accept and to adjust to their obvious dwarfism and also helping provide them with adequate education and vocational guidance so that they may pursue a meaningful and satisfying occupation.

Arachnodactyly (Hyperchondroplasia) (Marfan's Syndrome)

The most characteristic feature of *arachnodactyly* (which means "spider fingers") is the excessive length of the limbs and to a lesser extent of the trunk (Fig. 8.73). This is an autosomal dominant disorder, and 15% of patients have a spontaneous new mutation. The abnormal protein is fibrillin, for which a gene has been identified. The underlying abnormality is excessive longitudinal growth in the cartilage of the epiphyseal plate (*hyperchondroplasia*), and in this sense, it is the antithesis of achondroplasia. The child is always considerably taller and thinner than average, is generally weak, and exhibits marked joint laxity. Associated skeletal deformities may include a resistant and progressive type of scoliosis, depressed sternum (pectus excavatum), and very long, extremely flexible flat feet. In addition, there is a high incidence of associated congenital heart disease and congenital dislocation of the lens. The orthopaedic *treatment* of arach-

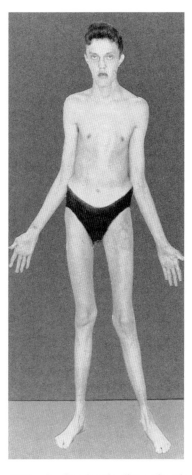

Figure 8.73. Arachnodactyly (hyperchondroplasia, Marfan's syndrome) in a 13-year-old boy is seen in this figure. Note the excessively long and slender limbs relative to the length of the trunk. This boy also demonstrates poor chest development, genu valgum, and hypermobile feet.

nodactyly involves operative correction of the associated skeletal deformities if and when they begin to interfere with the child's function. Before any orthopaedic treatment is undertaken, however, thorough assessment of the child's cardiovascular system should be conducted and any defects corrected if possible.

Enchondromatosis (Multiple Enchondromata) (Ollier's Dyschondroplasia)

Enchondromatosis is a relatively uncommon congenital abnormality that is associated with defective longitudinal growth of some long bones; the involvement tends to be predominantly unilateral. The condition is not usually detected at birth but presents itself in early childhood as a problem of limb length discrepancy and deformity. It is not genetically determined. The underlying defect is the persistence of epiphyseal plate cartilage cells that, instead of undergoing endochondral ossification to form metaphyseal bone, remain as a large cartilage mass (*enchondroma*) within the metaphysis. Irregular ossification and calcification in the radiolucent cartilage account for the typical radiographic appearance in the widened metaphysis of involved bones (Fig. 8.74). In the small long bones of the hands and feet, the enchondromata may expand the cortex significantly (Fig. 8.75). However, the lesions stop growing at skeletal maturity. A rare complication in adult life is the malignant change of an enchondroma to a chondrosarcoma. Angular deformities and relative shortening may develop in the involved limbs as a result of unequal or premature cessation of epiphyseal plate growth. *Treatment* includes the operative correction of bony deformity by osteotomy through the area of abnormal cartilage (which always heals), surgical correction of severe leg length discrepancy, and surgical trimming of grossly expanded metacarpals and phalanges.

Multiple Hereditary Exostoses (Diaphyseal Aclasis)

The characteristic feature of multiple hereditary exostoses, which is a relatively common and deforming abnormality, is the gradual de-

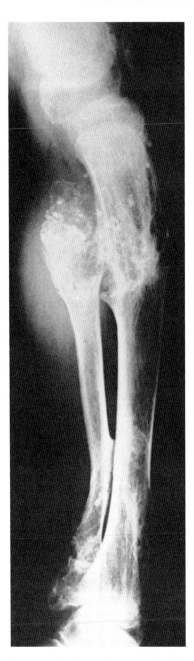

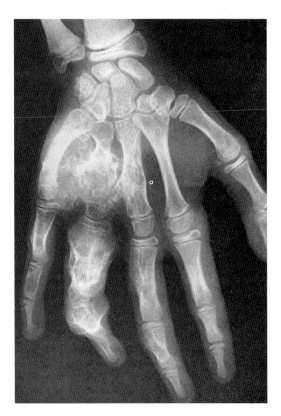

Figure 8.75. Enchondromatosis (multiple enchondromata, Ollier's dyschondroplasia) in a 13-year-old child is seen. The radiograph of the hand reveals multiple radiolucent cartilaginous lesions (enchondromata), some of which have expanded the overlying cortex.

Figure 8.74. This figure shows enchondromatosis (multiple enchondromata, Ollier's dyschondroplasia) in a 12-year-old child. The radiograph reveals irregular replacement of the proximal third of the tibia and fibula with radiolucent cartilaginous lesions (enchondromata). Note also the deformity in these involved bones.

velopment of multiple outgrowths of bone and cartilage (*osteocartilaginous exostoses*) from the abnormally broad metaphyseal region of long bones (Fig. 8.76). The abnormality is transmitted by an autosomal dominant gene, with 30% of the cases being due to a new mutation. The underlying defect is a lack of the normal osteoclastic activity (*aclasis*) in the process of remodeling of the metaphysis during longitudinal growth.

As a result, the metaphysis, rather than becoming trumpet-shaped, persists as a broad cylinder. Bony outgrowths, each capped by cartilage and a type of growth plate, develop during early childhood and always point away from the neighboring epiphysis. Each exostosis is clinically (both visibly and palpably) larger than it appears radiographically because of the radiolucent cartilaginous cap. It is not unusual for a given patient to have 20 or more such osteocartilaginous exostoses. They stop growing larger at the time of skeletal maturity. A rare complication in 2% of patients during adult life is the malignant change of one of the osteocartilaginous exostoses to a chondrosarcoma, which is always associated with a rapid increase in its size and radiographic evidence of calcification. The longitudinal growth in the long bones is somewhat decreased but never strikingly so. However, bony deformities sometimes develop as a result of uneven epiphyseal plate growth.

The exostoses may become sufficiently large in superficial locations that their mere presence causes deformity (Fig. 8.77). They may cause symptoms, either from pressure on soft tissues or by interference with the gliding of tendons, particularly in the region of the

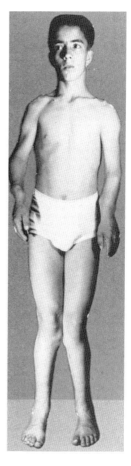

Figure 8.77. Multiple hereditary exostoses (diaphyseal aclasis) in a 14-year-old boy are seen. Some of the exostoses are sufficiently large that they produce obvious local deformities, particularly in the region of the wrists and knees. Each exostosis, being covered by a cap of cartilage, is always larger clinically than it appears radiographically.

knee. Operative *treatment* is indicated only for exostoses that are causing symptoms, producing a significant deformity, or enlarging rapidly. Treatment involves excision of the exostosis along with its periosteal covering and its cartilaginous cap.

Generalized Abnormalities of Nerve and Muscle

Neurofibromatosis (von Recklinghausen's Disease)

A discussion of neurofibromatosis, a generalized congenital abnormality of peripheral nerves, is included here because it involves

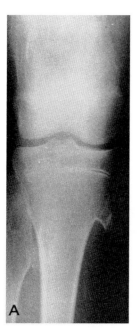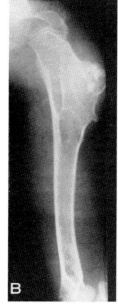

Figure 8.76. This figure demonstrates multiple hereditary exostoses (diaphyseal aclasis). **A.** There are multiple osteocartilaginous exostoses arising from the abnormally broad metaphyseal regions of the long bones in the area of the knee. The exostoses always point away from the neighboring epiphysis. **B.** There is a large osteocartilaginous exostosis arising from the upper end of the humerus.

mesodermal as well as ectodermal structures, and one half of afflicted children develop related skeletal abnormalities. The condition is transmitted by an autosomal dominant gene. The relationship between neurofibromatosis and the associated skeletal abnormalities is not clear, but the latter include congenital pseudarthrosis of the tibia (as discussed in a preceding section of this chapter), local gigantism of part or all of a limb (Fig. 8.78), and a particularly serious and progressive type of scoliosis that requires early spinal fusion (Fig. 8.79). The skin manifestations, which serve as useful clues in the diagnosis, include areas of light brown pigmentation (café-au-lait spots) as well as elevated cutaneous neurofibromata, the latter being more noticeable in later years (Fig. 8.80)

Additional musculoskeletal manifestations of neurofibromatosis result from the pressure of an enlarging neurofibroma on normal nervous tissue. For example, a neurofibroma arising in a nerve root may extend into the spinal canal and compress the spinal cord, thereby simulating a spinal cord tumor. Furthermore, a neurofibroma may cause pressure on the nerve root from which it is arising and thereby produce radiating pain in the lower limb (sciatica) or in the upper limb (brachialgia). Treatment of neurofibromatosis involves operative correction of the associated skeletal deformities and excision of a neurofibroma that is causing symptoms.

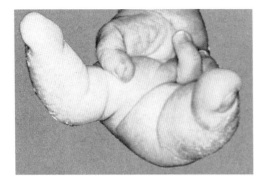

Figure 8.78. Local gigantism of the index and middle fingers resulting from local neurofibromatosis in the hand of a two-year-old child.

Hypotonia of Neuromuscular Origin (Amyotonia Congenita, Spinal Muscular Atrophy)

Hypotonia of neuromuscular origin is a generalized congenital abnormality of muscle that is characterized at birth by an extreme lack of muscle tone (*hypotonia, amyotonia*), which gives the infant the appearance and feel of a floppy rag doll (Fig. 8.81). Associated with the decreased muscle tone are decreased tendon reflexes and generalized muscle weakness. The child has difficulty learning to hold his or her head up, to sit up, and to stand up; therefore, these milestones of musculoskeletal development are delayed. There is usually a marked degree of coexistent joint laxity and when the child does manage to stand up, flexible flat feet and knock knees are exhibited. The prognosis in the more severe forms of hypotonia of neuromuscular origin is poor. Treatment is limited to the support of weak and floppy limbs and trunk by appropriate braces.

Amyoplasia Congenita (Arthrogryposis Multiplex Congenita) (Myodystrophia Fetalis)

Amyoplasia congenita is a crippling congenital abnormality of muscle development that is characterized by marked stiffness and severe deformity in many joints of the limbs (hence the term *arthrogryposis,* which means "bent joints"). The abnormality, which is immediately apparent at birth, gives the infant the appearance and feel of a wooden doll (Fig. 8.82). It is not genetically determined. The underlying defect is aplasia and hypoplasia of many muscle groups during embryonic development (*amyoplasia*) and is sometimes secondary to a defect in the anterior horn cells of the spinal cord. Thus, there is a marked decrease in the amount of muscle in the spindly limbs. Microscopically, fatty and fibrous infiltration is seen between the scant muscle fibers. As a result, the joints that are controlled by involved muscles have never moved normally *in utero* and consequently, they fail to develop normally, not only before birth but also after. Excessive fibrous tissue infiltration is found in the periarticular soft tissues as well as in the subcutaneous fat, and even the skin is tight

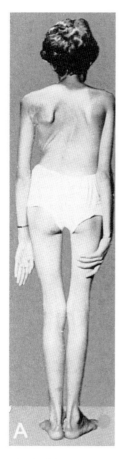
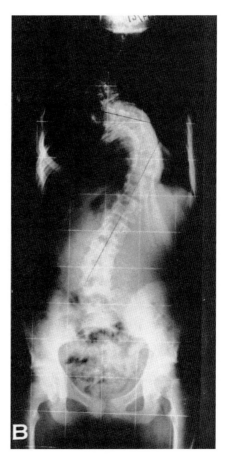

Figure 8.79.   A. Neurofibromatosis (von Recklinghausen's disease) complicated by severe and progressive lateral curvature of the spine (scoliosis) is seen in a 14-year-old girl. Note the café-au-lait pigmentation on the posterior aspect of this girl's left shoulder. **B.** The radiograph of this girl reveals the severe type of scoliosis seen in association with neurofibromatosis.

and inelastic. The muscle abnormality is static rather than progressive, but the secondary changes in and around the joints tend to become more severe during the growing years.

The more common clinical deformities that result from amyoplasia congenita include severe and extremely resistant clubfeet, knee flexion or knee extension deformity (sometimes with resultant dislocation of the knee), a severe and irreducible prenatal (teratologic) type of congenital dislocation of the hip, flexion deformity of the fingers and wrists, extension deformities of the elbows, and adduction deformity of the shoulders. The trunk is usually spared, but when it is involved, scoliosis

may be present. Occasionally, the deformities are limited to the hands and feet. The child's mentality is within normal limits.

Treatment of the joint deformities associated with amyoplasia congenita represents one of the most difficult problems in the musculoskeletal system and demands all the patience, ingenuity, and skill of the most experienced orthopaedic surgeon. Daily passive stretching of the stiff and deformed joints by a physiotherapist and by the parents may improve the passive joint motion somewhat, but any gain is seldom maintained because of lack of muscle power. In this abnormality, there is a vicious tendency to form excessive amounts of dense

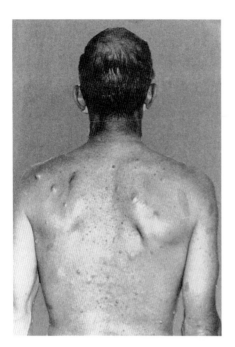

Figure 8.80. Neurofibromatosis (von Recklinghausen's disease) in the father of the girl shown at left. Note the multiple areas of pigmentation (café-au-lait spots) as well as the elevated cutaneous neurofibromata.

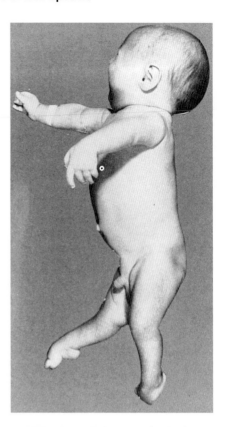

Figure 8.82. Amyoplasia congenita (arthrogryposis multiplex congenita, myodystrophia fetalis) is seen in a newborn infant. The limbs are deformed and rigid giving the child the appearance and the feel of a wooden doll. Note the associated clubfeet and the congenital hyperextension of the right knee.

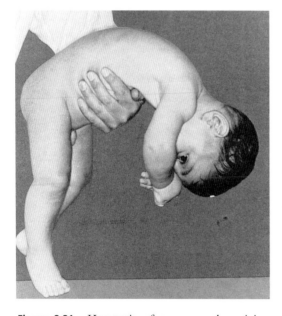

Figure 8.81. Hypotonia of neuromuscular origin (amyotonia congenita, infantile spinal muscular atrophy) seen in a 1-year-old boy. The extreme lack of muscle tone prevented this child from sitting up or even holding his head up. The child looks and feels like a floppy rag doll.

fibrous scar tissue around the joints following soft tissue operations such as capsulotomy and tendon lengthening and, as might be expected, the results of such procedures are disappointing. Bony operations such as osteotomy and arthrodesis are more effective and the results more permanent. Sound orthopaedic judgment is required in the planning of operative treatment for these severely disabled children so that after a given operation, the child may be better, and not just different.

Perhaps one of *you* will accept the challenge of working—through clinical and experimental investigation—to solve the perplexing problems posed by these generalized congenital abnormalities of the musculoskeletal system.

SUGGESTED ADDITIONAL READING

Aronsson DD, Goldberg MJ, Kling TF Jr, Roy DR. Developmental dysplasia of the hip. Pediatrics 1994;94:201–208.

Atar D, Lehman WD, Tenenbaum Y, et al. Pavlik harness versus Frejka splint in treatment of developmental dysplasia of the hip: bicenter study. J Pediatr Orthop 1993;13:311–313.

Bailey RW. Further experience with the extensible nail (for osteogenesis imperfecta). Clin Orthop 1981;159:171–176.

Barlow TG. Early diagnosis and treatment of congenital dislocation of the hip. J Bone Joint Surg 1962;44B:292.

Beaty JH, Canale ST. Orthopaedic aspects of myelomeningocele. J Bone Joint Surg 1990;72A:626–630.

Bennett GL, Weiner DS, Leighley B. Surgical treatment of symptomatic accessory tarsal scaphoid. J Pediatr Orthop 1990;10:445–449.

Benson MKD, Fixen JA, Macnichol MF. Children's orthopaedics and fractures. Edinburgh: Churchill-Livingstone, 1994.

Boeree NR, Clarke NMP. Ultrasound imaging and secondary screening for congenital dislocation of the hip. J Bone Joint Surg (Br) 1994;76B:525–533.

Brown LM, Robson MJ, Sharrard WJW. The pathophysiology of arthrogryposis multiplex congenita neurologica. J Bone Joint Surg 1980;62B:291–296.

Camp J, Herring JA, Dworezynski C. Comparison of inpatient and outpatient traction in developmental dislocation of the hip. J Pediatr Orthop 1994;14:9–12.

Campbell CC, Waters PM, Emans JB. Excision of the radial head for congenital dislocation. J Bone Joint Surg 1993;74A:726–733.

Carroll NC, McMurtry R, Leete, SF. The pathoanatomy of congenital club foot. Orthop Clin North Am 1978;9:225–232.

Cheng JCY, Au AWY. Infantile torticollis: a review of 624 cases. J Pediatr Orthop 1994;14:802–808.

Cole WG. Genetics, embryology and pathology. Curr Opin Orthop 1992;3:647–650.

Cole WG. Bone, cartilage and fibrous tissue disorders. In: Benson MKD, Fixen JA, Macnichol MF, eds. Children's Orthopaedics and Fractures. Chapter 3. Edinburgh: Churchill Livingstone, 1994; 35–71.

Cole WG. Genetic aspects of orthopaedic conditions. In: Morrissy RT, Weinstein SL, eds. Lovell and Winter's pediatric orthopaedics. 4th ed. Chapter 5. Philadelphia: Lippincott-Raven, 1996.

Coleman SS. Congenital dysplasia and dislocation of the hip. St. Louis: CV Mosby, 1978.

Cowell HR. The management of club foot. Editorial. J Bone Joint Surg 1985;67A:991–992.

Cowell HR. Genetic aspects of orthopaedic conditions. In: Lovell WW, Winter RB, eds. Paediatric orthopaedics. 2nd ed. Philadelphia: JB Lippincott, 1986;147–179.

Crawford AH Jr, Bagamery N. Osseous manifestations of neurofibromatosis in childhood. J Pediatr Orthop 1986;6:72–88.

Czeizel A, Dundas I. Prevention of the first occurrence of neural tube defects by periconceptual vitamin supplementation. N Engl J Med 1992;327:1823.

De Puy J, Drennan JC. Correction of idiopathic clubfoot. A comparison of results of early versus delayed posteromedial release. J Pediatr Orthop 1989;9:44–48.

Desai SS, Johnson LO. Long term results of valgus osteotomy for congenital coxa vara. Clin Orthop 1993;294:204–210.

Drennan JC. Congenital vertical talus. J Bone Joint Surg 1995;77A:1916–1923.

Dubé ID, Cournoyer D. Gene therapy: here to stay. Can Med Assoc J 1995;152:1605.

Farsetti P, Weinstein SL, Ponseti IV, et al. The long-term functional and radiographic outcomes of untreated and non-operatively treated metatarsus adductus. J Bone Joint Surg 1994;76A:257–265.

Forman R, Singal N, Perelman V, Chow S, Hoffman L, Parkin P, Koren G. Folic acid and prevention of neural tube defects: a study of Canadian women giving birth to children with spina bifida. Clin Invest Med 1996;19:195–201.

Fukuhara K, Schollmeier G, Uhthoff HK. The pathogenesis of club foot: A histomorphometric and immunohistochemical study of fetuses. J Bone Joint Surg (Br) 1994;76B:450–457.

Gamble JG, Strudwick WJ, Rinsky, LA, et al. Complications of intramedullary rods in osteogenesis imperfecta: Bailey-Dubow rods versus nonelongating rods. J Pediatr Orthop 1988;8:645–649.

Goldberg MJ. The dysmorphic child: an orthopaedic perspective. New York: Raven Press, 1987.

Gonzalez P, Kumar SJ. Calcaneonavicular coalition treated by resection and interposition of the extensor brevis muscle. J Bone Joint Surg 1990;72A:71–77.

Graf R. New possibilities for the diagnosis of congenital hip joint dislocation by ultrasonography. J Pediatr Orthop 1983;3:354–359.

Greitemann B, Rondhuis JJ, Kaerbowski A. A treatment of congenital elevation of the scapula: ten (2–18) year follow up of 37 cases of Sprengel's deformity. Acta Orthop Scand 1993;64:365–368.

Handelsman JE, Badalamente MA. Neuromuscular studies in club foot. Pediatr Orthop 1981;1:23–32.

Harcke HT, Kumar SJ. The role of ultrasound in the diagnosis and management of congenital dislocation and dysplasia of the hip (current concepts review). J Bone Joint Surg 1991;73-A: 622–628.

Harris IE, Dickens R, Menelaus MB. Use of the Pavlik harness for hip displacements: when to abandon treatment. Clin Orthop Rel Res 1992; 281:29–33.

Herzenberg JE, Carroll NC, Christopherson MR. Clubfoot analysis with three-dimensional computer modeling. J Pediatr Orthop 1988;3: 257–262.

Howard CB, Benson MK. Clubfoot: its pathological anatomy. J Pediatr Orthop 1993;13: 654–659.

Joseph KN, Bowen JR, MacEwen GD. Unusual orthopaedic manifestations of neurofibromatosis. Clin Orthop 1992;278:17–28.

Klisic PJ. Congenital dislocation of the hip. A misleading term: brief report. J Bone Joint Surg (Br) 1989;71-B:136.

Koren G, Forman R, Chow S, Parkin P, Koren G, ed. Folic acid and the prevention of neural tube defects. Toronto: The Motherisk Program at the Hospital for Sick Children 1997.

Kruger L, Fishman S. Myoelectric and body-powered prosthesis. J Pediatr Orthop 1993;3: 68–75.

Lee MS, Harcke HT, Kumar SJ, Bassett GS. Subtalar joint coalition in children: new observations. Radiology 1989;172:635–639.

Lloyd-Roberts GC, Fixen JA. Orthopaedics in infancy and childhood. London: Butterworth-Heineman, 1990.

Manske PR, Rotman MB, Dactey LA. Long term functional results after pollicization for the congenitally deficient thumb. J Hand Surg 1992; 17-A:1064–1072.

McKusick VA. Mendelian inheritance in man. 7th ed. Baltimore: Johns Hopkins University Press, 1986.

Miller LS, Bell DF. Management of congenital fibular deficiency by Ilizarov technique. J Pediatr Orthop 1992;12:651–657.

Morrissy RT, Weinstein SL. Developmental hip dysplasia. In: Morrisy RT, Weinstein SL, eds. Lovell and Winter's Pediatric Orthopaedics. 4th ed. Vol 2. Chapter 23. Philadelphia: Lippincott-Raven, 1996.

O'Brien TM (Guest Editor). Idiopathic hip dysplasia: Clinical Orthopaedic Baillière's International Practice and Research Vol 1 No 1 London, Baillière, Tindall, 1996.

O'Hara JN. Congenital dislocation of the hip: acetabular deficiency in adolescence (absence of the lateral acetabular epiphysis) after limbectomy in infancy. J Pediatr Orthop 1989;9:640–648.

Paley D, Catagni M, Argnani F, et al. Treatment of congenital pseudarthrosis of the tibia using the Ilizarov technique. Clin Orthop 1992;280: 81–93.

Paterson DC, Simonis RB. Electrical stimulation in the treatment of congenital pseudarthrosis of the tibia. J Bone Joint Surg 1985;67B:454–462.

Salter RB. Innominate osteotomy in the treatment of congenital dislocation and subluxation of the hip. J Bone Joint Surg 1961;43B:518–539.

Salter RB. Etiology, pathogenesis and possible prevention of congenital dislocation of the hip. Can Med Assoc J 1968;98:933–945.

Salter RB. Osteotomy of the pelvis (editorial comment). Clin Orthop 1974;98:2–4.

Salter RB, Dubos JP. The first 15 years' personal experience with innominate osteotomy in the treatment of congenital dislocation and subluxation of the hip. Clin Orthop 1974;98:72–103.

Salter RB, Kostuik J, Dallas S. Avascular necrosis of the femoral head as a complication of treatment for congenital dislocation of the hip in young children: a clinical and experimental investigation. Can J Surg 1969;12:44–60.

Sarwark JF, MacEwen GD, Scott CI Jr. Amyoplasia: a common form of arthrogryposis. J Bone Joint Surg 1990;72A:465–469.

Slate RK, Posnick JC, Armstrong DC, Buncic JR. Cervical spine subluxation associated with congenital muscular torticollis and craniofacial asymmetry. Plast Reconstr Surg 1993;91: 1187–1197.

Sofield HA, Millar EA. Fragmentation, realignment and intramedullary rod fixation of deformities of long bones in children. J Bone Joint Surg 1959;41A:1371–1392.

Staheli LT. Fundamentals of pediatric orthopaedics. New York: Raven Press, 1992.

Tredwell SJ, Bell HM. Efficacy of neonatal hip examination. J Paediatr Orthop 1981;1:61–65.

Wald N (MRC Vitamin Study Research Group). Prevention of neural tube defects. Results of the MRC vitamin study. Lancet 1991;338:131.

Watson JD. The human genome project: past, present, and future. Science 1990;278:44–49.

Weiland AJ, Weiss A-PC, Moore JR, Tolo VT. Vascularized fibular grafts in the treatment of congenital pseudarthrosis of the tibia. J Hand Surg 1990;72-A:654–662.

Wenger DR, Rang M. The art and practice of children's orthopaedics. New York: Raven Press, 1993.

Williams PF, Cole WG. Orthopaedic management in childhood. 2nd ed. London: Chapman and Hall, 1991.

Worton RG. The era of genetic medicine. Can Med Assoc J 1993;148:1455.

Wright J, Dormans J, Rang M. Pseudarthrosis of the rat tibia: a model for congenital pseudarthrosis? J Paediatr Orthop 1991;11: 277–283.

Wynne-Davies R, Hall CM, Apley AG. Atlas of skeletal dysplasias. Edinburgh: Churchill Livingstone, 1985.

9 Generalized and Disseminated Disorders of Bone

You will recall from the discussions in Chapter 2, that although each *individual bone* of the skeleton may be considered as a *structure, bone* of the entire skeleton may be considered as an *organ.* Bone, as an organ, is the major storehouse for calcium and phosphorus and is normally the site of active *turnover* at a cellular level in relation to its physiology. You may find it helpful at this stage to review the brief description of *biochemistry and physiology of bone* in Chapter 2, as well as the *reactions of bone to disorders and injuries* in Chapter 3.

Bone reacts to a wide variety of diseases, many of which have their origin outside the skeletal system. These reactions of bone serve as a *mirror of disease* in that they *reflect* the nature of the underlying abnormality. These bony reflections, or *manifestations,* of disease are of practical importance because they can be detected by clinical and radiographic methods; furthermore, they are often serious in themselves because they may cause pain, deformity, and disability in patients. Therefore, the reactions of bone as an organ and as a structure are equally important to you in the diagnosis and treatment of patients. Without an understanding of bone in both these capacities, you run the risk, as a surgeon, of becoming a mere carpenter of cortical bone and, as a physician, of becoming a mere purveyor of pills. Indeed, as you will see, the problems presented by many bone diseases require the combined efforts of both physician and surgeon.

It will be apparent to you that any abnormal metabolic disturbance affecting bone as an organ will be reflected by a *generalized* reaction in *all* bones of the skeleton and that the result will be a *generalized disease of bone.* The generalized disease of osteoporosis is not actually a "metabolic" disease but, rather, is probably the result of "intrinsic" abnormalities of bone cell function, bone cell-cell communication, or bone gene expression. Other, and less clearly understood, disturbances are reflected by a *localized* reaction in parts of a number of bones. Since the unaffected bones, as well as the uninvolved parts of the affected bones, are completely normal, the widely scattered lesions constitute a *disseminated disease of bone.*

GENERALIZED BONE DISORDERS CAUSED BY METABOLIC DISTURBANCES (METABOLIC BONE DISEASE)

The generalized reactions of bone include alterations (an increase or decrease) in either bone deposition or bone resorption, or both. Bone deposition, however, involves the two major processes of osteoblastic formation of organic matrix (osteoid) and calcification of the matrix to form bone. Bone resorption involves osteoclastic removal of formed bone and the release of bone minerals. In some metabolic disturbances, such as *rickets* and *osteomalacia,* the generalized reaction of bone is inadequate calcification of matrix (hypocalcification). In others, such as *scurvy* and *osteoporosis,* the generalized reaction is either a decreased osteoblastic formation of matrix or an increased osteoclastic bone resorption (or both), with a resultant decrease in the total amount of bone. In addition, combinations of these reactions may appear together as seen in the osteoporosis that coexists with hypocalcification in certain types of refractory rickets. It is important to appreciate that one third of the total amount of bone mineral may be lost before the resultant decrease in radiographic density of the bones is readily detectable by ordinary radiographic techniques. However, the modern, sophisticated noninvasive radiographic technique of bone densitometry can quantitate bone density accurately. The equipment currently of choice is DEXA (dual energy x-ray absorptiometry).

In some of these generalized disorders, the causative factor is either nutritional or hormonal, and the disorder is said to be metabolic, whereas in other disorders, a combination of factors, including physical stresses and strains, are responsible. Nevertheless, in all these disorders, there is a disturbance of the *metabolism of bone* and, accordingly, they are best considered together in the broad category of *metabolic bone disease*.

Rickets

Rickets may be defined as a generalized disease of *growing* bone characterized by a failure of calcium salts to be deposited promptly in organic bone matrix (osteoid) as well as in the preosseous cartilage of the epiphyseal plate at the zone of calcifying cartilage. The normal deposition of calcium in osteoid and preosseous cartilage is largely dependent on the maintenance of physiological levels of calcium and phosphorus in the serum which, in turn, is dependent on a balance among the three factors of 1) *absorption* of each element from the intestine, 2) their *excretion* by the kidneys and intestine, and 3) their *rates of movement* into and out of bone. Important factors in maintaining this balance are vitamin D and parathyroid hormone. Thus, several types of disturbances are capable of causing the one generalized bone reaction of rickets. The various clinical forms of rickets are best classified on the basis of their cause; the three main causes of rickets are vitamin D deficiency, chronic renal insufficiency, and renal tubular insufficiency. The dietary deficiency type of rickets has become much less common since the fortification of dairy products with vitamin D. The latter two forms of rickets do not respond to *normal* amounts of vitamin D and are therefore "vitamin D-refractory."

Pathology

The pathological changes in rickets include a *generalized decrease in calcified matrix (bone)* and an *increase in uncalcified matrix (osteoid)*. In addition, a wide zone of *uncalcified preosseous cartilage* forms at the usual site of calcifying cartilage in the epiphyseal plate (Fig.

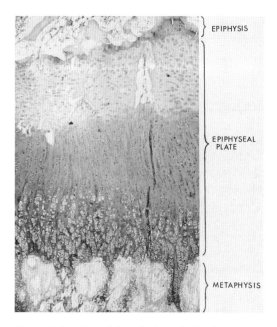

Figure 9.1.   An epiphyseal plate obtained postmortem from a 1-year-old child with rickets. (He died of an unrelated condition.) Note the wide zone of uncalcified preosseous cartilage and the disorganized columns of hypertrophic cartilage cells in the epiphyseal plate, as well as the uncalcified bone matrix (osteoid) in the metaphyseal region.

9.1). Since calcium provides the "hardness" of bone, the uncalcified areas are "soft" and consequently, progressive deformities occur not only in the substance of bones but also through their epiphyseal plates (Fig. 9.2).

Diagnosis

In infants, the possibility of rickets must be considered in the presence of convulsions, tetany, irritability, delayed physical development (including skeletal growth), weakness, and failure to thrive. In children who have started to walk, the possibility of rickets must also be considered in the presence of deformities of the lower limbs (particularly severe genu valgum, genu varum, and torsional deformities) and a small stature (Fig. 9.2).

The diagnosis of rickets, whatever the cause, is *suggested* by clinical enlargement at the sites of epiphyseal plates, particularly at the distal end of each radius and at the costochondral junctions, the latter being known as a "rachitic rosary" (Fig. 9.3). However, the diag-

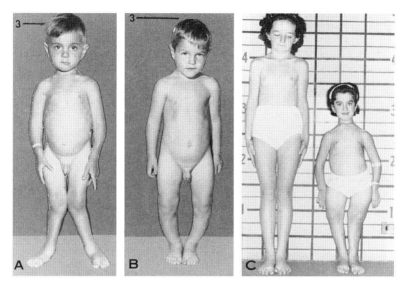

Figure 9.2. Clinical deformities caused by rickets are seen. **A.** Genu valgum in a 5-year-old boy with vitamin D-refractory rickets. Note also the enlargement of the sites of epiphyseal plates, particularly at the ankles, knees, wrists, and costochondral junctions. **B.** Genu varum with internal tibial torsion and external femoral torsion in a 4-year-old boy with vitamin D-refractory rickets. **C.** Small stature, genu varum of the right lower limb, and genu valgum of the left lower limb in an 11-year-old girl with vitamin D-refractory rickets. The 11-year-old girl on the left is normal.

nosis is *established* by the typical radiographic changes in the growing ends of long bones, which demonstrate a widened radiolucent zone in the epiphyseal plate (resulting from uncalcified preosseous cartilage) and also by the generalized coarse appearance of trabeculation resulting from the mineralization defect of all the areas of bone (Fig. 9.4). The serum alkaline phosphatase level is elevated in most types of rickets, but in one type of hereditary rickets—hypophosphatasia—it is normal. However, the differentiation between the various types of rickets necessitates the use of a number of standard diagnostic methods. For

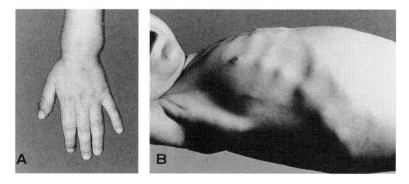

Figure 9.3. Clinical enlargement at the sites of epiphyseal plates. **A.** Enlargement at the sites of the distal radial and distal ulnar epiphyseal plates in a 11-year-old boy with vitamin D-refractory rickets. **B.** Enlargement at the sites of the epiphyseal plates at the costochondral junctions in the same child. Because of the beaded appearance, this is known as a "rachitic rosary."

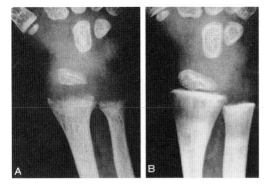

Figure 9.4.   A. The wrist of a 3-year-old child with rickets. Note the widened radiolucent zone in the epiphyseal plate (caused by uncalcified preosseous cartilage and osteoid), the generalized rarefaction of the bones, and the coarse trabecular pattern of cancellous bone. **B.** The same patient after treatment with vitamin D. Note the normal ossification in the metaphyseal regions and the normal generalized density of the bones.

example, elevated blood creatinine and serum inorganic phosphorus levels indicate a renal *glomerular* lesion, whereas normal blood creatinine and lowered serum inorganic phosphorus (hypophosphatemia) levels, in the absence of vitamin D deficiency, indicate a renal *tubular* defect.

Clinical Aspects of the Three Main Forms of Rickets

Vitamin D Deficiency Rickets (Nutritional Rickets). Although the incidence of vitamin D deficiency rickets has diminished greatly since the recognition of the importance of sunlight and vitamin D, it is still seen in clinical practice. A typical history is that the child, who is usually around the age of 1 year, has been breastfed since birth, has not received supplementary vitamins, and has not been taken outdoors for exposure to sunlight. The aforementioned clinical and radiographic signs are readily detected. This type of rickets responds well to treatment, which includes normal doses of vitamin D and improvement in diet. In the early stages of vitamin D deficiency, the child may develop severe hypocalcemia, with resultant tetany or even convulsions but minimal radiographic changes. Vitamin D deficiency can also be caused by its defective ab-

sorption from the intestinal tract because of steatorrhea caused by chronic intestinal or hepatic disorders.

Renal Osteodystrophy (Azotemic Osteodystrophy). Renal osteodystrophy is a relatively uncommon type of rickets that was formerly called *renal rickets*. It is complex in that chronic renal disease produces not only the bony lesion of rickets already described but also a secondary hyperparathyroidism that results in the superimposition of hyperparathyroid bone lesions (irregular disintegration of metaphyses and erosion of cortical bone) (Fig. 9.5). This type of rickets is understandably refractory to ordinary doses of vitamin D.

Treatment is directed toward the renal insufficiency, the rickets, and the secondary hy-

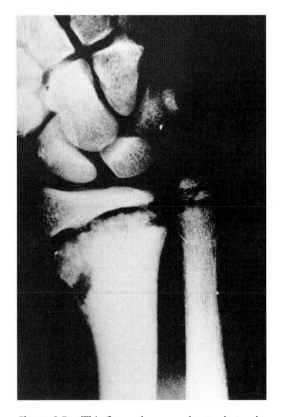

Figure 9.5. This figure shows renal osteodystrophy caused by chronic renal insufficiency in a 14-year-old boy. Note the widened radiolucent zone in the epiphyseal plates (resulting from rickets) and, in addition, the irregular disintegration of metaphyses and the erosion of cortical bone (resulting from secondary hyperparathyroidism).

perparathyroidism. Both the hyperparathyroidism and the rickets are treated with an active metabolite of vitamin D, namely, 1,25-dihydroxyvitamin D_3.

Rickets Caused by a Renal Tubular Defect. The mechanism by which the various renal tubular dysfunctions cause the bony reaction of rickets is defective tubular reabsorption of phosphate and consequent excess loss of phosphate in the urine, with resultant hypophosphatemia. The most common type of such rickets is designated *hypophosphatemic vitamin D-refractory (resistant) rickets* (also known as familial hypophosphatemic rickets or X-linked hypophosphatemia). This form of rickets is usually inherited as an X-linked dominant trait, but occasionally autosomal dominant inheritance is observed. The child exhibits the clinical and radiographic signs already described but is otherwise healthy and has a normal life expectancy.

The medical treatment of the various types of vitamin D-refractory rickets includes the oral administration of phosphates and 1,25-dihydroxyvitamin D_3. Careful monitoring of the patient's progress is required to achieve an optimal therapeutic response as well as to avoid the harmful effects of vitamin D intoxication.

Other less common types of rickets caused by renal tubular insufficiency include the following: vitamin D dependency rickets, type I and type II; Fanconi syndrome; cystinosis; and the oculocerebrorenal syndrome of Lowe. In addition, renal tubular acidosis may result in rickets.

The Orthopaedic Management of Deformities in Rickets

The recognition of rickets as the underlying cause of the deformity is essential because correction of such a deformity, without controlling the rickets, invariably leads to its recurrence. Furthermore, once the rickets has been controlled, bony deformities tend to regress somewhat. This improvement can often be enhanced by the use of appropriate night splints of the type described for torsional deformities, genu varum, and genu valgum in Chapter 7. If, despite adequate medical therapy and nonoperative orthopaedic measures,

severe rachitic deformities persist, operative correction by osteotomy is indicated. Under these circumstances, vitamin D therapy should be discontinued 1 month before operation to avoid the risk of severe hypercalcemia, which would otherwise occur during the postoperative period of immobilization.

Osteomalacia

Osteomalacia, which means "soft bones," is a generalized disease of *adult* bone characterized by a failure of calcium salts to be deposited promptly in newly formed organic bone matrix (osteoid). It is, in effect, "adult rickets," but the absence of epiphyseal plates in adults, of course, precludes the epiphyseal plate changes seen in rickets. The causes and types of osteomalacia are comparable to those already described for rickets, that is, vitamin D deficiency, chronic renal insufficiency, and renal tubular insufficiency. The dietary deficiency type of osteomalacia has been eradicated to a large extent by the widespread supplementation of dairy products with vitamin D. However, osteomalacia does occur in the malnourished elderly who may be exposed to sunlight less often.

Pathology

The pathological changes in osteomalacia, like those in rickets, include a generalized *decrease in calcified matrix (bone)* and an *increase in uncalcified matrix (osteoid)*. Thus, there is too little (calcified) bone and, hence, osteomalacia is one form of *osteopenia*, which means "too little bone." The bone changes may become severe, with the result that the significantly weak and "soft" bones gradually bend and become progressively deformed. Microscopically, wide *osteoid seams* are seen adjacent to the relatively sparse areas of calcified bone (Fig. 9.6). In addition, *pseudofractures,* known as Looser's zones, may develop from the healing of multiple microstress fractures with osteomalacic bone in the moderately severe form of osteomalacia known as *Milkman's syndrome* (an eponym rather than an occupational hazard in milkmen).

Diagnosis

The *possibility* of osteomalacia should be considered in the presence of anorexia, weight

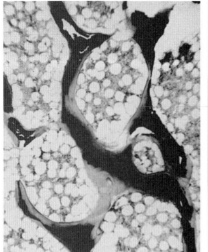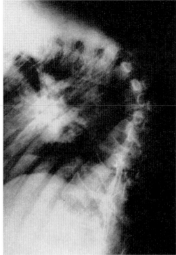

Figure 9.6.   Left. In this case of osteomalacia, undecalcified histological section of cancellous bone reveals a decrease in the amount of calcified matrix, or bone (dark areas), and an increase in the amount of uncalcified matrix, or osteoid (light areas), the latter forming wide "osteoid seams" on sparse areas of bone.

Figure 9.7.   Right. This is a progressive kyphosis of the thoracic spine caused by compression of vertebral bodies in a 23-year-old woman with osteomalacia. Note also the generalized rarefaction of all the bones.

loss, muscle weakness, and widespread bone pain as well as bone tenderness and progressive bony deformity of the spine and limbs (Fig. 9.7). The diagnosis is *established* by the typical radiographic changes of gross skeletal deformity (compression of vertebral bodies, distortion of the pelvis, and bending of the long bones) and the prominence of trabeculation of bone. In Milkman's syndrome, pseudofractures may be seen in the ribs, pelvis, upper ends of the femora, and elsewhere (Fig. 9.8). The serum alkaline phosphatase level is usually elevated, and the serum phosphate concentration is lowered. Serum assays of calcium, phosphorus, parathyroid hormone, and vitamin D metabolites are helpful, but an iliac crest bone biopsy may be necessary to confirm the diagnosis (Fig. 9.6).

Treatment

As with rickets, the underlying cause of osteomalacia must be corrected insofar as is possible. In vitamin D deficiency osteomalacia, the administration of vitamin D and a high calcium diet usually improve the calcification of

the organic matrix and thereby result in healing of the pseudofractures, as well as in a general strengthening of the bones. Hypophosphatemic forms of osteomalacia may require therapy with phosphorus and 1,25-dihydroxyvitamin D. The latter may also be useful therapy for other forms of vitamin D-resistant osteomalacia. Following adequate medical treatment of the osteomalacia, residual bony deformities may require correction by appropriate osteotomies.

Scurvy (Avitaminosis C)

Scurvy is a generalized disease characterized by a failure of osteoblastic formation of bone matrix, with a resultant decrease in the total amount of bone (osteoporosis), and accompanied by subperiosteal and submucous hemorrhages. This disease, which is caused by a lack of vitamin C (ascorbic acid) and the associated defect in the synthesis of collagen, occurs in children between the ages of 6 months and 1 year. Severe scurvy is now relatively uncommon; nevertheless, mild scurvy can occur, not

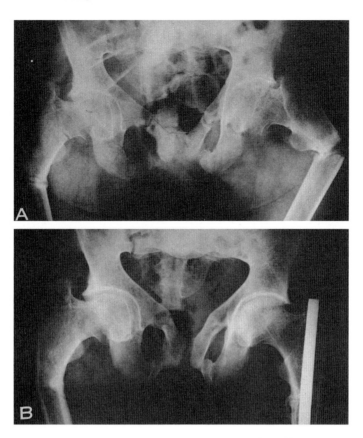

Figure 9.8.   This figure demonstrates Milkman's syndrome in a 25-year-old woman. **A.** A deformity of the pelvis and femora with multiple pseudofractures in the right femur as well as a displaced pathological fracture in the subtrochanteric region of the left femur. **B.** The same patient after treatment with vitamin D and a high-calcium diet. The pathological fracture has been treated by means of a large intramedullary nail. Note the healing of the fracture and of the pseudofractures as well as the improvement in the generalized density of all the bones.

only in children but also in the elderly who tend to eat too little food containing vitamin C.

Pathology
The decreased osteoblastic formation of bone matrix in the presence of normal osteoclastic resorption of bone accounts for the generalized osteoporosis. Because bone matrix is not being formed on the calcified cores of cartilage in the epiphyseal plate, the zone of calcifying cartilage persists and becomes thicker. Avitaminosis C, however, also increases capillary fragility and consequently, spontaneous hemorrhages occur, not only under the loosely attached periosteum but also under the mucous membrane of the gums and intestine. When the subperiosteal hemorrhage is massive, the normal attachment of the epiphysis and its epiphyseal plate to the metaphysis is disrupted and an epiphyseal separation ensues.

Clinical Features
The child with scurvy appears undernourished and experiences the fairly rapid onset of irritability, swelling of the limbs (particularly the thighs), and pain that may be so severe that he or she refuses to move the limbs (pseudoparalysis). Examination reveals marked swell-

ing, warmth, and exquisite tenderness over the affected bones as well as evidence of hemorrhage elsewhere, especially in the gums.

Radiographic Features

The typical radiographic signs of severe scurvy include a generalized rarefaction of all bones (osteoporosis), a dense white line on the metaphyseal side of the epiphyseal plates and a similar line ringing the epiphyses (both of which represent thick zones of calcifying cartilage), and evidence of epiphyseal separations (Fig. 9.9). Soft tissue shadows surrounding the long bones represent the subperiosteal hematomata, which become ossified with remarkable rapidity following treatment with vitamin C (Fig. 9.10).

Differential Diagnosis

Although severe scurvy is not readily confused with other conditions, less severe degrees of the condition must be differentiated from paralysis, osteomyelitis, congenital syphilis, and "child abuse" with multiple epiphyseal separations. In untreated scurvy, the blood ascorbic acid concentration is always significantly decreased.

Treatment

The administration of vitamin C (ascorbic acid) leads to rapid and complete correction of all aspects of the disease. Ossification of the subperiosteal hematomata secures the epiphyseal separations, and the prognosis for subsequent epiphyseal plate growth is excellent.

Osteoporosis

Osteoporosis, which means "porous bone," is a generalized disease of bone characterized by a combination of decreased osteoblastic formation of matrix and increased osteoclastic resorption of bone, with a resultant decrease in the total amount of bone in the skeleton. Thus, osteoporosis is one form of *osteopenia,* which means "too little bone." Another form of osteopenia is osteomalacia, in which there is inadequate calcification of matrix and, therefore, too little calcified bone, as discussed in a previous section of this chapter. Although the bone in osteoporosis is thin and porous, the bone that is present is well calcified and

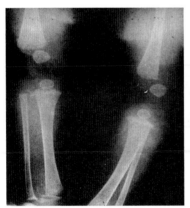 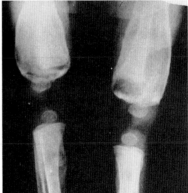

Figure 9.9.   Left. Scurvy in a 1-year-old girl is seen. The lower limbs reveal generalized rarefaction of all bones (indicating osteoporosis), a dense white line on the metaphyseal side of the epiphyseal plates, and a similar line ringing the epiphyses (both of which represent thick zones of calcified cartilage), as well as separation of both lower femoral epiphyses and both lower tibial epiphyses.

Figure 9.10.   Right. Treated scurvy in the same 1-year-old girl seen in Figure 9.9 after 10 days of therapy with vitamin C (ascorbic acid). Note the ossification of the massive subperiosteal hematomata and the increased generalized density of the bones. The epiphyseal separations are now securely healed, and the prognosis for subsequent epiphyseal plate growth is excellent.

its microscopic appearance is normal (in contradistinction to osteomalacia). Although decreased bone deposition has long been considered the major factor in the imbalance that leads to osteoporosis, it is now recognized that increased bone resorption may be the more important factor. The decreased bone mass in osteoporosis is associated with increased fragility or brittleness and, consequently, increased susceptibility to fracture.

Osteoporosis is a common form of metabolic bone disease. Indeed, it has been estimated that, at any given time, there are 22 million adults with osteoporosis in North America alone and that, in a given year, 1.5 million of these adults will sustain at least one fracture. Furthermore, the annual costs involved with osteoporosis in North America amount to more than $10 billion. With the increasing longevity of the population in North America, these figures are certain to increase significantly. In fact, the World Health Organization estimates that there will be a fourfold increase in osteoporosis worldwide by the year 2050. Therefore, it is not surprising that during the past decade there has been greater than ever emphasis on the basic and epidemiological research relevant to the prevention, quantitative diagnosis, and treatment of osteoporosis.

Etiological Factors

Since generalized osteoporosis represents a disturbance not only in bone deposition but also in bone resorption, there are several types of osteoporosis based on the most prominent causative factor, even though the resultant skeletal lesion is the same. Osteogenesis imperfecta, a congenital type of osteoporosis, has been described in Chapter 8. The many causative factors in the production of osteoporosis include endocrine diseases, disuse, a postmenopausal state, and senility, although in any given patient, two or more factors may be combined. Furthermore, the importance of genetic factors is becoming increasingly recognized.

Risk factors for the development of osteoporosis include the following: gender (one in four females compared with one in eight males older than 50 years of age acquire osteopo-

rosis); amenorrhea, either postmenopausal or artificially induced; insufficient calcium in the diet; eating disorders; smoking; excessive use of caffeine or alcohol; and inadequate physical exercise.

Hormonal Osteoporosis (Endocrine Osteoporosis)

In some patients with osteoporosis, the underlying cause is hormonal imbalance in that there is an increased secretion of antianabolic hormones relative to the secretion of anabolic hormones. Thus, osteoporosis is a feature of hyperparathyroidism, hyperpituitarism, hyperthyroidism, and hyperadrenocorticism (either from adrenal cortical hyperactivity or prolonged cortisone therapy). Disorders resulting from various types of hormonal, or endocrine, disturbances are discussed in a subsequent section of this chapter.

Disuse Osteoporosis

All tissues of the body atrophy when they are not used, and bone is no exception. The intermittent pressures of weightbearing and the tensions of muscle pull transmitted to the skeleton exert stresses and strains that create a piezoelectric current that, along with Wolff's law, stimulate bone deposition by osteoblastic activity. In a person who, for any reason, is either confined to bed or grossly restricted in his or her activities, decreased bone deposition is soon overbalanced by increased bone resorption, and the result is disuse atrophy of bone (disuse osteoporosis). The weightlessness experienced by astronauts in space also causes such osteoporosis. This type of osteoporosis, of course, is most marked in those parts of the skeleton that are being used the least, namely, the lower limbs and spine. Indeed, in a single limb, prolonged immobilization, relief of weightbearing, and paralysis can all produce a *localized* disuse osteoporosis limited to the bones that are not being used.

Postmenopausal and Senile Osteoporosis

Postmenopausal and senile osteoporosis are two types of generalized osteoporosis that are considered together because they have so much in common. The distinction is somewhat arbitrary in that when women develop osteoporosis between menopause and the age of 65 years (during which there is an estrogen deficiency), the osteoporosis is termed *post-menopausal,* whereas when either men or women develop the condition after the age of 65 years, it is termed *senile.* Postmenopausal and senile osteoporosis represent by far the most common generalized bone disease that you will see in patients. It has been estimated to be radiographically detectable to some extent in 50% of all persons older than 65 years of age, and when you realize that the total amount of bone must be decreased by one third before the decrease can be readily detected radiographically, you will appreciate that less severe degrees of postmenopausal and senile osteoporosis are very common indeed. Hypogonadism in the elderly, as well as an inadequate dietary intake of calcium, would seem to be factors in the cause of this type of osteoporosis and, furthermore, the condition may well be aggravated by a superimposed "disuse osteoporosis" associated with the usual decline in physical activity of the elderly.

Pathology

Bone deposition and bone resorption are both surface phenomena, and since trabecular, or cancellous, bone has a much larger surface area than cortical bone, it is understandable that osteoporosis, which represents an imbalance between bone deposition and bone resorption affects trabecular bone more than cortical bone and that the calcified trabeculae become both thin and sparse (Fig. 9.11**A**). Thus, the osteoporosis is most severe in the vertebral bodies and the metaphyses of long bones, both of which normally consist largely of cancellous bone. The cortical bone eventually becomes thin and porous as well. As a result, the individual bones, rather than becoming "soft" as in osteomalacia, become fragile, or brittle, and are susceptible to pathological fractures of either the gross or microscopic type from even the most trivial trauma. Gross pathological fractures are very common, particularly in the predominantly cancellous metaphyses of long bones (neck of femur, neck of humerus, distal end of radius) and in the predominantly cancellous vertebral bodies of the spine. In addition, repeated microscopic fractures in the spine produce a gradual wedge-shaped deformity of the vertebral bodies, with a resultant slowly progressive dorsal kyphosis and loss of total height. The pressure of the resilient intervertebral discs gradually deforms the less resilient bone of the subjacent

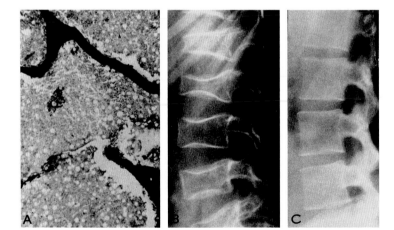

Figure 9.11.   Osteoporosis is seen in this figure. **A.** Undecalcified histological section of cancellous bone from a 75-year-old woman with senile osteoporosis. Note the sparse and thin trabeculae of bone, which are normally calcified. **B.** Lateral radiograph of the lumbar spine of an adult with osteoporosis. Note the compressed, biconcave vertebral bodies with "ballooning" of the intervertebral discs, as well as the generalized rarefaction of all the bones. **C.** Normal lumbar spine of a 45-year-old man shown for comparison.

surface of each vertebral body, and as a result the vertebral bodies become biconcave as the intervertebral discs become biconvex or balloon-shaped (Fig. 9.11**B**).

Clinical Diagnosis

The symptoms of generalized osteoporosis include chronic and intermittent back pain (which is probably related to repeated microscopic fractures) as well as bone pain at other sites, loss of both standing and sitting height, and reduction in physical performance, including respiratory function. The patient with advanced osteoporosis usually looks frail and exhibits an abnormal degree of dorsal kyphosis (the so-called dowager's hump) (Fig. 9.12). Gross pathological fractures in the aforementioned sites are a very common clinical complication.

Radiographic Diagnosis

The radiographic features include a generalized rarefaction of all bones (but most marked in cancellous bone), thin cortices, and evidence of deformity, particularly in the vertebral bodies (Figs. 9.11 and 9.13).

A relatively recent development is *bone densitometry* to quantitate accurately the *bone mineral density* of a given patient. As previously stated, the current method of choice is dual energy X-ray absorptiometry (DEXA). Determination of bone mineral density by bone densitometry is of great value in the precise diagnosis of osteoporosis, a given patient's response to treatment, and the estimation of the risk of fracture for a given patient. The fracture risk doubles with every standard deviation decrease in bone mineral density below the normal young person mean control.

Laboratory Diagnosis

In postmenopausal and senile osteoporosis, the serum calcium, phosphorus, and alkaline phosphatase levels are all normal, but metabolic studies may reveal a negative calcium balance. Any endocrinopathy or osteomalacia can be ruled out by appropriate laboratory investigations, as discussed in other sections of this chapter.

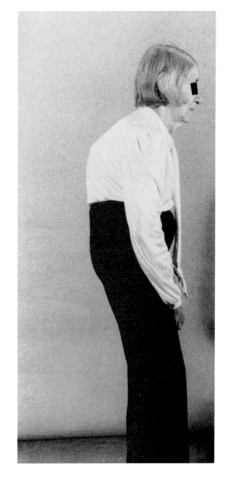

Figure 9.12.   Postmenopausal osteoporosis in a 60-year-old woman who complained of intermittent pain in her back. Note this patient's frail appearance and the increased dorsal (thoracic) kyphosis.

Treatment

The treatment of the various types of osteoporosis has become so sophisticated that consultation with a metabolic bone physician should be obtained, at least for the purposes of establishing an accurate diagnosis, assessment of severity, and establishment of a treatment regimen. The main purpose of treatment is the prevention of further bone loss. Reversal of osteoporosis in a given patient is extremely difficult to achieve.

Because of the magnitude of the morbidity related to postmenopausal and senile osteoporosis (especially gross and microscopic pathological fractures), it is not surprising that metabolic bone physicians have striven for many

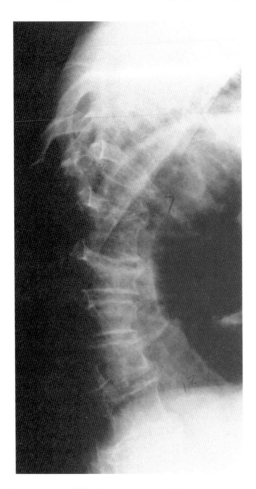

Figure 9.13.   The thoracic spine of the patient shown in Figure 9.12. Note the compression of the vertebral bodies with resultant kyphosis. The osteophyte formation at the edges of the vertebral bodies indicates secondary degenerative joint disease of the spine. Note also the generalized rarefaction of all the bones.

years to prevent, arrest, or even reverse such osteoporosis by medical treatment, that is, therapeutic agents. The many agents investigated to date (either alone or in various combinations) include estrogens (for women only), anabolic hormones, bisphosphonates, calcitonin, vitamin D (or its active metabolites), calcium, and sodium fluoride. Each of these agents in high doses may produce undesirable side effects in some patients and, hence, must be administered with caution and only with regular supervision.

Estrogen is the most effective form of hormone replacement therapy (HRT) for the pre-vention of progressive postmenopausal osteoporosis. Calcium supplements are of value both in the prevention and treatment of osteoporosis. Calcitonin (which was discovered by Copp of Canada) decreases the number and activity of osteoclasts and thereby decreases bone resorption. Of the various bisphosphonates, alendronate (Fosamax*trade*) is currently considered to be the most efficacious in inhibiting osteoclastic resorption of bone; it may actually increase bone mineral density as well and thereby decrease the incidence of fractures.

In many patients with osteoporosis, some degree of true osteomalacia coexists, and this component of the problem is correctable by adequate doses of vitamin D or one of its metabolites. Although much scientific investigation remains to be done in both animals and humans before widespread medical treatment of all osteoporotic patients with sodium fluoride is justifiable, the currently recommended combination of sodium fluoride and calcium seems to be promising in that, with proper supervision, an 80% response rate can be achieved, and this is comparable to the response rate to bisphosphonates. A program of regular and vigorous physical exercise has been shown to help overcome at least the disuse atrophy component of the osteoporosis that is secondary to the sedentary life of postmenopausal women as well as of the elderly, both men and women. The back pain caused by microfractures in osteoporotic vertebrae can be diminished by the use of a light, close-fitting brace. For all patients with osteoporosis of whatever type, the orthopaedic management of their fractures (which in reality are pathological fractures) should include early ambulation and resumption of other physical activities as soon as possible to prevent the problem of disuse osteoporosis being superimposed upon the pre-existent osteoporosis.

Hyperparathyroidism (Parathyroid Osteodystrophy) (Osteitis Fibrosa Cystica)

Parathyroid osteodystrophy is a rare generalized bone disease resulting from hyperparathyroidism and characterized by a combination of generalized and localized excessive osteoclastic resorption of bone with marrow fibrosis. The resultant bone disease, therefore, consists not only of a generalized hormonal, or endocrine, form of osteoporosis but also of disseminated osteolytic lesions.

Etiology and Pathology

Primary hyperparathyroidism is the result of a parathyroid adenoma in one or more glands; occasionally, the involved gland is abnormally situated (aberrant). Although clinical hyperparathyroidism, with hypercalcemia, is common, most cases of primary hyperparathyroidism are asymptomatic in modern practice, and symptomatic bone disease is uncommon (less than 2% of cases). Rarely, the hyperparathyroidism results from primary hyperplasia of all four glands. The associated excessive bone resorption liberates both calcium and phosphorus into the bloodstream, but the phosphorus is more readily excreted in the urine; the calcium-phosphorus product remains constant and therefore there is hypercalcemia and hypophosphatemia.

Secondary hyperparathyroidism is secondary to the hypocalcemia associated with chronic renal insufficiency, in which case neither calcium nor phosphorus is readily excreted by the kidneys. Secondary hyperparathyroidism also occurs in association with the osteomalacia that is seen with intestinal malabsorption or vitamin D deficiency. The generalized bone lesion, which is a form of hormonal osteoporosis, is exemplified by thin trabeculae and cortices.

The disseminated osteolytic lesions vary greatly in that they may be *solid* and filled with vascular fibrous tissue, hemosiderin, and giant cells ("brown tumors"), or they may be truly *cystic* and filled with old blood. In either case, the bone is greatly weakened by the disseminated lesions through which pathological fractures may occur. The hypercalcemia associated with hyperparathyroidism leads to the complication of renal calculi of the calcium type.

Diagnosis

The patient with hyperparathyroidism experiences two types of clinical manifestations: those caused by the hypercalcemia (anorexia, lethargy, weakness, and symptoms of renal calculi) and those caused by the associated bone disease (bone pain, progressive bony deformity, pathological fractures, and loosening of the teeth). The radiographic changes include generalized rarefaction of all bones and disseminated osteolytic lesions of multiple bones (Fig. 9.14). The earliest radiographic change is resorption of the lamina dura of the tooth sockets and of the cortical bone in the phalanges. The serum calcium level is always

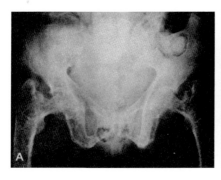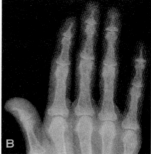

Figure 9.14.   This figure demonstrates hyperparathyroidism caused by a parathyroid adenoma in a 60-year-old woman. **A.** There is generalized rarefaction of the bones, coarse trabeculae of cancellous bone (caused by loss of minor trabeculae and preservation of major trabeculae), cystic lesions of the pelvis and femora, deformity of the pelvis, bilateral coxa vara, and subperiosteal absorption of bone in the femoral necks. **B.** Note the generalized rarefaction of all the bones and the coarse trabeculae of cancellous bone and subperiosteal absorption of cortical bone in the phalanges.

elevated and, indeed, primary hyperparathyroidism is frequently diagnosed today because of an elevated serum calcium level in an asymptomatic individual. Usually the urinary calcium concentration is also elevated. The serum phosphorus level is lowered, but the urinary phosphorus concentration is elevated (except in secondary hyperparathyroidism in which the reverse is true). The serum alkaline phosphatase level is elevated. An important advance in the diagnosis of hyperparathyroidism has been the demonstration of an elevated serum level of parathyroid hormone (PTH) by means of radioimmunoassay.

Treatment

Patients who have primary hyperparathyroidism with significant osseous, renal, gastrointestinal, or neuromuscular symptoms require parathyroidectomy to remove the causative adenoma or adenomata. Postoperatively, considerable improvement may be expected in the bone disease. Residual deformity may require surgical correction by osteotomy. However, patients who have asymptomatic primary hyperparathyroidism with only mild hypercalcemia and no evidence of damage to a target organ (bone, kidney, stomach, intestine, muscle, or nerve) may be managed medically. In secondary hyperparathyroidism, treatment is directed toward the underlying chronic renal insufficiency; the associated bone disease may be improved by high doses of vitamin D and, in carefully selected cases, by parathyroidectomy.

Hyperpituitarism

Excessive hormone secretion by the anterior lobe of the pituitary gland exerts a variety of profound generalized effects on bone depending on the state of skeletal growth at the time, as well as on the type of abnormal cell in the gland. Thus, an eosinophil (chromophil) adenoma during the growth period produces *gigantism*, whereas the same neoplasm after growth, produces *acromegaly*. By contrast, a basophil adenoma at any age produces *Cushing's syndrome* (which can also be caused by hyperadrenocorticism).

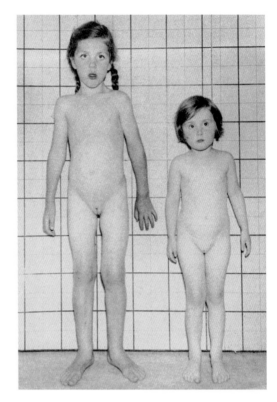

Figure 9.15.   Gigantism caused by hyperpituitarism in a 5-year-old girl is seen. Note the long limbs and somewhat coarse features compared with those of the normal 5-year-old girl on the right.

Gigantism

During *childhood*, excessive hormone secretion from an eosinophil adenoma stimulates epiphyseal plate growth to a remarkable degree, with the result that the affected child reaches an unusual height, sometimes more than 7 feet (Fig. 9.15). The condition is usually associated with subnormal sexual development and is occasionally complicated by slipping of the upper femoral epiphysis (adolescent coxa vara), which is described in Chapter 13. If the hyperpituitarism persists, the adult counterpart, acromegaly, is superimposed upon the gigantism in adult life.

Acromegaly

During *adulthood*, excessive hormone secretion from an eosinophil adenoma cannot affect longitudinal growth, but it does stimulate circumferential growth from periosteal intra-

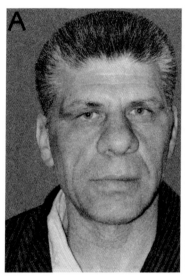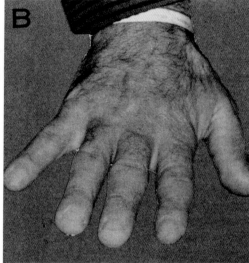

Figure 9.16.   This figure shows acromegaly resulting from hyperpituitarism in a 40-year-old man. **A.** The facial features are coarse because of enlargement of the jaw, nose, and supraorbital ridges as a result of excessive periosteal intramembranous ossification. **B.** The fingers are coarse and unduly thick.

membranous ossification so that the bones become progressively thicker. The clinical disorder is easily recognized by the coarse facial features (enlargement of the jaw, nose, and supraorbital ridges) and the thick fingers (Fig. 9.16). The patient may be unusually strong in the early stages, but general weakness frequently supervenes.

Cushing's Syndrome

The generalized bone disease that is associated with Cushing's syndrome is a severe and progressive *osteoporosis*, with all the previously described features of that disorder. In addition, the patient exhibits obesity, particularly of the face ("moon face"), increased body hair, and hypertension (Fig. 9.17). This syndrome is the result of *hyperadrenocorticism*, which, in turn, may be *primary*, resulting from either hyperplasia or a neoplasm of the adrenal cortex, or *secondary*, resulting from either a basophil adenoma of the anterior lobe of the pituitary gland or prolonged cortisone therapy. The neurosurgical removal of pituitary adenomas has been made possible by the development of the operating microscope and the use of the transsphenoidal approach. Cortisone

therapy is currently the most common cause of Cushing's syndrome and is a disturbing example of "iatrogenic disease." In Cushing's syndrome, the diagnosis is usually suggested by measurement of an unsuppressed plasma cortisol after the administration of dexamethasone as a screening test the previous night or by measurement of an elevated level of urinary free cortisol. Serum adrenocorticotropic hormone (ACTH) levels are also useful in the diagnosis. The complications of gross and microscopic pathological fractures with progressive bone deformity are common because of the severe degree of generalized osteoporosis.

Hypopituitarism

A deficient amount of anterior pituitary hormone during *childhood* retards epiphyseal growth and thereby results in a perfectly proportioned *Lorain type of dwarfism* (Fig. 9.18). Hypopituitarism may also produce various degrees of *dystrophia adiposogenitalis* (*Fröhlich's syndrome*) characterized by prominent obesity, subnormal sexual development, relatively normal growth, and a predisposition to slipping of the upper femoral epiphysis (adoles-

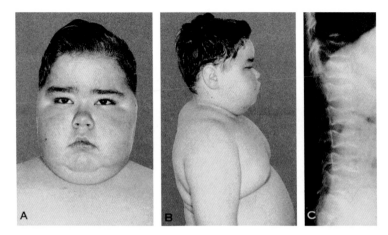

Figure 9.17.   Cushing's syndrome resulting from hyperadrenocorticism from prolonged cortisone therapy in a 10-year-old boy is seen. **A** and **B.** Note the obesity, particularly of the face ("moon face"). **C.** The spine reveals compressed, biconcave vertebral bodies, "ballooning" of the intervertebral discs, and generalized rarefaction of all the bones because of osteoporosis.

cent coxa vara), which is described in Chapter 13 (Fig. 9.19).

Hypothyroidism in Childhood (Cretinism)

Congenital deficiency of thyroid function is manifested in children by delayed epiphyseal plate growth as well as by delayed, irregular ossification of epiphyses (which may mimic the appearance of avascular necrosis). Mental impairment is usual, and the child exhibits a large tongue, dry skin, and a dull facial expression. The significance of cretinism lies in the fact that if it is recognized early and treated by thyroid extract for life, great improvement in all aspects of the disorder can be achieved. Fortunately, because of widespread neonatal screening programs to determine the level of thyroid-stimulating hormone (TSH), even mild forms of hypothyroidism can be diagnosed and, hence, treated early so that the full-blown clinical picture of cretinism is becoming progressively less common.

DISSEMINATED BONE DISORDERS

The heterogenous group of disorders included in this section are manifested in the skeleton by widely disseminated, but discrete, lesions in bone. They are not associated with generalized bone disease in that the uninvolved bone is completely normal. These disorders include *polyostotic fibrous dysplasia, Paget's disease (osteitis deformans), Langerhans cell histiocytosis* and *Gaucher's disease.*

Polyostotic Fibrous Dysplasia

Polyostotic fibrous dysplasia is a curious disseminated disorder of bone that is probably a developmental fault of bony development resulting from somatic cell mutations of genes coding for the α-subunit of the guanyl nucleotide regulatory protein, G_s, which is the protein that mediates parathyroid hormone action in bone. It is characterized by multiple areas of fibrous tissue replacement within multiple bones without any evidence of generalized osteoporosis.

Pathology

The slowly progressive lesions appear in early childhood and consist of fibrous tissue accumulations within the marrow spaces. The lesions gradually expand the host bone from within as they erode and replace bone, but they are always confined by at least a thin layer of cortical bone because periosteal intramembranous ossification is not involved. The lo-

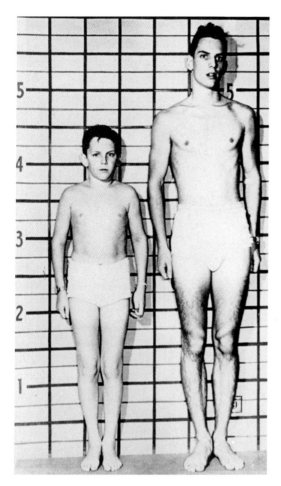

Figure 9.18. This is the Lorain type of dwarfism caused by hypopituitarism. These 15-year-old boys are identical twins. Note that the hypopituitary twin, although very short, is normally proportioned.

mity or a pathological fracture. The progressive radiographic changes include expanded osteolytic lesions enclosed by a thin shell of cortical bone and frequently severe bony deformities, particularly in the upper end of the femur where the deformity may resemble a "shepherd's crook" (Fig. 9.20). The blood chemistry profile is normal, which helps differentiate this condition from the generalized disease of hyperparathyroidism.

Treatment

There is, as yet, no specific treatment for polyostotic fibrous dysplasia. The complications of pathological fracture and severe bony deformities may necessitate operative procedures such as currettement of a fibrous tissue lesion followed by packing of the defect with bone grafts; osteotomy may be indicated to correct residual deformity.

Paget's Disease (Osteitis Deformans)

The disseminated bone disorder of *Paget's disease* is characterized by slowly progressive enlargement and deformity of multiple bones associated with unexplained acceleration of both deposition and resorption of bone. This condition, particularly in its milder forms, is extremely common, affecting approximately 4% of all persons older than 55 years of age. Since first-degree relatives of patients with Paget's disease have an increased risk of contracting the disease, there would seem to be a genetic predisposition.

Etiology

Although the precise cause of Paget's disease is not proved, it is now thought that a "slow virus" affecting primarily osteoclasts may be involved.

Pathology

The pathological process of Paget's disease (which was originally thought to be inflammatory) involves a significantly accelerated bone turnover, with excessive osteoclastic resorption and excessive osteoblastic deposition taking place simultaneously. The involved areas of bone are extremely vascular and may even

cally destructive lesions weaken the bone considerably, resulting in pathological fractures, but these usually unite well. Microscopically, there is dense fibrous tissue in which spicules of bone are embedded. Rarely, the condition may be limited to one bone (*monostotic* fibrous dysplasia). An unusual variant is *McCune-Albright syndrome,* which occurs in girls and in which there is a combination of sexual precocity, skin pigmentation, and polyostotic fibrous dysplasia.

Diagnosis

Polyostotic fibrous dysplasia is usually detected in early childhood because of a defor-

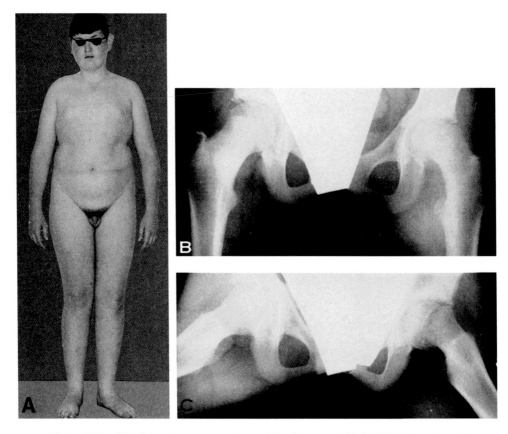

Figure 9.19. This figure demonstrates dystrophia adiposogenitalis (Fröhlich's syndrome). **A.** This 14-year-old boy is obese. His stature is normal for his age, but his sexual development is subnormal. Note that his left lower limb is externally rotated. He complained of pain in his left knee (referred from the hip) because of a slipped left upper femoral epiphysis. **B.** The anteroposterior radiograph reveals a posteromedial slip of the left upper femoral epiphysis. **C.** The lateral radiograph (frog position) reveals the slip of the left upper femoral epiphysis more clearly.

exhibit arteriovenous shunts. During the early and more active phase, resorption exceeds deposition and the bone, although enlarged, becomes spongelike, weakened, and deformed. This *osteolytic phase* is followed by an *osteosclerotic phase* in which the balance swings in favor of deposition, with the result that the enlarged bones become thick and dense, and they remain so even though the disease eventually becomes burned out. The bones most commonly involved are the tibia, femur, pelvis, vertebral bodies, and skull. Although the disease is usually polyostotic, it is occasionally limited to one bone (*monostotic* osteitis deformans). Microscopically, the normal lamellar pattern of bone is lost and is replaced by an irregular mosaic pattern of alternating mature and immature bone. Complications of this bizarre process include progressive deformities resulting from the enlargement and bending of bones in the osteolytic phase, degenerative arthritis of nearby joints, pathological fractures (which are usually transverse and somewhat slow to unite), and occasionally malignant change in the hyperactive osteoblasts resulting in an exceedingly malignant and invariably fatal type of osteogenic sarcoma.

Diagnosis

Although Paget's disease is common, the milder forms (which constitute the majority) are subclinical in that they do not cause symp-

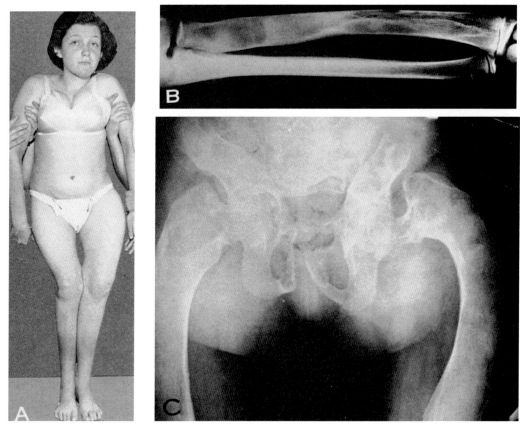

Figure 9.20. Polyostotic fibrous dysplasia is seen. **A.** This 14-year-old girl exhibits severe deformities, particularly of her lower limbs and is unable to stand without support. **B.** The forearm reveals expanded osteolytic lesions in the radius enclosed by a thin shell of cortical bone. **C.** The hips reveal severe deformities of the pelvis and femora with multiple expanded osteolytic lesions enclosed by a thin shell of cortical bone. Note the evidence of previous pathological fractures that have led to the development of a "shepherd's crook" deformity of both femora.

toms and are discovered only incidentally. The more severe forms cause bone pain that may be distressingly severe. The patients observe that their lower limbs are becoming progressively bowed, their heads are becoming gradually larger (their hats seem too small), and they are becoming shorter (Fig. 9.21). A technetium bone scan is useful in localizing the areas involved. The radiographic changes include enlargement, deformity and porosity of involved bones during the osteolytic phase and increased, but irregular, density of the bones in the osteosclerotic phase (Fig. 9.22). The serum alkaline phosphatase and urinary hydroxyproline levels are always significantly elevated when the disease is disseminated, but they are not always elevated when the disease is localized.

Treatment

As yet there is no medical treatment that is specific for Paget's disease. However, considerable success can be realized using antiresorptive treatments such as the bisphosphonates and calcitonin, which inactivate osteoclasts. For most mild cases, etidronate will reduce alkaline phosphatase activity and ameliorate bone pain not associated with mechanical joint abnormalities that result from Paget's disease. However, for more severe

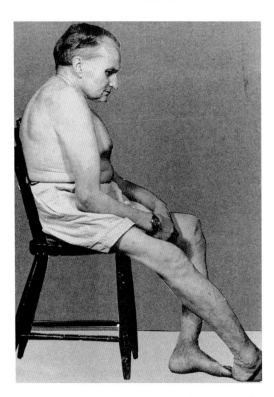

Figure 9.21.   This 60-year-old man has Paget's disease (osteitis deformans). He complained of severe pain in his lower limbs, which were becoming progressively bowed. He also has deformities in his upper limbs. He noticed that he was becoming shorter but that his head was becoming larger.

cases, newer bisphosphonates such as pamidronate or alendronate are preferred; these drugs result in a greater degree of disease suppression. Calcitonin can also be used and may be more effective for lytic disease. Plicamycin, an antitumor antibiotic, also has antiosteoclastic activity and may be used in resistant cases.

The Histiocytoses

Proliferation of the cells of the reticuloendothelial system within bone occurs in a number of poorly understood granulomatous conditions. Although these conditions differ considerably, they are all capable of producing disseminated lesions in bone and are referred to collectively as *the histiocytoses*. The nonlipid histiocytoses include the following conditions that were previously known as *Letterer-Siwe's disease, Hand-Schüller-Christian disease,* and

eosinophilic granuloma. Since the predominant cell is the histiocyte, these three conditions were also designated *histiocytosis X*. Currently, however, the most acceptable term for histiocytosis X is *Langerhans cell histiocytosis*. The lipid histiocytosis known as *Gaucher's disease* is a manifestation of abnormal lipid metabolism and is, in fact, a lipid storage disease.

Langerhans Cell Histiocytosis (Histiocytosis X)

The three conditions that were formerly known as Letterer-Siwe's disease, Hand-Schüller-Christian disease, and eosinophilic granuloma are now considered to be different presentations of the same disease (Langerhans cell histiocytosis) because they share the same abnormal cell. In the rare but extremely serious type of Langerhans cell histiocytosis (known previously as Letterer-Siwe's disease), the onset is in infancy and the progress is extremely rapid. The clinical manifestations involve mainly soft tissues (enlarged spleen, liver, and lymph nodes) and are accompanied by thrombocytopenic purpura with petechial hemorrhages. The condition usually results in early death before significant bone lesions have developed.

In the variety of Langerhans cell histiocytosis, known previously as Hand-Schüller-Christian disease, proliferation of histiocytes within the bone causes disseminated, but discrete, destructive lesions, particularly in the skull but also in other bones. Deposits of similar cells around the pituitary gland result in diabetes insipidus. The onset is in early childhood, and the progress of the condition is moderately rapid. Microscopically, the lesions in bone contain histiocytes (which become secondarily laden with lipids eventually), eosinophils, and giant cells. Radiographically, the lesions in the skull are seen as clearly demarcated osteolytic defects, whereas the lesions elsewhere are osteolytic but less clearly defined (Fig. 9.23). Radiotherapy causes the skeletal lesions to heal, at least temporarily, but when the involvement is extensive, the prognosis is unfavorable.

The less serious and more localized variety of Langerhans cell histiocytosis was formerly known as *eosinophilic granuloma*, which is en-

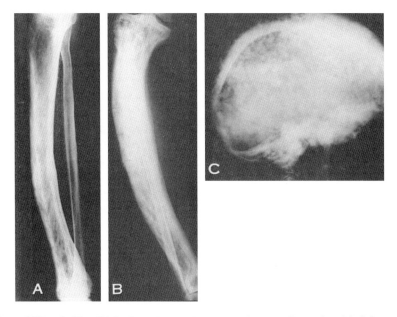

Figure 9.22.   A. The tibia in the early osteolytic stage of Paget's disease (osteitis deformans) is seen in this figure. The lesion, which is most marked in the distal half of the tibia, is advancing proximally. **B.** The tibia is seen in the late osteosclerotic phase. The tibia is thickened and bowed. Horizontal pseudofractures can be seen on the convex side of the deformed tibia. **C.** The skull reveals irregular sclerosis of bone. The new bone formation on the outer surface of the skull accounts for the increasing size of the head.

countered in children and young adults. The osteolytic lesion, which is usually single, is composed of histiocytes as well as an impressive accumulation of eosinophils. Pathological fractures may occur through the osteolytic lesions, but they always heal. When a vertebral body is involved, the primary center of ossification becomes dense and thin, but it is subsequently reconstituted to a large extent. (This type of vertebral lesion, originally described by Calvé, was formerly thought to represent avascular necrosis.) The osteolytic lesions de-

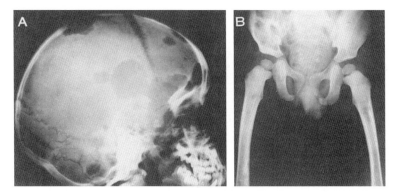

Figure 9.23. This figure shows the variety of Langerhans cell histiocytosis previously known as Hand-Schüller-Christian disease. **A.** The skull in a 4-year-old boy showing numerous round, clearly demarcated osteolytic defects. Note also the spreading of the suture lines. **B.** The hips of the same boy showing numerous osteolytic lesions of the right innominate bone and the right femur.

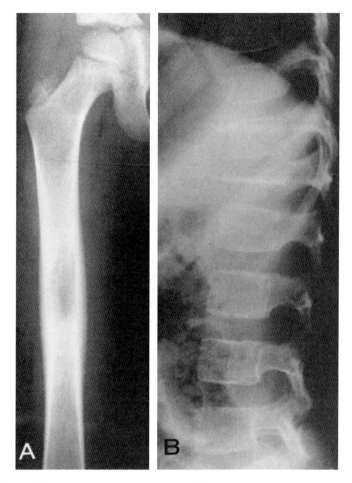

Figure 9.24.   This is the variety of Langerhans cell histiocytosis previously known as eosinophilic granuloma. **A.** This shows the femur of a 10-year-old boy who complained of pain in his thigh. The osteolytic defect is associated with subperiosteal new bone formation (reactive bone) and is frequently difficult to differentiate from other bone lesions radiographically. **B.** This is the spine of a 7-year boy who complained of back pain. The first lumbar vertebra has collapsed. Formerly this radiographic appearance was invariably thought to represent avascular necrosis of the primary center of ossification (Calvé's disease).

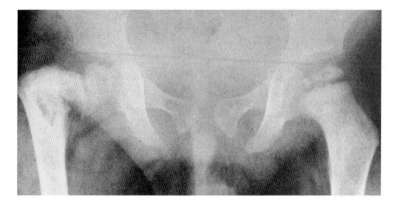

Figure 9.25.   Gaucher's disease. This 3-year-old boy's hips reveal a pathological fracture at the base of the neck of the right femur (through a localized osteolytic lesion) and avascular necrosis of the left femoral head.

velop rapidly and are accompanied by periosteal new bone formation.

Clinically and radiographically, this localized variety of Langerhans cell histiocytosis is a great imitator of several bone diseases, including osteomyelitis, tuberculosis, simple bone cyst, fibrous dysplasia, and various malignant bone neoplasms (Fig. 9.24). Although the discrete lesions are similar to those of the other varieties of Langerhans cell histiocytosis, the prognosis of eosinophilic granuloma is extremely good in that it seems to be a self-limiting condition in which the bony lesions gradually heal spontaneously. However, the ominous clinical and radiographic features usually merit biopsy to exclude a more serious lesion. Curettement of the lesion at the time of biopsy seems to accelerate healing.

Diagnostic markers for all of the Langerhans cell histiocytoses include the C-100 protein and Burbeck bodies: the latter can be demonstrated by electron microscopy.

Gaucher's Disease—Lipid Histiocytosis

Gaucher's disease is an uncommon genetically determined inborn error of lipid metabolism in which proliferating macrophages of the reticuloendothelial system in the bone marrow, spleen, and liver are filled with *glucocerebroside*. These cells, called Gaucher's cells, infiltrate the bone marrow and cause localized osteolytic lesions of bone. The hematopoetic changes that result from replacement of the bone marrow include anemia, leukopenia, and thrombocytopenia. The genetic defect is located on chromosome 1. The lesions in bone may be complicated by avascular necrosis of bone, particularly when they occur in the femoral head (Fig. 9.25). However, for demonstrating involvement of the bone marrow, magnetic resonance imaging (MRI) is more sensitive than radiographs. The more severe forms of Gaucher's disease, which become manifested in early childhood, have a poor prognosis; but the milder forms, which are encountered later, do not seem to shorten the patient's life expectancy. The diagnosis is established by the demonstration of Gaucher's cells in the bone marrow (obtained by either sternal or iliac crest puncture). Radiotherapy usually results in regression of the bony lesions, and splenectomy may be indicated solely to relieve local discomfort from the gross splenomegaly. More recently, bone marrow transplantation has been shown to be capable of curing the disease.

SUGGESTED ADDITIONAL READING

Apley AG, Solomon L. Apley's system of orthopaedics and fractures. 7th ed. Oxford: Butterworth-Heinemann, 1993.

Avioli LV, Krane SM. Metabolic bone disease and clinically related disorders. Philadelphia: WB Saunders, 1990.

Beutler E. Gaucher's disease. N Engl J Med 1991; 325:1354–1360.

Bronner F, Worrell RV. A basic science primer in orthopaedics. Baltimore: Williams & Wilkins, 1991.

Einhorn TA. Bone metabolism and metabolic bone disease. In: Frymoyer JW, ed. Orthopaedic knowledge update 4. Rosemont, IL: American Academy of Orthopaedic Surgeons 1993; 69–88.

Einhorn TA. Bone metabolism and metabolic bone disease. In: Kasser JR. ed. Orthopaedic knowledge update 5. Rosemont, IL: American Academy of Orthopaedic Surgeons 1996;119–132.

Fraser D, Kooh SW. Disturbance of parathyroid hormone and calcitonin. In: Forfar JO, Arneil GC, eds. Textbook of paediatrics. 3rd ed. Edinburgh: Churchill Livingstone, 1984.

Fraser D, Salter RB. The diagnosis and management of the various types of rickets. Pediatr Clin North Am 1958;5:417–444.

Hadjipavlou A, Lander P. Paget's disease of the spine. J Bone Joint Surg 1991;73A:1376–1381.

Kaplan FS, Hayes WC, Keaveny TM. Form and function of bone. In: Simon SR, ed. Orthopaedic basic science. Rosemont IL: American Academy of Orthopaedic Surgeons, 1994;127–184.

Kaplan FS, Singer FR. Paget's disease of bone: pathophysiology, diagnosis, and management. J Am Acad Orthop Surg 1995;3:336–344.

Lane JM, ed. Metabolic bone disease. Curr Opin Orthop 1994;5:1–9.

Lane JM, Healey JH, eds. Diagnosis and management of pathological fractures. New York: Raven Press, 1993.

Lane JM, Riley EH, Wirganowicz PZ. Osteoporosis: diagnosis and treatment. An instructional course lecture. The American Academy of Orthopaedic Surgeons. J Bone Joint Surg 1996; 78-A:618–632.

Liberman UA, Weiss SR, Bröll J, et al. Effect of oral alendronate on bone mineral density and the incidence of fractures in postmenopausal osteoporosis. N Engl J Med 1995;333: 1437–1443.

Lindsay R. Hormone replacement therapy for prevention and treatment of postmenopausal osteoporosis. Am J Med 1993;95:375–395.

Mankin HJ. Rickets, osteomalacia and renal osteodystrophy: an update. Orthop Clin North Am 1990;21:81–96.

Mankin HJ. Metabolic bone disease. In: Jackson DW, ed. Instructional course lectures 44. Rosemont, IL: American Academy of Orthopaedic Surgeons, 1994;3–29.

Pak CYC, Sakahee K, Adams-Huet B, et al. Treatment of postmenopausal osteoporosis with slow-release sodium fluoride. Ann Intern Med 1995; 123:401–408.

Riggs BL, Melton LJ. Osteoporosis: Etiology, diagnosis and management. New York: Raven Press, 1988.

Riggs BL, Melton LJ III. The prevention and treatment of osteoporosis. N Engl J Med 1993;327: 620–627.

Simon SR, ed. Orthopaedic basic science. Rosemont IL: American Academy of Orthopaedic Surgeons, 1994.

Siris ES, Ottman R, Flaster E, Kelsey JL. Familial aggregation of Paget's disease of bone. J Bone Miner Res 1991;6:495–500.

Zaleske DJ. Metabolic and endocrine abnormalities. In: Morrissy RT, Weinstein SL, eds. Lovell and Winter's Pediatric Orthopaedics. 4th ed. 1996;137–201.

10 Inflammatory Disorders of Bones and Joints

A wide variety of disorders of the musculoskeletal system are manifested clinically by the phenomenon of *inflammation* and are therefore best considered as a broad group in relation to this basic pathological process. For some of these clinical disorders, such as osteomyelitis and septic arthritis, a specific causative microorganism can be incriminated; however, for others, such as ankylosing spondylitis and rheumatoid arthritis, the exact cause remains an unsolved and challenging mystery.

Before learning about the various disorders as clinical entities, you will find it helpful to review some of the general features of the inflammatory process and the reactions of the musculoskeletal tissue to this process.

THE INFLAMMATORY PROCESS: GENERAL FEATURES

Inflammation, a process of biological events, is best defined as "the local reaction of living tissues to an irritant" (Boyd). In this reactive process, cells and exudates accumulate in the irritated tissue and usually (but not invariably) tend to protect them from further injury. Once considered a disease entity in itself, inflammation is now known to be a tissue response, or reaction, to any one of many types of irritants. The four clinical manifestations of inflammation originally described by Celsus are *rubor, tumor, calor* et *dolor* (redness, swelling, heat, and pain). To these Galen later added a fifth—*functio laesa* (loss of function). These five clinical manifestations are readily explained by the nature of the inflammatory process.

The *redness* and the *heat* are caused by the vascular response, namely, a dilatation of local blood vessels combined with an increased rate of flow. The *swelling* represents the formation of an exudate that results from the combination of increased hydrostatic pressure within the capillaries and increased capillary permeability. Added to this inflammatory exudate is the emigration of various types of leukocytes from the capillaries. The *pain*, which is most severe in the acute type of inflammatory process, is related to the marked increase in local pressure within the tissues. When the inflammatory process develops in a closed space, such as a bone or synovial joint, it is easy to understand why the pain may be severe. The initial *loss of function* of the involved part results from pain and swelling; however, subsequent loss of function may result from a combination of actual destruction of tissue, such as articular cartilage, and dense scar formation in soft tissues.

In the central zone of the inflammatory process, local tissue necrosis and liquefaction are frequently seen. By contrast, the reaction in the peripheral zone is hyperplasia of connective tissue cells, a reaction that initially serves to localize the process and subsequently aids in the repair of the inflammatory lesion.

REACTIONS OF THE MUSCULOSKELETAL TISSUES TO INFLAMMATION

Each specialized type of tissue in the body reacts in a characteristic way to the general process of inflammation. Thus, a knowledge of the characteristic reactions of the various musculoskeletal tissues will enhance your *understanding* not only of the clinical, radiographic, and laboratory *manifestations* of inflammatory musculoskeletal disorders in your patients but also of the underlying *reason* for the principles and methods of their treatment. The characteristic reactions to infection and other types of inflammation in bone, epiphyseal plate, articular cartilage, synovial membrane, capsule, and ligaments are discussed and illustrated in Chapter 3. They are of sufficient importance that you may wish to review these reactions in Chapter 3 before proceeding to a discussion of the various clinical disease entities that result from inflammation of musculoskeletal tissues.

TYPES OF INFLAMMATORY DISORDERS OF BONES AND JOINTS

The various musculoskeletal disorders discussed in this chapter have in common as their most prominent feature the phenomenon of inflammation. They are best considered in four broad groups.

First is the group of *specific infections* for which causative organisms can be detected. Of these, many are *pyogenic* (pus-producing) infections, such as osteomyelitis, septic arthritis, and tenosynovitis. Others are *granulomatous* (granuloma-producing) infections, such as tuberculous osteomyelitis and tuberculous arthritis.

A second broad group of inflammatory disorders includes the nonspecific and idiopathic *inflammatory types of rheumatic diseases,* which include entities such as rheumatic fever, transient synovitis, rheumatoid arthritis, and ankylosing spondylitis.

A third group includes inflammation of musculoskeletal tissue secondary to a chemical irritant, as seen in the form of *metabolic arthritis* known as gout.

A fourth group is characterized by chronic inflammation caused by *repeated physical injury*—now known as *chronic repetitive strain injury*—usually minor injury (microtrauma), or mechanical irritation. Bursitis and tenovaginitis stenosans, which are examples of this type of inflammation secondary to chronic repetitive strain injury, are described in Chapter 11.

Pyogenic Bacterial Infections

Pyogenic bacterial infections in bones and joints continue to represent a serious threat to both life and limb. Although chemotherapeutic and antibiotic drugs have dramatically reduced the mortality of the various pyogenic infections involving the musculoskeletal system, the incidence of these infections and their morbidity have been less dramatically reduced. Indeed, drug therapy may mask the clinical manifestations of infection without completely controlling the local lesion, thereby creating an altered clinical picture.

Principles of Antibacterial Therapy

Acute pyogenic infection is an exceedingly rapid process measured in hours and days. Thus, even a short delay in treatment may lead to serious consequences for the patient. Antibiotics such as tetracycline, chloramphenicol, and erythromycin exert their effect on the metabolism of bacteria and thereby greatly decrease their rate of multiplication; their action, therefore, is bacteriostatic. Other antibacterial drugs, such as the penicillins and cephalosporins, actually kill bacteria and hence are *bacteriocidal.*

To control an infection, the concentration of the appropriate antibiotic in the blood and at the site of infection must exceed the level necessary to kill the infecting organism. The ideal antibiotic is *bacteriocidal* (as opposed to *bacteriostatic*), should be known to be effective against the most likely infecting bacteria, must reach the infected tissues in high concentrations (which can be difficult in bone), should be nontoxic, and should have little effect on the normal flora. The parenteral (intravenous or intramuscular) route of administration is more effective than the oral route in achieving adequate serum and tissue levels of the antibiotic and is therefore preferable in the initial treatment, especially if the patient is unable to take medications by mouth.

Since patients vary in their response to antibiotics and since the infecting organisms vary in their resistance, both clinical and laboratory monitoring of the patient are essential. An effective laboratory method of such monitoring is the weekly determination of the serum bacterial titer.

Antibacterial therapy must be continued for a longer period to control infection in bone than in soft tissues in order to achieve a permanent cure and thereby prevent either chronic or recurrent infection. Empirically, this period is from 3 to 4 weeks.

The relatively slow diffusion of antibacterial agents into the area of bacterial inflammation is dependent on an intact local blood supply. When the local pressure within the inflamed tissues becomes excessive, with resultant is-chemia, the circulating antibacterial agents are no longer able to reach the causative organism to exert their effect. Likewise, accumulation of a purulent exudate *(pus)* in an abscess prevents the agents from reaching the bacteria. These facts emphasize the real value of surgical de-compression of the increased pressure within a closed space—such as bone or joint—and surgical evacuation of accumulated pus.

Acute Hematogenous Osteomyelitis

One of the most serious inflammatory disor-ders of the musculoskeletal system is *acute he-matogenous osteomyelitis,* a rapidly developing blood-borne bacterial infection of bone and its marrow in children.

Incidence

At the beginning of the era of specific antibac-terial drug therapy, there was a sharp fall in the incidence of acute hematogenous osteo-myelitis; indeed, some clinicians optimistically predicted the eradication of this disease. Sub-sequently, however, the incidence returned al-most to its former level. This phenome-non—which has been paralleled by bacterial infections involving other tissues—is ex-plained by a combination of the emergence of resistant strains of bacteria (especially staphy-lococci) and the failure of too many clinicians to understand and apply the principles of anti-bacterial and surgical therapy in relation to bone and joint infections.

Hematogenous osteomyelitis is primarily a disease of growing bones and, therefore, of children; boys are afflicted three times as often as girls. The long bones most frequently in-volved (in order of decreasing frequency) are the femur, tibia, humerus, radius, ulna, and fibula, and the characteristic site in any given bone is the metaphyseal region—possibly be-cause of the unique blood vessels and low-flow state to this part of the bone during child-hood.

Etiology

Staphylococcus aureus is by far the most com-mon causative organism, being responsible for at least 90% of acute hematogenous osteo-

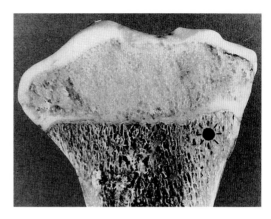

Figure 10.1.   Site of the initial focus of hematogenous osteomyelitis in the metaphyseal region of the upper end of the tibia showing the cut surface of the tibia; note the architectural arrangement of the cancellous bone in the metaphysis, which is different from that in the epiphysis.

myelitis cases. The *portal of entry* is usually through the skin secondary to infected scratches, abrasions, pimples, or boils; some-times it is through the mucous membranes of the upper respiratory tract as a complication of a nose or throat infection. Even vigorous brushing of the teeth in the presence of in-flamed gums can result in transient bacter-emia. In the presence of bacteremia, local trauma seems to play a significant role in de-termining the particular bone in which osteo-myelitis develops (perhaps because of local thrombosis and hence decreased resistance to infection); this may account, in part, for the higher incidence in boys and also in the lower extremities. *Streptococcus* or *Pneumococcus* may on occasion be the offending bacteria, particularly in infants. *Hemophilus influenzae* has almost been eliminated as a cause of osteo-myelitis by the development of an effective vaccine.

Pathogenesis and Pathology

The early and rapid development of untreated hematogenous osteomyelitis is characterized by an initially small focus of bacterial inflam-mation with early *hyperemia* and *edema* in the cancellous bone and marrow of the metaphy-seal region of a long bone (Fig. 10.1). Unlike soft tissues, which are capable of expanding

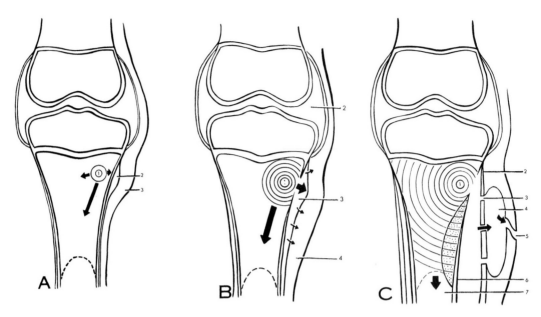

Figure 10.2.   Routes of spread of untreated acute hematogenous osteomyelitis in the upper end of the tibia. **A.** *(1)* Initially the infection spreads in three directions as shown by the arrows; *(2)* periosteal edema; *(3)* edema in the soft tissues. **B.** *(1)* Original focus of infection has increased in size; *(2)* there may be an inflammatory exudate in the knee joint but no direct extension of the infection; *(3)* subperiosteal abscess; *(4)* cellulitis in the overlying soft tissues. **C.** *(1)* The area of osteomyelitis has become extensive; *(2)* the periosteum has been elevated from the underlying bone over a large area; *(3)* infection has penetrated the periosteum to produce *(4)* a soft tissue abscess. *(5)* The abscess has drained onto the skin surface through a sinus; *(6)* an area of bone necrosis that will subsequently sequestrate; *(7)* continuing spread of the infection in the medullary cavity.

to accommodate swelling, the bone represents a rigid closed space; therefore, the early edema of the inflammatory process produces a sharp rise in the intraosseous pressure, which explains the symptom of severe and constant local pain. Pus forms, thereby increasing the local pressure even further with resultant compromise of the local circulation which, in turn, leads to vascular thrombosis and consequent *necrosis of bone*.

The untreated infection rapidly spreads by several routes, destroying bone in its path by *osteolysis* (Fig. 10.2). Through damaged vessels in the local lesion, large numbers of bacteria reinvade the bloodstream; the clinically undetectable bacteremia becomes a *septicemia*, which is manifest by the onset of malaise, anorexia, and fever. Local spread of the infection by direct extension, aided by increased local pressure, penetrates the relatively thin cortex of the metaphyseal region and involves the highly

sensitive periosteum, which accounts for the exquisite local tenderness. The periosteum, being loosely attached to bone during childhood, is readily separated and elevated from the bone. The result is a *subperiosteal abscess* that may either remain localized or spread along and around the entire shaft of the bone; such elevation of the periosteum disrupts the blood supply to the underlying cortex, thereby increasing the extent of bone necrosis.

After the first few days, the infection penetrates the periosteum to produce a *cellulitis* and eventually a *soft tissue abscess*. In sites where the metaphyseal region is within the synovial joint, as in the upper end of the femur and the upper end of the radius, penetration of the periosteum carries the infection directly into the joint, with resultant *septic arthritis* (Fig. 10.3). In other sites where the metaphyseal region is outside but close to the joint, a sterile synovial effusion frequently develops.

Meanwhile, local spread of the infection within the medullary cavity further compromises the internal circulation. The resultant area of bone necrosis, which may vary in extent from a small spicule to the entire shaft, eventually becomes separated, or sequestrated, from the living bone, thereby forming a separated fragment of infected dead bone, a *sequestrum*. Extensive new bone formation from the deep layer of the elevated periosteum produces an enveloping bony tube, or *involucrum,* which maintains the continuity of the involved bone, even when large segments of the shaft have died and sequestrated (Fig. 10.2). The epiphyseal plate usually acts as a barrier to direct spread of infection, but if it is damaged in the process, a serious growth disturbance will become apparent at a later date.

If uncontrolled, the septicemia may produce metastatic foci of infection in other bones at any time; more important, it may produce these foci in other organs, particularly the lungs and the brain. Indeed, in the days before antibacterial drugs, 25% of all children with acute hematogenous osteomyelitis died of the associated septicemia. If the child survives the septicemia, the local bone lesion—unless adequately treated—gradually passes into a chronic state. Chronic osteomyelitis, which is perpetuated by the presence of infected dead bone, is discussed in a subsequent section of this chapter.

Clinical Features and Diagnosis

The clinical features of acute hematogenous osteomyelitis are readily correlated with the foregoing description of its pathogenesis. The onset is acute and the infection progresses with remarkable rapidity. There is a history of recent local injury in 50% of the children; frequently you will find evidence of a pre-existing bacterial infection either in the skin or in the upper respiratory tract.

The first and most significant symptom the afflicted child experiences is severe and constant pain near the end of the involved long bone; this is accompanied by exquisite local tenderness and the child's unwillingness to use the limb (Fig. 10.4). Within 24 hours, the associated septicemia is evidenced by malaise, anorexia, and fever; the child appears acutely ill. Increasing pain and local tenderness near the end of a long bone, combined with systemic manifestations of infection, in a child

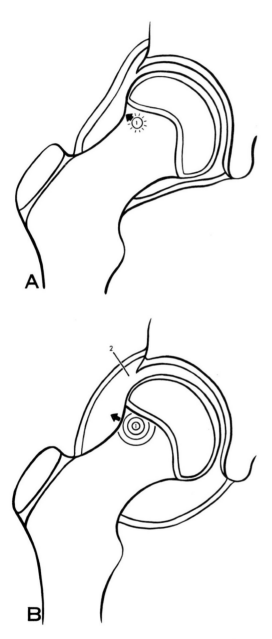

Figure 10.3. Acute hematogenous osteomyelitis of the upper end of the femur in a child. **A.** *(1)* Initial focus of infection in the metaphyseal region. **B.** *(1)* The focus of infection has spread through the metaphyseal cortex directly into *(2)* the synovial cavity of the hip joint.

always justify the *clinical* diagnosis of acute hematogenous osteomyelitis—at least until there is definite evidence to the contrary. Soft tissue swelling is a relatively late sign appearing only after a few days and indicating that the infection has already spread beyond the confines of the bone (Fig. 10.5).

It is extremely important for you to appreciate that the early diagnosis of acute hematogenous osteomyelitis must be made on *clinical* grounds alone. During at least the first week of illness, there is absolutely no concrete radiographic evidence of bone infection, despite severe local involvement of bone. There may be radiographic evidence of soft tissue

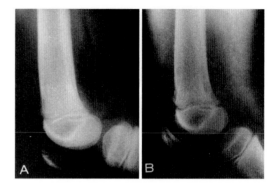

Figure 10.6. Radiographic evidence of soft tissue swelling secondary to acute hematogenous osteomyelitis. **A.** Normal lower end of the femur of a child. **B.** Soft tissue swelling posterior to the lower end of the opposite femur in the same child with acute hematogenous osteomyelitis 3 days after the onset of symptoms. At this stage there is no evidence of bone destruction.

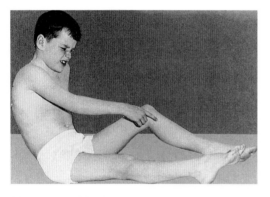

Figure 10.4. This boy has early acute hematogenous osteomyelitis of the upper end of the left tibia; he is unable to bear weight on his left foot and is unwilling to move his knee. He is able to localize the point of pain and tenderness very accurately.

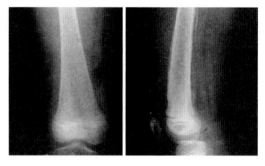

Figure 10.7. Radiographic evidence of bone destruction in the metaphyseal region of the lower end of the femur in a child with acute hematogenous osteomyelitis of 10 days' duration. Note also the evidence of subperiosteal new bone formation along the shaft of the femur in the lateral projection.

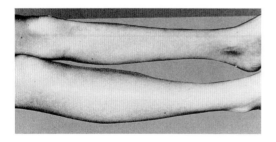

Figure 10.5. Soft tissue swelling secondary to osteomyelitis of the right tibia in a child. This child had severe pain in the right leg for 7 days prior to this photograph. The infection has already spread from the bone into the soft tissues to produce an extensive cellulitis.

swelling after the first few days (Fig. 10.6). Such swelling can also be detected by ultrasonography. However, only after the first week does the radiograph reveal the first evidence of destruction of bone in the metaphysis and the first signs of reactive new bone from the periosteum (Fig. 10.7). During this first week before radiographic changes become apparent, scintigraphy—that is, a bone scan—may be of value in establishing the diagnosis. With magnetic resonance imaging (MRI), the combination of a dark focus on T1-weighted images and a bright signal on T2-weighted images is consistent with osteomyelitis.

In infants, the systemic manifestations of infection are often less apparent than they are in children. Furthermore, the localization of the osteomyelitis is obviously more difficult because of the lack of communication and requires careful examination of all the major long bones and joints.

The white blood cell count and the sedimentation rate are usually elevated, but despite the underlying bacteremia, and the later septicemia, a single blood culture gives positive results in only about half of the patients.

The clinical manifestations of acute hematogenous osteomyelitis—particularly the systemic manifestations—may be masked during the first few days of the illness by the casual and speculative use of inadequate antibacterial therapy for what is loosely considered "a little infection." This deplorable type of management obscures the true diagnosis until irreparable changes in the bone have developed and the local infection has progressed relentlessly to chronic osteomyelitis (Fig. 10.8).

In its early stages, acute hematogenous osteomyelitis must be differentiated from rheumatic fever, cellulitis of soft tissues, and local trauma to soft tissues or bone. After the first week or more, particularly if the systemic manifestations have been masked by antibacterial drugs, the radiographic changes of irregular

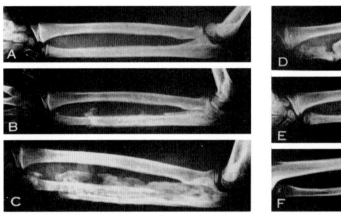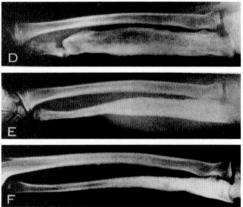

Figure 10.8. Relentless progression from acute hematogenous osteomyelitis to chronic osteomyelitis. This series of radiographs of a girl's forearm extends over a period of 10 years and demonstrates many of the radiographic changes of acute and chronic osteomyelitis of the ulna. **A.** One week after the onset of symptoms. There is soft tissue swelling, a small area of destruction in the metaphyseal region of the distal end of the ulna, and beginning new bone formation along the shaft of the ulna. This child had been thought to have a "a little infection" and had received a small amount of antibacterial therapy for a few days. At the end of 1 week her arm was significantly swollen and tender. The infection had already spread throughout the length of the ulna and at this stage even extensive therapy could not eradicate all the infection. **B.** Ten days later there is evidence of further destruction in the ulna and more subperiosteal new bone formation. **C.** One month later, there is involucrum formation and sequestration of the distal third of the ulna. At this stage, the child was still ill and in pain. Consequently, the large sequestrum was removed. **D.** Eight months later, there is still chronic osteomyelitis; there is a pathological fracture in that portion of the lower end of the ulna that has reformed from the deep surface of periosteum. **E.** Three years later, there is evidence of premature cessation of growth at the distal ulnar epiphyseal plate secondary to the infection. There is still marked thickening of the proximal two thirds of the ulna because of residual chronic osteomyelitis. **F.** Ten years after the onset of the osteomyelitis, there is a small abscess in the upper end of the ulna and additional evidence of chronic osteomyelitis in the entire upper third of the ulna. This relentless progression from acute hematogenous osteomyelitis to chronic osteomyelitis could have been prevented by early adequate treatment.

metaphyseal rarefaction and subperiosteal new bone formation can mimic bone lesions such as Langerhans cell histiocytosis (eosinophilic granuloma), Ewing's sarcoma, and osteosarcoma.

Treatment

Acute hematogenous osteomyelitis represents an extremely serious infection that demands urgent and vigorous treatment. As soon as the *clinical* diagnosis is strongly suspected on the basis of the previously mentioned symptoms and signs, the child should be admitted to hospital for intensive treatment. As soon as one blood sample has been taken for culture to seek the causative bacteria as well as its sensitivity to the various antibacterial drugs, antibacterial therapy is instituted. Since the incidence of bacterial resistance to antibiotics continues to increase and because the bacterial environment varies not only from one locality to another but also from year to year, the choice of the specific drug to be used initially will depend on existing conditions in your locale at the time. Nevertheless, general guidelines can be stated.

Currently, penicillin is still the safest antibiotic drug, but in many communities more than 70% of the staphylococci are penicillin-resistant. Therefore, at least initially, one of the newer antibiotics such as cloxacillin should be given for older children or, alternatively, one of the cephalosporins such as cefotaxime for neonates and cefuroxime for young children (all of which are effective in the presence of penicillinase). As soon as the culture and sensitivity results are known, antibiotic therapy can be modified appropriately if necessary. A consultant in the rapidly changing field of infectious diseases can be of much help in advising about the antibacterial therapy for these patients.

The following general plan of treatment has been found to be most effective:

1. Provide bed rest and analgesics for the child.
2. Supportive measures are given, including, when necessary, intravenous fluids.
3. Local rest for the involved extremity is provided by either a removable splint or trac-

tion to reduce pain, retard the spread of infection, and prevent soft tissue contractures.
4. For a child too sick to take drugs by mouth, immediate parenteral administration of appropriate antibacterial therapy (as soon as a blood sample has been taken for culture) is necessary, not only to control the bacteremia and septicemia but also to reach the area of osteomyelitis before it has become ischemic and therefore inaccessible to the circulating drug. For a child who is able to take drugs by mouth, oral administration of the antibiotic is an acceptable alternative from the beginning. After the first 2 weeks (provided that there has been a good clinical response), the antibiotic may be given orally (which has been proved effective and is certainly more comfortable for the child).
5. If local and systemic manifestations have not improved dramatically after 24 hours of intensive treatment, surgical decompression of the involved area of bone (evacuation of subperiosteal pus, drilling of bone) is performed to reduce the intraosseous pressure and to obtain pus for culture. Postoperatively, continuous local infusion of saline with an appropriate antibiotic, combined with drainage, may be required for severe infections for at least a few days (Fig. 10.9).
6. Antibacterial therapy is continued for a minimal period of 3 to 4 weeks, even if clinical improvement during the first few days has been satisfactory. (After 3 to 4 weeks, treatment is discontinued only when the sedimentation rate begins to approach a normal level.)

Prognosis

Four important factors determine the effectiveness of antibacterial treatment for acute hematogenous osteomyelitis and consequently its prognosis:

1. *The time interval between the onset of infection and the institution of treatment.* Treatment begun during the first 3 days of illness is ideal because at this stage the local area of osteomyelitis has not yet become

ischemic. Such early treatment, provided that the causative organism is sensitive to the drug chosen, usually controls the infection completely so that osteolysis, bone necrosis, and reactive new bone formation are prevented; under these circumstances, radiographic changes in the bone may not appear later (Fig. 10.10).

Treatment begun between 3 and 7 days usually attenuates the infection both systemically and locally, but is too late to prevent bone destruction (Fig. 10.11).

Treatment instituted after the first week of illness may control the septicemia and therefore still be lifesaving, but it has little effect on the relentless progression of the local pathological process within the bone (Fig. 10.8).

2. *The effectiveness of the antibacterial drug against the specific causative bacteria.* This depends on whether the bacteria is sensitive to the drug or resistant to it and emphasizes the importance of culture and sensitivity studies.

3. *The dosage of the antibacterial drug.* The local factor of compromised circulation within the area of bone infection necessi-

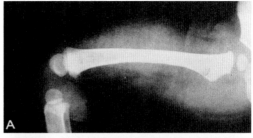
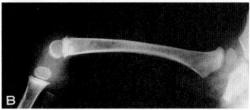

Figure 10.10.   Complete resolution of acute hematogenous osteomyelitis of the femur following early adequate treatment. **A.** Two days after the onset of pain in the lower end of the thigh of a young child. There is soft tissue swelling but no evidence of bone destruction. At this time, the child was acutely ill and exhibited the classic signs of acute hematogenous osteomyelitis. **B.** One month later there is no evidence of bony changes because the osteomyelitis had been completely controlled by effective antibacterial therapy that had been instituted within the first 3 days of its onset.

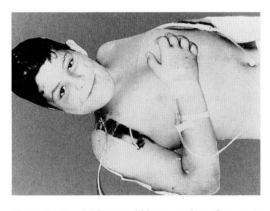

Figure 10.9.   A 10-year-old boy two days after surgical decompression of an extensive area of osteomyelitis of the upper end of the right humerus. You will observe from the boy's facial expression that he is completely comfortable. Note the continuous intravenous infusion in the right forearm, the plastic tube for infusion in the region of the shoulder, and the second plastic tube at the lower end of the wound for continuous drainage. The incision, which has been closed, is under the blood-stained dressing.

tates much larger doses of antibacterial drugs for osteomyelitis than for soft tissue infections.

4. *The duration of antibacterial therapy.* Premature cessation of therapy, especially less than 3 to 4 weeks, frequently results in either chronic or recurrent osteomyelitis.

Complications of Acute Hematogenous Osteomyelitis

The early complications of acute hematogenous osteomyelitis include 1) *death* from the associated septicemia, 2) *abscess formation,* and 3) *septic arthritis,* especially in the hip joint.

The *late complications* include 1) *chronic osteomyelitis,* either persistent or recurrent; 2) *pathological fracture* through a weakened area of bone; 3) *joint contracture;* 4) *local growth disturbance* of the involved bone, either overgrowth from the stimulation of prolonged hy-

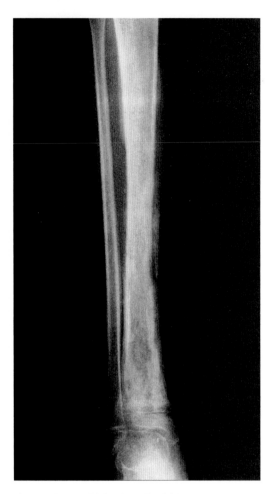

Figure 10.11.   Right tibia of a child with acute hematogenous osteomyelitis 5 weeks after the onset of infection. Treatment had been started 5 days after the onset of symptoms, and although the infection had been controlled systemically, the treatment was started too late to prevent bone destruction. Note evidence of destruction in the distal two thirds of the tibia and also the subperiosteal new bone formation.

peremia or premature cessation of growth from epiphyseal plate damage (Fig. 10.12).

Chronic Hematogenous Osteomyelitis

Inadequate treatment of the acute phase of hematogenous osteomyelitis allows the local pathological process either to persist and become chronic or to become relatively quiescent for a time, only to recur at a later date. Both the persistent chronic form and the re-

current chronic form of osteomyelitis are exceedingly difficult to eradicate.

Incidence

The continuing prevalence of chronic hematogenous osteomyelitis testifies to the frequent failure to diagnose acute osteomyelitis within the first few days of onset as well as the failure to provide effective antibacterial therapy and the failure to intervene surgically, when indicated, in the acute phase.

Pathogenesis and Pathology

The most significant pathological lesion in the chronic phase of hematogenous osteomyelitis, and the one that prevents its spontaneous resolution, is infected dead bone. Unlike a segment of sterile dead bone, which is gradually revascularized, resorbed, and replaced by living bone, infected dead bone always separates, or sequestrates, from the remaining living bone and thus becomes a sequestrum. Bacte-

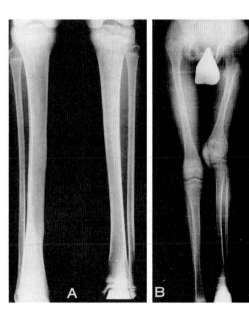

Figure 10.12.   Local growth disturbance in the involved bone complicating osteomyelitis. **A.** Overgrowth of the right tibia in a 14-year-old girl with chronic osteomyelitis involving the distal end of the tibia. The infection has been chronic for 5 years. **B.** Premature cessation of growth in the left lower femoral epiphysis complicating osteomyelitis in early childhood. In this full length radiograph (orthroentogenogram), a severe leg length discrepancy is apparent.

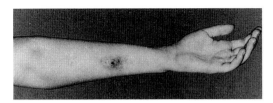

Figure 10.13.   Draining sinus in the forearm of a child with chronic osteomyelitis. This type of sinus will not heal until all infected bone (sequestra) has been removed.

ria are able to survive and continue to multiply within the tiny haversian canals and canaliculi of this island of avascular bone; the surrounding pond of pus prevents revascularization of the sequestrum and thereby protects its bacterial inhabitants not only from the living leukocytes of the defensive inflammatory reaction but also from the action of circulating antibacterial drugs. Furthermore, in the absence of revascularization, the living process of osteoclastic resorption of dead bone cannot reach the sequestrum. As a result, the sequestrum persists as a haven for bacteria and a source of either persistent or recurrent infection. Thus, the infection cannot be permanently eradicated until all sequestra have been eliminated, either by the natural process of spontaneous extrusion through an opening (*cloaca*) in the *involucrum* and thence through a *sinus track* to the exterior (Fig 10.13), or by surgical removal (*sequestrectomy*). An area of persistent infection within cancellous bone may eventually become walled off from the surrounding bone by fibrous tissue to form a chronic abscess (*Brodie's abscess*).

Clinical Features and Diagnosis

The child, having recovered from the septicemia of the acute phase, is no longer acutely ill but has a residual painful lesion in the involved long bone associated with swelling, tenderness, and loss of function of the limb; there may be one or more draining sinuses (Fig. 10.13).

The radiographic diagnosis is usually apparent, particularly in the presence of obvious

sequestra (Fig. 10.14). Nevertheless, the combination of local rarefaction, sclerosis, and periosteal new bone formation may mimic other bone lesions such as osteosarcoma, Ewing's sarcoma, and Langerhans cell histiocytosis (eosinophilic granuloma). The radiographic appearance of a Brodie's abscess is not unlike that of an osteolytic bone neoplasm (Fig. 10.14). In the presence of a draining sinus, a sinogram often helps locate the site of underlying infection (Fig. 10.15).

Persistent anemia and elevation of the sedimentation rate reflect the chronic infection.

Treatment

Chronic osteomyelitis can seldom be completely eradicated until all the infected dead bone has separated, or sequestrated, and has either been extruded spontaneously through a sinus track or been removed surgically (*sequestrectomy*). In the absence of clinical evidence of local and systemic infection, a small sequestrum may be resorbed.

Antibacterial therapy is required both systemically and locally. A residual abscess cavity within the bone usually necessitates an operation in which one surface of the tubular bone is removed to make it open like a saucer (*saucerization*). Following either sequestrectomy or saucerization, antibacterial drugs in saline solution are instilled into the area by continu-

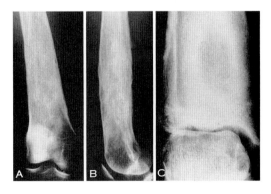

Figure 10.14.   **A** and **B.** Residual chronic osteomyelitis with several small sequestra in the lower end of the femur of a 40-year-old woman who had acute hematogenous osteomyelitis in this site at 10 years of age. **C.** Brodie's abscess in the distal end of the tibia in a young adult. The osteolytic lesion is not unlike that of an osteolytic bone neoplasm.

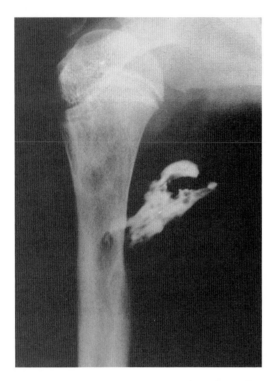

Figure 10.15. This sinogram was taken after radio-paque material had been injected into a draining sinus in the axilla. Note that the contrast medium tracks along the sinus to a small area of osteolysis in the shaft of the humerus. Note also a small sequestrum lying within the osteolytic area.

ous infusion, and pus is removed by drainage. Occasionally, reconstructive operations such as bone grafting and skin grafting are required later to overcome a residual defect in the bone and soft tissues.

Complications
The complications of persistent chronic osteo-myelitis include 1) *joint contracture,* 2) *patho-logical fracture,* 3) *amyloid disease,* and 4) ma-lignant changes in the epidermis (*epidermoid carcinoma*) of a sinus track in which infection has been allowed to persist for many years.

Acute Septic Arthritis (Pyogenic Arthritis)

When pyogenic bacteria invade a synovial joint, the result is acute septic (pyogenic) ar-thritis, a rapidly progressive infection that, un-less adequately treated, leads to severe de-struction of the joint.

Incidence
The incidence of septic arthritis parallels that of hematogenous osteomyelitis with which it is so frequently associated. Septic arthritis, therefore, is primarily a disease of childhood. Newborn infants are particularly susceptible, especially those who have an immunodefi-ciency, as suggested by Lloyd-Roberts. Dur-ing childhood, the most common sites are those in which the metaphysis of the bone is entirely intracapsular, namely, the hip and the elbow (Fig. 10.3). In adult life, septic arthritis can develop in any joint because it is unrelated to osteomyelitis.

Etiology
The spread of pyogenic bacteria from hema-togenous osteomyelitis in the metaphysis di-rectly into the joint is the most common source of septic arthritis in children. Conse-quently, as in osteomyelitis, the most frequent causative organism is *S. aureus.* However, bac-teria, particularly streptococci and pneumo-cocci and less commonly *Salmonella,* may reach the joint by the bloodstream to produce hematogenous septic arthritis. In adults, staphylococci, pneumonococci, and gono-cocci may also invade a synovial joint by the hematogenous route as a complication of sys-temic infection. Human immunodeficiency virus (HIV) and acquired immunodeficiency syndrome (AIDS), as well as intravenous drug use and prolonged adrenocorticosteroid ther-apy are risk factors for the development of sep-tic arthritis.

Pathogenesis and Pathology
Acute septic arthritis is an extremely serious infection because the purulent exudate—par-ticularly that of staphylococci—rapidly digests articular cartilage. The mechanism of initial cartilage destruction includes enzymatic digestion of the matrix by lysosomal enzymes from both polymorphonuclear leukocytes and bacteria. As a result, the collagen fibers lose their support and the cartilage disintegrates. Granulation tissue may creep over the articular cartilage as a *pannus,* blocking its nutrition from synovial fluid and thereby leading to even further destruction. Since cartilage is vir-tually incapable of regeneration under ordi-

nary circumstances, its destruction is not only devastating but also permanent. The inflamed synovial membrane becomes grossly swollen. As the joint becomes filled with pus, the fibrous capsule softens and stretches, with the result that a pathological dislocation may ensue, particularly in the hip joint of infants and children. Furthermore, in the hip joint, the increased intra-articular fluid pressure of the pus frequently occludes the precarious blood supply to the bone, with resultant avascular necrosis of the femoral head. The infantile femoral head, being entirely cartilaginous, may be completely destroyed. Late sequelae of inadequately treated septic arthritis include degenerative joint disease, fibrous ankylosis, and occasionally bony ankylosis.

Clinical Features and Diagnosis

The clinical manifestations of acute septic arthritis in infants are significantly different from those in older children or adults and consequently are best considered separately.

Septic Arthritis in Infants

During infancy, particularly in the newborn period, acute septic arthritis may develop with few clinical manifestations other than irritability and the infant's reluctance to move the affected joint, with resultant "pseudoparalysis." Local examination reveals tenderness over the joint and obviously painful restriction of joint motion (Fig. 10.16). Fever and elevation of the white blood cell count are misleadingly

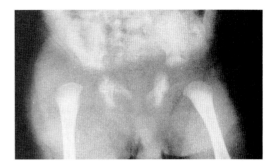

Figure 10.17. Acute septic arthritis and pathological dislocation of the right hip in an infant. Note the lateral and upward displacement of the ossified portion of the upper end of the right femur in contrast to the normal position of the left femur.

slight in this age group, and unless the major joints of the limbs are examined daily during any febrile illness, the diagnosis of septic arthritis may not be made sufficiently early to prevent avascular necrosis of the femoral head and irreparable damage to the joint. Clinical suspicion of acute septic arthritis is an urgent indication for immediate needle aspiration of the joint as a valuable diagnostic procedure and as a means of obtaining fluid from the joint for a Gram stain and culture.

Radiographic examination and also ultrasonography during the first week may reveal evidence of soft tissue swelling, but not until the second week is there evidence of a pathological dislocation (Fig. 10.17). Equally delayed are the radiographic changes of osteomyelitis in the intracapsular part of the metaphysis (Fig. 10.18).

Septic Arthritis in Older Children and Adults

Unlike the uncommunicative infant, the older child or adult with septic arthritis is able to tell you of severe pain in the region of the involved joint and, furthermore, that the pain is made much worse by even the slightest movement in the joint. Clinical signs include protective spasm in the muscles controlling the joint, marked tenderness and, when the involved joint is superficial, an obvious effusion. The systemic manifestations of infection and elevation of temperature, white blood cell count, and sedimentation rate are more

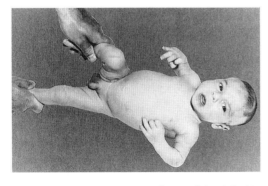

Figure 10.16. Acute septic arthritis of the right hip in an infant. The right hip is held in flexion and abduction and the infant resists passive movement of the hip because of pain.

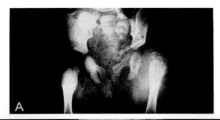

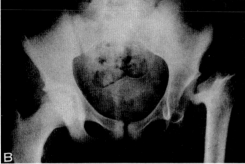

Figure 10.18. Late metaphyseal changes in the neck of the femur associated with septic arthritis of the hip. **A.** One month after the onset of septic arthritis of the left hip in an infant. Note the pathological dislocation of the left hip and marked metaphyseal changes in the neck of the femur. **B.** Sequelae of acute septic arthritis of the hip in a 14-year-old girl. Note the marked destruction of the upper end of the left femur that has resulted from acute septic arthritis of the hip in infancy. This girl's hip, which is also severely subluxated, is seriously damaged and will require reconstructive operations.

marked in this age group than in infants. Needle aspiration of the joint is equally important in both groups. A white blood cell count of greater than 100,000/mL in the synovial fluid is strongly suggestive of septic arthritis.

Radiographic findings in the older age group are comparable to those seen in infants, although pathological subluxation is more common than dislocation. Only after considerable destruction of articular cartilage is there evidence of a narrowed cartilage space (Fig. 10.19).

Treatment

Acute septic arthritis represents a surgical emergency that demands early and vigorous treatment to preserve normal joint function. The general plan of treatment, including antibacterial drugs, is similar to that described, in a previous section of this chapter, for acute hematogenous osteomyelitis, with the addition of specific local treatment for the joint itself. Although needle aspiration of an infected joint is of the utmost importance in establishing the diagnosis and obtaining the causative organism, the therapeutic regimen of repeated aspiration and instillation of antibacterial drugs is seldom sufficient to control septic arthritis; after the first few days, the pus has become too thick to be completely removed even through a large-bore needle. Nevertheless, arthroscopic lavage is effective for the knee joint.

Far more effective treatment for other joints (especially the hip joint) is the operation of opening and exploring the joint (*arthrotomy*) with complete removal of the pus and thorough irrigation of the joint. The wound may be closed, but continuous local infusion of saline with an appropriate antibacterial drug

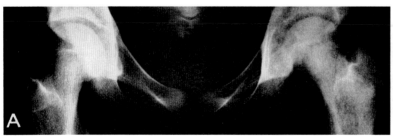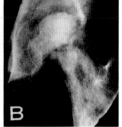

Figure 10.19. Septic arthritis of the left hip in a 13-year-old girl. **A.** This radiograph, taken 1 month after the onset of symptoms, shows that the cartilage space is narrowed and the hip has subluxated slightly. Note also the rarefaction in the neck of the femur. **B.** The same hip 2 months later shows further changes in the neck of the femur and radiographic evidence of avascular necrosis of the femoral head. This girl's hip is irreparably damaged.

should be combined with drainage for at least a few days, until the fluid being drained from the joint is sterile.

When septic arthritis of the hip in an infant is complicated by a pathological dislocation, the dislocated hip should be reduced and the hip immobilized in a stable position. In the absence of a pathological dislocation and in all other sites of septic arthritis, the infected joint should be allowed to move in an attempt to prevent complications such as intra-articular adhesions and progressive destruction of cartilage. Indeed, in an experimental model of acute septic arthritis of the knee in rabbits, we have found that continuous passive motion (CPM) has a protective effect on articular cartilage (Salter et al.).

Most gonococcal arthritis in adults is resistant to penicillin and requires a parenteral β-lactamose–resistant cephalosporin. Treatment of the late sequelae of septic arthritis involves various types of reconstructive operations. Often the residual damage of inadequately treated septic arthritis is so severe that surgical fusion (*arthrodesis*) of the joint is necessary to relieve pain, provide stability, and correct deformity—but at the cost of permanent loss of joint motion (Fig. 10.20).

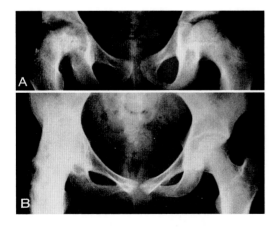

Figure 10.20. Chronic septic arthritis of the right hip in a 12-year-old girl. **A.** Two months after the onset of infection. Note the marked destruction of the femoral head and the incongruity of the joint surfaces. **B.** After a surgical fusion (arthrodesis) of the right hip, which was necessitated by persistent and progressive pain.

Prognosis

The four important factors that determine the effectiveness of treatment for acute septic arthritis are the same four factors outlined for acute hematogenous osteomyelitis in a previous section of this chapter.

You will appreciate, however, that inadequately treated septic arthritis of a major joint, especially the hip, leads to an even more significant and more permanent disability for the patient than does inadequately treated osteomyelitis.

Complications of Acute Septic Arthritis

The *early complications* of acute septic arthritis include 1) *death* from the associated septicemia, 2) *destruction of joint cartilage*, 3) *pathological dislocation* of the joint (especially in infants), and (4) *avascular necrosis of the epiphysis*, particularly in the hip.

The *late complications* are the sequelae of a destroyed joint and include 1) *degenerative joint disease*, 2) *permanent dislocation* with a false joint, 3) *fibrous ankylosis*, and 4) *bony ankylosis*.

Hematogenous Osteomyelitis of the Spine

Acute hematogenous osteomyelitis of the spine differs sufficiently from osteomyelitis of the long bones that it merits separate consideration.

The vertebrae may become involved by acute osteomyelitis at any age, but young children are afflicted more often than are older children or adults. In young children, the condition is sometimes referred to by the somewhat misleading term *benign osteitis of the spine* because the systemic manifestations of the disease are relatively mild and there is little suppuration. Another, more descriptive term is *spondylarthritis*, which signifies that in addition to the bone of the vertebral bodies, the adjacent intervertebral disc is invariably involved and partially destroyed.

The most common sites are the vertebrae of the lower thoracic and upper lumbar spine, which raises the suspicion that the route of infection may be via Batson's plexus of paravertebral veins. *Staphylococcus aureus* and *Escherichia coli* are the most frequent causative organisms.

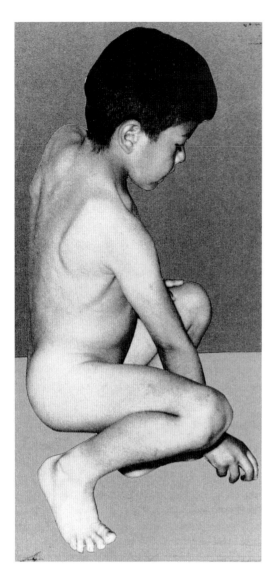

Figure 10.21. A boy with hematogenous osteomyelitis of the spine. On attempting to pick something up from the floor he keeps his spine perfectly straight because of pain and muscle spasm in the lumbar region, the site of osteomyelitis.

Clinical Features and Diagnosis

In childhood, the first symptom is poorly localized back pain accompanied by the physical signs of protective muscle spasm in the back and local deep tenderness. There may even be signs of meningeal irritation (painful limitation of neck flexion and straight-leg raising). The child is frequently reluctant to sit up or stand and is always reluctant to bend forward (Fig. 10.21).

Systemic manifestations include irritability and loss of appetite, but fever is usually mild. The white blood cell count is frequently normal, but the sedimentation rate is always elevated.

Radiographic examination of the spine within the first 2 weeks of illness fails to reveal any bony abnormality, but during this period a bone scan may be helpful (as discussed in Chapter 5). Subsequently, narrowing of the adjacent intervertebral disc space and osteolysis of the involved vertebrae become obvious (Fig. 10.22).

The most important differential diagnosis is spinal tuberculosis, which can be excluded if the tuberculin skin test result is negative. Vertebral punch biopsy (under anesthesia and with radiographic control) may be necessary

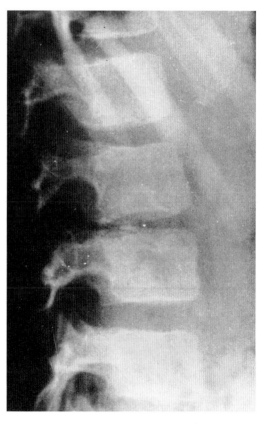

Figure 10.22. Hematogenous osteomyelitis of the lumbar spine in a 7-year-old child. Note the marked narrowing of the involved intervertebral disc space and the osteolytic lesions in the adjacent vertebral bodies.

Treatment and Prognosis

The general plan of treatment for acute hematogenous osteomyelitis of the spine is similar to that described for osteomyelitis of the long bones in a previous section of this chapter.

Bed rest for the patient is supplemented by local rest for the spine, which is provided by a body cast. Operative drainage of the vertebra and disc space is indicated only if nonoperative treatment fails to control the infection; it is seldom necessary.

In children, the involved disc space remains permanently narrow but seldom fuses spontaneously, whereas in adults, spontaneous fusion is more frequent. Occasionally, persistent or recurrent back pain arising from the abnormal segment necessitates local spinal fusion.

Osteomyelitis and Septic Arthritis Secondary to Wounds

Bone and joint infection secondary to wounds, whether accidental or surgical, is caused by pathogenic bacteria that have gained access to the skeletal tissues directly from the outside environment. This *exogenous* type of infection, in contradistinction to the hematogenous or endogenous type, can develop in any site and at any age. Patients affected by HIV and AIDS are particularly susceptible to exogenous bone and joint infections.

Pathogenic bacteria may reach a bone or joint through a variety of wounds, such as a penetrating wound produced by a high-velocity missile or even a small puncture wound produced by a sharp object (Fig. 10.24). Furthermore, all open (compound) fractures and joint injuries are obviously contaminated by exogenous bacteria and consequently carry the risk of serious infection. Likewise, closed (simple) fractures and joint injuries that are treated by operation (*open reduction and internal fixation*) may become infected. Indeed, any operation carries this risk, but it is particularly significant in the musculoskeletal system because the sequelae of bone and joint infection are so serious.

Synovial joints are particularly susceptible to infection and therefore even simple needle aspiration of a joint demands rigid aseptic pre-

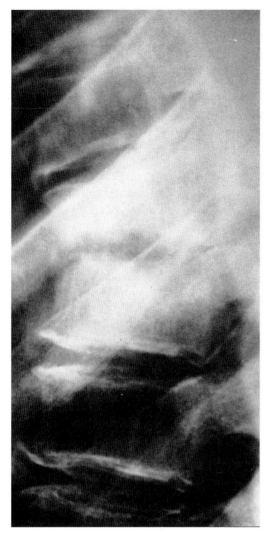

Figure 10.23. Osteomyelitis of the thoracic spine in a 41-year-old adult. Note the marked destruction of the intervertebral disc space and the destruction of the adjacent portions of the involved vertebral bodies.

to confirm the diagnosis of osteomyelitis, but it is safe in the lumbar region only.

In adults afflicted with osteomyelitis of the spine, severe back pain is a prominent feature. The physical signs are similar to those seen in children, but the systemic reaction to the infection is usually more marked. As with children, the radiographic findings of osteolysis of the vertebral body and narrowing of the intervertebral disc space become obvious only after the first 2 weeks of illness (Fig. 10.23).

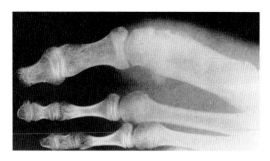

Figure 10.24. Osteomyelitis in the neck of the first metatarsal secondary to a puncture wound in the sole of the foot. This child's puncture wound had occurred 6 months previously and she had experienced recurring pain and swelling in the foot since that time. Note the areas of the osteolysis and sclerosis in the neck of the metatarsal. The most common infecting bacteria in puncture wounds of the foot is *Pseudomonas*.

cautions. In children with bacteremia, the practice of obtaining a blood sample by femoral artery or vein puncture directly over the hip joint is potentially dangerous because the needle may traverse the vessel, penetrate the joint, and thereby inoculate it with bacteria.

The pathological and clinical features of established exogenous infections of bones and joints are comparable to those of the hematogenous, or endogenous, variety and hence need not be repeated here. The preventive aspects of exogenous infection, however, merit emphasis. Since any wound, large or small, that communicates with skeletal tissues is potentially serious, the most important therapeutic aspect of such wounds is careful wound cleansing and, when necessary, débridement of devitalized tissues and delayed closure of the wound in an attempt to prevent bone and joint infection (Fig. 10.24).

Should infection develop despite preventive measures, you will be alert to the first manifestations and will be able to institute appropriate therapy at the earliest possible moment. This exogenous type of infection, once established, does not respond to antibacterial therapy alone and requires exploration of the wound, removal of necrotic tissue, adequate drainage of pus, local instillation of antibiotic drugs, and delayed wound closure.

Chronic Recurrent Multifocal Osteomyelitis

Although it resembles bacterial osteomyelitis in some ways, chronic recurrent multifocal osteomyelitis is distinctly different from either acute hematogenous osteomyelitis or subacute osteomyelitis. It is characterized by a series of recurrences and remissions of multifocal areas of bone pain in different sites at different times. The underlying bone lesions are somewhat similar radiographically to those of bacterial osteomyelitis. The striking difference, however, is that in chronic recurrent multifocal osteomyelitis (CRMO) no bacteria can be isolated from the lesions. Consequently, antibiotics are not indicated, but nonsteroidal anti-inflammatory drugs (NSAIDs) are helpful in relieving the pain of inflammation. It is probable that CRMO overlaps the seronegative spondyloarthropathies such as psoriatic arthritis. Fortunately, it is a self-limited disorder, although it may extend over a period of a few months to a few years before subsiding permanently with no significant sequelae.

Pyogenic Infections in the Hand

The soft tissues of the hand are frequently infected by pyogenic bacteria because of the high incidence of minor hand injuries such as lacerations and puncture wounds. Such infections are not only common but also potentially serious because they may spread to the bones, joints, or tendon sheaths.

Soft tissue infections in the hand include the following three groups: 1) those involving the nail fold (paronychia) (Fig. 10.25A); 2) those involving potential spaces in the hand—the pulp space (felon) (Fig. 10.25B), the thenar space (Fig. 10.26A), and the midpalmar space (Fig. 10.26B); and 3) those involving a tendon sheath (pyogenic tenosynovitis). Of these, pyogenic tenosynovitis is the most serious and deserves special mention.

Pyogenic Tenosynovitis
Etiology
Laceration and puncture wounds provide the portal of entry to the tendon sheath for patho-

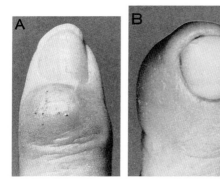

Figure 10.25.   A. Paronychia. **B.** Pulp space infection (Felon).

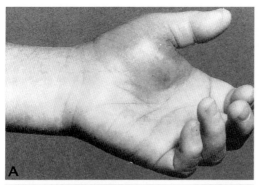

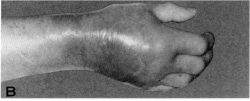

Figure 10.26.   A. Thenar space infection. **B.** Mid-palmar space infection. The swelling rapidly extends to the dorsum of the hand where the areolar planes are loosely arranged.

genic bacteria, the most common of which is *Staphylococcus aureus.*

Pathogenesis and Pathology

The synovial lining of a tendon sheath is comparable to the synovial lining of a joint and responds in the same manner to pyogenic infection, namely, by edema, hypertrophy, and production of a synovial effusion. The inflamed synovial sheath becomes progressively distended by pus under pressure, which ex-

plains the semiflexed position of the digit, a position in which the synovial sheath can accept the greatest volume of fluid. The blood supply to the tendon may be compromised, with resultant tendon necrosis. In the later stages of untreated tenosynovitis, fibrous adhesions between the tendon and its enveloping sheath lead to permanent loss of motion in the involved digit.

Clinical Features and Diagnosis

The symptom of severe local pain and the signs of local swelling, tenderness, and severe pain with any passive movement of the digit are readily understood on the basis of the underlying pathological process (Fig. 10.27). Elevation of temperature, white blood cell count, and sedimentation rate indicate the systemic reaction to infection.

Treatment

Pyogenic tenosynovitis requires the same plan of systemic and local treatment as that described for acute hematogenous osteomyelitis in a previous section of this chapter. Early operative treatment (through an incision along one side of the digit) is as important for tenosynovitis as for septic (pyogenic) arthritis; pus is evacuated and, in addition, continuous drainage and instillation of antibacterial drugs

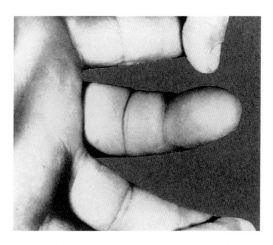

Figure 10.27. Pyogenic tenosynovitis of the ring finger. Note that the involved finger is swollen and tends to assume a flexed position because of the tension in the inflamed synovial sheath.

are instituted in an attempt to preserve the tendon as well as the motion between it and its sheath.

Necrotizing Fasciitis

Necrotizing fasciitis, a potentially lethal soft tissue infection, is caused by a particularly virulent strain of group A β-hemolytic streptococcus. Initially involving the deep fascia and subcutaneous fat, the infection spreads at an alarming rate, causing extensive necrosis and even gangrene with associated toxic shock and end organ failure. Understandably, the lay term for necrotizing fasciitis is *flesh-eating disease*. Vigorous antibiotic therapy combined with radical surgical débridement and, when necessary, amputation of an involved limb, along with treatment of shock, are required as lifesaving measures. Even with such aggressive treatment, however, the mortality rate is greater than 30%.

Meningococcal Septicemia

A meningococcal infection may progress inexorably to an overwhelming and potentially fatal meningococcal septicemia despite antibiotic therapy. A serious complication is a rapidly developing peripheral vascular occlusion that initially leads to distal areas of soft tissue necrosis and sometimes even to extensive gangrene of one or more limbs that require lifesaving amputation.

VIRAL INFECTIONS
Human Immunodeficiency Virus and Acquired Immunodeficiency Syndrome

During the last two decades of the twentieth century, the incidence of HIV infection and the resultant fatal disorder of AIDS have reached epidemic proportions. Since the normal human immune system helps to ward off conditions such as infections and neoplasms and because AIDS ravages an individual's immune system, it is understandable that these severely immunocompromised patients are at high risk for the development of a wide variety of infections, including the exogenous type of bacterial osteomyelitis and septic arthritis as well as tuberculous osteomyelitis, tuberculous

arthritis, and various rheumatic diseases. These are the disorders of the musculoskeletal system that you are most likely to see in patients who are HIV-positive and especially those who have full-blown AIDS. You will learn much about HIV and AIDS in other parts of your curriculum, including their relevance to other body systems and the "universal precautions" that must be taken by health care workers who are exposed to the hazards of penetrating injuries from needles and sharp surgical instruments while attending such patients.

GRANULOMATOUS BACTERIAL INFECTIONS

The terms *granulomatous* or *granuloma-producing* infections refer to a group of chronic inflammatory conditions, some of which are caused by *bacteria*, such as tuberculosis and syphilis, and others by *fungi*, such as actinomycosis.

The inflammatory reaction incited by these granulomatous infections is chronic from the onset because the *productive* element of inflammation exceeds the *exudative* element. Characteristic of this type of chronic inflammation is the reaction of the local tissue cells (histiocytes, including epithelioid cells), which collect to produce small discrete lesions about the size of a *granule* (1 to 2 mm); hence the terms *granulomatous* or *granuloma-producing* infections. As the inflammatory reaction progresses, more granules are produced, and these subsequently coalesce to form progressively larger lesions. Of the granulomatous infections involving the musculoskeletal system, the most important is *tuberculosis*.

Tuberculous Infections: General Features

Improved public health measures concerning prevention and early detection of tuberculosis and the development of effective antituberculous drugs have both been important factors in the striking reduction of *mortality* and *morbidity* of tuberculous infection. However, the *incidence* of this potentially serious infection has actually increased significantly in recent years, even in well-developed countries; indeed, in some of the developing countries of the world, tuberculosis continues to be a common and serious epidemic, with more than 10 million active cases at any time and 3 million deaths per year. Individuals who are infected by HIV or who have AIDS are definitely at risk for the development of potentially fatal tuberculosis.

Establishment of Infection

In the past, the bovine type of tubercle bacillus, present in the milk of tuberculous cows and ingested by children, was the main cause of tuberculosis involving bowel, lymph nodes, bones, and joints. Fortunately, in most areas, this has been well controlled by enforced inspection and tuberculin testing of dairy herds, as well as pasteurization of milk.

At present, the human type of tubercle bacillus is responsible for virtually all tuberculous infection in humans; the initial, or primary, lesion is in the lung. The mode of infection is inhalation of air and dust particles that contain bacilli released when a tuberculous patient with infected sputum coughs. The initial infection usually occurs during childhood in areas where tuberculosis is common; in areas of low incidence, the initial infection may occur in adult life.

Within the lung, the tubercle bacilli incite a granulomatous type of inflammatory reaction. A *miliary tubercle* is formed by histiocytes, which, being phagocytic macrophages, engulf the bacilli. Nevertheless, tubercle bacilli are able to survive and multiply even in this intracellular environment. Groups of macrophages may fuse to form *giant cells,* which are a characteristic part of the histological picture. Since the tubercle is relatively avascular, its central portion eventually becomes caseous (cheeselike) because of *coagulation necrosis.* Later, the caseous material *liquifies,* but all the while the tubercle bacilli continue to multiply.

The child's defense reactions may be sufficiently strong to heal the tubercle by fibrosis with subsequent calcification; indeed, radiographs of the lungs reveal evidence of such healed primary lesions in many apparently healthy individuals (Fig. 10.28). Nevertheless, even in healed tubercles, living tubercle bacilli tend to persist in a dormant state and are capable of *reactivation,* particularly if the defense

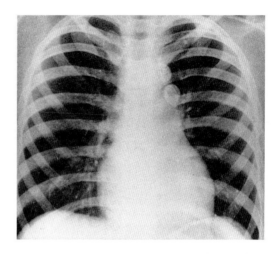

Figure 10.28. Healed primary lesions of tuberculosis in a young adult. Note the two calcified lesions in the left side of the chest along the left side of the arch of the aorta.

reaction, or resistance, of the patient is weakened by factors such as poor nutrition and chronic fatigue.

Principles of Antituberculous Therapy

For many years before the development of antituberculous chemotherapy, the traditional treatment of musculoskeletal tuberculosis centered on prolonged immobilization of the involved joint or joints and often total recumbency in a sanitorium. Fortunately, these unphysiological and demoralizing forms of nonspecific treatment have been replaced by aggressive chemotherapy, but such therapy must be continued for at least 1 year. Streptomycin was the first chemotherapeutic agent found to be effective against tuberculosis. Because of the emergence of resistant organisms, however, streptomycin was usually administered in combination with isonicotinic acid hydrazide (INH) and *para*-aminosalicylic acid (PAS). Currently, rifampicin is the most effective antituberculous agent and is usually used instead of PAS; indeed, it has almost replaced streptomycin also. Thus, rifampicin and pyrazinamide are given in combination with INH, with or without streptomycin. These antituberculous drugs are reasonably effective against early lesions, but once the tubercle bacilli are enclosed within an avascular caseous lesion, they are protected from the action of blood-borne drugs. Furthermore, an increasing percentage of tubercle bacilli have become drug-resistant. This fact emphasizes the importance of early diagnosis and the institution of antituberculous drug therapy in the earliest stages of the tuberculous infection. Because of the chronic nature of the infection, the combined antituberculous chemotherapy is continued for at least 1 full year.

The avascularity of well-established tuberculous lesions explains the necessity for bold surgical excision of diseased tissues and evacuation of the pus of "cold abscesses."

Tuberculous Osteomyelitis

Tuberculous osteomyelitis, or bone tuberculosis, is always secondary to a tuberculous lesion elsewhere in the body. Like hematogenous pyogenic osteomyelitis, it is a blood-borne infection and usually afflicts children; by contrast, however, tuberculous osteomyelitis, rather than developing in the metaphyseal region of long bones, develops most frequently in vertebral bodies (*tuberculous spondylitis*).

Hematogenous tuberculous osteomyelitis may also develop in the *epiphyses* of long bones and spread into the joint to produce a tuberculous arthritis; sometimes the reverse is true in that the infection in a tuberculous joint spreads into the epiphysis. (Tuberculous arthritis is discussed in a subsequent section of this chapter). Occasionally, particularly in young children, hematogenous tuberculous osteomyelitis involves the shaft, or diaphysis, of a phalanx (tuberculous dactylitis).

Tuberculosis of the spine merits special attention.

Tuberculous Osteomyelitis of the Spine (Tuberculous Spondylitis; Pott's Disease)

Tuberculosis of the spine, which accounts for more than half of all bone and joint tuberculosis, usually begins during early childhood. The most common sites are the lower thoracic and upper lumbar vertebrae; in these sites, it is probably secondary to urinary tract tuberculosis, the hematogenous route being Batson's plexus of paravertebral veins.

Pathogenesis and Pathology

The tuberculous infection, a specific type of granulomatous inflammation, is characterized by slowly progressive bone destruction (*local osteolysis*) in the anterior part of a vertebral body and is accompanied by regional osteoporosis. Spreading caseation prevents reactive new bone formation and at the same time renders segments of bone avascular, thereby producing *tuberculous sequestra,* particularly in the thoracic region.

Gradually, *tuberculous granulation tissue* penetrates the thin cortex of the vertebral body to produce a *paravertebral abscess* that spans several vertebrae. In addition, the infection spreads up and down the spine under the anterior and posterior longitudinal ligaments. The intervertebral discs, being avascular, are relatively resistant to tuberculous infection; initially, the adjacent disc becomes narrowed from dehydration, but eventually it may be partially destroyed by tuberculous granulation tissue. Progressive destruction of bone anteriorly and resultant anterior collapse of the involved vertebral bodies lead to progressive *kyphosis* (posterior angulation) of the spine (Fig. 10.29).

Clinical Features and Diagnosis

The patient, usually a child, experiences back pain and is reluctant to sit up, stand up, or bend forward, precisely like a child with hematogenous osteomyelitis of the spine (Fig. 10.21). Local deep tenderness is readily elicited, and protective muscle spasm is apparent. Systemic manifestations include chronic ill health and, usually, evidence of either pulmonary or urinary tract tuberculosis. The sedimentation rate is elevated and the tuberculin skin test result is positive.

Radiographic examination of the spine in the early stages reveals an osteolytic lesion in the anterior part of a vertebral body, regional osteoporosis, and narrowing of the adjacent intervertebral disc (Fig. 10.30). At a more advanced stage, there is evidence of extensive anterior destruction, involvement of other vertebrae, and a paravertebral abscess (Fig. 10.31).

The diagnosis can be confirmed by aspiration of paravertebral "pus," which is studied microscopically for tubercle bacilli and also in-

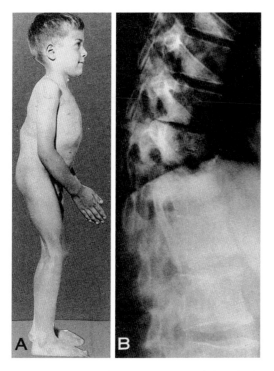

Figure 10.29. Tuberculous osteomyelitis of the spine. **A.** Posterior angulation (kyphosis) caused by collapse of the anterior portion of the vertebral bodies in the lumbar region of this boy. This type of deformity is sometimes referred to as a "gibbus." **B.** Tuberculous osteomyelitis of the spine in the lumbar region. Note the anterior destruction of adjacent vertebral bodies and the resultant anterior collapse with production of a kyphotic deformity. In this lateral radiograph there is also evidence of involvement of the two vertebral bodies above the major area of disease.

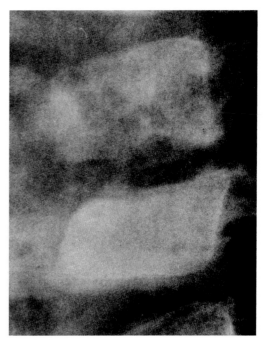

Figure 10.30. Early tuberculous osteomyelitis of the spine in a child. In the lateral radiograph there is narrowing of the intervertebral disc space and osteolytic lesions in the anterior portions of the adjacent vertebral bodies.

oculated into a guinea pig. The sensitivity of the causative tubercle bacillus to various antituberculous drugs should be determined. Tissue obtained either by closed punch biopsy or open surgical biopsy reveals the typical histological picture of tuberculous infection, including histiocytes and giant cells.

Treatment

The care of a patient with tuberculosis of the spine includes the treatment of generalized tuberculosis—antituberculous drugs, general rest, nourishing diet—as well as the treatment of the local disease in the spine by local rest on a turning frame or in a plaster bed. After 1 month of drug therapy and local rest, the

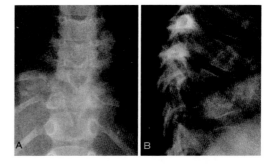

Figure 10.31. Extensive tuberculous osteomyelitis of the lower thoracic spine with a paravertebral abscess in a child. **A.** The bulbous soft tissue swelling on each side of the spine represents a paravertebral abscess. Note also the marked destruction of vertebral bodies. **B.** In the lateral radiograph there is evidence of destruction of two vertebral bodies, with resultant anterior collapse of the spine and a kyphotic deformity.

spinal lesion is most effectively treated by bold, direct open operation to evacuate the tuberculous "pus," to remove tuberculous sequestra as well as diseased bone, and to fuse the involved segments of the spine, preferably by anterior interbody fusion using autogenous bone grafts.

In countries where adequate surgical facilities are lacking, an acceptable alternative is prolonged antituberculous chemotherapy combined with a spinal brace or cast.

Complications of Tuberculous Spondylitis

The most serious complication of spinal tuberculosis is *paraplegia* (Pott's paraplegia), which may occur either early or late in the course of the disease. The *paraplegia of active disease* develops relatively early; it can result either from extradural pressure (tuberculous "pus," sequestra, sequestrated intervertebral disc) or from direct involvement of the spinal cord by tuberculous granulation tissue. Under the latter circumstances, the prognosis for recovery is poor. The *paraplegia of healed disease* always develops late; it can result either from the gradual development of a bony ridge that impinges on the spinal canal or from progressive fibrosis of tuberculous granulation tissue. Myelography and MRI are helpful in differentiating between the pressure type of paraplegia (which can be alleviated surgically) and paraplegia resulting from invasion of the dura and spinal cord.

The development of paraplegia caused by pressure during the course of spinal tuberculosis represents a relative emergency that should be treated by surgical decompression of the spinal cord and nerve roots.

A less common complication is rupture of a thoracic paravertebral abscess into the pleura to produce a *tuberculous empyema*. In the lumbar region, tuberculous "pus" may enter the iliopsoas muscle and spreads distally as a *psoas abscess*, which is an example of a "cold abscess."

Tuberculous Arthritis

Tubercle bacilli may infect a synovial joint by hematogenous spread from a distant tuberculous lesion. More commonly, however, tuberculous arthritis is caused by direct extension of infection into the joint from an area of tuberculous osteomyelitis in the epiphysis; although the underlying epiphyseal lesion may be too small to detect radiographically, it can usually be seen at operation.

Any synovial joint may be affected, but the two most common sites are the hip and the knee. As with tuberculosis in other tissues, the onset is nearly always in childhood.

Pathogenesis and Pathology

The synovial membrane responds to tuberculous infection by villous hypertrophy and an effusion, with resultant distension of the joint capsule. Small grayish *tubercles* may be seen on the inflamed synovial surface. Later, tuberculous granulation tissue creeps across the joint surfaces as a *tuberculous pannus*, which deprives the articular cartilage of its nutrition from the synovial fluid and thereby causes *cartilage necrosis*. In addition, tuberculous granulation tissue erodes subchondral bone to produce a local area of tuberculous osteomyelitis with subsequent collapse of bone. It also burrows under the articular cartilage, causing the cartilage to sequestrate. The combination of cartilage necrosis and destruction of the underlying bone leads to irreparable joint damage.

Clinical Features and Diagnosis

The patient, usually a child, presents with a chronically irritable joint; when the involved joint is in the lower limb, there is an obvious limp. Painful limitation of joint motion, protective muscle spasm, and muscle atrophy are apparent. The sedimentation rate is elevated and the tuberculin skin test result is positive.

Radiographic examination in the early stages reveals regional osteoporosis as well as evidence of soft tissue swelling around the joint. In the later stages, osteolytic lesions in the epiphysis become apparent (Fig. 10.32). Eventually, loss of the radiographic cartilage space indicates that the articular cartilage has been destroyed (Fig. 10.33).

The diagnosis can be proved by open surgical biopsy of the synovial membrane. The joint fluid obtained at the time of operation is studied microscopically and inoculated into a

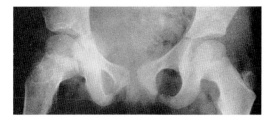

Figure 10.32. Tuberculous arthritis of the right hip in a child. Note the regional osteoporosis as well as small osteolytic lesions in the femoral epiphysis.

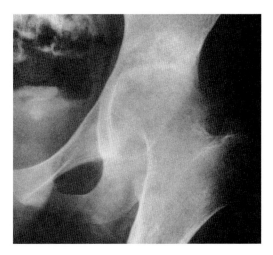

Figure 10.33. Advanced tuberculous arthritis of the left hip in a young adult. There has been considerable destruction of the femoral head. The cartilage space has almost disappeared, indicating destruction of articular cartilage.

guinea pig to isolate the causative tubercle bacillus and subsequently test its sensitivity to the various antituberculous drugs.

Treatment

The care of a patient with tuberculous arthritis involves the treatment of generalized tuberculosis—antituberculous drugs (as mentioned in the section entitled "Principles of Antituberculous Therapy"), general rest, nourishing diet—as well as the treatment of the local arthritis. During the early stages of tuberculous arthritis while the infection is predominantly synovial, adequate treatment, including synovectomy, can prevent damage to joint carti-

lage and underlying bone and can thereby preserve joint function, particularly in children.

Once the articular cartilage is destroyed, however, the joint is irreparably damaged and, consequently, surgical fusion (*arthrodesis*) of the joint is required not only to relieve the pain in the arthritic joint but also to bring about permanent healing of the tuberculous infection.

NONSPECIFIC INFLAMMATORY DISORDERS OF JOINTS

A wide variety of clinical conditions, all of which cause *pain and stiffness in the musculoskeletal system,* are commonly grouped under the broad heading of "*rheumatic disease.*" In the majority of these diseases, the predominant lesion is articular (*arthritis, articular rheumatism*), whereas in others it is extra-articular (*nonarticular rheumatism*). Although the venerable term *rheumatism* has no pathological significance, its use is so prevalent that, for want of a better term, it has persisted (rheumatism is derived from the Greek word *rheumatismos,* a "flowing of an evil body humor," that was thought to go from the brain to the joints and other parts of the body, producing pain). Thus, the clinical study of rheumatic diseases constitutes the medical specialty of *rheumatology* and specialists in internal medicine who devote themselves to the medical care of arthritis and allied conditions are known as *rheumatologists.*

Of course, many others, including family physicians, orthopaedic surgeons, rehabilitation physicians (physiatrists), physiotherapists, occupational therapists and social workers, also share an interest and a responsibility in the overall management of this group of patients.

Classification of Rheumatic Diseases

The large number and variety of clinical diseases that are capable of causing "pain and stiffness in the musculoskeletal system" make their classification difficult and somewhat unsatisfactory. An exhaustive—and exhausting—classification compiled by a committee of the American College of Rheumatology comprises 10 major headings and more than

190 subheadings and individual disorders. The major headings are presented here for the sake of standardized nomenclature.

1. Diffuse connective tissue disease
2. Arthritis associated with spondylitis
3. Osteoarthritis (degenerative joint disease)
4. Rheumatic syndromes associated with infectious agents
5. Metabolic and endocrine disorders associated with rheumatic states
6. Neoplasms
7. Neurovascular disorders
8. Bone and cartilage disorders
9. Extra-articular disorders
10. Miscellaneous disorders associated with articular manifestations

The diseases in which arthritis is the predominant feature can be grouped in the following simple working classification:

1. Inflammatory polyarthritis of unknown cause, including rheumatoid arthritis, ankylosing spondylitis, rheumatic fever
2. Degenerative joint disease, also called osteoarthritis and osteoarthrosis
3. Infectious arthritis, including septic (pyogenic) arthritis, tuberculous arthritis
4. Traumatic arthritis, secondary to fractures and joint injuries
5. Metabolic arthritis, including gout

From the onset you should appreciate that degenerative joint disease represents a slowly progressive deterioration of a given joint and can be secondary to *any* local disturbance of joint structure and function. Therefore, in a given joint, residual abnormalities from *any other* type of arthritis can initiate the process of degenerative joint disease, which is then superimposed on the original condition.

Prevalence of the Rheumatic Diseases

The rheumatic diseases lead all causes of crippling and economic loss in the general population and therefore represent a major health problem. For example, it has been estimated that more than 6% of all persons in North America suffer at some time from some form of arthritis or rheumatism. Since the overall incidence of rheumatic diseases increases with age, increasing longevity will render this particular health problem even more prevalent in the future than it has been in the past.

Adult Rheumatoid Arthritis

Rheumatoid arthritis, which is one type of inflammatory polyarthritis, is characterized by a variable but usually prolonged clinical course with exacerbations and remissions of joint pains and swelling that frequently lead to progressive deformities and may even lead to permanent disability. Indeed, after 5 years, fewer than one third of the patients can continue to work. The arthritis is the dominant clinical manifestation of a more generalized systemic disease of connective tissue (*rheumatoid disease*).

Buchanan has stated that although there is good historical evidence that *degenerative* joint disease (osteoarthritis) has afflicted humans for at least 40,000 years, and probably much longer, *rheumatoid* arthritis would seem to have appeared as a relatively new disease in humans only 200 years ago.

Incidence

Rheumatoid arthritis is relatively common; indeed, surveys have revealed that approximately 1.5% of the adult population in countries of temperate climate suffer from this disease. Women are afflicted three times more frequently than men, and although the disease may begin at almost any age, the peak period of onset is between the ages of 20 and 40 years. The peripheral joints, especially those of the hands, are the most frequent sites of initial involvement by rheumatoid arthritis, and the distribution in paired limbs tends to be symmetrical (Fig. 10.34).

Etiology

Despite intensive clinical and experimental research, the cause of rheumatoid arthritis has eluded discovery and remains a challenging mystery. However, the observation that this is a relatively new disease has sparked the speculation that the causative agent may be an oc-

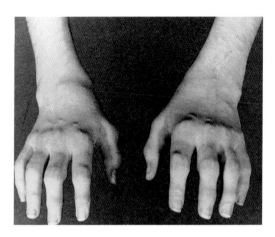

Figure 10.34.   Rheumatoid arthritis of the hands of a 30-year-old woman who has had symptoms for one year. Note the symmetrical involvement in the wrists, metacarpophalangeal joints and proximal interphalangeal joints.

cult mycobacterium or a relatively new microorganism, such as the ubiquitous Epstein-Barr retrovirus or some other virus. Former theories of foci of bacterial infection, vitamin deficiency, and hormonal imbalance have been discarded because of lack of scientific proof.

Some of the features of rheumatoid arthritis and the frequent coexistent lesions of rheumatoid disease suggest an exaggeration of normal immune mechanisms, or hypersensitivity—a continuous immunological response of an immunogenetically susceptible host. Affected individuals exhibit disease susceptibility markers on the major histocompatibility complex (MHC) on chromosome 6 to a persistent antigen. In 70% of patients, a *rheumatoid factor,* which is a macroglobulin, can be demonstrated by serological means, such as latex and sheep cell agglutinin tests. These tests produce negative results in the early phases of the disease and in most afflicted children but the results tend to become positive as the disease progresses. However, the presence of a rheumatoid factor not only is inconsistent in rheumatoid arthritis but also may occur in a variety of unrelated connective tissue diseases. This macroglobulin has been isolated from plasma cells of diseased synovial membrane as well as from regional lymph nodes, suggesting the possibility of an antigenic stimulus arising from an altered gamma globulin in the diseased joint, a type of autoimmune mechanism. Nevertheless, these immune responses could be a secondary phenomenon—the result rather than the cause of rheumatoid arthritis. Many of the patients who test positive for the rheumatoid factor possess the human leukocyte antigen (HLA-DR4 haplotype).

In the past, it was thought that psychological factors may predispose an individual to this disease. The anxiety-ridden and depressed person who tends to suppress feelings of hostility and aggression seemed more prone to acquire rheumatoid arthritis than the average, whereas the psychotic individual seemed less prone. However, the current consensus is that these psychological or personality traits are an understandable reaction to the disease, that is, an effect or result rather than a factor in its cause. Nevertheless, in a given patient, emotional stress is often followed by an exacerbation of rheumatoid activity.

Obviously much ongoing research is required before the significance and interrelationship of the various causative factors will be understood.

Pathogenesis and Pathology
The primary "target" of the disease is the synovial membrane of joints and tendon sheaths. This membrane, normally a thin syncitium of cells, reacts to the inflammation by congestion, edema, fibrin exudation, proliferation, and villous formation. Polymorphonuclear leukocytes, although present in large numbers in the synovial fluid, are not found in the membrane; the characteristic inflammatory cells in the synovial membrane in rheumatoid arthritis are monocytes (T and B lymphocytes, plasma cells, and macrophages), some of which are grouped in nodular formations with germinal centers.

It is now thought that the T lymphocytes are responsible for cell-mediated immunoregulatory functions, whereas the B lymphocytes become antibody-producing plasma cells. The resultant immune process within the diseased synovium produces immune complexes that, in turn, activate a multitude of chemical mediators of inflammation. In the acute inflammatory exudate in the synovial fluid, polymorphonuclear leukocytes engulf immune complexes, but in so doing, they extrude hydrolytic enzymes (neutral proteases such as cathepsin G, elastase, and collagenase) that are capable of degrading the proteoglycans and collagen of cartilage matrix and thereby inducing an autoimmune response that can lead to destruction of the joint.

Inflammatory granulation tissue infiltrates the subsynovial connective tissue, causing it to become swollen and boggy. Even the fibrous capsule and joint ligaments may be involved and, if they become sufficiently softened and stretched, the joint may become subluxated or even dislocated. As occurs in other types of inflammation, granulation tissue is eventually replaced by reparative fibrosis or scar formation, with resultant *joint contracture* and *deformity*.

The inflammatory granulation tissue also creeps across the joint surface to form a *pannus* (from the Latin word meaning "a rug"), which interferes with the normal nutrition of articular cartilage from synovial fluid and causes *cartilage necrosis* (Fig. 10.35). Furthermore, the same tissue erodes subchondral bone at the margins of the joint and burrows beneath the cartilage to produce local areas of *osteolysis* (erosions) in the bone. The remaining bone in the area of the joint exhibits *regional osteoporosis*. If the process continues over a period of months or years, fibrous adhesions eventually form between opposing joint

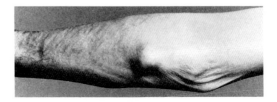

Figure 10.36. Subcutaneous rheumatoid nodule on the extensor aspect of the forearm just below the elbow joint. This is the most common site for such nodules.

surfaces with a resultant *fibrous ankylosis*. Indeed, the fibrous ankylosis may eventually ossify to become a *bony ankylosis*.

The synovial membrane, covering tendons and lining their sheaths, reacts in a similar manner with a corresponding disturbance of function. Even the connective tissue elements of the muscles that control the joint become involved by the inflammatory process. Thus, in addition to disuse atrophy of muscle, foci of monocellular infiltrations appear and are subsequently replaced by reparative fibrosis, with resultant *contracture* of the muscle, another factor in the pathogenesis of deformity.

Approximately 30% of patients exhibit subcutaneous *rheumatoid nodules* over areas subjected to pressure, particularly in the upper limbs (Fig. 10.36). These extra-articular lesions, which seem to begin as an area of rheumatoid vasculitis with subsequent necrosis, are composed of a central zone of fibrinoid material and cellular debris surrounded by a middle zone of mononuclear cells and an outer zone of granulation tissue.

Other extra-articular lesions of rheumatoid disease may occur in the connective tissue components of the cardiovascular system (pericardial adhesions, myocarditis, vasculitis), the reticuloendothelial system, and even the respiratory system (pulmonary fibrosis).

Clinical Features and Diagnosis

The clinical manifestations of rheumatoid arthritis are so variable in their mode of onset, distribution, degree of severity, and rate of progression that they almost defy brief description.

The onset is usually insidious but can be

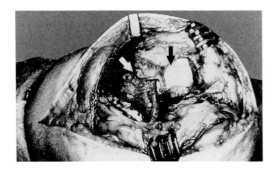

Figure 10.35. Anterior aspect of the left knee at the time of synovectomy. The black arrow points to part of the articular surface of the lateral condyle of the femur. The white arrow points to the inflammatory granulation tissue that is creeping across the articular cartilage. This pannus had already resulted in some destruction of the underlying cartilage.

episodic or even acute. The disease usually begins in several joints (*rheumatoid polyarthritis*) but can begin, and even remain for long periods, in a single joint (*monarticular rheumatoid arthritis*). The most common joints involved, in order of frequency and progression, are those of the hands, wrists, knees, elbows, feet, shoulders, and hips; the distribution of polyarthritis that is associated with periarticular soft tissue swelling tends to be bilaterally symmetrical (Fig. 10.34).

In the early stages of rheumatoid arthritis, the most characteristic distribution of involvement is in certain joints of the hands and feet—the metacarpophalangeal joints of the thumb, index, and middle fingers; the proximal interphalangeal joints of the index, middle, and ring fingers; and the metatarsophalangeal joints of the four small toes. Occasionally, the larger joints are involved before the small peripheral joints.

In the early phases of the disease, systemic manifestations such as malaise, fatigability, and weight loss are common, particularly among young and middle-aged patients. Less common is acute systemic toxicity with high fever, weakness, and anemia.

Initially, the most frequent local symptoms are vague pain and stiffness of involved joints; these symptoms are most noticeable as the patient rises each morning and begins to move inflamed joints that tend to "stiffen up" during sleep (referred to as "morning stiffness"). In the early phases, these symptoms tend to abate after the patient has "limbered up," but later they tend to become progressively more severe and more persistent.

In each involved active joint, four manifestations of inflammation (swelling, heat, pain, and loss of function) become progressively more marked. The joint swelling is caused by a combination of synovial thickening plus synovial effusion and its appearance is exaggerated by the rapidly developing atrophy of neighboring muscles (Fig. 10.37). The joints, which have a characteristic boggy feel, are tender to pressure and painful on movement, both active and passive, especially when the involved joint is passively nudged or "stressed" a little beyond the limits of its range of motion. Protective muscle spasm is

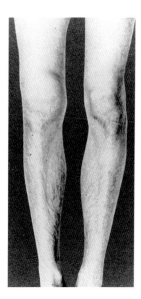

Figure 10.37.   Rheumatoid arthritis of the right knee in a young adult. There is thickening of the synovial membrane as well as a massive synovial effusion in the joint. After aspiration of the effusion, atrophy of the quadriceps muscle was obvious in the suprapatellar region.

apparent in the muscles that control the inflamed joints that soon become stiff if immobilized. Subcutaneous rheumatoid nodules become apparent in 30% of patients and are most common in the upper limbs (Fig. 10.36).

Deformities develop fairly rapidly with rheumatoid arthritis because of a combination of the following factors: 1) mu*scle spasm,* which maintains the joint in the least painful position, usually flexion; 2) *muscle atrophy,* with decreasing strength to move the joint; 3) *muscle contracture* resulting from fibrosis in the inflamed muscles; 4) *subluxation* and *dislocation* caused by a stretched joint capsule and ligaments; 5) late *capsular* and *ligamentous contracture* resulting from fibrosis; and 6) *rupture of tendons,* particularly in the hands, resulting from rheumatoid involvement plus friction against bony spurs. The typical deformities of rheumatoid arthritis are more effectively illustrated than described (Fig. 10.38).

Repeated exacerbations and remissions of the rheumatoid process typify the clinical

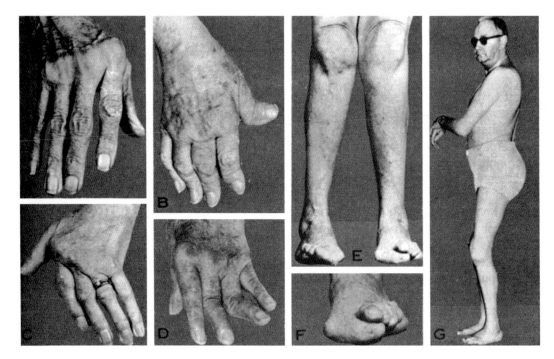

Figure 10.38.   Typical deformities of rheumatoid arthritis. **A.** Mild ulnar deviation of the fingers at the metacarpophalangeal joints. **B.** Subluxation of the interphalangeal joint of the thumb and the distal interphalangeal joint of the index finger. **C.** Marked ulnar deviation of the fingers at the metacarpophalangeal joints. Fusiform swelling of the proximal interphalangeal joints. **D.** Subluxation of the proximal interphalangeal joints of the middle and ring fingers. **E.** Genu valgum (knock knees) and hallux valgus. **F.** Severe hallux valgus and dorsal displacement of the second, third and fourth toes. **G.** Flexion deformities of the knees, hips, elbows, and wrists.

course for the majority of patients, the remissions being most frequent early in the disease. Nevertheless, 20% of patients have a complete remission following the initial episode with neither recurrent nor residual inflammation. In the remainder of patients, the rheumatoid process eventually becomes "burned out," but the functional state of the joints, as well as of the patient, depends on the amount of structural and irreversible joint damage that has occurred during the active phase of the disease.

Radiographic examination early in the disease reveals evidence of periarticular soft tissue swelling and joint effusion. Subsequently, regional osteoporosis, osteolytic erosions in subchondral bone, and narrowing of the cartilage space become apparent (Fig. 10.39). Subluxation and dislocation, which are most common in the hands and feet, are late features, whereas bony ankylosis, which is most

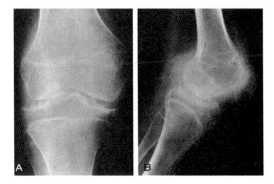

Figure 10.39.   **A** and **B.** Radiographic changes in rheumatoid arthritis of the knee in an adolescent girl. Note the regional osteoporosis, osteolytic areas in the subchondral bone (particularly in the upper end of the tibia), and narrowing of the cartilage space.

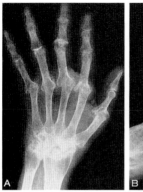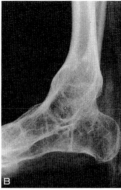

Figure 10.40. Late radiographic changes of rheumatoid arthritis. **A.** Note the dislocations of all five metacarpophalangeal joints. In addition, there is marked narrowing of the proximal interphalangeal joints of the fingers. The wrist joint has been almost completely obliterated. **B.** Spontaneous bony ankylosis of the ankle joint and tarsal joints.

common in the wrists and ankles, is seen only in advanced rheumatoid arthritis (Fig. 10.40).

Laboratory examinations are useful in the diagnosis and differential diagnosis of rheumatoid disease even though there is as yet no specific laboratory test. They are also of value in monitoring the activity of the disease in a given patient over a period of time. Anemia, an elevated white blood cell count and an elevated erythrocyte sedimentation rate (ESR) are characteristic findings, and the elevated erythrocyte sedimentation rate usually correlates with acute-phase reactants such as fibrinogen and C-reactive protein. Rheumatoid factor, which is an autoantibody to gamma globulin, is detectable because of its ability to agglutinate particles of latex coated with the human immunoglobulin IgG. Although rheumatoid factor may not be present in the earliest stages, its titer usually reflects the severity of the disease. Examination of the synovial fluid (synovianalysis) reveals it to be turbid because of excessive numbers of leukocytes (more than 2000/mm) and it is less viscous than normal. In addition, the synovial fluid exhibits a low glucose concentration, and its mucin clots poorly on addition of acetic acid.

Prognosis

It is estimated that in about 30% of patients, the disease is so mild that a physician is not consulted for treatment. However, in most patients, rheumatoid arthritis runs either a subacute or a chronic course over a period of many years with multiple exacerbations and remissions. As might be expected, the prognosis is least favorable in patients in whom the process remains active over several years or longer. Nevertheless, approximately 50% of treated patients recover sufficiently to be able to return to their previous occupations. Indeed, of all treated patients, only 10% are left severely disabled and largely confined to bed or a wheelchair (Fig. 10.41). Understandably, patients with severe and widespread systemic disease, such as cardiovascular and pulmonary involvement, have a somewhat shortened life expectancy.

Treatment

Although there is, as yet, no specific cure for rheumatoid arthritis or the associated rheuma-

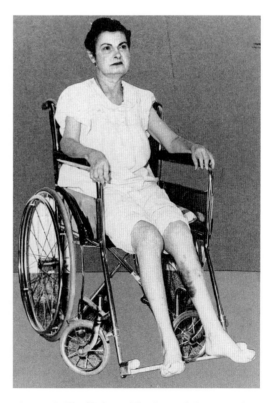

Figure 10.41. Patient with advanced rheumatoid arthritis who is severely handicapped and largely confined to a bed or a wheelchair. Note the multiple deformities of this patient's extremities.

toid disease and although, in a given patient, the rheumatoid process tends to run an almost predetermined course, much can be accomplished for rheumatoid patients therapeutically provided that the treatment, both general and local, is tailored to meet the specific needs of each afflicted individual.

The aims of treatment as well as the available methods of treatment must all be considered in planning a treatment program for each patient. Ideally, the complex treatment of patients with rheumatoid arthritis should be formulated and at least supervised by a rheumatologist. The initial complete assessment of a patient and the initiation of treatment for the early phase as well as for exacerbations are most effectively carried out in hospital. Aggressive medical treatment of rheumatoid arthritis early in the course of the disease is more effective than treatment later in the disease.

Aims of Treatment

The overall management of a given patient with rheumatoid arthritis is based on the following aims: 1) to help the patient understand the nature of the disease, 2) to provide psychological support, 3) to alleviate pain, 4) to suppress the inflammatory reaction, 5) to encourage the patient to remain as physically active as possible in order to maintain joint motion and prevent deformity, 6) to correct existing deformity, 7) to improve function, 8) to strengthen weak muscles, and 9) to rehabilitate the individual patient.

Methods of Treatment
Psychological Considerations

In any long-term, chronic illness such as rheumatoid arthritis, the relationship between physician and patient is particularly important; it must be developed by sympathetic understanding and free discussion of the nature of the disease, the prognosis, and the proposed treatment. These patients seldom require psychiatric care but are greatly helped by careful attention to their specific psychological needs, not the least of which is the need to have complete confidence in their physician.

Therapeutic Drugs

The multiplicity of drugs prescribed for patients with rheumatoid arthritis can be catego-

rized in the order of frequency of their administration: short- or fast-acting nonsteroidal anti-inflammatory drugs (NSAIDs), slow-acting antirheumatic drugs (SAARDs), corticosteroids, and immunosuppressive agents.

Of the NSAIDs, salicylates such as enteric-coated aspirin continue to be the most useful drugs in the first-line treatment of rheumatoid arthritis. They not only relieve pain but also have a definite anti-inflammatory effect when administered in sufficiently large doses to provide a blood level of 20 mg/100 mL. The goal is to reach a total dose of 12 to 24 (300 mg) tablets a day within the limits of toxic effects, which include gastrointestinal disturbance, tinnitus, and hearing loss.

During the last two decades, many new NSAIDs have been developed by medical scientists and the pharmaceutical industry—each drug having its specific beneficial effects as well as its specific undesirable side effects and none having been scientifically proven to be more effective than salicylates. Examples of these newer drugs include phenylalcanoic or proprionic acids (e.g., naproxen), pyrazolidinediones (e.g., phenylbutazone), indoleacetic acids (e.g., indomethacin). One of the more recently developed drugs, piroxicam, which is chemically unrelated to the NSAIDs, is longer acting and requires administration only once daily. These various newer NSAIDs and piroxicam are particularly useful for patients who, for various reasons, are unable to tolerate salicylates.

When the disease process progresses despite the use of salicylates or other NSAIDs, the second line of drugs, namely, the SAARDs are indicated. These more powerful, but also more toxic, disease-suppressing agents include methotrexate, gold salts (chrysotherapy), antimalarial agents (e.g., chloroquine), D-penicillamine, cyclosporine, and azathioprine. For some patients, two or more of these drugs may need to be combined.

The third line of therapeutic agents, that is, corticosteroids, which were at one time widely recommended, are now used more sparingly because their nonspecific beneficial anti-inflammatory effects must be weighed against their undesirable side effects, which include a decreased resistance to infection, generalized

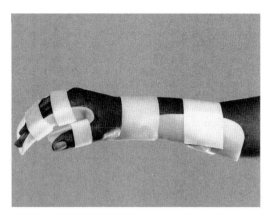

Figure 10.42. Removable splint designed to relieve pain and prevent deformity.

osteoporosis, deleterious metabolic effects, and steroid dependency. Thus, corticosteroids are usually reserved for extremely severe forms of rheumatoid arthritis and for serious complications of the disease.

For patients whose disease has been refractory to the preceding forms of medication and continues to progress, there is a place for immunosuppressive drugs and cytotoxic agents, preferably under the direction of a rheumatologist.

Suppressive measures for local disease include the intra-articular injection of corticosteroids, which should not be repeated frequently with short intervals in a given joint because of the harmful effects on articular cartilage (Salter et al.) and "radiation synovectomy" by means of the intra-articular injection of radioactive material such as yttrium-90.

The therapeutic hope for the future is the discovery of biological agents that block the pivotal steps in the pathogenesis of rheumatoid arthritis. Such "biologics" could be targeted to the specific cells that create the arthritis. Gene therapy of rheumatoid arthritis also has the potential for eradicating the disease process.

Orthopaedic Appliances

In addition to adequate general rest (bed rest), local rest of painfully inflamed joints by *removable splints* is of great value, not only in relieving pain but also in the prevention of deformity (Fig. 10.42). Remedial shoes often make it possible for a patient with painful feet to continue walking. Eventually, canes or crutches may become necessary.

Physical Therapy

Active movements of involved joints within the limits of pain are important in the attempt to preserve joint motion and maintain muscle strength. A program of physical therapy, although initiated in a hospital setting, must of course be carried out subsequently by the patient at home and, hence, the motivation of the patient is an important factor in the efficacy of physical therapy. When muscles have been affected by the rheumatoid process, the associated atrophy is understandably difficult to overcome by exercises alone.

Orthopaedic Surgical Operations

For many years it was thought that surgical operations for rheumatoid arthritis should not be performed during the active stage of the disease for fear of producing an exacerbation of both the local and systemic inflammatory process. Consequently, in the past, operations were performed only as a last resort and in the very late, "burned out" stage of the disease, by which time the joints had suffered irreparable damage. Such operations included fusion of joints (*arthrodesis*) and reconstruction of joints by various means (*arthroplasty*).

It is now known, however, that surgical operations can be performed with relative safety, even during the active stages of rheumatoid arthritis. Thus, when the rheumatologist and the orthopaedic surgeon work closely together in selecting the patient, as well as the type of operation, much can be accomplished early in the disease to prevent some of the joint and tendon damage as well as the associated deformities (Fig. 10.38). Severe chronic pain is the primary indication for surgical operations in these patients.

Excision of the grossly hypertrophied synovial membrane (*synovectomy*) of a severely swollen joint frequently results in an improved range of motion, decreased effusion, and less pannus formation; thus, some of the cartilage and subchondral bone destruction may be prevented, with resultant preservation of joint function. Postoperatively, the involved joint should be treated by continuous passive motion (CPM) as originated by Salter for at least 3 weeks. Although the synovial membrane regenerates following synovectomy, the newly formed membrane seldom becomes severely involved. For large joints, a preferable alternative to open synovectomy (through an arthrotomy) is arthroscopic synovectomy. Synovectomy of tendon sheaths has also proved helpful in preserving the gliding function of the tendons, particularly in the hand. Spontaneous tendon ruptures can be repaired by *tendon grafts*, or their action can be replaced by *tendon transfer*. Subluxations and dislocations of finger joints and displacement of their tendons can be treated surgically before secondary changes occur in articular cartilage.

A nodule within a flexor tendon can produce a "trigger finger" or "trigger thumb," necessitating surgical division of the tendon sheath. Rheumatoid tenosynovitis of the flexor tendon sheaths at the wrist may cause median nerve compression within the carpal tunnel, requiring surgical decompression.

Rheumatoid arthritis involving the synovial joints of the first and second cervical vertebrae may cause a potentially serious degree of spinal instability at this level, with the threat of spinal cord compression in which case a C1–C2 arthrodesis (fusion) is indicated.

Prosthetic joint replacement of either the cemented or the noncemented type can be useful in the surgical management of irreparably damaged hip joints. The reduced physical activity of patients with advanced rheumatoid arthritis means fewer complications, such as loosening of the prosthesis and, consequently, a longer "life" of the prosthetic joint. For rheumatoid arthritis involving only one half (one compartment) of the knee joint, a unicompartmental prosthesis has proved effective. For extensive damage involving both the medial and lateral compartments, a semiconstrained prosthetic joint replacement is indicated. In general, prosthetic joint replacements are of most value in the knee, hip, elbow, and metacarpophalangeal joints, whereas arthrodesis is most suitable for the ankle, wrist, and interphalangeal joints. When walking becomes painful because of depression of the metatarsal heads, excision of the metatarsophalangeal joints corrects the deformity and relieves the pain.

Diffuse Connective Tissue Diseases ("Collagen Diseases")

Chronic polyarthritis may develop in a variety of other diffuse connective diseases that are frequently referred to as the *collagen diseases*. These include *systemic lupus erythematosus* (formerly disseminated lupus erythematosus), *polyarteritis nodosa* (formerly periarteritis nodosa), *progressive systemic sclerosis* (formerly scleroderma), *polymyositis, dermatomyositis, and thrombotic thrombocytopenic purpura*.

Juvenile Rheumatoid Arthritis (Juvenile Chronic Arthritis)

In most children who acquire chronic arthritis involving one or more joints, the disease process is quite different—both genetically and immunologically—from that of rheumatoid arthritis in adults. Consequently, the term *juvenile rheumatoid arthritis*, although hallowed by tradition, is not entirely appropriate and in some countries has been replaced by the term *juvenile chronic arthritis* or simply *juvenile arthritis*. Thus, in 90% of children, this disease is not the beginning of the adult type of rheumatoid arthritis and, in general, it carries a better prognosis. Despite the fact that the disease is usually "seronegative" in these children (i.e., the rheumatoid factor is absent), the pathologic features of the synovium in a given joint are similar in the two age groups.

Clinical Varieties

During childhood, at least three varieties of chronic arthritis can be distinguished on the basis of the number of joints involved within the first 6 months of onset and extra-articular clinical features. Consequently, each of these varieties merits separate consideration.

Pauciarticular (Oligoarticular) Juvenile Arthritis. In one half to two thirds of children with chronic arthritis the disease affects only a paucity of joints (less than five); hence, this is known as the pauciarticular or oligoarticular variety, which includes, of course, single joint involvement, that is, monarticular arthritis. This form is more common in girls. The child's general health usually remains good. The most commonly affected joints are the knee, ankle, and elbow and less commonly the finger and toe joints. When the knee is involved, the associated hyperemia may cause local overgrowth through the distal femoral and proximal tibial epiphyseal plates. If the disease remains limited to one joint for at least 1 year, it is unlikely that other joints will become involved, but frequently a few joints are involved from the beginning. Although the clinical course is characterized by exacerbations and remissions over a period of years, the arthritis eventually resolves in most of the patients. Young children with the pauciarticular form of juvenile arthritis are prone to the development of the complication of iridocyclitis of the eye. Older children with a pauciarticular onset of arthritis may develop ankylosing spondylitis or a related spondyloarthropathy. This form is more common in boys.

Polyarticular Juvenile Arthritis. Polyarticular juvenile arthritis is a variety of chronic arthritis that can begin at any age during childhood and affects girls predominantly. Five or more joints are involved, the most frequent sites being the knees, ankles, feet, wrists, hands, and neck.

Usually the disease is limited to the joints. The onset may be either insidious or acute; in either case, the disease remains active for several years and may be complicated by general retardation of skeletal growth, a phenomenon that is aggravated by prolonged, and often inappropriate, administration of corticosteroids.

In one subvariety of polyarticular arthritis that primarily affects girls older than 10 years of age, the disease truly resembles the adult type of rheumatoid arthritis in that it runs a similar clinical course and the disease is seropositive. This type may be associated with classic rheumatoid nodules (Fig. 10.36).

Systemic Juvenile Arthritis. In systemic juvenile arthritis, the least common but most serious variety, the disease usually begins in young boys and girls younger than the age of 5 years and involves multiple body systems. It is this systemic variety that is known eponymously as *Still's disease*. The acute onset includes a high fever, an erythematous rash, anemia, generalized lymphadenopathy and, less

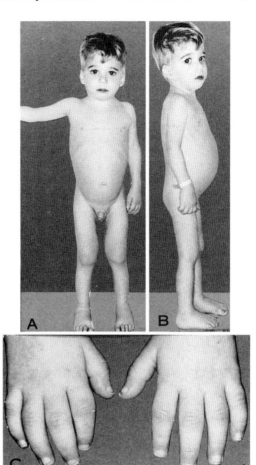

Figure 10.43. Rheumatoid polyarthritis and a visceral involvement (Still's disease) in a 2-year-old boy. **A** and **B.** Note the symmetrical swellings of the ankles, knees, fingers, and wrists as well as the generalized muscle atrophy. This boy's protruberant abdomen results, in part, from an enlarged spleen. **C.** The hands of the same boy, showing diffuse swelling in the region of the proximal interphalangeal joints.

frequently, hepatosplenomegaly and pericarditis. Indeed, the systemic component of the disease may precede the multiple joint involvement (Fig. 10.43). Exacerbations and remissions characterize the prolonged clinical course of the disease. Approximately 50% of the children experience severe destructive polyarthritis. An adult-onset type of Still's disease may also occur.

Laboratory Investigations

The erythrocyte sedimentation rate (ESR) is generally raised while the disease process is active, especially in the systemic variety, and it correlates with an elevated C-reactive protein level. The presence of antinuclear antibodies is usually seen in young patients with early onset pauciarticular juvenile arthritis and is associated with the complication of asymptomatic iridocyclitis, whereas the rheumatoid factor is found only in the aforementioned variety that resembles adult rheumatoid arthritis.

Treatment

The aims and methods of treatment already outlined in this chapter for adult rheumatoid arthritis are, for the most part, applicable to juvenile chronic (rheumatoid) arthritis. Temporary splints may be necessary to prevent joint deformities, but active exercises are essential to help maintain a useful range of joint motion. NSAIDs are still the first line of medical treatment because they relieve pain and decrease inflammation with relatively few side effects. The judicious use of intra-articular corticosteroid therapy is beneficial. Such intra-articular injections should not be repeated frequently with short intervals in a given joint because of the aforementioned harmful effects on articular cartilage (Salter et al.).

A poor response to NSAIDs and joint injections is an indication for second-line agents. In children, the most efficacious seem to be weekly methotrexate and sulfasalazine. Intramuscular gold salts are usually reserved for children with seropositive disease. Systemic corticosteroids have not been proven to improve the ultimate prognosis or to prevent complications of the disease, but their cautious use is indicated in the presence of severe systemic disease and in the child with relentless polyarticular arthritis that has not responded to other forms of medical treatment. Excessive corticosteroid therapy, however, decreases the child's resistance to infection, produces generalized osteoporosis and even generalized retardation of skeletal growth with resultant dwarfism.

Orthopaedic surgical operations including the release of muscle contractures, especially around the hips and knees, and sometimes even synovectomy (as discussed for the adult form of rheumatoid arthritis) may be required to help preserve joint function. However, for children, prosthetic joint replacement is contraindicated except in the case of skeletally mature adolescents with completely disabling involvement of both hip joints.

The poignant psychological needs of children and adolescents with persistent disability must be met by all those involved with their care as well as by their parents.

Ankylosing Spondylitis

The clinical entity of *ankylosing spondylitis* (Marie-Strumpell disease, Bechterew's disease, pelvospondylitis ossificans, "rheumatoid spondylitis") is a form of chronic seronegative spondyloarthritis characterized by progressive involvement of the sacroiliac and spinal joints with eventual ossification in and around these joints (*bony ankylosis*). The proximal joints of the extremities, particularly the hips, may be affected, as may the peripheral joints, especially in the lower extremities.

Ankylosing spondylitis differs sufficiently from rheumatoid arthritis in relation to its immunogenetics, age of onset, sex incidence, distribution, clinical and radiographic features, and response to therapy that it is currently believed to be a separate disease of connective tissue rather than an expression, or variant, of rheumatoid disease.

Incidence

Until the past decade, ankylosing spondylitis was considered a relatively uncommon rheumatic disease occurring predominantly in young males. It is now known, however, that when less severe forms of the disease are recognized and included, ankylosing spondylitis is almost as common as rheumatoid arthritis and young women are affected almost as often as young men. Typically, the onset is in the late teens and seldom after the age of 30 years. Nevertheless, a juvenile form of ankylosing spondylitis can begin as early as 10 years of age in association with pauciarticular arthritis.

Etiology

Although the precise cause is unknown, the importance of a genetic predisposing factor has been emphasized by the discovery that 96% of white persons suffering from ankylos-

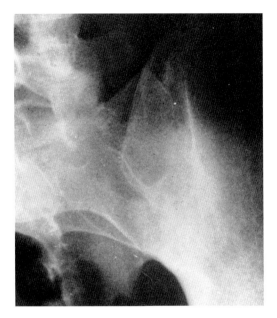

Figure 10.44. Ankylosing spondylitis, involving the left sacroiliac joint. The joint is gradually becoming ankylosed.

ticular tissues of the intervertebral joints, which are symphyses, are likewise affected. Eventually, the soft tissues of both types of joint ossify, thereby producing a bony ankylosis that may come to involve the entire spine, converting it to one rigid mass of bone (Fig. 10.45). The extraspinal joints became involved in one third of patients; the hips are particularly prone to becoming completely ankylosed. A systemic element of ankylosing spondylitis exists, as evidenced by lesions that may involve the eyes, lungs, heart, or prostate gland.

Clinical Features and Diagnosis
The patient, usually a young person, first experiences the gradual onset of vague low back pain that is aggravated by sudden movement but is not relieved by rest. Thus, night pain is characteristic. Morning stiffness of the spine persists well into the day and, in contrast to "mechanical" low back pain, the pain of anky-

ing spondylitis carry the inherited tissue antigen HLA-B27, which serves as a genetic marker. This particular antigen is found in 5 to 15% of all white persons, but of those who carry it, only 20% acquire ankylosing spondylitis. In certain races in whom HLA-B27 is extremely rare in the general population, ankylosing spondylitis is equally rare.

Pathogenesis and Pathology
In contrast to rheumatoid arthritis that attacks the synovial membrane, ankylosing spondylitis attacks the site of insertion of tendons, ligaments, fascia, and fibrous joint capsules—sites that have been named *entheses*. The pathological process is one of progressive fibrosis and ossification in these periarticular soft tissues; this process—*termed enthesopathy*—eventually leads to bony ankylosis of the entire joint (Fig. 10.44).

Beginning in the sacroiliac joints, the disease slowly spreads upward along the spine, where it affects the capsule of the posterior facet joints (apophyseal joints). The lumbar spine may be spared in the early stages but is eventually involved. Subsequently, the periar-

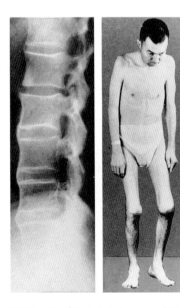

Figure 10.45. (Left). Ankylosing spondylitis involving the lumbar spine ("bamboo spine"). Note the ossification across the intervertebral disc spaces and also the ankylosis of the posterior joints.

Figure 10.46. (Right). Ankylosing spondylitis. This man has ankylosis of most of his spine and also his left hip. He is unable to look up or even to look straight ahead.

losing spondylitis improves with physical exercise. Physical examination reveals local deep tenderness over the sacroiliac joints and spine as well as spinal muscle spasm and a loss of the normal lumbar lordosis. The patient may also complain of pain in the back of the heel at the site of insertion of the Achilles tendon into the os calcis or under the heel at the site of insertion of the plantar fascia. These symptoms are accompanied by local tenderness. Progression of signs and symptoms is usually continuous but may be intermittent. After a year or more, by which time the disease has usually spread upward along the spine, the patient's back becomes progressively stiffer. Involvement of the costovertebral joints causes pain on deep breathing and, as these joints lose motion, there is a measurable decrease in the normal chest expansion.

In the more severe forms of ankylosing spondylitis, as the spinal column becomes progressively stiffer ("poker back") it also tends to become progressively flexed ("rocker back"). Furthermore, this progressive flexion deformity of the spine may be dramatically accelerated by a series of pathological vertebral fractures that result from trivial trauma. Eventually, the patient is no longer able to look straight ahead, a dangerous as well as embarrassing disability (Fig. 10.46). If, in addition, the hips become ankylosed, the unfortunate victim has extreme difficulty walking. Although the disease process may become arrested spontaneously at any stage, the more common course is one of slow but relentless progression.

Radiographic examination in the early stages reveals narrowing of the sacroiliac cartilage space and subchondral sclerosis (Fig. 10.44); a bone scan, although nonspecific, may be abnormal at an even earlier stage. Eventually these joints may ossify. Subsequently, ossification of the annulus fibrosus of the intervertebral joints produces the classic radiographic picture of the "bamboo spine" (Fig. 10.45). In later stages, a disuse type of osteoporosis may develop and lead to pathological compression fractures with a resultant increase in spinal deformity.

Clinical manifestations of systemic illness include fatigue, weight loss, and a low-grade fever. Laboratory examination may reveal anemia and an elevated erythrocyte sedimentation rate. Since only 20% of HLA-B27 positive individuals experience ankylosing spondylitis and since not *all* individuals with the disease carry this antigen, the HLA-B27 antigen is not of absolute diagnostic value. Hence, the diagnosis must be made primarily on clinical and radiographic grounds.

Treatment

The aims of treatment for ankylosing spondylitis are comparable to those already described for adult rheumatoid arthritis in a previous section of this chapter.

Psychological Considerations

These young, previously healthy patients need to be informed that less than one third of them will acquire the full-blown "classic" picture of ankylosing spondylitis. They also need psychological support in accepting the importance of developing good postural habits and of doing daily exercises for the rest of their lives.

Therapeutic Drugs

Although salicylates are the safest of the NSAIDs, they are not usually effective in ankylosing spondylitis. Of the many other NSAIDs available, indomethacin is currently the most appropriate, although it, in turn, may be replaced in the future by newer drugs. For patients in whom indomethacin is not well tolerated, phenylbutazone may be used, but with caution because of its long-term toxicity, including bone marrow depression and peptic ulceration. Neither corticosteroids nor gold salts are effective in this disease.

Radiation Therapy

Once a common modality of treatment for ankylosing spondylitis because it relieved the pain, radiation therapy is no longer widely recommended because it has been proved to have the potential for causing either radiation-induced aplastic anemia or leukemia.

Orthopaedic Appliances

Spinal braces are ineffectual in preventing the progressive flexion deformity of the spine, but a firm, flat mattress may help during sleep. A sudden increase in the flexion deformity is usually the result of one or more pathological fractures of the osteoporotic vertebral bodies and may necessitate reduction of the fracture or fractures and the temporary use of external fixation by means of a halopelvic device.

Physical Therapy

It is absolutely essential for these patients to exercise faithfully several times a day for the rest of their lives. Swimming and running are especially beneficial.

Orthopaedic Surgical Operations

Although one of the basic aims of treatment is the prevention of severe spinal deformity, those patients most severely involved may, nevertheless, experience disabling and permanent deformity (even more severe than that seen in Fig. 10.46). For such patients, spinal osteotomy is now feasible in either the lumbar or the cervical region (depending on the site of the major deformity) and produces dramatic improvement. Understandably, this type of major surgery carries a moderate risk but one that is minimized when the operation is performed under local anaesthesia as recommended by Simmons. Ankylosis of one or both hips is particularly disabling when combined with ankylosis of the spine, but fortunately this condition can be helped by prosthetic joint replacement of the conventional type ("total hip") even though in these patients such surgery may be complicated by some degree of heterotopic ossification in the surrounding soft tissues.

Many of the patients with severe ankylosing spondylitis require vocational rehabilitation.

Reiter's Syndrome

Reiter's syndrome consists of urethritis, conjunctivitis, and seronegative asymmetric arthritis. It is thought to be secondary either to a venereal type of infection or to bacillary dysentery. It afflicts mostly males, and the arthritis involves joints of the lower extremities predominantly. As with ankylosing spondylitis, there is a close correlation between Reiter's syndrome and the histocompatibility antigen HLA-B27.

Psoriasis

Although the skin disease psoriasis is relatively common, only 2% of patients, both male and female, exhibit an associated polyarthritis. The arthritis characteristically develops in the distal interphalangeal joints of the fingers and toes and seems to be related to psoriatic involvement of the nails.

Rheumatic Fever

Rheumatic fever is an acute inflammatory disease that attacks connective tissues in the heart, blood vessels, and joints of children. The heart lesions are particularly significant because they may be followed by serious and permanent scarring of the valves (chronic rheumatic heart disease). By contrast, the joint lesions are always transient.

Etiology

This disease, which usually afflicts children older than 5 years of age, is a sequel to infection with group A hemolytic streptococci; hence, its incidence parallels the incidence of such infections. Consequently, with improved health conditions and the use of effective antibiotics, rheumatic fever occurs less frequently now than in the past. Although the relationship to group A streptococcal infections has been well established immunologically by elevated titers of antibodies to streptococcal antigens, the pathogenesis of rheumatic fever is not yet understood.

Pathology

The acute inflammatory polyarthritis is characterized by an intense synovitis. However, the local inflammatory process is transient, and no pannus forms; hence, articular cartilage is spared and the joints always recover completely.

Clinical Features and Diagnosis

Rheumatic fever usually presents as an attack of acute febrile illness accompanied by acute polyarthritis. Although more than one joint may be involved at a given time, the transient inflammatory process tends to migrate from joint to joint (Fig. 10.47). The more serious heart lesions are manifest by heart murmurs and

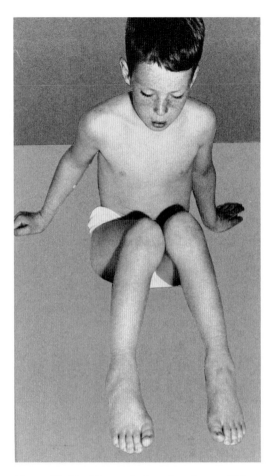

Figure 10.47.   Rheumatic fever in a 6-year-old boy. Note the symmetrical swelling of both ankle joints. Two days later the swelling on the left ankle subsided but the right elbow became swollen.

electrocardiographic changes (prolongation of the P-R interval). The acute phase of rheumatic fever seldom lasts more than 2 months.

Laboratory examination reveals an elevated erythrocyte sedimentation rate, but the diagnosis is strengthened by the demonstration of a changing antistreptolysin-O titer, which indicates a recent streptococcal infection. The mucin of the synovial fluid clots well on the addition of acetic acid.

Treatment

As with the other rheumatic diseases, there is no specific cure. The joint lesions, however,

are so transient that only symptomatic treatment is required. Salicylates in high doses tend to suppress the inflammatory reaction and are much safer than adrenocorticosteroids, although the latter may be required for some patients. Penicillin is administered orally in large doses during the acute phase and must be continued indefinitely in prophylactic doses in order to prevent recurrent attacks of rheumatic fever by preventing recurrent streptococcal infections. However, if after 5 years the child has neither a persistent heart murmur nor choreoathetosis (jerky involuntary movements), the prophylactic antibiotic may be discontinued.

Transient Synovitis of the Hip Joint in Children

The relatively common clinical entity *transient synovitis of the hip joint* in children (idiopathic monarticular synovitis) ("observation hip") is a nonbacterial inflammatory disorder of uncertain origin, although there is evidence to suggest that a virus may be the responsible organism. It develops most frequently in boys between the ages of 3 and 10 years.

Clinically, the synovitis is manifest by pain in the region of the hip, occasionally referred pain in the knee, a painful (antalgic) limp and restriction of hip joint motion with associated muscle spasm. The progressive synovial effusion bulges the hip joint capsule and as the intra-articular fluid pressure rises, the child comes to prefer lying down with the hip held in flexion, abduction, and external rotation, the position in which the capacity of the hip joint capsule is greatest (Fig. 10.48). Systemic manifestations of inflammation are minimal.

Radiographic examination reveals only evidence of an effusion in the involved hip joint (Fig. 10.49). Such an effusion can also be detected by ultrasonography. The diagnosis of transient synovitis of the hip can be suspected on clinical grounds alone but is established by exclusion of more serious conditions that mimic it—Legg-Perthes' disease, septic arthritis, rheumatic fever, monarticular rheumatoid arthritis and tuberculosis arthritis. Aspiration of the joint is of value when the diagnosis is in doubt.

Treatment consists of bed rest with the hip

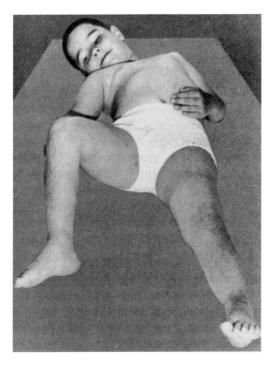

Figure 10.48. Transient synovitis of the right hip joint in a 6-year-old boy. The boy prefers to maintain the inflamed hip in position of flexion, abduction, and external rotation. This position, in which the capacity of the hip joint capsule is greatest, is the position of comfort.

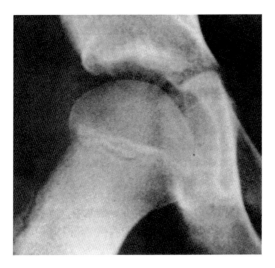

Figure 10.49. Evidence of an effusion in the right hip joint in a child with transient synovitis of the hip. The slightly denser shadow that is lateral to the femoral head and neck indicates a bulging of the hip joint capsule. Such an effusion in the hip joint can also be demonstrated by ultrasonography.

maintained in the most comfortable position of flexion, abduction, and external rotation until a full range of painless motion of the hip has returned, which is usually within 1 week. Relief of weightbearing on the involved hip by means of crutches is recommended for a further few weeks in an attempt to prevent recurrence.

Approximately 5% of children with transient synovitis of the hip exhibit radiographic evidence of Legg-Perthes' disease within the ensuing year. For this reason, all children who have such synovitis of the hip should be seen, and their hip joints radiographed, at 6 months and 1 year in order to detect the earliest evidence of this complication. The possible causative relationship of transient synovitis of the hip to Legg-Perthes' disease is discussed in Chapter 13.

Gout and Gouty Arthritis

The clinical condition of *gout,* which is the manifestation of a familial *inborn error of purine metabolism,* is characterized by an elevated serum uric acid level (*hyperuricemia*), recurrent attacks of *acute gouty arthritis* in peripheral joints and, eventually, *chronic gouty arthritis* associated with periarticular and subcutaneous deposits, or *tophi,* of urate salts; gout may also be associated with renal disease and uric acid nephrolithiasis.

Incidence

Although classic gout is relatively uncommon, milder forms of the disease, which often escape diagnosis, may be more prevalent than previously thought. Gout is predominantly a disease of males, the ratio being 20:1. It may present during adolescence, but the peak incidence is after the age of 40 years, and when females are afflicted, it is seldom before menopause. Gouty arthritis involves mainly the peripheral joints of the feet and hands, by far the most common site being the metatarsophalangeal joint of the great toe.

Etiology

In more than half the patients, there is a definite familial incidence of either clinical gout or hyperuricemia. The cause of the purine metabolic disorder is unknown, but presumably the hyperuricemia is caused by either excessive production or deficient urinary excretion of uric acid. Nevertheless, not all persons with hyperuricemia actually suffer from gout.

Attacks of acute gouty arthritis seem to be precipitated in a given patient by a variety of general factors, including infection, alcoholic or dietary indiscretion, and emotional factors, as well as by local factors, including injury and exposure to cold. In certain blood dyscrasias, such as leukemia and polycythemia, *secondary gout* can develop from overproduction of urates; in patients with chronic renal disease and in patients receiving diuretics, secondary gout can develop because of impaired urinary excretion of urates.

Pathogenesis and Pathology
Attacks of acute gouty arthritis are caused by the sudden deposition of sodium monourate crystals in the synovial membrane and therefore represent a type of *crystal-induced arthritis*. Leukocytes phagocytose the crystals and then disintegrate, releasing lysosomal enzymes that produce an acute and severe local inflammation.

Early in the disease, the urate crystals are usually absorbed after each attack and consequently the joint returns to normal. Several years later in the course of gout, however, nodular deposits, or *tophi* of urate crystals, eventually develop in one or more sites. In the involved joint, tophi develop in synovial membrane, articular cartilage, and even subchondral bone. In addition, they may form in the synovial membrane of bursae and tendon sheaths as well as in the cartilage of the external ear.

Eventually, the chronic inflammatory reaction to urate deposits in and around a given joint, plus associated destruction of cartilage and subchondral bone, leads to progressive degenerative changes in the joint, a type of degenerative joint disease.

Clinical Features
The clinical course of gout varies widely in relation to severity and rate of progression. The commonest pattern is a series of attacks of acute gouty arthritis over a period of years followed by the formation of tophi, both artic-

ular and extra-articular, and eventually the development of chronic gouty arthritis.

Acute Gouty Arthritis
During the early stages, attacks of acute gouty arthritis are usually monoarticular, and in at least half the patients the initial attack is in the metatarsophalangeal joint of the great toe ("podagra"); indeed, this particular joint is eventually affected in virtually every patient with gout, although other peripheral joints may also become involved.

Each episode may be preceded by forewarning symptoms, such as mood change, constipation, and diuresis. The actual attack, which develops with dramatic rapidity, is characterized by intense pain that progresses to the point of being excruciating; even the slightest movement of the joint is intolerable and local tenderness is exquisite. The joint becomes swollen within a few hours and is obviously acutely inflamed. Indeed, the clinical picture, which includes fever and leukocytosis, may simulate cellulitis or even acute septic arthritis (Fig. 10.50). Mild attacks of acute gouty arthritis last for several days, but more severe attacks may persist for as long as several weeks. However, once the attack is over, all signs of inflammation subside spontaneously and, at least in the early stages of the disease, the joint returns to normal.

At first the attacks tend to occur at infrequent intervals, even a few years apart, and between attacks the patient is completely free of symptoms. Later, however, the attacks not only occur more frequently but also are more severe and may even involve multiple joints.

Chronic Tophaceous Gout
After several years, half the patients develop tophaceous gout. Tophi, which consist of persistent deposits of urate crystals surrounded by chronic inflammatory tissue, develop in the synovial membrane and may become sufficiently large that they interfere with joint function. Tophi also develop in articular cartilage, where they cause local destruction, and in the subchondral bone, where they incite local osteoclastic resorption with cystlike lesions (Fig. 10.51). Extra-articular tophi form in bursae (the most common site being the

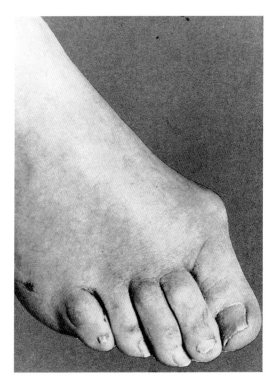

Figure 10.50.   Acute gouty arthritis involving the metatarsophalangeal joint of the great toe. The joint is greatly swollen and acutely inflamed.

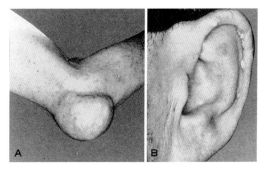

Figure 10.52.   Extra-articular gouty tophi in the olecranon bursa (**A**) and in the cartilage of the external ear (**B**).

olecranon bursa), in tendon sheaths, and in the cartilage of the external ear (Fig. 10.52). Since tophi form slowly, they are usually painless, but those that are subcutaneous may eventually ulcerate through the skin.

Chronic Gouty Arthritis

Articular and subchondral tophi lead to progressive degenerative arthritis with chronic joint pain, swelling, and stiffness. Nevertheless, even in this late stage, acute attacks may be superimposed on the chronic arthritis. Although pure urate deposits are radiolucent, subsequent secondary deposition of calcium in the soft tissues can be detected radiographically (Fig. 10.51).

Laboratory Diagnosis

Hyperuricemia is virtually always demonstrable in patients with gout both during and between attacks. (The normal serum uric acid level by colorimetric methods is 6 mg/100 mL for adult men and 5.5 mg/100 mL for adult women.) The demonstration of urate crystals from synovial fluid or from tophi by means of a polarizing microscope is diagnostic; however, tophi develop in only half of all patients with gout.

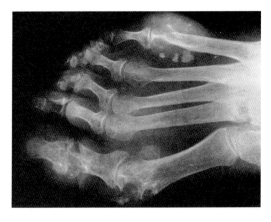

Figure 10.51.   Chronic gout in the foot of a 50-year-old man. Note the local osteoclastic resorption with cystlike lesions in the first metatarsal, the fifth metatarsal, and the phalanges of the great toe. Note also the areas of soft tissue calcification.

Treatment

By means of currently available drugs, most patients with gout are able to pursue their normal activities; acute attacks can be reasonably well controlled and tophaceous complications, including chronic gouty arthritis, can usually be prevented. However, the medical treatment of gout must continue for the rest of the patient's life and is ideally supervised by a rheumatologist.

Treatment of Acute Gouty Arthritis. *Colchicine*, which is of specific value in the treatment of acute attacks, is taken hourly from the onset until the severe pain is relieved, at least up to 12 hours, or until gastrointestinal symptoms develop. Alternatively, it may be given intravenously. *Indomethacin* is equally effective and does not upset the gastrointestinal tract. Subsequent acute attacks can often be prevented, or at least reduced in severity, by moderate dietary restrictions, particularly avoidance of purine-rich foods such as liver, kidney, and sweetbreads. Prophylactic administration of colchicine in small doses may also be helpful.

Treatment of Chronic Gout and Chronic Gouty Arthritis. In the chronic phase of gout, the hyperuricemia can be reduced by *uricosuric* drugs, which increase the urinary excretion of uric acid, presumably by blocking its reabsorption in the renal tubules. The currently limited indications for uricosuric drugs, which must be continued for the rest of the patient's life, are the presence of tophi, a persistent elevation of serum uric acid levels to greater than 8 mg/100 mL and the failure of other drugs to prevent frequent attacks. Two of the more effective uricosuric agents are *probenecid* and *sulphinpyrazone*. At present, the drug of choice as a uric acid–lowering agent is *allopurinol*, which helps to inhibit the production of uric acid and is therefore of particular value for patients with uric acid nephrolithiasis. This drug is required for the rest of the patient's life.

Pseudogout

Like true gout, its imitator *pseudogout* is a form of crystal-induced arthritis, but the deposited crystals are composed of calcium pyrophosphate dihydrate (CPPD) rather than uric acid. A relatively common type of metabolic arthritis, it primarily afflicts the elderly and is characterized by recurrent painful attacks of acute arthritis that may be triggered by either trauma or illness. The joints most frequently involved are those of the hand and wrist as well as the knee and hip, but there also is a high incidence of pre-existing degenerative arthritis. In the majority of patients, radiographic examination reveals calcium deposits within the hyaline articular cartilage and the fibrocartilage of menisci (*chondrocalcinosis*) and even calcification of periarticular soft tissues such as joint capsules and ligaments. One third of the patients experience a rapidly progressive and devastatingly destructive degenerative arthritis called *pyrophosphate arthropathy*. Although the diagnosis can be suspected on the basis of clinical and radiographic data, it can be confirmed only by the detection of the typical crystals of calcium pyrophosphate dihydrate within neutrophils in the synovial fluid using polarizing microscopy. This type of crystal-induced arthritis is usually idiopathic, but it can be secondary to an underlying metabolic disorder such as hyperparathyroidism. Phenylbutazone and indomethacin are equally effective in controlling the acute attacks of pseudogout. Although there is no effective prophylactic treatment, joint lavage may provide temporary improvement by reducing the number of crystals in the synovial fluid, and the intra-articular injection of steroids may help to reduce the synovitis but should be used only infrequently.

Rheumatic Disease Unit

The variety and complexity of the rheumatic diseases, which present many problems of diagnosis and treatment, justify the establishment of special *rheumatic disease units* in large general hospitals. In such units, the combined team efforts of rheumatologists, family physicians, orthopaedic surgeons, rehabilitation physicians, physical and occupational therapists, and medical social workers can most effectively improve the outlook for this unfortunate group of patients. Furthermore, a rheumatic disease unit is a splendid setting for both undergraduate and postgraduate teaching. In addition, such units provide a powerful stimulus for both clinical and experimental investigation, which hopefully will lead to a better understanding of this baffling group of diseases.

Hemophilic Arthritis

Classic *hemophilia and Christmas disease*,[1] *which are defects of the first-stage clotting mechanism of blood, are frequently complicated by repeated joint hemorrhages (hemarthroses)*, which, in turn, lead to progressive joint damage (*hemophilic arthritis, hemophilic arthropathy*). Other bleeding disorders are seldom complicated by hemarthrosis.

Incidence

Classic hemophilia, that is, hemophilia A, (a deficiency of antihemophilic factor, or factor VIII) is relatively uncommon, and Christmas disease, that is, hemophilia B, (a deficiency of plasma thromboplastin, or factor IX) is even less common. Nevertheless, in each of these bleeding disorders, hemarthrosis is the most frequent hemorrhagic event, since it occurs in most of the patients at some time. By far the most frequent site of hemarthrosis is the knee, followed by the ankle, hip, and the elbow. The first hemarthrosis usually occurs between the time the child starts to walk and the age of 5 years. Since hemophilia and Christmas disease are both inherited by boys (by a sex-linked recessive gene carried by the mother), hemophilic arthritis is limited to males. In one third of patients, the hemophilia is the result of a new mutation.

Pathogenesis and Pathology

Blood in a synovial joint does not clot even in a normal individual, although a clot does form in the torn vessels. In hemophilia, by contrast, a clot fails to form readily in the torn vessels and consequently bleeding into the joint tends to continue until it is stopped by the raised pressure of the hemarthrosis. In hemophilia, joint hemorrhage is probably always caused by trauma even though the initiating trauma may seem insignificant.

The synovial membrane reacts to the irritation of blood in the joint by an inflammatory proliferation and villous formation. Phagocytes transport the red blood cells from the joint cavity to the synovial membrane where they are broken down, with resultant formation of *hemosiderin deposits*, which constitute a further source of irritation. Inflammatory granulation tissue creeps across the surface as a *pannus* that interferes with the nutrition of cartilage from the synovial fluid. Furthermore, hemorrhages and inflammatory granulation tissue burrow under the cartilage with subsequent collapse of the joint surface.

After repeated hemarthroses, the grossly thickened synovial membrane tends to become fibrotic, with resultant joint adhesions, limitation of motion, contractures, and joint deformity. Consequently, the stage is set for progressive degenerative changes in the joint that, in turn, render the joint even more vulnerable to trivial trauma and lead to repeated hemarthroses; thus, a vicious repeating cycle is established.

Clinical Features and Diagnosis

The hemophilic patient and his parents are usually suspicious of the underlying diagnosis because of a family history of hemophilia or because of previous episodes of abnormal bruising or excessive bleeding from minor cuts or needle punctures; in some hemophilic children, the diagnosis is established after excessive bleeding at the time of circumcision.

Usually, the patient learns to recognize a vague feeling of joint discomfort, which heralds a major hemarthrosis. This is probably caused by a minor subsynovial hemorrhage that has not yet penetrated the synovial membrane to enter the joint. Once a progressive hemarthrosis begins, the joint becomes swollen, warm, painful, and limited in motion. After repeated hemarthroses in a given joint, the clinical picture is that of superimposed chronic arthritis with persistent swelling of the joint and atrophy of the surrounding muscles (Fig. 10.53).

Radiographic examination at the time of the first few hemarthroses reveals only soft tissue swelling. However, after repeated episodes of bleeding into a given joint, there is radiographic evidence of regional osteoporosis, subchondral defects in the bone, and narrowing of the cartilage space (Fig. 10.54). Ultrasonography, computed tomography (CT), and magnetic resonance imaging

---

[1] **The term** *Christmas disease* comes from the surname of the first boy in whom the disease was discovered.

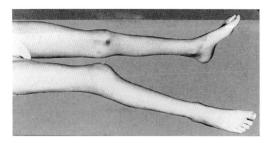

Figure 10.53. Hemophilic arthritis in the right knee of a 10-year-old boy. Note the gross swelling of the right knee joint and the atrophy of the quadriceps muscle. Note also a recent bruise over the medial aspect of the left knee.

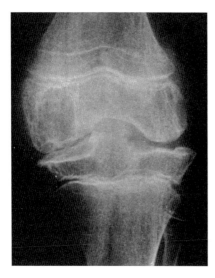

Figure 10.54. (**Left**). Chronic hemophilic arthritis. Note the regional osteoporosis, subchondral defects in the bone, and narrowing of the cartilage space.

(MRI) are useful in detecting the early changes of hemophilia.

Laboratory examination reveals a normal bleeding time but a prolonged partial thromboplastin time (PTT). The exact diagnosis is established by hematological assay of factor VIII (classic hemophilia) and factor IX (Christmas disease). For classic hemophilia, the severity of the disease is classified on the basis of the level of functional factor VIII activity as follows: severe—less than 1% activity (less than 0.01 international units/mL plasma), moderate—1 to 5% activity, mild—more than 5% activity.

Treatment

Hemarthrosis in a hemophilic patient constitutes an emergency because immediate treatment can prevent many of the late sequelae. The overall management should ideally be under the supervision of a hematologist. As soon as the patient experiences the forewarning symptoms of a joint hemorrhage, he should be given intravenous therapy with the appropriate concentrate of human factor (VIII or IX depending on the diagnosis) to prevent the development of a massive hemarthrosis.

Prior to 1984, more than half the hemophiliacs who received clotting factors from pooled plasma became HIV-positive and in many of these individuals, full-blown AIDS developed. Since 1984, however, all factor concentrates have been treated during preparation by methods known to be effective in killing the fatty-coated HIV organism.

One of the most important advances in the management of hemophiliacs during the past decade—and especially in the prevention of major hemarthroses—has been the development of "home care programs." Hemophiliacs are taught to recognize the previously mentioned "vague feeling of joint discomfort that heralds a major hemarthrosis." The appropriate factor as well as sterile needles and syringes are kept in the patient's home, and as soon as this warning signal is felt either the patient immediately gives himself an intravenous injection of the factor or one of his relatives does it for him. A hemarthrosis is thereby prevented. Many patients, as well as their relatives, master the management of home care, including the technique of intravenous injections, remarkably well.

If the patient is not seen until after the hemarthrosis has developed, his clotting mechanism should be corrected by the same measures and the affected joint splinted. Once the bleeding has stopped and the level of antihemophilic globulin has been raised adequately—and only then—the joint should be aspirated under sterile precautions if it is still distended to prevent the chronic synovial reaction to persistent blood in the joint.

Physiotherapy is necessary to improve joint motion and muscle strength and should be

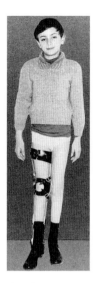

Figure 10.55.   (Right). A boy with chronic hemophilic arthritis involving the right knee. He is wearing a brace to protect the badly damaged right knee joint from further hemarthroses.

continued at least until previous motion is restored; during this time, the joint should be protected from weightbearing to prevent early recurrence of bleeding. In more severe cases, continuing prevention of recurrent hemarthroses may be prevented by the use of appropriate braces (Fig. 10.55).

During the early stages of hemophilic arthritis or arthropathy in a given joint that occurs secondary to several hemarthroses, surgical synovectomy (either open or arthroscopic) is indicated in an attempt to prevent subsequent hemarthroses and thereby prevent progression of the joint pathologic condition. Postoperatively, the patient's involved joint should be managed by continuous passive motion (CPM) as originated by the author to minimize reaction in the joint and maintain good joint motion. A reasonable alternative is "radiation synovectomy" by means of the intra-articular injection of radioactive material such as yttrium-90.

In the later stages of hemophilic arthritis, or arthropathy, reconstructive operations, including synovectomy, osteotomy, and prosthetic joint replacements, may be required and can be performed with relative safety provided that the patient's clotting mechanism is cor-

rected by appropriate treatment before, during, and for a period of at least 2 weeks after the operation. However, those patients known to have "inhibitors" to factor VIII should not undergo elective orthopaedic operations.

The future hope for hemophilic individuals lies in the continuing prevention of abnormal bleeding by means of daily prophylactic treatment with maintenance doses of the appropriate concentrate of human factor—especially the genetically engineered recombinant factor VIII. At present, the practical application of prevention is limited by the fact that the human factor must be given intravenously each day. The implantation of subcutaneous ports greatly facilitates the technique of self-treatment.

SUGGESTED ADDITIONAL READING

Abrams RA, Botte MJ. Hand infections: treatment recommendations for specific types. J Am Acad Orthop Surg 1996;4:219–230.

Apley AG, Solomon L. Apley's system of orthopaedics and fractures. 7th ed. Oxford: Butterworth-Heinemann, 1993.

Benson MKD, Fixen JA, Macnicol MF. Children's orthopaedics and fractures. Edinburgh: Churchill Livingstone, 1994.

Benson WJ, Benson W, Adachi JD, et al. Remodelling the pyramid: the therapeutic target of rheumatoid arthritis. J Rheum 1990;17:987–989.

Betz RR, Cooperman DR, Wopperer JM, Sutherland RD, White JJ, Schaaf HW, Aschliman RW, Choi IH, Bowen JR, Gillespie R. Late sequelae of septic arthritis of the hip in infancy and childhood. J Paediatr Orthop 1990;10:365–372.

Bisno AL. Group A streptococcal infections and rheumatic fever. N Engl J Med 1991;325:783–793.

Bloom BR, Murray CJ. Tuberculosis: commentary on a reemergent killer. Science 1992;257:1055–1064.

Boyd W, Sheldon H. Introduction to the study of disease. 8th ed. Philadelphia: Lea & Febiger, 1980.

Bradford WZ, Martin JN, Reingold AN, Schecter GF, Hopewell PC, Small PM. The changing epidemiology of acquired drug-resistant tuberculosis in San Francisco, U.S.A. Lancet 1996;348:928–931.

Brooks PM, Day RO. Nonsteroidal anti-inflammatory drugs: differences and similarities. N Engl J Med 1991;324:1716–1725.

Broughton N, ed. A textbook of paediatric orthopaedics, London: WB Saunders, 1997.

Buchanan WW. Rheumatoid arthritis: modern

medicine's major enigma. Ann R Coll Phys Surg Can 1982;15:93–97.

Bullough PG. Bullough and Vigorita's orthopaedic pathology. 3rd ed. London: CV Mosby, 1996.

Dagan R. Management of acute hematogenous osteomyelitis and septic arthritis in the pediatric patient. Pediatr Infect Dis J 1993;12: 88–92.

Duthie RB, Bentley G. Mercer's orthopaedic surgery. 9th ed. London, UK: Arnold, 1996.

Espinoza LR, Aguilar JL, Berman A, et al. Rheumatic manifestations associated with human immunodeficiency virus (H.I.V.) infection. Arthritis Rheum 1989;32:1615–1622.

Esterhai JL Jr. Infection. In: Frymoyer JW, ed. Orthopaedic knowledge update 4. Rosemont IL: American Academy of Orthopaedic Surgeons, 1993;155–168.

Esterhai JL Jr, Hughes TB. Infection. In: Kasser JR, ed. Orthopaedic knowledge update 5. Rosemont IL: American Academy of Orthopaedic Surgeons 1966;149–161.

Evanchick CC, Davis DE, Harrington TM. Tuberculosis of peripheral joints: an often missed diagnosis. J Rheum 1986;13:187–189.

Gamble JG, Rinsky LA. Chronic recurrent multifocal osteomyelitis: a distinct clinical entity. J Pediatr Orthop 1986;6:579–584.

Gatter RA, Schumacher HR. A practical handbook of joint fluid analysis. 2nd ed. Philadelphia: Lea & Febiger, 1991.

Gordon DA, ed. Rheumatoid arthritis. 2nd ed. Contemporary patient management series. New York: Elsevier Science, 1985.

Hamdy RC, Babyn PS, Krajbich JI. Use of bone scan in management of patients with peripheral gangrene due to fulminant meningococcemia. J Pediatr Orthop 1993;13:447–451.

Harris ED Jr. Mechanisms of disease: rheumatoid arthritis—pathophysiology and implications for therapy. N Engl J Med 1990;322: 1277–1289.

Harris WH, Sledge CB. Total hip and total knee replacement (second of two parts). N Engl J Med 1990;323:801–807.

Hedden DM. The current management of hemophilic arthropathy. Curr Opin Orthop 1993;4: 62–65.

Herrera R, Hobar PC, Ginsburg CM. Surgical intervention for the complications of meningococcal-induced purpura fulminans. Pediatr Infect Dis J 1994;13:734–737.

Houghton GR, Duthie RB. Orthopaedic problems in hemophilia. Clin Orthop 1979;138: 197–216.

Isomaki H. Long-term outcome of rheumatoid arthritis. Scand J Rheumatol 1992;95(Suppl): 3–8.

Kaiser S, Rosenborg M. Early detection of subperiosteal abscesses by ultrasonography: a means for further successful treatment in paediatric osteomyelitis. Pediatr Radiol 1994;24:336–339.

Khan MA. Ankylosing spondylitis. In: Klippel JH, Dieppe D, eds. Rheumatology. London: CV Mosby, 1994.

Kuettner DE. Biochemistry of articular cartilage in health and disease. Clin Biochem 1992;25: 155–163.

Lang BA, Shore A. A review of current concepts on the pathogenesis of juvenile rheumatoid arthritis. J Rheumatol 1990; 21(Suppl)17:1–15.

Levine SE, Esterhai JL Jr, Heppenstal RB, et al. Diagnosis and staging: osteomyelitis and prosthetic joint infections. Clin Orthop 1993;295: 77–86.

Levinson D, Becker MA. Clinical gout and pathogenesis of hyperuricemia. In: McCarty DJ, Koopman WJ, eds. Arthritis and allied conditions. 12th ed. Philadelphia: Lea & Febiger, 1993;1773–1805.

Lindgren JV. Arthritis. In: Kasser JR, ed. Orthopaedic knowledge update 5. Rosemont IL: American Academy of Orthopaedic Surgeons, 1996;163–175.

Lloyd-Roberts GC. Some aspects of orthopaedic surgery in childhood. Ann R Coll Surg Engl 1974;57:25–32.

Madhock R, York J, Sturrock RD. Haemophilic arthritis. Ann Rheum Dis 1991;50:588–591.

Mah ET, Le Quesne GW, Gent RJ, Paterson DC. Ultrasound features of acute osteomyelitis in children. J Bone Joint Surg (Br) 1994;76B: 969–974.

Malin JK, Patel NJ. Arthropathy and HIV infection: a muddle of mimicry. Postgrad Med 1993; 93:143–146, 149–150.

McCarty DJ, Koopman WJ. Arthritis and allied conditions. A textbook of rheumatology. 12th ed. Philadelphia: Lea & Febiger, 1992.

Morrissy RT, Weinstein SL, eds. Lovell and Winter's pediatric orthopaedics. Vol. 1. 4th ed. Philadelphia: Lippincott-Raven, 1996.

Pinsk MN, Simor NE. Necrotizing fasciitis: a mean strain of strep. Univ Toronto Med J 1995;72: 134–138.

Salter RB, Bell RS, Keeley FW. The protective effect of continuous passive motion on living articular cartilage in acute septic arthritis—an experimental investigation in the rabbit. Clin Orthop 1981;159:223–247.

Salter RB, Gross A, Hall JH. Hydrocortisone arthropathy—an experimental investigation. Can Med Assoc J 1967;97:374–377.

Schawecker DS. The scintigraphic diagnosis of osteomyelitis. Am J Roentgenol 1992;158: 9–18.

Schumacher HR, ed. Primer on the rheumatic diseases. 10th ed. Atlanta, GA: The Arthritis Foundation,1993.

Scopelitis E, Martinez-Osuna P. Gonococcal arthritis. Rheum Dis Clin North Am 1993;19:363–377.

Shaw BA, Kasser JR. Acute septic arthritis in infancy and childhood. Clin Orthop 1990;257:212–225.

Simmons EH. Arthritic spinal deformity—ankylosing spondylitis. In: White AW, ed. Spine Care. Vol. 2: Operative Technique. St. Louis: CV Mosby, 1995;1652–1719.

Soren A. Arthritis and related afflictions. Berlin: Springer-Verlag, 1993.

Staheli LT. Fundamentals of pediatric orthopedics. New York: Raven Press, 1992.

Stanford JL, Grange JM. New concepts for the control of tuberculosis in the twenty first century. J R Coll Phys Lond 1993;27:218–223.

Tehranzadeh J, Wang F, Mesgarzadeh M. Magnetic resonance imaging of osteomyelitis. Crit Rev Diagn Imaging 1992;33:495–534.

Thiery JA. Arthroscopic drainage in septic arthritis of the knee: a multicentre study. Arthroscopy 1989;5:65–69.

Thornhill TS, Schaffer JL. Arthritis. In: Frymoyer JW, ed. Orthopaedic knowledge update 4. Rosemont IL: American Academy of Orthopaedic Surgeons 1993;89–106.

Walker LG, Sledge CB. Total hip arthroplasty in ankylosing spondylitis. Clin Orthop 1991;262:198–204.

Walport MJ, Ollier WER, Silman AJ. Immunogenetics of rheumatoid arthritis and the Arthritis and Rheumatism Council's National Repository. Br J Rheumatol 1992;31:701–705.

Weinstein SL, Buckwalter JA, eds. Turek's orthopaedics: principles and their applications. 5th ed. Philadelphia: JB Lippincott, 1994.

Wenger DR, Rang M. The art and practice of children's orthopaedics. New York: Raven Press, 1993.

Whalen JL, Fitzgerald RH Jr, Morrisy RT. A histologic study of acute hematogenous osteomyelitis following physeal injuries in rabbits. J Bone Joint Surg 1988;70A:1383–1392.

Williams PF, Cole WG. Orthopaedic management in childhood 2nd ed. London: Chapman and Hall, 1991.

Winchester R, ed. AIDS and rheumatic disease. Rheum Dis Clin North Am 1991;17:1.

Wingstrand H. Transient synovitis of the hip in the child. Acta Orthop Scand 1986;57(Suppl 219):1–61.

Yelin E, Fells W. A summary of the impact of the musculoskeletal conditions in the United States. Arthritis Rheum 1990;33:750–755.

Yu L, Kasser JR, O'Rourke E, Kozakewich H. Chronic recurrent multifocal osteomyelitis. J Bone Joint Surg. 1989;71A:105–112.

11 Degenerative Disorders of Joints and Related Tissues

The various "rheumatic diseases" discussed in the preceding chapter are predominantly *inflammatory;* by contrast, the rheumatic diseases discussed in this chapter are predominantly *degenerative.* You will appreciate, however, that the division is somewhat arbitrary because some inflammatory reaction is incited in soft tissues even by the degenerative types of disorders of joints and related structures. This chapter includes a discussion of the degenerative types of arthritis (*degenerative joint disease* or *chronic articular rheumatism*) and also various rheumatic diseases of extra-articular, or nonarticular, structures such as tendons, muscles, and bursae (*nonarticular rheumatism*). Many aspects of these diseases are related to normal aging, a process that merits separate consideration.

NORMAL AGING OF ARTICULAR CARTILAGE

Although most joints may be expected to last a lifetime, at least as far as reasonable function is concerned, the normal aging process, which begins in early adult life and slowly progresses throughout the remainder of life, gradually changes the smooth, glistening surface of youthful articular cartilage to a granular, dull surface in old age. Furthermore, because of the very limited ability of articular cartilage to regenerate, the degenerative changes tend to be irreversible and progressive.

Biochemically, there is a gradual loss of proteoglycan, a basic component of the cartilage matrix; as the matrix deteriorates, the collagen fibrils lose their support and the cartilage tends to become shredded (*fibrillation*). Thus, with advancing years, articular cartilage becomes less effective, not only as a "shock absorber" but also as a lubricated surface; consequently, it becomes more vulnerable to the intermittent load-bearing and repeated friction of normal function.

These changes of age in articular cartilage are present to some degree in all adults; however, because these changes do not usually cause significant symptoms, they may be considered variations of normal. When these changes in a given joint are either premature or excessive and cause pain, however, the condition becomes clinically significant, and is known as *degenerative joint disease.*

DEGENERATIVE JOINT DISEASE (OSTEOARTHRITIS)

Degenerative joint disease, a common disorder of one or more joints, is initiated by a local deterioration of articular cartilage and is characterized by progressive degeneration of the cartilage, hypertrophy, remodeling of the subchondral bone, and secondary inflammation of the synovial membrane. It is a localized disorder with no systemic effects.

The currently accepted term *degenerative joint disease* is synonymous with the terms *osteoarthritis, osteoarthrosis, degenerative arthritis, senescent arthritis,* and *hypertrophic arthritis.* Nevertheless, many clinicians prefer the term *osteoarthritis* to the term *degenerative joint disease.*

Incidence

Degenerative joint disease is by far the most common type of arthritis, much more common than the more dramatic condition of rheumatoid arthritis and exerting a 30 times greater economic impact in North America. Indeed, it has been estimated that after the age of 60 years, 25% of women and 15% of men have symptoms related to degenerative joint disease. After the age of 75 years, more than 80% of women and men are affected.

The *primary, or idiopathic,* type, which is somewhat more common in adult women, develops spontaneously in middle age and progresses slowly as an exaggeration of the normal aging process of joints. The *secondary* type, which is more common in adult men, develops at any age as a result of any injury, deformity, or disease that damages articular cartilage. Because the "wear and tear" of continuing friction aggravates the underlying pathological process, degenerative joint disease is most common in weight-bearing synovial joints, such as the hip and knee, as well as in the intervertebral disc joints of the lower lumbar spine. However, degenerative joint disease frequently involves joints of the hands as well as of the cervical spine, and all joints are susceptible.

Etiology

Primary Idiopathic Degenerative Joint Disease

The normal aging process in cartilage, just as the normal graying of hair, may be premature and accelerated in some individuals on a genetic basis; there may even be some unknown constitutional factor. In such individuals, the resultant degenerative joint disease involves many joints without any known pre-existing abnormality and is said to be *primary or idiopathic*. Continued use—and especially abuse—of a given joint accelerates the local degenerative process. Obesity, although not an initiating factor, aggravates any existing degeneration in weight-bearing joints, especially the knee joints.

Secondary Degenerative Joint Disease

The secondary type of degenerative joint disease is much more common than the primary, or idiopathic, type. Many types of injury, deformity, and disease are capable of producing the initial cartilage lesion that leads to the development of progressive secondary degenerative joint disease. It will be obvious to you that such etiological factors will have a greater effect on aging cartilage than on young cartilage; however, any age group may be affected. Understandably, secondary degenerative joint disease is more common in the weight-bearing joints of the lower limb than in the non-weight-bearing joints of the upper limb.

The following conditions are all capable of initiating the progressive degeneration in this secondary type of chronic arthritis:

- Congenital abnormalities of joints: for example, congenital dislocation of the hip (developmental dysplasia of the hip), clubfeet
- Infections of joints: for example, septic (pyogenic) arthritis, tuberculous arthritis
- Nonspecific inflammatory disorders of joints: for example, rheumatoid arthritis, ankylosing spondylitis
- Metabolic arthritis: for example, gout, pseudogout, ochronosis
- Repeated hemarthroses: for example, hemophilia
- Injury: 1) major trauma—intra-articular fractures, torn menisci; 2) microtrauma—occupational stresses
- Acquired incongruity of joint surfaces: for example, avascular necrosis, slipped capital femoral epiphysis
- Extra-articular deformities with malalignment of joints: for example, genu valgum (knock knee), genu varum (bow leg)
- Joint instability: for example, lax or torn ligaments, stretched capsule, subluxation
- Iatrogenic damage to cartilage: for example, continuous compression of joint surfaces during orthopaedic treatment of deformities (Salter).

Pathogenesis and Pathology in Synovial Joints

Whether degenerative joint disease is primary, secondary, or a combination of the two, the pathological process in the early stages is similar and represents a significant exaggeration of the previously described aging process. The local pathological process is best considered in relation to the various tissue components of the joint.

Articular Cartilage

The earliest biochemical change of degenerative joint disease is always in the articular cartilage and consists of a loss of proteoglycan from the matrix. The resultant change in the physical, or biomechanical, properties of the cartilage is softening (*chondromalacia*) and loss of the normal elastic resilience that gives cartilage its shock-absorbing ability. Thus, the collagen fibrils of the cartilage, having lost some of their support and having become "unmasked," are rendered more susceptible to the friction of joint function. As a result, shredding of the tangential surface layers of cartilage is accelerated and the deeper vertical layers split, with consequent *fissuring* and *fibrillation* (Fig. 11.1). The joint surface, which is normally bluish-white, smooth, and glistening, becomes yellowish, granular, and dull (Fig. 11.2).

As Mankin has stressed, the pathogenesis of osteoarthritis, far from being a passive "wear and tear" phenomenon, is characterized by much cellular and metabolic activity within the articular cartilage. Not only does the cartilage become more cellular, but the adult chondrocytes (which normally no longer divide) begin once again to divide as evidenced by clustering of cells and even cell mitoses. These activated chondrocytes synthesize proteoglycans and collagen at a greatly accelerated rate. Despite this valiant effort, however, the proteoglycan content is diminished because of the progressive destruction by lysosomal proteases (cathepsins) and neu-

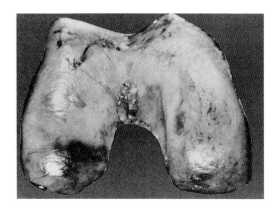

Figure 11.2. Degenerative arthritis as seen in the cartilage of the articular surface of the lower end of the femur (axial view from below). The cartilage was yellowish, granular and dull; in some areas it felt soft rather than rubbery. These abnormalities are most marked over the pressure areas: the weight-bearing surfaces of the femoral condyles and the load-bearing surfaces of the patellar groove.

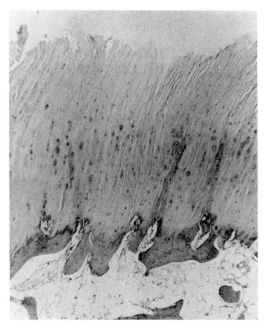

Figure 11.1. Fissuring and fibrillation of articular cartilage. This articular cartilage from a human arthritic joint exhibits a decreased number of chondrocytes in superficial layers, several deep vertical splits (fissuring) and innumerable superficial vertical splints (fibrillation).

tral metalloproteinases such as collagenase. Vascular invasion of the abnormal cartilage by vessels from the subchondral bone exposes the normally avascular cartilage to the systemic circulation for the first time and may lead to a type of self-perpetuating autoimmune disease that causes even further damage.

In the central area of the joint surface, which is exposed to the most friction, the softened, fibrillated cartilage is gradually abraded down to subchondral bone, which then serves as the articulating surface and gradually becomes as smooth as polished ivory (*eburnation*) (Fig. 11.3). The loss of articular cartilage is evidenced radiographically by a narrowing of the cartilage space (Fig. 11.4).

In the peripheral areas of the joint, the cartilage responds by hypertrophy and hyperplasia to form a thickened rim of cartilage around the joint margin. This outgrowth of cartilage (*chondrophyte*) subsequently undergoes endochondral ossification to become a bony outgrowth (*osteophyte*), also referred to as "osteoarthritic lipping" or "a bony spur." Osteophytes may become sufficiently large that they actually restrict joint motion (Figs. 11.3 and 11.4).

The loss of cartilage centrally and the building up of cartilage and bone peripherally pro-

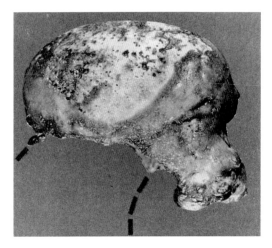

Figure 11.3. Advanced degenerative arthritis of the right hip as seen in the femoral head. The articular cartilage over the weight-bearing area as has been abraded down to subchondral bone which, in turn, has become eburnated to resemble polished ivory. The multiple pits in the eburnated surface represent arthritic cysts. The mass of bone growing out from the under-surface of the medial margin of the femoral head is a large osteophyte. This femoral head was excised at the time of prosthetic joint replacement arthroplasty in a 60-year-old man who had experienced increasing pain and loss of motion in the hip for 12 years.

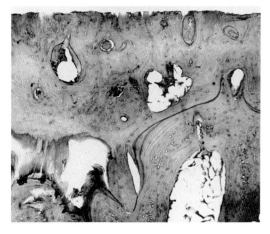

Figure 11.5. Hypertrophy of subchondral bone in an area of eburnation. This dense (sclerotic) bone has come to be the articulating surface and now resembles cortical bone. A similar type of bone is seen at the site labeled *B* in Figure 11.6.

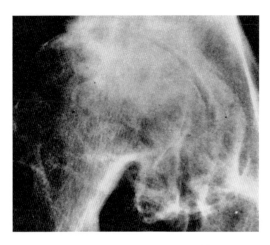

Figure 11.4. Preoperative radiograph of the same hip as that from which the femoral head shown in Figure 11.3 was excised. Narrowing of the cartilage space indicates loss of articular cartilage. Note the increased radiographic density (sclerosis) in the weight-bearing area on both sides of the joint; note also the large osteophyte growing out from the under-surface of the medial margin of the femoral head.

duce incongruity of the joint surfaces which, in turn, alters both the distribution and the magnitude of the biomechanical stresses on the joint. Some areas are subjected to much more stress than normal, whereas others are subjected to less than normal stress. Thus, the pathological process is self-perpetuating and a vicious cycle is established.

Subchondral Bone

Normal subchondral cancellous bone is stiffer than cartilage but much more resilient than dense cortical bone. As such, like cartilage, it also serves as a shock-absorber. The striking reaction of the subchondral bone in degenerative joint disease accounts for the synonyms *osteoarthritis* and *osteoarthrosis*. In the central area of maximum stress and friction, the subchondral bone, in addition to becoming eburnated, hypertrophies to the extent that it becomes radiographically dense (*sclerotic*) (Fig. 11.5). In the peripheral areas, however, where there is minimal stress, the subchondral bone atrophies and becomes radiographically less dense (*rarefied, i.e., osteoporotic*) (Fig. 11.6). Excessive pressure, particularly in weight-bearing joints such as the hip, leads to the development of *cystic lesions* within the subchondral bone marrow, possibly because of mucoid and fibrinous degeneration in the local tissues

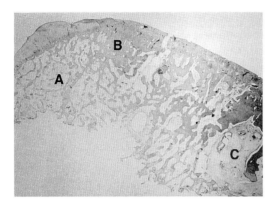

Figure 11.6. Low-power photomicrograph of part of a femoral head excised at operation. In the peripheral, non-weight-bearing area (**A**), the cancellous bone has atrophied. In the weight-bearing area (**B**), the cancellous bone has responded to excessive pressures by becoming hypertrophied. Note also the large cystic lesion (**C**) under an area of weight-bearing. This arthritic "cyst" contained fibrous tissue.

secondary to microfractures of trabeculae. These "cysts" may even communicate with the joint surface through defects in the subchondral bone, in which case they contain either fibrous tissue (Fig. 11.6) or synovial fluid (Fig. 11.7). The increased vascularity associated with these bony reactions in a closed space within the bone may be a factor in the production of pain.

The redistribution of biomechanical stresses on the joint leads to a *remodeling* of the subchondral bone; bone is worn away centrally but deposited (by endochondral ossification of the deep layer of cartilage) peripherally. Such remodeling accentuates the previously mentioned joint incongruity and contributes to the vicious cycle of degeneration (Fig. 11.8).

Synovial Membrane and Fibrous Capsule
Small fragments of abraded dead cartilage may float in the synovial fluid as loose bodies but tend to become incorporated in the synovial membrane which, in turn, reacts by undergoing hypertrophy and producing a moderate synovial effusion. The synovial fluid of such an effusion has an increased mucin content and consequently exhibits increased viscosity.

The fibrous capsule becomes greatly thick-

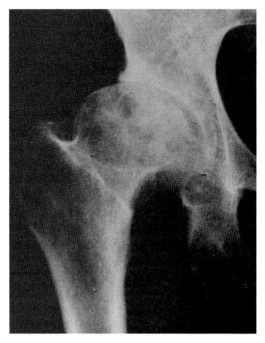

Figure 11.7. Right hip of a 65-year-old woman with degenerative arthritis. Note the large cystic lesion under the weight-bearing area of the femoral head. At operation this cyst was found to communicate with the joint cavity; it contained synovial fluid.

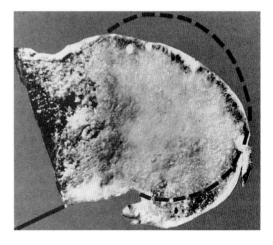

Figure 11.8. Cut surface of the femoral head from the arthritic hip of a 54-year-old man. The present shape of the femoral head is the result of gradual remodeling from the original shape (dotted lines). Such remodeling accentuates incongruity of the joint and contributes to the vicious cycle of degeneration.

ened and fibrotic, thereby further limiting joint motion. In the joints of the fingers, especially the distal interphalangeal joints, small areas of mucoid degeneration in the fibrous capsule at the joint margin form small subcutaneous protuberances which subsequently ossify and are known as *Heberden's nodes* (Fig. 11.9). Nevertheless, Heberden's nodes are not necessarily a manifestation of degenerative joint disease because the cartilage of the subjacent joint is usually normal.

Muscles

The muscles controlling the affected joint develop spasm in response to pain and eventually the stronger muscles (usually the flexors) undergo *contracture* with resultant joint deformity and further restriction of joint motion. With limited joint motion the excessive stresses are applied to a limited area of joint cartilage; this is another factor in the process of degeneration. The late result may be a *fibrous ankylosis* of the joint, but *bony ankylosis* seldom occurs spontaneously in degenerative joint disease.

Clinical Features and Diagnosis

Because there are no systemic manifestations of degenerative joint disease, the symptoms and signs are confined to individual joints.

Although articular cartilage has no nerve fibers, and hence no sensation, the predominant symptom in degenerative joint disease is *pain* that arises from bone and from the synovial membrane, fibrous capsule, and the spasm of surrounding muscles. The pain is at first a dull ache and later is more severe; it is intermittent and aggravated by joint movement ("friction effect") and relieved by rest. Eventually, however, the patient may even experience "*resting pain*," which is probably related to the hyperemia and consequent "intraosseous hypertension" in the subchondral bone. Characteristically, the pain is worse when the barometric pressure falls just before a period of inclement weather. Paradoxically, the severity of the patient's pain is not necessarily related to the severity of the degenerative joint disease as evidenced by radiographic changes, but this may be caused by individual differences in pain threshold as well as by differences in joint motion and the amount the joint is being used. Injuries, such as sudden strains or sprains, in an arthritic joint always aggravate the pre-existing symptoms.

The patient may become aware that the joint motion is no longer smooth and that it is associated with various types of *joint crepitus* such as squeaking, creaking, and grating. The joint tends to become stiff after a period of rest, a phenomenon referred to as *articular gelling*. Gradually, the involved joint loses more and more motion and eventually may even become so stiff that the pain (which is associated with motion) is decreased.

Physical examination reveals swelling of the joint caused by a moderate effusion but there is relatively little synovial thickening; the joint swelling is more obvious because of the atrophy of surrounding muscles. There is no increased warmth of the overlying skin. Both active and passive joint motion are restricted and associated with joint crepitus, as well as pain and muscle spasm at the extremes of the existing range of motion. In the primary, or idiopathic, type of degenerative joint disease, Heberden's nodes are frequently seen at the distal interphalangeal joints (Fig. 11.9); they are more common in women but their exact relationship to degenerative joint disease is not clearly understood. Similar nodular lesions in the proximal interphalangeal joints are known as Bouchard's nodes.

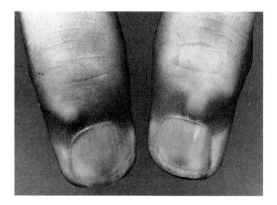

Figure 11.9. Heberden's nodes, which arise from the fibrous capsule at the margin of the distal interphalangeal joints.

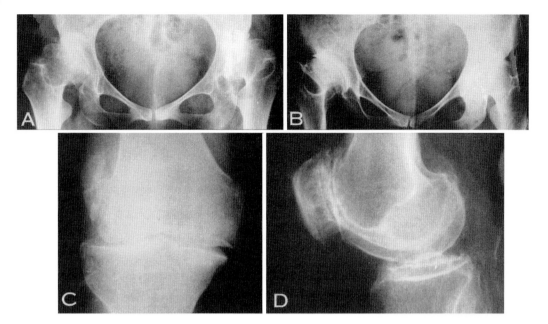

Figure 11.10. Radiographic changes of degenerative arthritis. **A.** Bilateral degenerative arthritis of the hips in a 36-year-old woman who had been treated for congenital dislocation of the hips at the age of 3 years. Both hips are subluxated, the left more so than the right. Note the joint incongruity, sclerosis, osteophytes, cysts, and narrowing of the cartilage space in both hip joints. **B.** Bilateral degenerative arthritis of the hips in a 40-year-old woman who had been treated for congenital dislocation of the hips at the age of 4 years. The right femoral head had undergone avascular necrosis. Note the joint incongruity, subchondral sclerosis and remodeling. C and D, degenerative arthritis of the knee of a 75-year-old man. Note the large osteophytes, subchondral sclerosis, and narrowing of the cartilage space of the knee joint, including the patella-femoral component.

Radiographic examination reveals changes that are readily correlated with the pathological process. They include narrowing of the cartilage space, subchondral sclerosis and cysts, osteophyte formation, joint remodeling, and incongruity (Figs. 11.4, 11.7, 11.10).

Laboratory examination does not reveal any evidence of systemic disease, but the synovial fluid exhibits an increased mucin content and increased viscosity.

In each individual patient with degenerative joint disease, you should attempt to determine whether the disease is primary—that is, idiopathic—or secondary; if it is secondary, you should diagnose the underlying condition.

Prognosis

Although virtually every person who reaches old age has some degree of degenerative disease in one or more joints, many experience only mild, annoying discomfort that they ascribe, quite rightly, to "getting old" or to "a touch of rheumatism." When a given joint is severely involved, however, and the patient continues to use that joint, the course is one of progressive deterioration with increasing pain and loss of motion, unless the joint eventually becomes so stiff that the pain is decreased. Such stiffness is more likely to develop in the joints of the upper limbs and spine; indeed, low back pain caused by degenerative joint disease is much less common in the elderly than in the middle aged, presumably because the arthritic spine eventually becomes relatively stiff and stable and also fewer demands are made on it.

In the lower limbs, degenerative joint disease has a relatively bad prognosis because of the continuing demands put on the affected joint with ordinary walking. This is particularly true in the hip joint, and when both hip joints are arthritic, the disability is very severe indeed.

Treatment

Although there is, as yet, no specific cure for degenerative joint disease and although the pathological lesions, being related to the aging process, tend to be permanent and progressive, much can be accomplished therapeutically for afflicted patients provided that the treatment, both general and local, is tailored to fit the needs of each involved joint and each patient. Indeed, by means of local treatment, there is some hope of at least retarding, if not reversing, the pathological process.

Aims of Treatment

The overall management of a patient with degenerative joint disease is based on the same general aims for rheumatoid arthritis outlined in the preceding chapter, although the methods used to achieve these aims are somewhat different. The aims are as follows: 1) to help the patient understand the nature of the disease; 2) to provide psychological support; 3) to alleviate pain; 4) to suppress the inflammatory reaction (in the synovial membrane); 5) to encourage the patient to remain as physically active as possible in order to maintain joint function and prevent deformity; 6) to correct existing deformity; 7) to improve function; 8) to strengthen weak muscles; and 9) to rehabilitate the individual patient.

Methods of Treatment
Psychological Considerations

The patient with degenerative joint disease needs to be reassured that the local condition of his or her joint or joints is simply an exaggeration of the normal aging process, or "wearing out" of joints, with increasing age and furthermore that he or she does not have a generalized disease such as the generalized rheumatoid disease associated with rheumatoid arthritis (as described in Chapter 10). The patient is then better prepared to live within the limits imposed by the painful joints. This implies a combination of rest and exercise, with avoidance of long periods of either. Overweight patients with degenerative disease in a weight-bearing joint must be encouraged to lose weight, with the understanding that

this will decrease the load on the affected joint and thereby help to retard the progression of the arthritic process.

Therapeutic Drugs

Salicylates, either in the form of aspirin or sodium salicylate, are the most useful drugs in the treatment of degenerative joint disease, not only because they relieve pain in moderate doses but also because they may inhibit cartilage deterioration and may even exert a beneficial effect on the regeneration of cartilage. More powerful (and more dangerous) nonsteroidal, anti-inflammatory drugs (NSAIDs) such as indomethacin and phenylbutazone are effective in relieving severe pain for some patients, but their toxic effects tend to outweigh their beneficial effects. Nevertheless, phenylbutazone and related drugs can often be administered by experienced physicians with much benefit to the patient. Narcotics should not be prescribed. The systemic administration of adrenocorticosteroids is of no value. Local intra-articular injections of corticosteroids, such as hydrocortisone, may produce temporary relief of joint pain but should not be repeated at frequent intervals in a given joint because of harmful effects on articular cartilage (Salter).

Investigators are continuing to seek therapeutic agents that inhibit cartilage degradation, stimulate cartilage regeneration, or both, with the aim of retarding or even reversing the disease process.

Orthopaedic Appliances

In addition to adequate periods of general rest, local rest of degenerated joints using removable splints is of value, not only in relieving pain but also in preventing deformity. Day braces are of limited value. When the hip is affected, the patient can take much weight off the joint by walking with a cane held in the hand of side opposite the affected hip (Fig. 11.11). When both hips are affected, the patient may need to use two canes or even crutches (Fig. 11.12). The same is true when one or both knees are affected.

Physical Therapy

Active movements of involved joints within the limits of pain are important in an attempt to preserve joint motion and maintain muscle

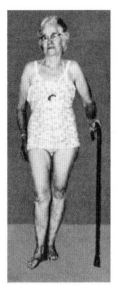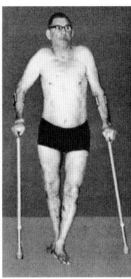

Figure 11.11. This woman with degenerative arthritis of the right hip is taking weight off the hip joint by taking some weight on a cane on the opposite side. Note the adduction, external rotation contracture of the right hip. Her cane should be shortened to enable her to almost completely extend her elbow and thereby take more weight through the cane.

Figure 11.12. This man with bilateral degenerative arthritis of the hips is taking weight off both hip joints by putting some weight on two crutches. His left crutch is the correct length but his right crutch is too long. Note the adduction and external rotation contracture of both hips.

strength; excessive exercising (especially against resistance), however, tends to aggravate the condition. Local heat by any means, including heating pads and infrared lamps, frequently provides temporary relief of pain.

Orthopaedic Surgical Operations

Prophylactic. Arthroscopic débridement and irrigation of large joints, primarily the knee, as recommended by Aichroth and colleagues, seems to provide at least temporary relief of pain in many patients. Degenerative changes can often be prevented, or at least delayed and sometimes even reversed, by surgical correction of joint conditions that are destined to cause the secondary type of degenerative joint disease—conditions such as marked genu valgum (knock knee) (Fig. 11.18), marked genu varum (bow leg) (Fig. 11.20), and residual congenital subluxation of the hip (Figs. 11.24 and 11.25).

Therapeutic Procedures. Surgical operations for the treatment of degenerative joint disease should be considered at a relatively early stage and not as a last resort because once the degenerative changes have become severe, only destructive operations can be expected to improve the situation. Nevertheless, considerable surgical judgment is required to assess the needs of each patient accurately and to choose the most effective method of surgical treatment as well as the optimal timing for such intervention. (For illustrations of the various bone and joint operations, please see Chapter 6, Figures 6.9 to 6.31).

Surgical operations that are effective for one joint may not be practical for another, but in general the types of operation that are performed for degenerative joint disease are the following:

1. *Osteotomy* near the joint: this is performed to improve the biomechanics of the joint, especially the alignment, and to bring a different area of joint cartilage into function (Figs. 11.19 and 11.21).
2. *Arthroplasty* (reconstruction of a joint): this consists of *resection arthroplasty* and replacement arthroplasty, that is, prosthetic joint replacement of either one or both sides of the joint using either cemented or noncemented prostheses (Figs. 11.22 and 11.27).
3. *Arthrodesis* (fusion of a joint): this provides permanent relief of pain but at the expense of permanent loss of all motion.
4. *Soft tissue operations:* release of tight muscles and excision of contracted capsule are usually performed in conjunction with an arthroplasty; these operations are occasionally performed to correct a severe joint contracture, but by themselves tend to provide only temporary relief of pain.
5. *Transplantation of partial joints:* this involves the transplantation of osteocartilaginous allografts for post-traumatic arthritis in young adults as recommended by Gross.
6. *Experimental methods:* A number of experimental investigations designed to produce a "biological resurfacing" of a full-thickness defect in articular cartilage have been reported including the use of autogenous

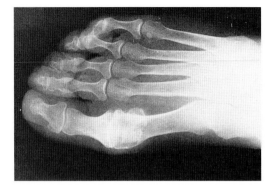

Figure 11.13. Hallux rigidus—degenerative arthritis in the metacarpophalangeal joint of the great toe. Note the narrowed cartilage space, cyst formation, osteophytes, and sclerosis.

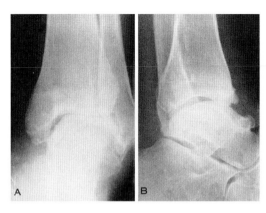

Figure 11.16. Traumatic arthritis of the left ankle in a 57-year-old man who had injured his ankle 25 years previously. Note the joint incongruity and the osteophytes.

periosteal grafts in the author's laboratory (O'Driscoll and colleagues) and cultured chondrocytes covered by periosteal grafts (Brittberg and colleagues).

Surgical Treatment of Degenerative Joint Disease in Specific Synovial Joints

Foot and Ankle

Degenerative joint disease in the metatarsophalangeal joint of the great toe, without deformity, is called *hallux rigidus* (Fig. 11.13).

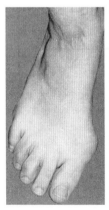
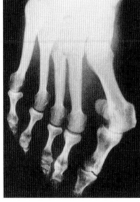

Figure 11.14. Hallux valgus of long duration in a 52-year-old woman who complained of increasing pain in the toe.

Figure 11.15. Supero-inferior radiograph of the same foot as shown in 11.14; note the narrowing of the metatarsophalangeal joint, which is subluxated.

Local treatment is either arthrodesis or resection arthroplasty (usually resection of the proximal half of the proximal phalanx). Degenerative changes can also develop secondary to a long standing deformity such as *hallux valgus* (Figs. 11.14 and 11.15), in which case the treatment is usually resection of the proximal half of the proximal phalanx (the Keller operation) combined with excision of the prominent medial portion of the metatarsal head. For the most severe degrees of osteoarthritis secondary to hallux valgus, arthrodesis may be required.

Involvement of the tarsal joints, which is usually secondary to residual deformity, may require arthrodesis of the involved joints. Likewise, degenerative joint disease of the ankle, which is most frequently secondary to trauma (Fig. 11.16), is best treated by arthrodesis.

Knee

The initial site of degenerative joint disease in the knee is frequently the articular cartilage of the posterior surface of the patella (which is a sesamoid bone in the quadriceps mechanism). Characterized by softening (malacia), fissuring and fibrillation of the cartilage, this common disorder is referred to as *chondromalacia patellae* (Fig. 11.17). The most typical symptom is retropatellar pain that is aggravated by going up or down stairs and by running. Al-

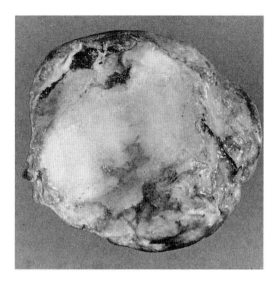

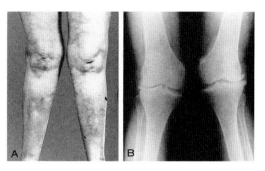

Figure 11.18. **A.** Bilateral genu valgum in a 61-year-old woman who complained of pain on the lateral aspect of both knees. **B.** The radiograph reveals degenerative arthritis of the lateral compartment of both knees secondary to the excessive pressures related to genu valgum.

Figure 11.17. Articular surface of an excised patella with severe and extensive chondromalacia. The cartilage is not only irregular, but also soft.

though the patella is certainly the most frequent site of chondromalacia, this disorder tends to be over-diagnosed, especially in adolescent girls. Non-operative treatment includes regular quadriceps exercise and salicylates. When true chondromalacia has been diagnosed by arthroscopic examination and when there is definite evidence of patellar malalignment (usually lateral "tracking"), a soft tissue procedure such as surgical release of the tight lateral retinaculum may provide relief of symptoms—at least for a few years. Surgical

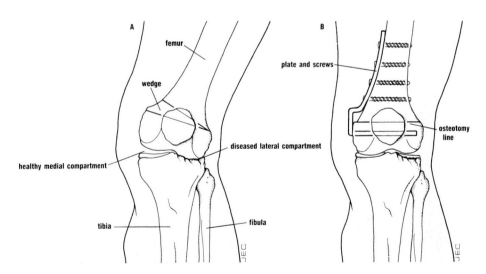

Figure 11.19. **A.** Genu valgum with secondary degenerative arthritis in the lateral compartment of the knee due to excessive load-bearing. The site and size of the wedge to be removed from the lower end of the femur are shown. **B.** Post-supracondylar osteotomy of the femur. The wedge of bone has been removed and the gap has been closed (a "closed-wedge" osteotomy) to correct the genu valgum. The osteotomy site has been secured by "internal fixation" using a blade plate and screws. Note that the lateral compartment of the knee joint has been unloaded.

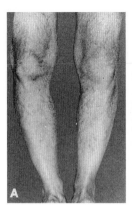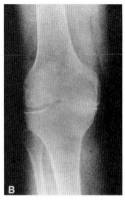

Figure 11.20. **A.** Genu varum of the right knee in a 65-year-old man who complained of pain on the medial aspect of the knee. **B.** The radiograph reveals degenerative arthritis of the medial compartment of the knee secondary to the excessive pressures related to the genu varum.

surface of the patella and that of the patellar groove of the femur.

McLaren and colleagues have reported that arthroscopic débridement and irrigation of an osteoarthritic knee joint provides relief of pain in 60% of patients for at least 2 years.

Although both chondral shaving and subchondral abrasion of the abnormal cartilage—either at open operation or through the arthroscope—smooth the joint surface and often decrease the patient's symptoms, mature hyaline articular cartilage is unable to regenerate unless the subchondral bone is entered to provide access to the pluripotential mesenchymal cells as demonstrated in the rabbit by the author and his colleagues (Kim et al.). In the middle-aged and the elderly, chondromalacia of the patella may lead to patellofemoral arthritis of sufficient severity that excision of the patella (patellectomy) is required.

Degenerative joint disease of the lateral compartment of the knee joint, secondary to long-standing genu valgum, can be improved by a closed-wedge supracondylar osteotomy of the femur (Figs. 11.18 and 11.19). Such

elevation of the tibial tubercle (i.e., the insertion of the patellar tendon) as recommended by Maquet may also relieve pain by decreasing the pressure and friction between the cartilage

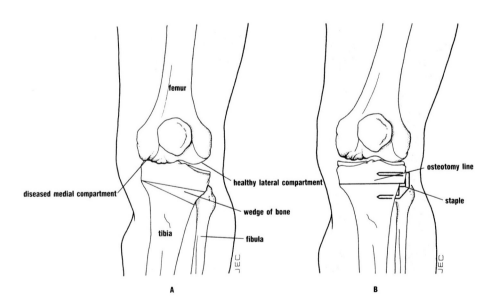

Figure 11.21. **A.** Genu varum with secondary degenerative arthritis in the medial compartment of the knee due to excessive load-bearing. The site and size of the wedge to be removed from the upper end of the tibia are shown. **B.** Post-high tibial osteotomy. The wedge of bone has been removed and the gap has been closed (a "closed-wedge" osteotomy) to correct the genu varum. The osteotomy site has been secured by "internal fixation" using a staple. Note that the medial compartment of the knee joint has been unloaded.

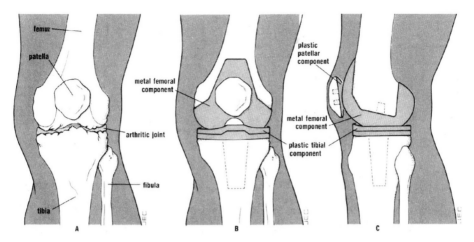

Figure 11.22. **A.** Severe, irreversible arthritis of both the medial and lateral compartments of the knee. **B** and **C.** A total prosthetic knee joint replacement for the femoral and the tibial joint surfaces of both the medial and the lateral compartments and also the patellar joint surface.

disease of the medial compartment secondary to long standing genu varum can be improved by a closed-wedge osteotomy of the upper end of the tibia (Figs. 11.20 and 21). These operations are designed to improve the joint alignment and thereby redistribute the biomechanical forces to the more normal side of the joint. When severe cartilage destruction involves either the medial compartment or the lateral compartment alone, a unicompartmental replacement arthroplasty is required. When the joint is irreparably damaged, however, a total prosthetic knee joint replacement is indicated (Fig. 11.22). McInnes and colleagues have reported that the use of continuous passive motion (CPM) after total prosthetic knee joint replacement (arthroplasty) improved the range of knee joint motion, decreased swelling, reduced the need for postoperative manipulation of the knee under anesthetic and was more cost effective than conventional postoperative treatment.

Hip

Degenerative joint disease of the hip represents one of the most challenging clinical problems for even the most experienced orthopaedic surgeon and taxes both clinical judgment and surgical skill. The disease may

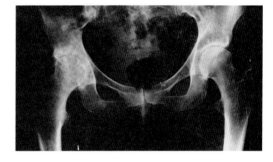

Figure 11.23. Primary (idiopathic) degenerative arthritis of the right hip (malum coxae senilis) in a 60-year-old woman who had no known preexisting abnormality of the hip. She required a total prosthetic joint replacement.

be *primary* (i.e., idiopathic), in which case it is sometimes referred to as *malum coxae senilis* (Fig. 11.23). Much more often, however, the disease is *secondary* to the sequelae of conditions such as avascular necrosis, slipped femoral epiphysis, and congenital dislocation of the hip (Fig. 11.24). Because of the complex biomechanics of the hip joint and the magnitude of stresses and forces to which a subluxated hip is subjected, the secondary degenerative hip joint disease is relentlessly progressive and

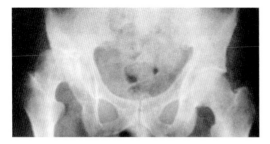

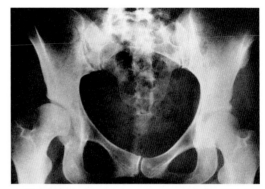

Figure 11.24.   Degenerative arthritis of the right hip in a 32-year-old woman secondary to treated congenital dislocation. She was too young for a total prosthetic joint replacement but gained relief of pain from a medial displacement (Chiari) type of pelvic osteotomy.

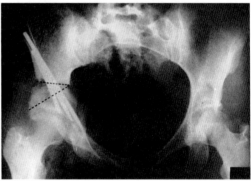

disabling (Fig. 11.25). For a young adult with residual congenital subluxation of the hip and early, hence mild, secondary degenerative arthritis, a femoral osteotomy or an innominate (Salter) osteotomy (Fig. 11.26), or a combination of the two, have been proven effective. A variety of other pelvic osteotomies for adults have been described by a number of surgeons including Chiari, Steel, Eppright, Wagner, and Ganz. For an older patient with either primary or secondary degenerative arthritis that is severe, and hence irreversible, total excision of the joint and prosthetic joint replace-

Figure 11.26.   Above. A-P radiograph of the pelvis and hip joints of a 34-year-old woman who complained of pain in the area of the right hip associated with a limp. Note the residual congenital subluxation of the right hip and the abnormal direction of the right acetabulum compared to the normal left hip. **Below.** The A-P radiograph of the same patient's pelvis and hips immediately after a single innominate osteotomy of the right hip (Salter) that has redirected the acetabulum and thereby corrected the subluxation. The site of the wedge-shaped bone graft in this "open-wedge" type of osteotomy is indicated by the dotted line. The three large threaded pins will maintain the position of the osteotomy and the graft and will subsequently be removed when bony union is solid.

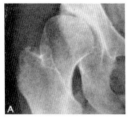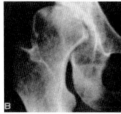

Figure 11.25.   A. Early degenerative arthritis of the right hip secondary to residual congenital subluxation of the hip in a 38-year-old woman. Symptoms at this stage were minimal but she could have been treated at this stage with the combination of a femoral and innominate (Salter) osteotomy to prevent progression of the disease. **B.** The same hip only 2 years later (without treatment) reveals that the degenerative joint disease has been relentlessly progressive. Note that the subluxation has increased. The symptoms at this time were more severe.

ment (Charnley), that is, a "total hip" (Fig. 11.27) is indicated. Indeed, this highly successful operation is one of the most cost-effective of all surgical procedures.

In general it may be stated that an osteotomy should be performed before the disease is far advanced, that prosthetic joint replacement is better restricted to the older patient (preferably older than 55 years) and that arthrodesis is most useful when only one hip is irreversibly affected in an adolescent or a relatively young adult.

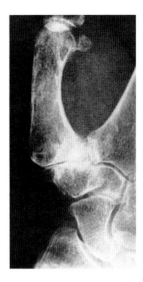

Figure 11.28.   Degenerative arthritis of the carpometacarpal joint at the base of the thumb in a 33-year-old man who had sustained a fracture dislocation of this joint 10 years earlier.

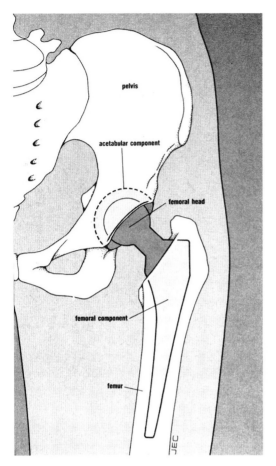

Figure 11.27.   Total prosthetic hip joint replacement for both the acetabular and the femoral joint surfaces after total excision of a severely arthritic hip joint (Charnley).

Hand and Wrist

Despite the obvious deformity caused by Heberden's nodes (Fig. 11.9), surgical treatment is seldom required for the hand and wrist. However, degenerative joint disease of the first carpometacarpal joint at the base of the thumb (Fig. 11.28) may be sufficiently disabling to require arthrodesis.

Involvement of the wrist is usually secondary to trauma (Fig. 11.29) and less commonly to avascular necrosis of the lunate bone (Kienböck's disease). If the arthritis does not respond to nonoperative methods of treatment, it is best treated by arthrodesis of the wrist in the functional position of slight dorsiflexion.

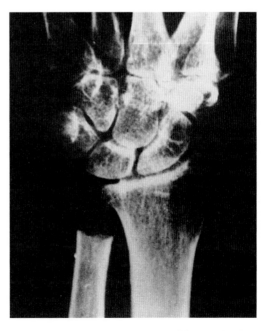

Figure 11.29.   Traumatic arthritis of the wrist in a 50-year-old man who had sustained a fracture of the distal end of the radius and ulna 8 years earlier. The distal end of the ulna had already been resected to relieve pain.

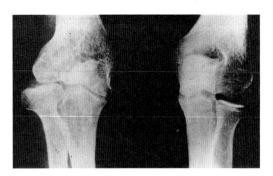

Figure 11.30.   Traumatic arthritis of the right radio-humeral joint in a 16-year-old boy who had sustained a fracture of the lateral condyle of the humerus at the age of 5 with a subsequent growth disturbance and secondary overgrowth of the radial head.

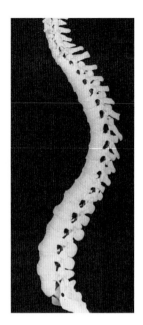

Figure 11.31.   Lateral view of the human spinal column. The lumbar and cervical segments of the spine are lordotic and mobile, whereas the thoracic segment is kyphotic and relatively immobile.

Elbow

Degenerative joint disease of the elbow is almost always of the secondary type and is frequently post-traumatic (Fig. 11.30). When the disease is limited to the radiohumeral joint, excision of the radial head is effective. When the entire joint is destroyed, prosthetic joint replacement may be necessary.

Shoulder

Osteoarthritis of the shoulder (glenohumeral) joint is not common, but it can be disabling. In the early stages, a soft tissue operation consisting of division of the coracoacromial ligament, transection of the subscapularis muscle, and capsulotomy of the joint often suffices to restore painless mobility of the shoulder. For more severe degrees of osteoarthritis, a prosthetic joint replacement may be required. Involvement of the acromioclavicular joint responds well to excision arthroplasty.

DEGENERATIVE JOINT DISEASE IN THE SPINE

Degenerative joint disease is even more common in the spinal column than in the limbs. This is not surprising when you consider the magnitude of the stresses and strains (partly related to the human upright position) that are applied to the spine during both work and play throughout a lifetime. Furthermore, the number of spinal joints is large—23 intervertebral disc joints and 46 posterior facet (apophyseal) joints. In addition, the intervertebral disc is the first structure in the musculoskeletal system to become affected by the degenerative changes of the normal aging process. Understandably, the incidence of such changes is higher in the more mobile lordotic segments of the lumbar and cervical spine than in the less mobile kyphotic segments of the thoracic spine (Fig. 11.31).

Form and Function of the Spinal Joints

The spine is an articulated column of vertebrae, each "couplet" of which is able to move through an intervertebral disc joint and two posterior facet joints. An abnormality of either type of joint has a deleterious effect on the other, a point of great importance in understanding the development of degenerative joint disease in the spine.

Intervertebral Disc Joints

Each intervertebral disc joint is a *symphysis* that forms a "coupling unit" between two vertebral bodies; it is comprised of three parts: the *nucleus pulposus*, the *annulus fibrosis*, and the *hyaline cartilage end plates* of the opposing surfaces of each vertebral body (Fig. 11.32).

In youth, the obliquely interlacing bands of fibrous tissue in the annulus fibrosus provide the annulus with *elasticity* that opposes the *turgor* of the nucleus pulposus, an incompressible gel containing proteoglycans. Normally, with flexion, extension, and lateral bending, the vertebral bodies roll over the turgid nucleus pulposus, which thus behaves like a ball bearing. The normal nucleus pulposus contains neither nerves nor blood vessels and is nourished by diffusion of tissue fluids through minute channels in the cartilage end plates of the vertebral bodies. The nucleus is much more resilient, and therefore more resistant to injury, than the subchondral cancellous bone of the vertebral body.

Posterior Facet Joints

The posterior facet (apophyseal) joints are of the *diarthrodial*, or *synovial*, type; they serve to guide, steady, and limit the movements of the vertebral bodies on one another. Being true synovial joints, they are composed of a *fibrous capsule*, *synovial membrane*, and *articular cartilage surfaces* (Fig. 11.33).

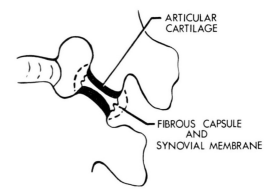

Figure 11.33. Lateral view of a normal posterior facet joint.

DEGENERATIVE JOINT DISEASE IN THE LUMBAR SPINE

Degenerative disease in the lumbar spine includes two interrelated conditions; one involves the intervertebral disc joints (*degenerative disc disease*), and the other, the posterior facet joints (*degenerative joint disease, osteoarthritis*). The latter condition is comparable to the degenerative disease of synovial joints in the limbs already described in this chapter. Both degenerative disc disease and degenerative joint disease represent an exaggeration of the normal aging process and may be aggravated by injury, deformity, and pre-existing disease of the spine. The resultant low back pain is the most common of all musculoskeletal symptoms. It has been estimated that 80% of adults, at least once in their lives, will suffer one or more episodes of back pain severe enough to stop them from working temporarily. Indeed, in young adult workers, back pain is the number one cause of disability that lasts more than 2 weeks and in older adults it is the number two cause after arthritis and nonarticular rheumatism combined.

Etiology

There are many causes of acute and chronic low back pain, including:

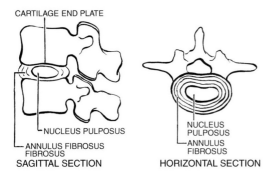

Figure 11.32. Components of the normal intervertebral disc joint in the human as seen in sagittal and horizontal sections.

- Mechanical factors: weakness of trunk muscles from inadequate physical exercise, obesity, poor posture, poor working habits

- Chemical factors: epidemiological investigations have revealed that the incidence of acute and chronic low back pain is three times greater in smokers than in non-smokers
- Specific injury: falls, motor vehicle accidents, sports injuries, lifting heavy objects from the floor without bending the knees (a preventable injury)
- Spondylolisthesis (as described in Chapter 13)
- Infection: hematogenous osteomyelitis of the spine, that is, spondylarthritis (as described in Chapter 10)
- Neoplasm: benign or malignant, primary or secondary (as described in Chapter 14)

Pathogenesis and Pathology

The interrelated degenerative processes of intervertebral disc disease and posterior facet joint disease in the lumbar spine are best considered under the headings of *disc degeneration, segmental instability, segmental hyperextension, segmental narrowing,* and *herniation of the intervertebral disc.*

Disc Degeneration

The initial degeneration in the human spinal column occurs in the nucleus pulposus. Beginning in early adult life and progressing slowly thereafter, this degeneration is characterized by a gradual loss of chondroitin sulfate and water content, with a resultant loss of turgor and resilience as well as a loss of actual height, or thickness, of the disc space. As the nucleus pulposus loses fluid, that is, becomes inspissated, its gelatinous ground substance loses its homogeneous texture and becomes somewhat lumpy. Although all of these degenerative changes may be considered within normal limits in an individual older than 60 years of age, they are considered abnormal if they develop to an advanced stage prematurely in a young person.

With increasing age, the annulus fibrosus gradually loses some of its elasticity, particularly posteriorly where it is relatively thin. Thus, its posterior fibers become more easily separated, or even torn, and this is one site of weakness in the annulus through which the nucleus pulposus may protrude or herniate. A

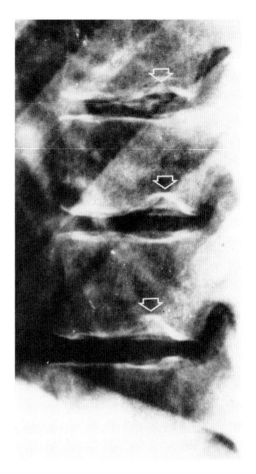

Figure 11.34.   Lateral radiograph of a portion of the thoracic spine showing Schmorl's nodes in three vertebral bodies (*arrows*).

second site of weakness is the thin cartilage end plate through which nuclear material may protrude into the underlying cancellous bone of the vertebral body and thereby form a *Schmorl's node* (Fig. 11.34). Schmorl's nodes are common radiographic findings but are of little clinical significance. Protrusion of the nucleus pulposus and annulus into the spinal canal, by contrast, is clinically very significant. It occurs more readily in relatively young individuals in whom the nucleus pulposus still exhibits considerable turgor; it is rare in persons older than 50 years of age.

Segmental Instability

As a result of degenerative changes in the intervertebral disc joints, smooth motion in

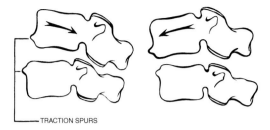

Figure 11.35. Lateral view of segmental instability at an intervertebral disc joint with resultant "traction spurs."

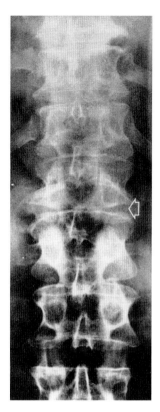

Figure 11.37. Spine of a 63-year-old man showing segmental narrowing at the intervertebral disc between the first and second lumbar vertebrae (*arrow*). Note the osteophytes arising from the bony margins of the adjoining vertebrae.

each involved segment of the spine is lost and is replaced by motion that is not only uneven, but also excessive. In this stage of segmental instability, the joint margins react by forming small "traction spurs," which are a form of osteophyte (Fig. 11.35). The unstable segments become more susceptible to injury, which, in turn, may produce a sprain or even a subluxation of the posterior facet joints.

Segmental Hyperextension

Normal extension of the lumbar spine is limited by the anterior fibers of the annulus fibrosus as well as by the abdominal muscles. However, the combination of degenerative changes in the annulus fibrosis, flabbiness of the abdominal muscles and obesity, leads to persistent hyperextension of the lumbar spine through the intervertebral joints. Consequently, the posterior facet joints are chronically strained and may even subluxate posteriorly (Fig. 11.36). Such malalignment causes degenerative joint disease (osteoarthritis) in these synovial joints, with loss of articular car-

tilage, eburnation of subchondral bone, formation of osteophytes, and resultant pain.

Segmental Narrowing

Progressive narrowing of the intervertebral disc space with increasing age leads not only to degenerative changes in the posterior facet joints, but also to bulging of the annulus fibrosus, which causes large osteophytes to develop from the bony margins of the adjoining vertebral bodies (*spondylosis, spinal osteophytosis*) (Fig. 11.37). Such osteophytes are detectable radiographically in 90% of individuals older than 60 years of age. At this stage, the narrowed intervertebral joint has lost much of its motion; thus, the joint, having become relatively stiff, is less likely to be painful. This explains the high incidence of low back pain in early adult life and middle age,

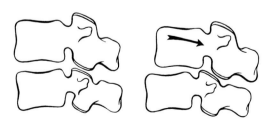

Figure 11.36. Lateral view of segmental hyperextension at an intervertebral disc joint with resultant posterior subluxation of the posterior facet joint.

when radiographic changes are minimal, and the low incidence of low back pain in the elderly, when radiographic changes are maximal.

Herniation of the Intervertebral Disc

Herniation (prolapse, protrusion, extrusion, rupture) of the intervertebral disc is not synonymous with degeneration of the disc; rather, it is a specific event that occurs as a complication of disc degeneration. The layman refers to it as a "slipped disc." Disc herniation is most frequent in relatively young individuals, particularly males, and the most common sites in the lumbar region are L-4–5, L-5–S-1 and L-3–4, in that order.

The nucleus pulposus, having no nerves, is insensitive, but as it begins to herniate posteriorly, it stretches the sensitive annulus fibrosus and causes pain. Subsequently, the stretched and degenerated fibers of the annulus separate and part of the nucleus herniates. Because the posterior longitudinal ligament covers the annulus in the midline, the herniation tends to be posterolateral (Fig. 11.38). A posterolateral herniation either compresses or stretches the nerve root that leaves the intervertebral foramen distal to the disc; thus, a herniation of the L-4–5 disc affects the fifth lumbar nerve root, whereas a herniation of the L-5–S-1 disc affects the first sacral nerve root. The clinical manifestation of such nerve root irritation is *sciatica*, pain that radiates down the lower limb in the distribution of the sciatic nerve. A large herniation in the midline of the lumbar spine compresses the cauda equina.

The herniated portion of the nucleus pulposus becomes dehydrated and firm. Previously avascular, it may even become vascularized, in which case the reaction to it might be in the nature of an autoimmune response. Eventually, several weeks after the event, the herniated portion of the nucleus undergoes fibrosis, shrinks, and thereby relieves the pressure on the nerve root. Occasionally, however, the herniated portion becomes separated, or sequestrated, and may even migrate either proximally or distally.

Spinal Stenosis

A bony narrowing of the spinal canal either centrally or in its lateral recesses (including the intervertebral foramina) is referred to as *spinal stenosis*. When the stenosis is central, the cauda equina is compressed, whereas when the stenosis is lateral, it is the emerging nerve roots and their blood supply that are compressed. In either case, the collective synonym *bony nerve root entrapment syndromes* is frequently used. Spinal stenosis may be congenital (as seen in association with achondroplastic dwarfism) or it may be acquired (as seen secondary to advanced disc degeneration, segmental narrowing, subluxation of the posterior facet joints or even secondary to a previous spinal fusion).

Clinical Features and Diagnosis of Various Syndromes in the Lumbar Spine

The various clinical manifestations of degenerative joint disease in the lumbar spine are best considered in relation to the phases of its pathogenesis described earlier. Disc degeneration, by itself, causes neither symptoms nor signs; indeed, the clinical syndromes in the lumbar spine are caused by the secondary effects of disc degeneration; namely, segmental instability, segmental hyperextension, segmental narrowing, disc herniation, and spinal stenosis.

Segmental Instability

The patient with instability of one or more lumbar segments is often aware of a chronic

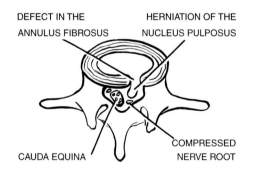

DEFECT IN THE ANNULUS FIBROSUS

HERNIATION OF THE NUCLEUS PULPOSUS

CAUDA EQUINA

COMPRESSED NERVE ROOT

HORIZONTAL SECTION

Figure 11.38.   Posterolateral herniation of the intervertebral disc (nucleus pulposus).

and intermittent backache that is aggravated by excessive activity and relieved by rest. The ache, which is deep, may be felt locally over the unstable segment, or it may be referred to the buttocks. There may be protective muscle spasm in the lumbar region.

Radiographic examination of the spine in both flexion and extension (after the pain has been controlled) provides evidence of the segmental instability, or hypermobility, as well as the associated "traction spurs" (Fig. 11.35).

Segmental Hyperextension

Chronic, persistent segmental hyperextension causes chronic and intermittent low back pain (*lumbago*) that may be felt locally, or may be referred over the buttocks and occasionally down the back of the thigh, but never below the knee. The low back pain is aggravated by any activity that involves active extension of the lumbar spine, such as lifting an object from the floor with the spine in a flexed position. During the painful episode, protective muscle spasm is apparent in the lumbar region. The patient obtains relief of the back pain by resting with the lumbar spine in flexion.

Radiographic examination of the spine in the standing position reveals posterior subluxation of the posterior facet joints (Fig. 11.36). Radiographic examination after injection of a radio-opaque material into the involved disc (*discography*) reveals evidence of degenerative changes and, in addition, the increased intradiscal pressure may reproduce the patient's symptoms. Discography continues to be a more specific imaging technique than magnetic resonance imaging (MRI) for this condition.

Segmental Narrowing

Permanent narrowing of the intervertebral disc space represents a late stage in degenerative disc disease; the involved segment, being relatively stiff and stable, is less likely to be a source of acute pain. The patient, who is usually beyond middle age, is aware of stiffness in the back, but complains of pain only after excessive activity. Loss of the normal mobility in the lumbar spine is detectable clinically.

Radiographic examination reveals spinal osteophytes in addition to narrowing of the involved disc space (Fig. 11.37).

Herniation of the Intervertebral Disc

When the nucleus pulposus suddenly herniates as a complication of degenerative disc disease (Fig. 11.38), the symptoms are often dramatic. For reasons already mentioned, this complication is most common during early adult life and middle age. The most frequent history is that a few days after some excessive activity, or mild injury, the patient experiences the sudden onset of severe, agonizing low back pain (*acute lumbago*) during some simple act such as sneezing, coughing, twisting, reaching, or stooping. Indeed, the pain may be so severe that even a stoical person is unable to move and has to be helped to a bed. Usually within a short time, a completely different type of pain is superimposed—severe pain radiating down one lower limb (buttock, thigh, calf, or foot) in the distribution of one or more roots of the sciatic nerve (*acute sciatica*).

In an epidemiological investigation of 11,000 patients with intervertebral disc herniation, Hall and associates have discovered that of those who had no reason to report a responsible injury, 67% considered their condition to have been of spontaneous onset. By contrast, of those patients who did have some reason to report a responsible injury, only 9% considered their condition to have been of spontaneous onset.

Physical examination reveals muscle spasm in the lumbar region with loss of the normal lumbar lordosis; in addition, the patient may stand with the trunk shifted to one side (*sciatic scoliosis*) in a subconscious effort to relieve pressure of the herniated disc on the nerve root (Fig. 11.39). Active flexion and extension of the spine are significantly restricted.

The diagnosis of disc herniation with compression of a nerve root depends on the clinical demonstration of *nerve root irritation* and, to a lesser extent, *impaired nerve root conduction*. Limitation of straight leg raising (*Lasègue's sign*) is not sufficient evidence of nerve root irritation; more accurate is a positive *bowstring test,* which specifically increases tension on the sciatic nerve (Fig. 11.40). Evidence of impaired conduction in the nerve

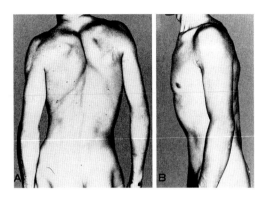

Figure 11.39. A. Sciatic scoliosis in a 30-year-old man who has an acute intervertebral disc protrusion. The longitudinal muscles are in spasm. **B.** In the lateral view there is loss of the normal lumbar lordosis as a result of the muscle spasm.

root is provided by decreased skin sensation and muscle weakness in the distribution of the involved nerve root. For example, impaired conduction in the fifth lumbar nerve root is evidenced by sensory loss over the dorsum of the foot and weakness of the dorsiflexor muscles of the ankles and toes; impaired conduction in the first sacral nerve root is accompanied by sensory loss over the lateral aspect of the foot, a decreased or absent ankle reflex, and weakness of the plantar flexor muscles of the ankle and toes. Accurate localization of the level of a disc herniation is usually possible by clinical examination alone.

Routine radiographic examination does not contribute to the diagnosis of disc herniation but does help to exclude other causes of low back pain and sciatica. A disc herniation

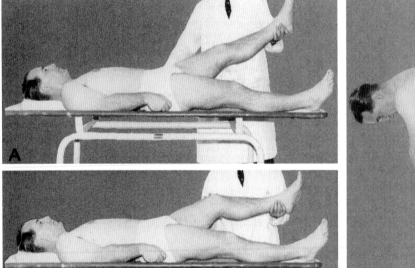

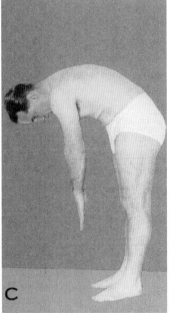

Figure 11.40.   Tests for sciatic nerve root irritation. **A.** Painful limitation of straight leg raising, in the absence of hip disease (Lasègue's sign), suggests irritation of the sciatic nerve root because this test increases the tension on the sciatic nerve and thereby aggravates the pain from any lesion, such as a herniated intervertebral disc, that is already stretching the nerve root. The normal range of passive straight leg raising is almost 90°. **B.** Further evidence of sciatic nerve root pain is then provided by the bowstring test. After reaching the limitation of straight leg raising, the knee is flexed slightly to take tension off the sciatic nerve. At this point, pressure of the examiner's thumb on the medical popliteal nerve as it "bowstrings" across the popliteal fossa increases the tension on the sciatic nerve and reproduces the pain. **C.** Forward bending with knees kept straight may be limited by sciatic nerve tension, spasm in the longitudinal muscles of the lumbar region, or a combination of the two.

may be present with a radiographically normal disc space, whereas there may be radiographic narrowing of the disc space without a disc herniation. Radiographic examination after injection of a water-soluble nonionic radiopaque contrast agent, such as metrizamide and, more recently, iohexol or iopamidol, into the subarachnoid space (*myelography*) is indicated if a spinal cord neoplasm is suspected, or if operative treatment is planned for a clinically diagnosed disc herniation (Fig. 11.41). Such lesions are even more accurately demonstrated

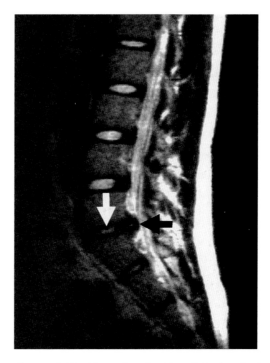

Figure 11.42.   Fast spin echo T_2-weighted sagittal MRI of the lumbar spine of a 24-year-old man with a clinical history and physical signs consistent with an L5–S1 intervertebral disc herniation. Note the degenerative changes in the disc (*white arrow*) and the posterior herniation of this disc (*black arrow*).

by either computed tomography (CT) combined with myelography or by MRI. The latter, which is non-invasive, is especially helpful in demonstrating soft tissue lesions such as disc degeneration and protrusion (Fig. 11.42).

Spinal Stenosis

The central type of spinal stenosis that compresses the cauda equina may produce diffuse back pain whereas the lateral type of spinal stenosis causes nerve root compression and hence radicular pain (such as sciatica). The radicular pain from spinal stenosis, however, differs from that caused by herniation of the intervertebral disc in that it mimics the lower limb intermittent claudication type of pain associated with muscle ischemia. Thus, the pain, which is caused in part by nerve root ischemia, is likely to be brought on by walking. Unlike intermittent claudication, however, the neu-

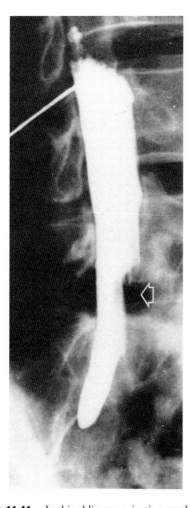

Figure 11.41.   In this oblique-projection myelogram, indentation of the column of a water-soluble, nonionic contrast medium at the level of the L-5–S-1 intervertebral disc indicates a space-occupying lesion such as a herniated intervertebral disc (*arrow*). The diagnosis of herniated disc was confirmed at the time of laminectomy.

rologic claudication type of pain associated with spinal stenosis is not relieved by cessation of walking; it is relieved only by sitting or lying down. You will appreciate that the various forms of spinal stenosis are best seen in cross-section and hence are best demonstrated radiographically by means of CT combined with myelography.

Differential Diagnosis of Low Back Pain

Pain in the lower part of the back is experienced at some time by virtually every adult and is therefore the most common symptom related to the musculoskeletal system. By no means, however, is all low back pain caused by degenerative joint disease or by degenerative disc disease, let alone disc herniation. Therefore, each patient who reports low back pain, with or without sciatica, merits careful assessment on the basis of the history, physical examination, examination by diagnostic imaging and laboratory investigation. You should be aware of the many possible sources of low back pain lest you fall into the ever-present trap of erroneous diagnosis.

The following *classification of the causes of low back pain*, developed by Macnab, is most helpful:

1. *Viscerogenic:* lesions of the genitourinary tract and pelvic organs as well as lesions, either intraperitoneal or retroperitoneal, that irritate the posterior peritoneum may cause low back pain. Characteristically, however, pain from such conditions is neither aggravated by activity nor relieved by rest.
2. *Vasculogenic:* abnormalities of the descending aorta and iliac arteries, such as vascular occlusion and expanding or dissecting aneurysms, may cause pain that is referred to the back.
3. *Neurogenic:* infections and neoplasms that involve either the spinal cord or the cauda equina may mimic disc herniation.
4. *Spondylogenic.* The most common causes of low back pain, with or without sciatica, are disorders of the bony components of the vertebral column (*osseous lesions*) and related structures (*soft tissue lesions*).

a. *Osseous lesions*
Trauma: residual effects of fractures and dislocations
Infection: pyogenic osteomyelitis, tuberculous osteomyelitis
Non-specific inflammation: ankylosing spondylitis
Neoplasm: primary and secondary
Disseminated bone disorders: eosinophilic granuloma, Paget's disease
Metabolic bone disease: osteoporosis, osteomalacia, ochronosis
Bony deformities: spondylolysis, spondylolisthesis, scoliosis, adolescent kyphosis
b. *Soft tissue lesions*
Myofascial lesions: muscle strains, tendinitis
Sacroiliac strain: usually related to childbirth
Intervertebral disc lesions: segmental instability, segmental hyperextension, segmental narrowing, disc herniation
Facet joint lesions: degenerative joint disease (osteoarthritis)
5. *Psychogenic:* the fact that a given patient who complains of low back pain is emotionally unstable or "neurotic" does not mean that his or her pain is imagined; indeed, in such a patient there is often an underlying organic basis for the pain, combined with a psychogenic exaggeration of its severity and significance (*functional overlay*). Thus, although low back pain is sometimes a manifestation of psychosomatic illness, an underlying organic cause of the pain must always be sought. The psychological needs of the patient, however, must always be met as well.

Treatment of Degenerative Joint Disease in the Lumbar Spine

Aims of Treatment

As with degenerative joint disease in the limbs, there is as yet no specific cure for this disorder in the spine. Nevertheless, much can be accomplished therapeutically for afflicted patients provided that the treatment is tailored to meet the specific needs of each patient. The overall treatment of patients with degenerative joint disease in the lumbar spine is based on the following six aims: 1) to alleviate pain; 2) to help the patient understand the nature of the disease; 3) to provide psychological support; 4) to strengthen weak trunk muscles; 5) to improve function; and 6) to rehabilitate the individual patient.

These aims can be achieved by the individual treating orthopaedic surgeon with the assistance of a physiotherapist but are particularly effectively achieved by the multidisciplinary staff of an established "Back Education Program" as recommended by Hall and others.

Methods of Treatment
Psychological Considerations
The patient needs to be reassured that the condition in his or her back represents an exaggeration of the normal aging process and that with non-operative methods of treatment, 90% of patients are relieved of their pain within 6 weeks. Patients must be prepared to live within the limits imposed by the disorder in their backs. Because no organic cause can be readily detected in a large percentage of patients with low back pain, it is important to ascertain not only what kind of back disorder the person has but also what kind of person has the back disorder (a concept first articulated in the nineteenth century by Osler).

Therapeutic Drugs
For the symptomatic relief of either severe or acute back pain (lumbago) or sciatica, the patient requires strong analgesics over a relatively short period; the continued use of narcotics, however, should be avoided. Muscle relaxants are of little value. Because of the inflammatory response to intervertebral disc herniation, NSAIDs, such as enteric coated aspirin, are indicated. Other NSAIDs, including naproxen, phenylbutazone, and indomethacin, should be used with caution because of their harmful side effects.

Bed Rest
All patients with degenerative joint disease in the lumbar spine are helped, at least to some degree, by adequate local rest of the spine, but the period of bed rest should be kept as short as possible—even as short as 2 days. Patients with segmental instability, segmental narrowing, and intervertebral disc herniation should rest in bed on a firm mattress supported by rigid boards. For acute attacks of either lumbago (back pain) or sciatica (radicular pain), complete bed rest should be continued until at least 2 days after the pain has been relieved. If neither sciatic pain nor straight leg raising have improved after several weeks, it is likely that operative treatment will be required. (The indications for such treatment are listed further on in this chapter.) Patients with segmental hyperextension and spinal stenosis are much more comfortable lying on their back with the mattress elevated at each end to keep the lumbar spine flexed or, alternatively, lying curled up on either side.

Orthopaedic Apparatus and Appliances
After a period of bed rest, the patient may require a temporary spinal support such as a plaster of Paris body jacket, a firmly applied canvas jacket (Fig. 11.43), a surgical corset, or a more permanent support such as a metal back brace (Fig. 11.44). The more permanent type of spinal support may have to be worn, at least during the day, for many months. Patients with segmental hyperextension require a spinal support that maintains their lumbar spine in flexion.

Physical Therapy
Local heat may give temporary relief during an acute attack of pain, but the most important function of physical therapy is to strengthen spinal and abdominal muscles after the acute attack through a program of regular low back exercises in an attempt to improve spinal posture and to prevent recurrence of pain.

Spinal Manipulation
Manipulation of the spine for low back pain has for many years been a controversial procedure, but it is gradually becoming more widely accepted and has even become very popular in some centers. It should be performed only by a specially trained expert. Spinal manipulation is designed to stretch the capsules of the posterior (apophyseal) joints and thereby temporarily separate the joint surfaces. This phe-

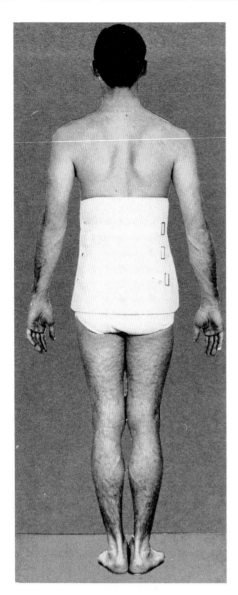

Figure 11.43.   Left. Temporary spinal support by means of a firmly applied canvas jacket.

for less than 6 weeks than in those with symptoms of longer duration. Spinal manipulation is at least potentially dangerous, however, in the presence of a suspected disc herniation with a neurological deficit because of the definite risk of aggravating the situation. This is particularly important in the presence of a cauda equina syndrome, in which circumstance, spinal manipulation is definitely con-

nomenon is accompanied by an audible "snap." Careful clinical assessment of the patient should be conducted and documented immediately before and after every spinal manipulation. It is best reserved for patients with acute lumbago, that is, low back pain secondary to segmental instability and segmental hyperextension in whom an acute subluxation of a posterior facet joint is suspected. It is more effective in patients who have had symptoms

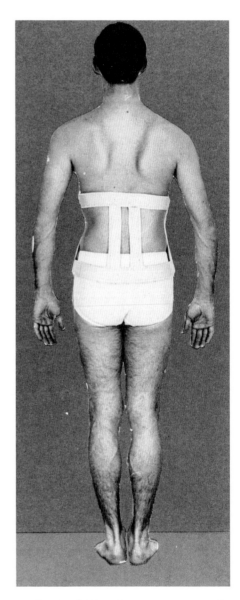

Figure 11.44.   Right. More permanent spinal support by means of a leather covered metallic back brace (Harris type).

tra-indicated and emergency surgical treatment is essential.

Chemonucleolysis

The enzymatic dissolution of the nucleus pulposus by the transcutaneous intradiscal injection of chymopapain is known as *chemonucleolysis,* a somewhat controversial form of treatment that has been used in many countries throughout the world. Chymopapain, a peptidase derived from papaya fruit, digests the polypeptide core of the proteoglycan molecules of the matrix of the nucleus pulposus. The resultant hydrolysis and shrinkage of the nucleus relieves the pressure of a protruded intervertebral disc on a nerve root and thereby relieves the sciatic pain. Thus, for patients with clear-cut evidence of herniation of an intervertebral disc in the lumbar region (the diagnostic features of which are outlined in an earlier section of this chapter), chemonucleolysis is a reasonable last step in the non-operative treatment when the other methods of non-operative treatment have failed and operative treatment seems inevitable. McCulloch, from an experience with more than 2000 such patients, has stated that when chemonucleolysis is used *only* for this particular and precisely diagnosed indication and only in adolescents and young adults, 80% of the patients are relieved of their pain and are thereby spared surgical exploration and excision of the disc (discectomy) by laminectomy. If, however, chemonucleolysis is used indiscriminately for spinal disorders other than nerve root irritation or compression from herniation of an intervertebral disc (such as spinal stenosis or psychogenic pain) the results are predictably disappointing. Chemonucleolysis, which is combined with discography, can be performed under local anesthesia; the procedure necessitates only a short hospital stay and can even be done on an outpatient basis. The most serious complication is an anaphylactic reaction to chymopapain, which fortunately is very rare and, furthermore, sensitivity to chymopapain can be detected pre-operatively by specific skin testing. Nevertheless, in some centers, chemonucleolysis has been associated with serious complications, mostly the results of technical problems (such as inadvertent injection of chymopapain into the subarachnoid space).

In an international clinical investigation, Tregonning and colleagues found that the long-term (10-year) results of chemonucleolysis were slightly inferior to those of open surgical discectomy. For all these reasons, chemonucleolysis is used less frequently in the 1990s than it was in the 1970s.

Surgical Operation

At least 90% of patients with degenerative joint disease and degenerative disc disease in the lumbar spine recover without a surgical operation. Therefore, unless there is a cauda equina syndrome as evidenced by loss of bladder or bowel function and saddle anaesthesia (which represents a surgical emergency), the *initial* treatment should always be non-operative. CT with myelography and MRI should be reserved for those patients in whom surgical operation is deemed necessary (Figs. 11.41, 11.42).

The indications for laminectomy and removal of a herniated disc (discectomy) are as follows: 1) a cauda equina syndrome: a surgical emergency; 2) persistent, unbearable pain that is not relieved even by strong analgesics; 3) persistent, severe pain and evidence of persistent nerve root irritation or impairment of nerve conduction after 3 weeks of complete bed rest; 4) evidence of progression of neurological changes even while the patient is still confined to bed; 5) recurrent episodes of incapacitating back pain or sciatica; 6) spinal canal stenosis (SCS) with claudicant leg pain that limits walking to one city block and standing to 15 minutes. The operation for SCS is an open laminectomy and excision of sufficient bone to decompress the compressed cauda equina or nerve root or roots.

When only discectomy is required, it used to be performed through the traditional operation that includes laminectomy and involves a wide surgical exposure. Currently, however, it is achieved by a small laminotomy and excision of the disc through a very limited surgical exposure combined with the use of an operating microscope. This procedure, which is known as *microdiscectomy,* is associated with less postoperative morbidity and a shorter hospital stay. For selected patients, it can even be performed on an out-patient basis. Although technically demanding, microdiscectomy is currently the standard technique for a patient with sciatica in whom nonoperative treatment has failed and the site of the disc protrusion has been confirmed by diagnostic imaging. The results of microdiscectomy are excellent in more than 90% of such patients.

An even more recent procedure, *percutaneous discectomy,* involves aspiration of herniated intervertebral disc material by means of powerful suction through a cannulated probe that is inserted percutaneously into the correct site with the guidance of three-dimensional diagnostic imaging. This procedure, which is still considered to be *investigational,* seems unlikely to replace the standard operation of microdiscectomy.

The operation of arthrodesis of one or more segments of the spine (spinal fusion) does not completely immobilize the intervertebral disc and cannot be expected to provide complete relief of pain. Furthermore, solid fusion is difficult to obtain, even in the hands of experienced orthopaedic surgeons. Modern methods of spinal fusion, including the bilateral intertransverse process fusion, have a higher percentage of success, but even with this technique, localized failure of fusion (pseudarthrosis) can still occur and can be a continuing source of pain. The relatively new technique of pedicle screw fixation has produced better results than former methods. Spinal fusion is most effective for the treatment of back pain caused by segmental instability and segmental hyperextension with degenerative joint disease (osteoarthritis) in the posterior facet joints; however, spinal fusion should not be undertaken unless extensive non-operative methods have failed to obtain relief of pain and unless the patient is willing to avoid heavy manual labor in the future.

Rehabilitation

Approximately 5% of all patients with degenerative joint disease in the lumbar spine remain severely disabled despite extensive treatment. For some of these unfortunate individuals the functional or emotional component of their disability is greater than the organic component, yet they need help. The future for this relatively small group of permanently disabled patients with degenerative joint disease in the lumbar spine, just as the future of other severely disabled persons, lies not so much in the development of better surgical operations, as in the development of more effective facilities for retraining them, and the development of more opportunities for gainful light work, either in sheltered workshops or in industry.

DEGENERATIVE JOINT DISEASE IN THE CERVICAL SPINE

Degenerative disease in the cervical spine (*cervical spondylosis*), which includes both degenerative disc disease and degenerative joint disease, although relatively common, is not so common as degenerative joint disease in the lumbar spine.

Pathogenesis and Pathology

Much of what has been written previously concerning the pathogenesis and pathology of degenerative disc disease and degenerative joint disease in the lumbar spine is equally applicable to the cervical spine—that is, the initial degeneration in the nucleus pulposus, the segmental instability, the segmental narrowing, the subsequent development of degenerative joint disease in the posterior facet joints with osteophyte formation and finally, herniation of the intervertebral disc. Thus, the details need not be repeated here.

The most common segments to be affected by such degenerative changes in the cervical spine are C-5–6 and C-6–7 which, like the lower lumbar segments, are particularly mobile and in the area of maximal lordosis. In the cervical spine, there is little room in the intervertebral foramina for exit of the nerve roots; consequently, subluxation and osteophyte formation in the posterior facet joints readily compress these roots, particularly after injury with its associated soft tissue swelling.

Herniation of the intervertebral disc, although much less common in the cervical spine than in the lumbar spine, may occur as a dramatic event in the degenerative process for the same reasons and in the same manner as previously described for the lumbar segments. The more common type of herniation, which is posterolateral, compresses a nerve root; the relatively uncommon, but more serious, central herniation compresses the spinal cord.

Clinical Features and Diagnosis

Most persons older than 60 years of age exhibit some radiographic evidence of degenerative disc disease and degenerative joint disease in the cervical spine, but in many the condition causes no symptoms apart from mild stiffness in the neck. When the cervical spondylosis is more severe, however, it may cause vague neck pain as well as pain that is referred to the shoulder, or arms, even without nerve root compression.

Cervical nerve root irritation, either from encroachment of osteophytes in the intervertebral foramina, or from intervertebral disc herniation, produces a variety of clinical syndromes, including pain in the neck and shoulder as well as pain radiating down the arm in the distribution of the involved nerve root (*brachialgia*). This radicular type of pain may be accompanied by paresthesia in the form of numbness or tingling. The onset of symptoms is often insidious but can be acute, particularly when an injury is added to the pre-existing degenerative changes.

Compression of the sixth cervical nerve root (from either osteophytes or disc herniation at the C-5–6 level) produces weakness of the deltoid and biceps muscles, diminished biceps reflex and diminished skin sensation in the thumb and index finger. Compression of the seventh cervical nerve root (either from osteophytes or from disc herniation at the C-6–7 level) produces weakness of the triceps muscle, diminished triceps reflex, and diminished skin sensation in the index and middle fingers. When the spinal cord is compressed by a central herniation of the disc, the clinical picture is indistinguishable from a spinal cord neoplasm and requires immediate investigation. A neurosurgeon should always be consulted forthwith.

Examination of the neck in the presence of pain may reveal limitation of motion, particularly lateral flexion, but there is relatively little

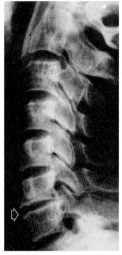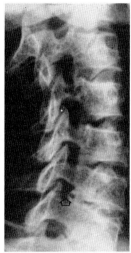

Figure 11.45.   Left. Lateral radiograph of the cervical spine in a 60-year-old man with cervical degenerative joint disease (cervical spondylosis). Note the narrowing of the C6–7 intervertebral disc space and the associated osteophytes arising from the adjoining vertebral bodies (*arrow*).

Figure 11.46.   Right. Oblique radiograph of the cervical spine in the same patient whose lateral radiograph is shown at left. Note the osteophytic encroachment on the intervertebral foramen (*arrow*).

muscle spasm; in a quiescent phase, there may be few clinical findings other than crepitus in the cervical spine during active movement. Complete neurological examination of the upper limbs is always indicated.

Radiographic examination reveals disc space narrowing and osteophyte formation, both of which are best seen in the lateral projection (Fig. 11.45). Because of the oblique direction of the intervertebral foramina, however, an oblique projection is required to demonstrate the osteophytic encroachment (Fig. 11.46). If a central herniation of the disc is suspected, CT combined with myelography is indicated. MRI is an excellent alternative to demonstrate the spinal cord and nerve roots.

Differential Diagnosis of Neck and Arm Pain

As with low back pain and sciatica, each of the many possible causes must also be considered in a given patient with neck and arm pain (brachialgia). The following general classification developed by Macnab is equally applicable in the cervical and lumbar region—only the specific details differ.

1. *Viscerogenic:* lesions of the pharynx, larynx and the upper part of the trachea and esophagus may cause neck pain.
2. *Vasculogenic:* angina pectoris and the pain of myocardial infarction from coronary artery occlusion may be referred to the neck as well as to the shoulder and down one or both arms. Likewise, occlusion of a carotid artery may produce neck pain.
3. *Neurogenic:* a spinal cord neoplasm mimics central herniation of a cervical disc. A neoplasm at the apex of the lung (*Pancoast's tumor*), or a cervical rib can cause pressure on the brachial plexus with resulting radicular pain and can therefore mimic nerve root compression from cervical spondylosis with nerve root compression. Even involvement of peripheral nerves, such as irritation of the ulnar nerve at the level of a deformed elbow and compression of the median nerve in the carpal tunnel, must be differentiated from cervical spondylosis and cervical disc herniation.
4. *Spondylogenic*
    a. *Osseous lesions*
        Trauma: residual effects of fractures and dislocations
        Infection: pyogenic osteomyelitis, tuberculous osteomyelitis
        Non-specific inflammation: ankylosing spondylitis
        Neoplasm: primary and secondary
        Disseminated bone disorders: eosinophilic granuloma
        Metabolic bone disease: osteoporosis, osteomalacia, ochronosis
    b. *Soft tissue lesions*
        Myofascial lesions: muscle strains, tendinitis
        Intervertebral disc lesions: segmental instability, segmental narrowing, disc herniation
        Facet joint lesions: degenerative joint disease (cervical spondylosis)
5. *Psychogenic:* The fact that a given patient who reports neck and arm pain is emotionally unstable, or "neurotic," does not mean that his or her pain is imagined; indeed, in such a patient there is nearly always an underlying organic basis for the pain combined with a psychogenic exaggeration of its severity and significance (*functional overlay*). Thus, although neck pain, with or without arm pain, is sometimes a manifestation of psychosomatic illness, the underlying organic cause of the pain must always be sought. In addition, however, the psychological needs of the patient must also be met.

Treatment of Degenerative Joint Disease in the Cervical Spine

The aims and methods of treatment for degenerative joint disease in the cervical spine are comparable to those already described in relation to the lumbar spine with only a few minor differences. Therefore, only the differences will be discussed here.

Local rest for the neck, which helps to relieve pain, is achieved by means of a cervical "ruff" (Fig. 11.47) or, when the symptoms are more protracted, a cervical brace or collar (Fig. 11.48). Intermittent traction on the cervical spine through a halter may also provide considerable relief of pain. The majority of patients can be managed effectively by nonoperative methods of treatment.

Surgical arthrodesis (fusion) of one or

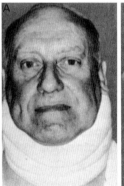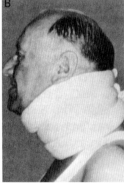

Figure 11.47.   Local rest for the cervical spine is provided by means of a firmly applied cervical "ruff," a series of three rolls of stockinette filled with cotton wool.

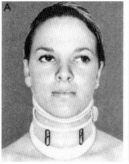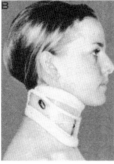

Figure 11.48. Local rest for the cervical spine is provided by means of an adjustable plastic cervical collar.

more segments of the cervical spine anteriorly (*anterior interbody fusion*) may be necessary to control the persistent pain of cervical spondylosis; the rate of successful spinal fusion is much higher in the cervical spine than in the lumbar spine. Laminectomy and removal of a herniated cervical disc (discectomy) is seldom necessary for a posterolateral herniation but is always indicated for a central herniation with compression of the spinal cord. Under these circumstances, laminectomy and decompression of the cord should usually be performed by a neurosurgeon; subsequently, it may be necessary for an orthopaedic surgeon to stabilize the decompressed segments by means of an anterior interbody fusion.

NEUROPATHIC JOINT DISEASE (CHARCOT'S JOINT)

The relatively uncommon condition of *neuropathic joint disease (Charcot's joint)* is characterized by severe and rapidly progressive destruction of one or more joints in which there is a pre-existing loss of normal sensation, particularly deep pain and position sense.

Incidence and Etiology

Any extensive disease or injury of the sensory elements of either the spinal cord or peripheral nerves may lead to neuropathic joint disease in the distribution of the sensory loss; yet, not all persons with sensory loss develop a neuropathic joint. Although the most common underlying disorder is *syphilitic tabes dorsalis* (locomotor ataxia), only a small percentage of

tabetics develop a Charcot joint, and it is usually a major joint in the lower limb or joints of the lumbar spine. *Diabetic neuropathy*, which is becoming more common because of the increased lifespan of diabetics, may result in neuropathic disease in the peripheral joints of the foot. *Syringomyelia*, which affects primarily the upper part of the spinal cord, is frequently complicated by neuropathic joint disease in one of the major joints of the upper limb. Other neurological disorders, such as *paraplegia, leprosy (Hansen's disease)*, and *congenital indifference to pain*, are less commonly the underlying cause of this unusual type of joint disease.

It is difficult to explain why neuropathic joint disease seldom involves more than one joint in a given patient despite the fact that other joints are equally insensitive. Also difficult to explain is the fact that many persons with sensory deficits escape this complication.

Pathogenesis and Pathology

The development of localized neuropathic joint disease is probably precipitated by an injury, the significance of which is not appreciated by the patient who continues to use—and abuse—the injured, but insensitive, joint. Initially, the pathological process resembles a severe traumatic arthritis but it progresses relentlessly at an alarming rate and soon the joint is completely disorganized. Articular cartilage is destroyed, the subchondral bone is absorbed in some areas and deposited excessively in others, fragments of bone and cartilage break off and become loose bodies in the joint, the fibrous capsule and ligaments are severely stretched by a massive synovial effusion, and the joint eventually becomes so unstable that it may subluxate or even dislocate.

Clinical Features and Diagnosis

The patient, usually over the age of 40, notices progressive swelling and instability of the involved joint. At first the rapid distention of the joint may be somewhat painful, but soon the patient becomes unaware of the devastating destruction in the joint except for crepitus and progressive loss of joint stability.

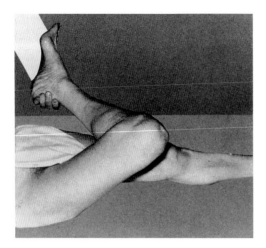

Figure 11.49. Neuropathic joint disease (Charcot's joint) of the right hip in a patient with syphilitic tabes dorsalis. Note the remarkably increased range of passive movement. This excessive movement was associated with crepitus but was completely painless.

Examination reveals gross swelling of the joint and a remarkably increased range of passive motion in almost all directions (Fig. 11.49). Joint aspiration yields a large amount of synovial fluid that may contain blood. Neurological examination provides evidence of the underlying neurological disorder.

The bizarre radiographic appearance of neuropathic joint disease, which is characteristic, reveals irregular areas of rarefaction and sclerosis, loose bodies in the joint, subluxation, and even dislocation; the entire joint is obviously completely disorganized and destroyed (Fig. 11.50).

Treatment

Because the massive and persistent effusion stretches both the fibrous capsule and ligaments and leads to joint instability, repeated aspiration of the joint is indicated. Recently, intra-articular injection of radioactive colloidal gold (which is taken up by the synovial cells) has proved effective in controlling the effusion in neuropathic joints.

Severe instability of a major joint in the lower limb necessitates a weight-relieving brace and the use of crutches, not only to permit walking but also to minimize further damage to the insensitive joint.

Surgical treatment of a neuropathic joint is fraught with frustration for both the patient and the surgeon. Successful arthrodesis (fusion) is difficult, although not impossible, to obtain. Total prosthetic joint replacement (i.e., arthroplasty) of a neuropathic joint is doomed to failure because it tends to accelerate the destructive process and therefore should be avoided.

NONARTICULAR RHEUMATISM

A variety of "rheumatic diseases" affect musculoskeletal tissues other than joints; these include disorders of muscles, fasciae, tendons, ligaments, synovial sheaths, and bursae, all of which may be grouped under the general heading of nonarticular rheumatism (extra-articular rheumatism or regional rheumatic pain syndromes).

Myofascial Pain Syndrome ("Fibrositis")

The number of different terms applied to this common but poorly understood and somewhat controversial clinical disorder (*fibromyalgia syndrome, sensitive deposits, muscular rheumatism, tension rheumatism, fibrositis*) reflect the lack of scientific knowledge concerning both its etiology and its pathology. However, because it does not seem to be an inflammatory disorder, the term *fibrositis* has been abandoned by many clinicians. Of the

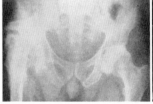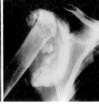

Figure 11.50. Neuropathic joint disease (Charcot's joint). **Left.** Hip joints of the patient shown in Figure 11.49. Note the complete disorganization of the right hip joint with irregular areas of rarefaction and sclerosis, loose bodies in the joint and dislocation. The left hip is an earlier stage of evolution of the same pathological process. **Right.** A Charcot shoulder joint of a patient with syringomyelia. The radiographic changes of neuropathic joint disease are comparable to those shown at left.

many theories proposed to explain this syndrome, not one has been proven. Nevertheless, the lack of understanding does not deny the existence of a clinical syndrome that is not only common and characteristic, but also very troublesome to those afflicted.

Clinical Features

Myofascial pain syndrome is characterized by deep pain in the region of various muscles and their fascial attachments to bone, most commonly in the neck and back; it is both chronic and recurrent but does not necessarily remain confined to one muscle group. Involved muscles and fasciae may be hypersensitive to direct pressure and squeezing, particularly at certain fairly constant "trigger points"; at these sites, small areas of induration in the muscle or fascia may or may not be palpable. Pain may be felt locally, but more often it is a referred type of pain and is thus felt elsewhere. Characteristically, the pain is aggravated by emotional tension, immobility, and chilling; it is relieved by equanimity, activity, and local heat. There is a plethora of symptoms but a paucity of physical signs. Studies by Smythe and Moldofsky have revealed a definite relationship between so-called fibrositis syndrome and disturbed sleep patterns with particular reference to non-REM (rapid eye movement) sleep. The patient reports insomnia, weariness, and fatigue, and yet there is neither clinical nor laboratory evidence of systemic disease; the patient reports joint stiffness, and yet there is neither clinical nor radiographic evidence of joint disease.

The psychogenic aspects of myofascial pain syndrome are apparent in these patients, most of whom exhibit a chronic anxiety state as well as a low pain threshold. Nevertheless, the pain, although exaggerated, is not imaginary. Indeed, the excessive muscle tension that accompanies the chronic emotional tension of a chronic anxiety state may, in itself, be a cause of pain either in the muscles or in their fascial attachments to bone. Unlike the complaints of purely psychogenic origin, which also tend to vary with the patient's emotional state, or "internal climate," the complaints of myofascial pain syndrome (like those of many other rheumatic diseases) tend to be aggravated by changes in the weather, or "external climate."

The diagnosis of myofascial pain syndrome can be suspected on the basis of the characteristic clinical features, but it can be established only after other, more serious, causes of musculoskeletal pain have been excluded.

Treatment

Patients who suffer from myofascial pain syndrome present a challenge to the physician because their condition represents a curious combination of psychological and somatic manifestations. Reassurances that the disorder is neither deforming nor life threatening and that the pain is related to tension, both emotional and muscular, are most helpful. Local pain and tenderness may be relieved, at least temporarily, by heat, massage, mild analgesics and, if necessary, local injections of hydrocortisone and a local anesthetic agent. In general, NSAIDs are not effective in this disorder. From a long-term point of view, however, these anxious patients need sound advice concerning a more appropriate lifestyle with less tension and more equanimity.

Degenerative Tendon and Capsule Disease

Although the weight-bearing joints of the lower limbs are frequently afflicted by degenerative joint disease, the non-weight-bearing joints of the upper limbs are more frequently afflicted by degenerative disease in the periarticular tissues, such as *degenerative tendon and capsule disease*.

Incidence and Etiology

The periarticular tissues of the shoulder are particularly prone to the development of this type of nonarticular rheumatism. Indeed, in individuals older than 40 years of age, shoulder pain is one of the most common musculoskeletal complaints. With both degenerative joint disease and degenerative tendon and capsule disease, many causative factors are superimposed on the progressive changes of the normal aging process in these tissues. With aging, the blood supply of tendons and joint capsules becomes less adequate; as a result of decreased diffusion of nutrients through the intercellular tissues, local degenerative changes are inevitable.

Pathogenesis and Pathology

The basic underlying pathological change in degenerative tendon and capsule disease is *local necrosis* of varying extent in a tendon or joint capsule. Subsequently, these areas of necrosis tend to become calcified (*dystrophic calcification*), and this can cause a chemical and physical inflammation (*calcific tendinitis*). Furthermore, local areas of degeneration in tendons so weaken their structure that they may rupture, or tear, with little trauma (*pathological tear*).

Degenerative Tendon and Capsule Disease in the Shoulder

The wide range of circumduction motion between the arm and the trunk occurs at several sites: 1) the glenohumeral (shoulder) joint; 2) the acromioclavicular joint; 3) the sternoclavicular joint; and 4) between the scapula and the thorax. Normally, smooth motion is possible between the under surface of the acromion and the upper surface of the musculotendinous cuff because of the large intervening subacromial (subdeltoid) bursa. The musculotendinous cuff ("rotator cuff") is composed of the conjoined tendinous attachments of four muscles (subscapularis, supraspinatus, infraspinatus and teres minor) and the capsular attachment into the upper end of the humerus.

Degenerative disease in the musculotendinous cuff of the shoulder is usually most marked in the supraspinatus portion, possibly because the blood supply in this area is least adequate and, hence, most vulnerable to pressure. Frequently, the degenerative changes and their sequelae produce either an acute or a chronic inflammatory reaction in the tissues, hence the clinical terms *tendinitis, bursitis,* and *capsulitis*. The more common clinical syndromes, all of which represent complications of degenerative tendon and capsule disease, are the following: *calcific tendinitis, subacromial bursitis, bicipital tendinitis, tear of the musculotendinous cuff,* and *adhesive capsulitis* or *"frozen shoulder."*

Shoulder pain is a common symptom, but it is not always a manifestation of intrinsic shoulder disease. The pain, although felt in the shoulder, may be either referred or radiating from a variety of extrinsic disorders, including cervical spondylosis, cervical disc herniation, angina pectoris, myocardial infarction, basal pleurisy, and subphrenic (subdiaphragmatic) inflammation from conditions such as cholecystitis, abscess, and even a ruptured spleen.

Calcific Supraspinatus Tendinitis (Rotator Cuff Tendinitis)

Dystrophic calcification in the supraspinatus portion of the musculotendinous cuff is common (3% of the adult population). Such calcium deposits may cause no symptoms. When symptoms do arise, however, the clinical condition is *calcific supraspinatus tendinitis,* which may be either acute or chronic. It is also referred to as *rotator cuff tendinitis* and *impingement syndrome.*

Acute Calcific Supraspinatus Tendinitis. Rapid deposition of calcium in a closed space within the substance of the supraspinatus tendon causes excruciating pain that, being caused by increased local pressure, is throbbing in nature and is not relieved by rest. At this stage, the calcium deposit has the consistency of toothpaste and behaves like a "chemical boil"; as it expands, it irritates the undersurface of the subacromial bursa and produces a secondary *subacromial bursitis* with aggravation of the pain. If, however, the calcium deposit bursts into the subacromial bursa, which has a good blood supply, the calcium is gradually absorbed and the symptoms subside.

The clinical picture is characteristic. The patient, more often a male and usually of middle age or older, may previously have experienced mild symptoms caused by degenerative changes in the musculotendinous cuff with or without calcium deposits. After unusual or excessive use of the shoulder, the patient experiences the rapid onset of extremely severe shoulder pain that necessitates immediate relief; the pain may radiate distally as far as the hand. The patient maintains the shoulder in a slightly abducted position, which keeps the painful lesion away from the undersurface of the acromion; there is exquisite local tenderness just lateral to the acromion. Abduction of the shoulder, both active and passive, is most painful during one arc of the normal range of motion, the arc from approximately 50° to 130°. This is known as the *painful arc syndrome*, which is explained by the anatomical fact that during this arc of abduction, the involved area of the supraspinatus tendon is in intimate contact with the undersurface of the acromion and impinges against it (Fig. 11.51). Radiographic examination with the shoulder externally rotated reveals deposits of calcium in the region of the musculotendinous cuff close to its insertion into the humerus (Fig. 11.52).

Treatment depends on the severity and duration of the acute episode. Local rest with an arm sling, combined with analgesics and adrenocorticosteroid therapy, bring relief of pain for some patients. In others, however, the pain is so severe and so disabling that these measures are inadequate. Under such circumstances, *aspiration* of the semi-fluid calcium

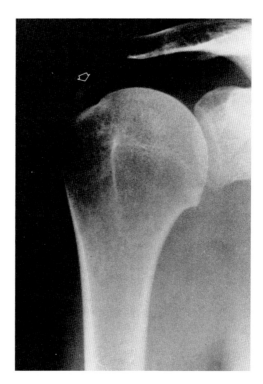

Figure 11.52. Chronic calcific supraspinatus tendinitis. Note the calcium deposits in the region of the musculotendinous cuff close to its insertion into the humerus (*arrow*).

in the "chemical boil" is justified. The aspiration, which is performed under local anesthesia and accompanied by local injection of hydrocortisone, does not always yield calcium, but usually the multiple punctures in the deposit allow the calcium to be dispersed into the subacromial bursa where it can be absorbed. Occasionally, aspiration may have to be repeated. If these methods of treatment fail to relieve the severe pain, surgical removal of the calcium is indicated. After the acute symptoms have subsided, active exercises help to prevent prolonged stiffness of the shoulder.

Chronic Calcific Supraspinatus Tendinitis. Even when calcium is deposited slowly in degenerated areas of the supraspinatus tendon, the lesion may become sufficiently large that it causes symptoms. Deposits of long duration tend to become semi-solid and to have a gritty sensation because of desiccation.

The clinical picture is less dramatic than that described for the acute episode. The pa-

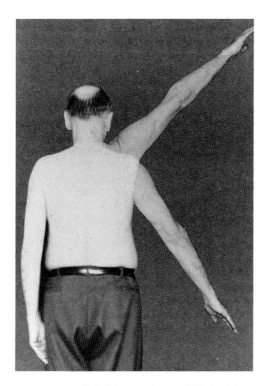

Figure 11.51. Painful arc syndrome. This double exposure photograph demonstrates the limits of the painful arc of abduction (approximately 50° to 130°).

tient experiences chronic pain that, although not severe, is annoying during the day and interferes with sleep at night. Examination reveals mild local tenderness just lateral to the acromion; the *painful arc syndrome* can also be demonstrated (Fig. 11.51). The pain is also aggravated when the patient, or the examiner, moves the adducted and externally rotated shoulder into a position of abduction and internal rotation at which time the greater tuberosity of the humerus impinges against the under surface of the acromion (a positive "impingement test").

Treatment with NSAIDs as well as local injection of corticosteroids may relieve the pain but attempts at aspiration of chronic, desiccated calcium deposits are usually unsuccessful, and even surgical removal of the deposit may be followed by recurrence. For patients with persistent pain, it may become necessary to eliminate friction between the degenerated area of the tendon and the acromion by excising the under surface of the acromion (acromioplasty) or by lowering the glenoid cavity through an osteotomy of the neck of the scapula.

Tears of the Musculotendinous Cuff

Pre-existing changes of aging and deficient blood supply in the musculotendinous cuff weaken it sufficiently that with a superimposed injury such as a fall it is prone to tear (rupture). Thus, tears of the musculotendinous cuff are most common during middle age and beyond; they may be either *partial* or *complete* and are twice as common in males as in females.

Partial Tear of the Musculotendinous Cuff. The supraspinatus component of the musculotendinous cuff, being the most common site of degenerative changes and also being subjected to the greatest strains, is the most frequent site of a tear. Indeed, in postmortem studies of the shoulder, such tears are seen as an incidental finding in one quarter of elderly persons, most of whom had not complained about the shoulder.

The patient is usually able to initiate abduction, but experiences pain in doing so; the *painful arc syndrome* can be demonstrated (Fig. 11.51). After injection of a local anes-

thetic agent, active abduction becomes more comfortable. These observations help to differentiate between a *partial* tear and a *complete* tear.

Treatment consists of active exercises under the supervision of a physiotherapist to prevent prolonged stiffness in the shoulder joint. Steroid injections into the area may relieve the pain. Occasionally, division of the coracoacromial ligament and acromioplasty are necessary.

Complete Tear of the Musculotendinous Cuff. An injury such as a fall on the shoulder, may completely tear a previously degenerated musculotendinous cuff, including the capsule. Nevertheless, in half the patients, a progressive tear occurs gradually without a significant injury. The proximal part of the cuff retracts and the glenohumeral (shoulder) joint then communicates with the subacromial bursa. The patient complains of pain in the shoulder that may be most severe at night.

The patient with a complete tear of the musculotendinous cuff, usually a male past the age of 60 years, cannot initiate abduction of the arm and on attempting to do so, merely shrugs the shoulder (Fig. 11.53). If, however, the arm is passively abducted to 90°, he is able to maintain this position of abduction by means of the deltoid muscle.

Radiographic examination after injection of radio-opaque material into the shoulder joint (arthrography) reveals that the material spreads from the joint into the bursa and confirms the presence of a complete tear. Ultrasonography and MRI are also useful in demonstrating a tear. Arthroscopy of the shoulder may be of help in determining its extent.

Treatment of complete tears of the musculotendinous cuff by surgical repair is somewhat unsatisfactory because of degenerative changes in the torn edges. Thus, in the elderly, the best treatment consists of simple exercises to prevent shoulder stiffness. In more active persons, however, extensive surgical repair of the completely torn cuff through an open operation is justified; postoperatively, the patient's shoulder is immobilized in a position of abduction for 3 weeks after which active exercises are begun.

Bicipital Tendinitis and Tenosynovitis

Degenerative changes in the tendon of the long head of the biceps muscle, combined with chronic inflammation of its enveloping synovial sheath within the bicipital groove of the humerus, can be a source of shoulder pain, particularly in females. The pain, which is felt anteriorly, is aggravated by active supination of the forearm against resistance with the elbow flexed and without the shoulder moving; this phenomenon is sometimes referred to as the *palm-up pain sign* or *Yergason's sign*. Local tenderness over the bicipital groove can be detected. There are no radiographic signs of the disorder.

Treatment of this relatively mild but irritating condition consists of local rest with an arm sling plus NSAIDs. One or more local injections of hydrocortisone may be required to

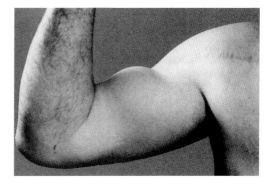

Figure 11.54.   Rupture of the long head of the biceps tendon in a 52-year-old man who is flexing his elbow. The muscle belly of the long head of the biceps can be seen in a position that is more distal than normal.

relieve the pain. Occasionally, the symptoms are sufficiently severe and persistent that operative treatment is indicated; the degenerated tendon is divided and the distal stump is sutured to the bicipital groove.

Rupture of the Biceps Tendon

Pre-existing degenerative changes in the proximal tendon of the long head of the biceps muscle may weaken it sufficiently that it may rupture during active flexion of the elbow against resistance as in lifting a heavy object.

The patient experiences immediate pain and is aware that something has "given way." Examination reveals that when the patient flexes the elbow (using the short head of biceps, brachialis, and brachioradialis muscles), the muscle belly of the long head of the biceps contracts into a "ball" that is more distal than normal (Fig. 11.54).

The resultant disability is not particularly severe in an elderly person, but for a person who requires strong elbow flexion to work, it may be necessary to suture the distal stump of the ruptured tendon into the bicipital groove.

Rupture of the distal tendon of the biceps muscle is less common. It is associated with weakness of supination of the forearm and flexion of the elbow. In this injury, the muscle belly contracts into a "ball" that is more proximal than normal. For a young laborer, surgical repair is indicated.

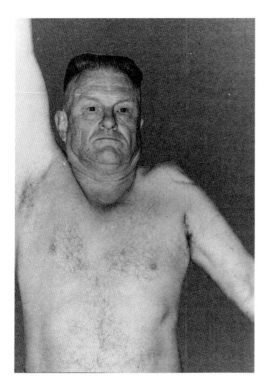

Figure 11.53.   Complete tear of the musculotendinous cuff of the left shoulder in a 65-year-old man who is attempting to abduct the shoulder. He is able to obtain only slight abduction as he shrugs his shoulder and rotates the scapula. If, however, his arm were passively abducted to 90°, he would be able to maintain this position with his deltoid muscle.

Adhesive Capsulitis of the Shoulder (Frozen Shoulder)

A variety of disorders, not only in the shoulder (intrinsic) but also outside the shoulder (extrinsic), may lead to the development of diffuse capsulitis of the glenohumeral joint, particularly in older persons. Subsequently, the inflamed capsule becomes adherent to the humeral head rather like adhesive tape (*adhesive capsulitis or pericapsulitis*) and undergoes contracture: the adherent, shrunken capsule prevents motion in the glenohumeral joint, which becomes "frozen" usually in the neutral, that is, anatomical position (*frozen shoulder*).

Intrinsic disorders that may initiate this process include calcific supraspinatus tendinitis, a partial tear of the musculotendinous cuff, and bicipital tendinitis. Even prolonged immobilization of the shoulder in a cast or a sling may lead to adhesive capsulitis. Extrinsic disorders capable of producing this condition are those that cause pain in the region of the shoulder and that therefore cause the patient to keep the shoulder still. These disorders include cervical spondylosis, cervical disc herniation, myocardial infarction, basal pleurisy, and subphrenic inflammation such as cholecystitis, abscess, or ruptured spleen.

The onset of adhesive capsulitis is usually gradual. Initially, in the inflammatory phase, the patient experiences shoulder pain, and examination reveals muscle spasm in all the muscles about the shoulder. After a few weeks the inflammation becomes subacute, the shoulder joint becomes stiff, or "frozen," in all directions, and the acute pain subsides. Thus, when the patient attempts to abduct the arm he or she does so by elevating and rotating the scapula (Fig. 11.55). Because of the lack of virtually all motion in the glenohumeral joint, additional strain is applied to the acromioclavicular joint, which may become painful; the pain radiates proximally from the shoulder and may be felt as high as the ear. Arthrography reveals a decreased volume of the shoulder joint.

The prognosis for adhesive capsulitis is quite good in that the pathological process tends to be self-limiting. It may take from 12 to 24 months, however, for the shrunken, ad-

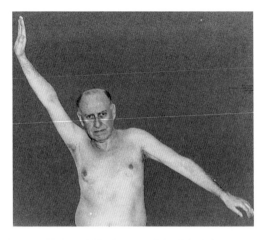

Figure 11.55.   Adhesive capsulitis of the left shoulder (frozen shoulder) in a 63-year-old man who is attempting to abduct his shoulder. He can obtain 45° of apparent abduction by elevating and rotating his scapula.

herent capsule to become separated from the humeral head and for reasonable motion to return; the frozen shoulder usually "thaws" slowly.

Treatment of adhesive capsulitis in the early, painful stage includes local rest with the arm in a sling, local heat, and analgesics. Forcing motion at this stage aggravates the situation. Approximately half the patients are improved significantly by NSAIDs or by the systemic administration of adrenocorticosteroids. Inflation of the glenohumeral joint with saline injected through a needle is sometimes successful in separating the adherent capsule from the humeral head.

In the later stages if motion is not returning at a reasonable rate, surgical manipulation, or even operative treatment such as arthroscopic surgery, is occasionally required to release the contracture of the subscapularis muscle and to separate the adherent capsule from the articular cartilage of the humeral head. After manipulation, the patient's shoulder should be managed in a continuous passive motion (CPM) device as recommended by the author.

Shoulder-Hand Syndrome

The shoulder-hand syndrome is a distressing, but poorly understood, disorder affecting the upper limb, particularly the shoulder and hand. It is an example of *reflex sympathetic dystrophy*. Although the cause of the shoulder-hand syndrome is not known, it can be initiated by any disorder, either intrinsic or extrinsic, associated with pain in the upper limb.

This syndrome usually afflicts persons past the age of 50 years, especially those who have a low pain threshold. It is characterized by disabling pain in the shoulder and hand accompanied by local neurovascular disturbances, moisture and hyperesthesia of the skin, atrophy of subcutaneous tissues, chronic edema, and eventually regional disuse atrophy of bone (disuse osteoporosis) (Fig. 11.56).

Because the limb is painful, the fearful patient refuses to use it; absence of muscle action in the dependent limb results in chronic edema of the hand which, in turn, makes joint motion in the fingers more painful. Eventually joint contractures develop, disuse atrophy becomes progressive, and a vicious cycle is established. Therefore, prompt recognition of shoulder-hand syndrome and immediate initiation of treatment are essential.

Treatment of the shoulder-hand syndrome includes psychological measures to support and encourage the patient, analgesics, systemic adrenocorticosteroids, local heat, and active exercises. Injection of the stellate ganglion with a local anesthetic agent to produce a sympathetic nerve block may improve the local blood supply and help to reverse the process by providing temporary relief of pain. After such an injection, the patient's hand

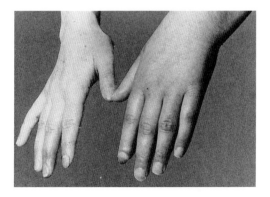

Figure 11.56. Shoulder-hand syndrome, a form of reflex sympathetic dystrophy. The left hand of this 54-year-old woman is swollen, cool, and moist.

should be managed in a CPM device to reduce the swelling and increase the range of finger joint motion.

Degenerative Tendon Disease in the Elbow

As in the shoulder, the tendinous and fascial attachments of muscles to bone (i.e., at the tendon-bone junction) in the elbow may degenerate, with subsequent local necrosis, dystrophic calcification, and pathological rupture. Many causative factors, including local trauma and excessive activity, are superimposed upon the progressive degenerative changes of the normal aging process.

Tennis Elbow (Lateral Epicondylitis). The most common example of degenerative tendon disease in the elbow is "*tennis elbow,*" also called *lateral epicondylitis*. Although proof of the pathogenesis of this disorder is lacking, it is thought to be a premature degeneration in the flat tendinous origin of the *forearm extensor muscles* from the lateral epicondyle of the humerus.

Tennis elbow is by no means limited to those who play tennis; indeed, it can develop as a sequel to local injury and to any repetitive overuse activity that involves the forearm extensor muscles. Patients with cervical spondylosis may exhibit referred hyperesthesia and tenderness just distal to the lateral epicondyle, a phenomenon that is easily confused with tennis elbow.

Clinically, tennis elbow is characterized by pain over the lateral aspect of the elbow and radiation of the pain down the forearm. The pain is aggravated by any activity that puts tension on the forearm extensor muscle origin, such as active dorsiflexion of the wrist while grasping an object, and passive flexion of the wrist against resistance. A discrete point of local tenderness is detectable just distal to the lateral epicondyle (Fig. 11.57).

Radiographic examination may reveal dystrophic calcification in the area of degeneration in the extensor muscle origin, but the elbow joint itself appears normal.

Treatment of this chronic and recurrent form of nonarticular rheumatism includes local rest, heat, NSAIDs, and one or more injections of hydrocortisone with a local anes-

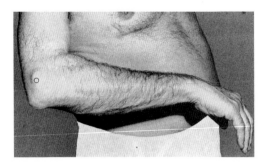

Figure 11.57.   Tennis elbow (lateral epicondylitis). The circle marks the discrete point of local tenderness.

thetic agent into the precise area of local tenderness. A broad snug band around the proximal area of the forearm decreases the pull on the affected muscles and frequently relieves symptoms during related activities. For those patients in whom troublesome symptoms persist despite these measures, it may become necessary to immobilize the wrist in a cast for several weeks (to rest the wrist extensor muscles). On rare occasions, it is necessary to resort to operative treatment in which the fascial attachment of the extensor muscles to the lateral epicondyle is divided and allowed to retract distally or is repaired. This is combined with an epicondylectomy.

Golfer's Elbow (Medial Epicondylitis). A comparable example of degenerative tendon disease involves the medial epicondyle (medial epicondylitis). Its symptoms and signs are similar to those of tennis elbow, as is its treatment.

Degenerative Tendon Disease in the Wrist and Hand

The most common form of nonarticular rheumatism in the wrist and hand is that associated with thickening of the fibrous sheath of a tendon with resultant narrowing of the tunnel (*tenovaginitis stenosans*). Two definite clinical entities are readily recognized—one at the wrist and the other in the fingers. Although tenovaginitis stenosans usually develops in otherwise normal persons, occasionally it is a manifestation of early rheumatoid arthritis.

de Quervain's Tenovaginitis Stenosans. At the level of the lower end of the radius, the tendons of the abductor policis longus and extensor pollicis brevis share a common fibrous sheath. Excessive friction between those tendons and their common sheath, caused by repeated forceful use of the hands in typing, in gripping objects, or in wringing clothes, probably account for the abnormal thickening of the fibrous sheath and the resultant constriction, or stenosis, of the tunnel.

This fairly common clinical disorder, which is seen more frequently in women, is characterized by wrist pain that radiates proximally up the forearm and distally toward the thumb. Examination reveals a firm local tenderness in the area of the common fibrous sheath over the radial styloid (Fig. 11.58). Forceful passive adduction (ulnar deviation) of the patient's wrist with the thumb held completely flexed puts tension on the involved tendons and reproduces the pain (Finklestein's test).

Treatment of de Quervain's tenovaginitis stenosans by local injection of hydrocortisone into the tendon sheath usually brings temporary relief. Immobilization of the thumb or wrist in a plastic splint in a position to take tension off the involved tendons for 6 weeks is often effective. If this proves ineffective, operative division of the stenosed tendon sheath is required to provide permanent relief of pain.

Digital Tenovaginitis Stenosans (Trigger Finger or Snapping Finger). In the palm of the hand, the deep (profundus) and superficial (sublimus) flexor tendons to each finger are enclosed by a common fibrous sheath. Excessive thickening of this fibrous sheath may develop spontaneously for no apparent reason, particularly in middle-aged women. It may

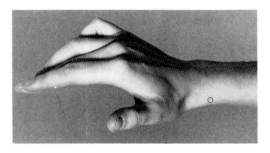

Figure 11.58.   de Quervain's tenovaginitis stenosans. The circle marks the site of local tenderness over the common fibrous sheath for the tendons of the abductor pollicis longus and extensor pollicis brevis.

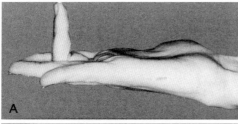

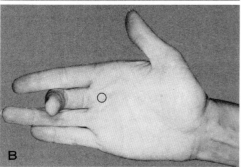

Figure 11.59. Tenovaginitis stenosans involving the right middle finger in a 43-year-old woman. **A.** The patient is attempting to extend the finger but is unable to do so. The finger can be extended passively and the extension occurs with a "snapping" motion. The patient is then able to flex the finger actively, but again with a snapping action similar to the action of a trigger. **B.** The circle marks the site of the palpable nodular enlargement in the flexor tendons.

also occur, however, as a complication of rheumatoid synovitis in the hand.

Thickening of the fibrous sheath produces a stenosis, or constriction, in the tunnel and, as a result, free gliding of the flexor tendons is impeded. The tendons become secondarily enlarged proximal to the tunnel, presumably because of repeated friction. The patient is unable to extend the involved finger actively (Fig. 11.59). The finger can be extended passively and the extension occurs with a "snapping" motion. The patient is then able to flex the finger actively, but again with a "snapping" action similar to the action of a trigger. The nodular enlargement in the flexor tendons can be palpated just proximal to the base of the finger.

Treatment by means of immobilization of the finger in complete extension and one or more injections of hydrocortisone may relieve the snapping phenomenon. Sometimes, however, operative division of the fibrous sheath

is required to provide permanent relief of the symptoms.

A congenital type of fibrous tunnel stenosis involving the thumb of infants and young children (trigger thumb) is discussed in Chapter 8.

Dupuytren's Contracture of the Palmar Fascia

Progressive fibrous tissue contracture of the palmar fascia (*Dupuytren's contracture*) on the medial (ulnar) side of the hand is not uncommon in men past the age of 50 years. The cause is unknown, but there is evidence of a hereditary predisposition. The involved fascia exhibits abnormal collagen composition and fibroblast activity as well as altered levels of some enzymes, but the pathogenesis is not understood.

The disorder is frequently bilateral; it may even involve the plantar fascia of the feet. The initial manifestation of this insidious and painless process is nodular thickening in the palmar fascia, which becomes adherent to the overlying skin. Over the ensuing years, a slowly progressive contracture of thick cordlike fibrous tissue of the palmar fascia gradually pulls the ring and little fingers into flexion at the metacarpophalangeal and proximal interphalangeal joints (Fig. 11.60). Although the synovial joints are not involved primarily, they eventually develop secondary capsular contractures and degeneration of articular car-

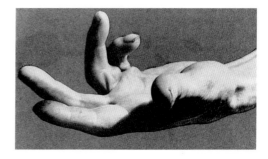

Figure 11.60. Dupuytren's contracture of the palmar fascia involving the ring and little fingers of the hand of a 56-year-old man. Note the flexion deformity of the metacarpophalangeal and proximal interphalangeal joints as well as the local adherence of the puckered skin to the palmar fascia.

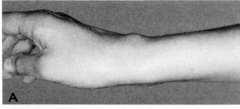

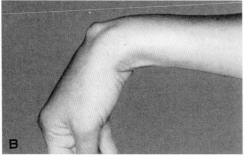

Figure 11.61.   A. Ganglion on the dorsum of the hand of a 26-year-old woman. **B.** The cystic swelling is more apparent when the wrist is flexed.

tilage secondary to the persistent restriction of motion.

Treatment of Dupuytren's contracture involves surgical excision of all the abnormal palmar fascia when the fingers have begun to develop a significant flexion deformity (more than 30° at the metacarpophalangeal joint and 10° at the interphalangeal joints). Less complete operations, such as multiple subcutaneous division of fibrous bands, are frequently followed by recurrence of the contracture. The postoperative use of a CPM hand device helps to maintain the finger joint motion gained at operation.

Ganglion

A *ganglion* is a thin-walled, cystic, synovial-lined lesion containing thick, clear, mucinous fluid. Its origin is as yet unknown, but it arises in relation to periarticular tissues, joint capsules, and tendon sheaths, possibly because of mucoid degeneration. Ganglia are limited to the hands and feet, by far the most common site being the dorsum of the hand (Fig. 11.61).

The patient notices a soft swelling that tends to enlarge gradually but may vary in size from time to time. Occasionally, the ganglion

causes local discomfort, but usually the patient is more concerned about its appearance. A ganglion on the palmar aspect of the hand may even cause pressure on either the median or ulnar nerve with resultant disturbance of nerve function.

Ganglia tend to regress spontaneously over a long period of time, but usually the patient wishes to be rid of the unsightly swelling. If a ganglion is deliberately ruptured by firm pressure, with or without needling, it tends to recur. Some ganglia respond to aspiration, but usually complete operative excision of the ganglion is necessary to achieve a permanently satisfactory result.

Popliteal Cyst (Baker's Cyst)

A cyst that is somewhat similar to a ganglion may develop in the popliteal region, usually in relation to the semimembranous bursa. Such popliteal cysts (Baker's cysts) are common in childhood, in which case they seldom cause symptoms (Fig. 11.62). A popliteal cyst usually regresses spontaneously during childhood.

In adults, popliteal cysts are secondary to disease in the knee joint with which they communicate through a hollow stalk, and in a sense they represent a "synovial hernia." Thus, in the presence of a synovial effusion in the knee, caused by either rheumatoid arthritis or degenerative joint disease, the popliteal cyst becomes distended by the effusion and may extend distally even as far as the mid-calf. A large popliteal cyst in an adult may even rupture and produce a clinical picture somewhat similar to a deep calf vein thrombosis.

If a popliteal cyst becomes sufficiently enlarged that it interferes with knee function, operative excision of the cyst and exploration of the joint are indicated.

Meniscal Cyst

A fluid-filled cyst of a meniscus may develop in childhood and produce a tender swelling at the joint line; it is more often the lateral meniscus that is involved. Barrie has demonstrated that such cysts usually communicate with a meniscal tear and are "fueled" by syno-

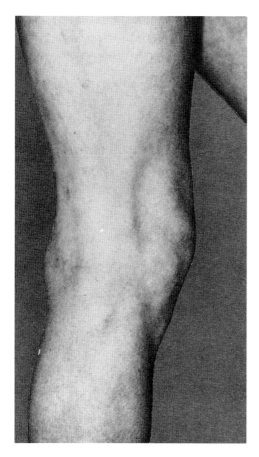

Figure 11.62.   Popliteal cyst (Baker's cyst) behind the right knee of a 10-year-old child. The cyst caused no symptoms.

friction bursitis is that caused by the pressure and friction of tight shoes over the prominence of the first metatarsal head, especially in the presence of a hallux valgus deformity; this particular example of friction bursitis is referred to as a *bunion* (Fig. 11.63). The friction type of bursitis may be related to excessive friction associated with specific occupations. The following are examples of this type of bursitis: *prepatellar   bursitis*   ("housemaid's knee") (Fig. 11.64), ischial bursitis (*weaver's bottom*), and olecranon bursitis ("student's elbow") (Fig. 11.65).

Degenerative changes and calcification in a subjacent tendon may irritate the overlying bursa and cause a *chemical bursitis;* subacromial bursitis secondary to calcific supraspinatus tendinitis is an example of chemical bursitis. In addition, a chemical bursitis may develop secondary to the tophaceous deposits of urate crystals in gout.

Infection of a bursa, by either pyogenic or granulomatous organisms, results in an *infective,* or *septic, bursitis,* which although initially acute, may later become chronic.

Treatment of bursitis is directed toward the underlying cause. Friction bursitis usually resolves after cessation of the friction, but if the bursa has become sufficiently large, it may re-

vial fluid. When it causes symptoms, such a cyst may have to be excised.

Bursitis

Bursae are lined with synovium and synovial fluid containing sacs that exist normally at sites of friction between tendons and bone as well as between these structures and the overlying skin. In addition, pluripotential connective tissue cells are capable of creating "adventitious bursae" at sites of friction caused by abnormalities such as pathological bony prominence and protruding parts of metallic inserts.

As a result of repeated excessive friction, a bursa may become inflamed (*friction bursitis*); the wall of the bursa thickens and a bursal effusion develops. The most common example of

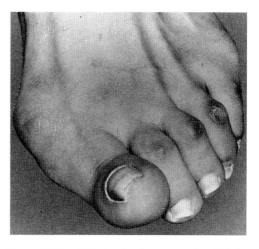

Figure 11.63.   This bunion is an example of friction bursitis over the head of the first metatarsal in association with a hallux valgus deformity. Note also the corns overlying the proximal interphalangeal joints of the four small toes.

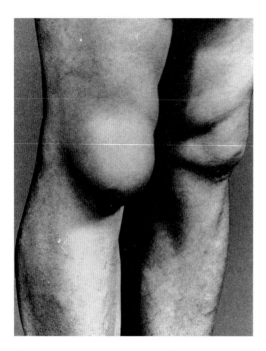

Figure 11.64. Prepatellar bursitis (housemaid's knee)—an example of friction bursitis in a 45-year-old woman. In this patient, the amount of fluid in the bursa is greater than is usually seen in prepatellar bursitis.

quire excision. Chemical bursitis responds to removal of the responsible irritant (calcium or urate crystals) and the local injection of hydrocortisone. Acute septic bursitis requires surgical drainage, but chronic septic bursitis necessitates operative excision of the bursa.

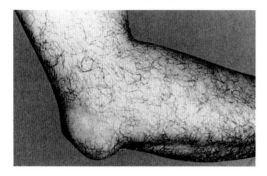

Figure 11.65. Olecranon bursitis (student's elbow) is an example of bursitis that may be caused either by the repeated microtrauma of friction (as against a desk top) or by a single direct trauma.

SUGGESTED ADDITIONAL READING

Aichroth PM, Cannon WD, Patel DV. Knee surgery. Current practice. New York: Raven Press, Martin Dunitz Ltd., 1992.

Aichroth PM, Patel DV, Moyes ST. A prospective review of arthroscopic debridement for degenerative joint disease of the knee. Int Orthop 1991; 15:351–355.

Apley AG, Solomon L. Apley's system of orthopaedics and fractures. 7th ed. Oxford: Butterworth-Heinemann, 1993.

Barrie HJ. The pathogenesis and significance of meniscal cysts. J Bone Joint Surg 1979;61B: 184–189.

Bennett RM. Fibromyalgia and the disability dilemma. A new era in understanding a complex, multidimensional pain syndrome. Arthritis Rheum 1996;39:1627–1634.

Boden SD, Wiesel SW. Lumbar spine imaging: role in clinical decision making. J Am Acad Orthop Surg 1996; 4:238–248.

Boden SW. The use of radiographic imaging studies in the evaluation of patients who have degenerative disorders of the lumbar spine. Current Concepts Review. J Bone Joint Surg 1996;78A: 114–124.

Brandt KD, Shemenda CW. Osteoarthritis. A. Epidemiology, pathology and pathogenesis. In: Schumacher HR Jr, ed. Primer on the rheumatic diseases. 10th ed. Atlanta: Arthritis Foundation, 1993:184–188.

Brittberg M, Lindahl A, Ohlsson C, et al. Treatment of deep cartilage defects in the knee with autologous chondrocyte transplantation. N Engl J Med 1994;331:889–895.

Brower AC. Arthritis in black and white. Philadelphia: WB Saunders, 1988.

Buckwalter JA. Operative treatment of osteoarthritis. Current practice and future development. Current Concepts Review. J Bone Joint Surg 1994;76A:1405–1418.

Buckwalter JA, Goldberg VM, Woo, Savio L-Y, eds. Musculoskeletal soft-tissue aging: impact on mobility. Rosemont, IL: American Academy of Orthopaedic Surgeons, 1992.

Charnley J. Low friction arthroplasty of the hip. Theory and practice. Berlin: Springer-Verlag, 1976.

Chiari K. Iliac osteotomy in young adults. In: Sledge CB, ed. The hip. Proceedings of the Seventh Open Scientific Meeting of the Hip Society. St. Louis: CV Mosby, 1979:260–277.

Clark CR, Bonfiglio M, eds. Orthopaedics. Essentials of diagnosis and treatment. New York: Churchill Livingstone, 1994.

Cohen J, Bonfiglio M, Campbell CJ. Orthopaedic pathophysiology in diagnosis and treatment. New York: Churchill Livingstone, 1990.

Coventry MB, Ilstrup DM, Wallricks SL. Proximal tibial osteotomy: a critical long-term study of eighty-seven cases. J Bone Joint Surg 1993;75A: 196–201.

Curl WW. Popliteal cysts: historical background and current knowledge. J Am Acad Orthop Surg 1996;4:129–133.

Czitrom AA, Gross AE, eds. Allografts in orthopaedic practice. Baltimore: Williams & Wilkins, 1992.

Dandy DJ. Essential orthopaedics and trauma. 2nd ed. Edinburgh: Churchill-Livingstone, 1993.

Duncan CP, Spangehl M, Beauchamp C, McGraw R. Hip arthrodesis. An important option for advanced disease in the young adult. Can J Surg 1995;38(Suppl 1):S39-S46.

Duncan CP, Waddell JP. Hip disease in the young adult. A social as well as a medical dilemma. Can J Surg 1995;38(Suppl 1)55–56.

Duthie RB, Bentley G, eds. Mercer's orthopaedic surgery. 9th ed. London: Arnold, 1996.

Ejeskar A, Nachemson A, Herberts P, et al. Surgery versus chemonucleolysis for herniated lumbar discs. Clin Orthop 1982;171:252–259.

Eppright RH. Dial osteotomy of the acetabulum in the treatment of dysplasia of the hip (abstract). J Bone Joint Surg 1975;57A:1172.

Finklestein JA, Gross AE, Davis A. Varus osteotomy of the distal part of the femur. A survivorship analysis. J Bone Joint Surg 1996;78A: 1348–1352.

Frymoyer JW, ed. The adult spine. 2nd ed. Hagerstown: Lippincott-Raven Publishers, 1996.

Frymoyer JW. Back pain and sciatica: medical progress. N Engl J Med 1988;318:291–300.

Ganz R, Klave K, Vinh TS, et al. A new periacetabular osteotomy for the treatment of hip dysplasias: technique and preliminary results. Clin Orthop 1988;232:260–277.

Hall HJ, McIntosh G, Melles T. A different approach to back pain diagnosis: identifying a pattern of pain. Can J CME 1994;6(2):31–43.

Hochberg MC, Altman RD, Brandt KD et al. Guidelines for the medical management of osteoarthritis. Part I. Osteoarthritis of the hip. Arthritis Rheum 1995;38:1535–1541.

Hochberg MC, Altman RD, Brandt KD, et al. Guidelines for the medical management of osteoarthritis. Part II. Osteoarthritis of the knee. Arthritis Rheum 1995;38:1541–1547.

Jobe FW, Chiccotti MG. Lateral and medial epicondylitis of the elbow. J Am Acad Orthop Surg 1994;2:1–8.

Kasser JR, ed. Orthopaedic knowledge update 5. Home study syllabus. Rosemont IL: American Academy of Orthopaedic Surgeons, 1996.

Kim HKW, Moran ME, Salter RB. The potential for the regeneration of articular cartilage created by chondral shaving and subchondral abrasion. An experimental investigation in the rabbit. J Bone Joint Surg 1991;73A:1301–1315.

Kirkaldy-Willis WH. Managing low back pain. 3rd ed. New York: Churchill Livingstone, 1992.

Kuettner KE, Schleyerbach R, Hascall VC. Articular cartilage biochemistry. New York: Raven Press, 1986.

Laupacis A, Bourne R, Rorabeck C, et al. The effect of elective total hip replacement on health-related quality of life. J Bone Joint Surg 1993;75A: 1619–1626.

Mankin JH. The reaction of articular cartilage to injury and to osteoarthritis. Part I. N Engl J Med 1974;291:1285.

Mankin JH. The reaction of articular cartilage to injury and to osteoarthritis. Part II. N Engl J Med 1974;291:1335.

Mankin HJ, Buckwalter JA. Restoration of the osteoarthritic joint (Editorial). J Bone Joint Surg 1996;78A:1–2.

Maquet P. The biomechanics of the knee and surgical possibilities of healing osteoarthritic knee joints. Clin Orthop 1980;146:102.

Mattsson E, Broström LA. The physical and psychosocial effect of moderate osteoarthrosis of the knee. Scand J Rehab Med 1991;23:215–218.

McCulloch JA. Chemonucleolysis: experience with 2000 cases. Clin Orthop Related Res 1980;146: 128–135.

McCulloch JA. Principles of microsurgery for lumbar disc disease. New York: Raven Press, 1989.

McCulloch JA, Transfeldt EE. Macnab's backache. 3rd ed. Baltimore: Williams & Wilkins, 1997.

McInness J, Larson MG, Daltroy LH, et al. A controlled evaluation of continuous passive motion in patients undergoing total knee arthroplasty. JAMA 1992;268:1423–1428.

McLaren AC, Blokker CP, Fowler PS, et al. Arthroscopic débridement of the knee for osteoarthrosis. Can J Surg 1991;34:595–598.

Meyers MH, Chatterjee SN. Osteochondral transplantation. Surg Clin North Am 1978;58: 429–434.

Morrey BF. The elbow and its disorders. 2nd ed. Philadelphia: WB Saunders, 1993.

Moskowitz RW, Goldberg VM. Osteoarthritis B. Clinical features and treatment. In: Schumacher HR Jr, ed. Primer on the rheumatic diseases. 10th ed. Atlanta: Arthritis Foundation, 1993: 188–190.

Moskowitz RW, Howell DS, Goldberg M, Mankin HJ, eds. Osteoarthritis. Diagnosis and medical/surgical management. Philadelphia: WB Saunders, 1992.

Nachemson AL. Advances in low-back pain. Clin Orthop 1985;200:266–278.

Nagel A, Insall JN, Scuderi GR. Proximal tibial osteotomy. A subjective outcome study. J Bone Joint Surg 1996;78A:1353–1358.

O'Driscoll SW, Keeley FW, Salter RB. The chondrogenic potential of free autogenous periosteal grafts for biological resurfacing of full-thickness defects in joint surfaces under the influence of continuous passive motion: An experimental investigation in the rabbit. J Bone Joint Surg 1986;68A:1017–1035.

Postacchini F. Management of lumbar spinal stenosis (instructional course lecture). J Bone Joint Surg 1996;78B:154–164.

Radin EL, Paul IL. Does cartilage compliance reduce skeletal impact loads? The relative force attenuating properties of articular cartilage, synovial fluid, peri-articular soft tissues and bone. Arthritis Rheum 1970;13:139–144.

Radin EL, Yang KH, Riegger C, et al. Relationship between lower limb dynamics and knee joint pain. J Orthop Res 1991;9:398–405.

Richards RR. Soft tissue reconstruction in the upper extremity. New York: Churchill Livingstone, 1995.

Salter RB. Continuous passive motion—CPM—a biological concept for the healing and regeneration of articular cartilage, ligaments, and tendons: from origination to research to clinical applications. Baltimore: Williams & Wilkins, 1993.

Salter RB, Field P. The effects of continuous compression on living articular cartilage. An experimental investigation. J Bone Joint Surg 1960;42A:31–49.

Salter RB, Gross A, Hall JH. Hydrocortisone arthroplasty: an experimental investigation. Can Med Assoc J 1967;97:374–377.

Salter RB, Hansson G, Thompson GH. Innominate osteotomy in the management of residual congenital subluxation of the hip in young adults. Clin Orthop Related Res 1994;182:53–68.

Salter RB, McNeill OR, Carbin R. The pathological changes in articular cartilage associated with persistent joint deformity. An experimental investigation. In: Studies of rheumatoid disease. Proceedings of the Third Canadian Conference in Rheumatic Diseases. Toronto: University of Toronto Press, 1965:33–47.

Santore RF, Dabezies EJ Jr. Femoral osteotomy for secondary arthritis of the hip in young adults. Can J Surg 1995;38(Suppl 15):S35–S39.

Schumacher HR Jr, ed. Primer on the rheumatic diseases. 10th ed. Atlanta: Arthritis Foundation, 1993.

Sledge CB, ed. The 1993 year book of orthopaedics. St. Louis: Mosby, 1993.

Sledge CG, ed. The 1995 year book of orthopaedics. St. Louis: Mosby, 1995.

Smythe HA, Moldofsky H. Two contributions to the understanding of the "fibrositis syndrome." Bull Rheum Dis 1977;28:929–931.

Soren A. Arthritis and related affections: clinic, pathology, treatment. Berlin: Springer-Verlag, 1993.

Steel HH. Triple osteotomy of the innominate bone. J Bone Joint Surg 1973;55A:343–350.

Swank M, Stulberg SD, Jiganti J, Machairas S. The natural history of unicompartmental arthroplasty: an eight-year follow-up study with survivorship analysis. Clin Orthop 1993;286:130–142.

Tregonning GD, Transfeldt EE, McCulloch JA, et al. Chymopapain versus conventional surgery for lumbar disc herniation. 10-year results of treatment. J Bone Joint Surg 1991;73B:3:481–486.

Wagner H. Osteotomies for congenital hip dislocation. In: Evarts CM, ed. The hip: proceedings of the fourth open scientific meeting of the hip society. St. Louis: CV Mosby, 1976:45–66.

Warner JJP, Answorth A, Marks PH, Wong P. Arthroscopic release for chronic refractory adhesive capsulitis of the shoulder. J Bone Joint Surg 1996;78A:1808–1816.

Wedge JH. Osteotomy of the pelvis for the management of hip disease in young adults. Can J Surg 1995;38(Suppl 1):S25-S33.

Wedge JH, Salter RB. Innominate osteotomy: its role in the arrest of secondary degenerative arthritis of the hip in the adult. Clin Orthop 1974;98:214–224.

Weinstein JN, Gordon SL. Low back pain: a scientific and clinical overview. Rosemont, IL: American Academy of Orthopaedic Surgeons, 1996.

Weinstein SL, Buckwalter JA, eds. Turek's orthopaedics, principles and their application. 5th ed. Philadelphia: JB Lippincott, 1994.

12 Neuromuscular Disorders

In other chapters of this textbook concerning the musculoskeletal system, most of the emphasis is placed on the skeletal components, that is, the bones that provide the rigid framework for the body and the joints that permit movement between the bones. The musculoskeletal system (sometimes called the *motorskeletal* or *locomotor* system) relies on its voluntary muscles, or motors, to provide active coordinated movement. The muscles in turn depend on the nervous system for the innervation that provides the stimulus for contraction. Indeed, this interrelationship is so close that together they are thought of as the neuromusculoskeletal system.

A wide variety of clinical disorders and injuries of the nervous system appear as disturbances of both form and function of the musculoskeletal system; the more significant of these are considered in this textbook. You will learn much about these neurological disorders and injuries from others; the present chapter, however, will emphasize their musculoskeletal manifestations, as well as the principles of their orthopaedic treatment and the rehabilitation of patients so afflicted.

CLINICAL MANIFESTATIONS OF NEUROLOGICAL DISORDERS AND INJURIES

The human brain, spinal cord, and peripheral nerves comprise a complex system. Diagnosis based on the clinical manifestations of neurological disorders and injuries requires precise detective work. The data, or clues, obtained from a detailed history and a complete neurological examination enable the clinician to narrow the possible diagnoses down to a few suspects, or differential diagnoses. Often they provide sufficient evidence to at least postulate a diagnosis of the anatomical site(s) and nature of the disorder or injury. These methods of investigation, of course, are available to every clinician. Diagnostic imaging and laboratory investigations are sometimes necessary,

either to confirm or disprove the postulated diagnosis by determining the precise location of a lesion as well as its pathological nature.

To appreciate the significance of the clinical manifestations of neurological disorders and injuries, you must be aware of their underlying pathological, anatomical and physiological factors.

Pathological Factors

Nervous tissue is affected by disease and injury in only four ways; therefore, all neurological signs and symptoms are manifestations of one or more of these four modes of disturbed function:

1. Destruction of nerve cells with permanent loss of their function, as in the destruction of motor cells (anterior horn cells) in poliomyelitis.
2. Transient disturbance of nerve cells with temporary loss of their function, as in cerebral shock and spinal shock, seen only in lesions of sudden development as occur in acute injury.
3. Unlimited action (usually overaction) of intact mechanisms of the nervous system that have been "released" from the normal inhibitory control of higher centers. An example of this phenomenon is the spasticity that develops after a lesion in the cerebral motor cortex.
4. Irritation phenomena caused by a lesion that stimulates nerve cells to excessive activity. Examples are excessive pain that may follow a peripheral nerve injury (causalgia) and epilepsy.

Clinical Manifestations of Lesions in Specific Systems of Neurons

Being equipped with the foregoing knowledge of the normal functions of the major neuron systems of the central and peripheral nervous system you will understand the following clinical manifestations of neurological lesions.

Upper Motor Neuron (Corticospinal) Lesions

In humans the upper motor neuron, or corticospinal, system and the extrapyramidal system are so closely related anatomically throughout most of their respective courses that, in most sites, a given lesion tends to affect both systems. The term *corticospinal* is currently preferred over the term, *pyramidal*. A cerebrovascular lesion involving the internal capsule, for example, affects both corticospinal and extrapyramidal tracts. Nevertheless, for clarity, it is wise to consider these two systems separately.

Corticospinal Lesions

1. *Weakness (paresis) of voluntary movements:* The paresis, which is a flaccid type at first because of cerebral shock, involves patterns of movement rather than movement by individual muscles. Paresis is not a true paralysis of all movement, because the corticospinal system is not the only mediator of movement. The remaining intact part of the motor cerebral cortex can compensate to a remarkable degree for the weakness of extensors of the upper limb and flexors of the lower limb.
2. *Increased muscle tone:* Several weeks after the loss of initiating impulses from the corticospinal system, other reflexes, having been "released" from higher control, take over and produce increased muscle tone that, in turn, is manifest by spasticity, increased stretch reflex, exaggerated deep tendon reflexes, and clonus.
3. *Muscle contractures:* The spastic muscles develop permanent shortening (contracture) due to increased fibrosis.
4. *Loss of abdominal cutaneous reflexes.*
5. *Extensor-type plantar cutaneous reflex* (Babinski response).

Extrapyramidal System Lesions

1. *Increased muscle tone:* Loss of the inhibitory, or relaxing, function of the extrapyramidal system leads to the development of increased muscle tone with manifestations similar to those of corticospinal system lesions, described above.
2. *Muscle contractures:* The spastic muscles develop permanent shortening.
3. *Involuntary movements:* Lesions of the basal ganglia may lead to uncontrolled, purposeless movements that are aggravated by emotional tension and attempts at voluntary control. These "mobile spasms," called *athetosis,* are seen in the athetoid type of cerebral palsy. Another type of involuntary movement due to lesions of certain basal ganglia is the tremor seen in paralysis agitans (Parkinson's disease).
4. *Rigidity:* Lesions of certain basal ganglia may cause rigidity of a limb due to uninhibited simultaneous stimulation of all muscles that move a given part.

Cerebellar Lesions

1. *Loss of coordination of muscle action:* The resultant jerky, halting, uncoordinated movements of a limb are manifest by the inability to perform the finger-to-nose test accurately.
2. *Disturbed sense of balance:* As a result, the gait is unsteady and stumbling (cerebellar ataxia).
3. *Decreased muscle tone:* The loss of cerebellar regulation of posture results in decreased muscle tone with diminution of deep tendon reflexes. Muscle contractures do not develop with pure cerebellar lesions.
4. *Slow slurred speech* (ataxic dysarthria).
5. *Nystagmus.*

Spinal Cord Lesions

Lesions of the spinal cord often produce a combined upper and lower motor deficit; damage to the upper motor neurons at a given level in the cord may also affect the lower motor neurons in the spinal nerve roots arising from a higher level. A lesion that develops suddenly, such as a spinal cord injury or hemorrhage, is followed by a transient state of "spinal shock" in which the innervated muscles demonstrate a flaccid paralysis. This flaccidity is superseded within a few weeks by spasticity of the paralyzed muscles, because the spinal cord reflexes take over in the absence of the normal inhibitory impulses from higher centers. The paralysis may involve both lower limbs (paraplegia, diplegia) or all four limbs (quadriplegia, tetraplegia). Depending on the precise site of the spinal cord lesion, there may be an associated sensory loss distal to the level of that lesion.

The reflex response to any stimulation is greatly exaggerated and, indeed, mass reflexes may occur in the paralyzed segments, with total flexion of the limbs and trunk (paraplegia-in-flexion). These troublesome spasms may even cause the bladder to empty. When the responsible lesion is in the brain stem, the paralysis involves rigidity of all muscle groups (akin to decerebrate rigidity). The attitude of the limbs and trunk under these circumstances is one of persistent extension (paraplegia-in-extension).

Lower Motor Neuron Lesions

1. *Flaccid paralysis:* complete loss of contraction in some or all of the fibers of the affected muscle or muscles, depending on the number of lower motor neurons involved by the lesion.
2. *Absence of muscle tone:* and therefore absence of deep tendon reflexes.
3. *Progressive atrophy of muscle:* This type of neurogenic atrophy of muscle is referred to as *amyotrophy*. During the period of atrophy, there may be twitching of muscle fascicles (fasciculation) within the paralyzed muscle, particularly if the lesion is due to a subacute or chronic process.
4. *Muscle contracture:* Permanent shortening (contracture) may develop in the unopposed normal muscles that are no longer being passively extended to their full length.
5. *Sensory loss:* A lesion involving the spinal nerve root or the peripheral nerve, both of which carry sensory as well as motor fibers, will produce a corresponding loss of sensation in addition to the flaccid paralysis.

Examples of lower motor neuron lesions at various levels in the final common pathway are as follows: 1) destruction of the anterior horn

cells of the spinal cord by a virus as in poliomyelitis; 2) compression of a spinal nerve root by a herniated intervertebral disc; 3) traumatic division of a peripheral nerve.

Diagnostic Imaging of the Nervous System

Before the development of CT, radiographic examination of the nervous system was indirect in that it could demonstrate only the skull, cerebral blood vessels (by cerebral arteriography), and fluid-filled spaces of the brain, such as the ventricles (by pneumoencephalography). By contrast, CT imaging depicts the brain and spinal cord directly, and MRI can even distinguish between gray and white matter. With MRI, T_1-weighted images reveal clear resolution of anatomical details, and T_2-weighted images, which are high contrast, demonstrate fluid (either edema or cerebrospinal fluid). Positron-emission tomography (PET) and single-proton-emission computed tomography (SPECT) depict not only structure of the brain but also some of its hemodynamic and metabolic functions.

PATHOGENESIS OF NEUROGENIC DEFORMITIES OF THE MUSCULOSKELETAL SYSTEM

A serious sequela to many disorders and injuries of the nervous system is the development of progressive musculoskeletal deformities over time, particularly during the growing years. These secondary deformities, which frequently add significantly to the patient's disability, are caused by the following factors:

1. *Muscle imbalance.* The continuing unequal pull of muscles in the presence of paralysis, whether because of excessive pull of spastic muscles or the inadequate pull of flaccid muscles, leads eventually to the development of a persistent joint deformity.
2. *Muscle contracture.* In any muscle that is not repeatedly extended to its full length many times a day, as in spastic muscles or normal muscles lacking opposition from flaccid partners or opponents, fibrosis of

the muscle leads to permanent shortening (contracture). Thus, muscle imbalance and muscle contracture are equally important in the pathogenesis of paralytic joint deformities. Examples of such deformities include paralytic equinus at the ankle, paralytic hip flexion deformity, and paralytic scoliosis. The combination of muscle imbalance and contracture can even cause a major joint such as the hip to dislocate (paralytic dislocation).

3. *Muscle atrophy.* Neurogenic atrophy of muscle (amyotrophy) leads to an obvious deformity by altering the normal contour of a limb.

4. *Retardation of bone growth.* The combination of paralysis, disuse, and decreased blood supply in an involved limb causes a retardation of longitudinal bone growth. When the paralysis involves either the lower or upper pair of limbs unequally during childhood, the inevitable result is a progressive limb-length discrepancy.

PRINCIPLES OF ORTHOPAEDIC TREATMENT OF NEUROLOGICAL DISORDERS AND INJURIES

The orthopaedic treatment of the residual sequelae of neurological disorders and injuries is based upon the following aims or principles:

1. *Prevention of musculoskeletal deformity:* Paralytic deformities of joints can be prevented partially by passively moving each involved joint through a full range of motion for at least several minutes each day.

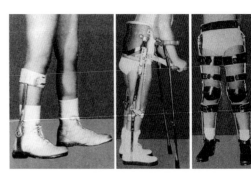

Figure 12.2. Lower limb braces that prevent unwanted motion while permitting desired motion in weak or unstable limbs.

Other means of preventing paralytic deformity include the use of removable splints (Fig. 12.1) and day braces (Fig. 12.2). Correction of the underlying muscle imbalance is often possible by means of tendon transfer (Fig. 12.3).

2. *Correction of existing musculoskeletal deformity:* Passive stretching of a muscle contracture may be enough to correct an existing deformity. More often, however, permanent correction of a paralytic deformity requires surgical procedures such as tendon lengthening (Fig. 12.4), tenodesis (Fig. 12.5), osteotomy (Fig. 12.6), or arthrodesis (Fig. 12.7).

3. *Improvement of muscle balance:* This requires the judicious use of muscle and tendon transfers (Fig. 12.3).

4. *Improvement of function:* Even when function in a limb cannot be helped by surgery,

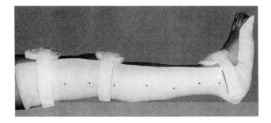

Figure 12.1. Removable splint to maintain the joints of a paralyzed limb in the optimal position in an attempt to prevent paralytic deformity.

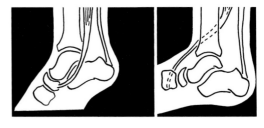

Figure 12.3. Tendon transfer. In this example the tendon of the tibialis posterior muscle has been rerouted through the interosseous membrane and transferred to the lateral cuneiform bone on the dorsum of the foot. In its new position, it will serve as a dorsiflexor of the ankle and an evertor of the foot.

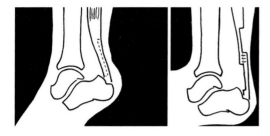

Figure 12.4. Tendon lengthening. After the long step-cut in this Achilles tendon, the ends are allowed to shift in relation to each other, then sutured in the elongated position.

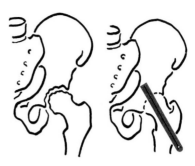

Figure 12.7. Arthrodesis. In this example, the cartilaginous joint surfaces are excised from each joint surface and the raw bony surfaces are encouraged to join each other (fuse). Internal fixation and bone grafts may be required. The completely fused (arthrodesed) joint is immobile, but stable and painless.

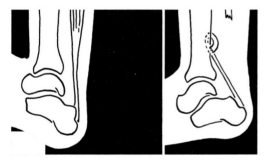

Figure 12.5. Tenodesis. In this example, the Achilles tendon of the paralyzed calf muscle is separated from the muscle and transplanted into the tibia where it will serve as a check rein, or ligament, thereby limiting passive dorsiflexion.

functional braces may be useful (Fig. 12.8).

5. *Improvement of gait or appearance:* A lower limb-length discrepancy may require surgery on the shorter leg (surgical stimulation, surgical lengthening) or on the longer leg (epiphyseal arrest, surgical shortening), as depicted in Chapter 6. The appearance of an atrophied limb can be improved by a suitably designed cosmetic prosthesis (Fig. 12.9).

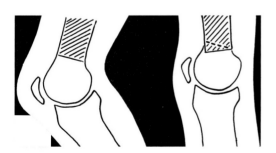

Figure 12.6. Osteotomy to deal with a joint deformity by producing a compensatory bony deformity near the joint. In this example, the knee flexion deformity persists, but the limb is made straight by the compensatory osteotomy in the supracondylar region of the femur.

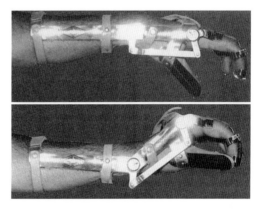

Figure 12.8. Functional brace, used to compensate for loss of power in the finger flexors. It is designed so that active dorsiflexion of the wrist will cause the paralyzed fingers to flex and the thumb to oppose them.

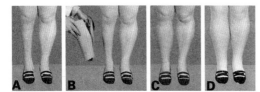

Figure 12.9. Cosmetic prosthesis for atrophy of the leg. **A.** Marked residual atrophy from poliomyelitis in the leg of a 19-year-old woman, who was embarrassed by the appearance of her leg. **B.** A custom-made foam prosthesis (produced from a reverse mold of the normal leg) is about to be applied. **C.** The flesh-colored prosthesis in place; it closes with a hidden zipper on the inner side. The patient then puts a flesh colored stocking on both legs before putting on dress stockings. **D.** The appearance is greatly improved.

6. *Rehabilitation—a philosophy in action:* The philosophy of total care *of* your patient as well as continuing care *for* your patient is vital, as outlined at the end of Chapter 6.

DISORDERS OF THE BRAIN
Cerebral Palsy

The broad term *cerebral palsy* ("spastic paralysis," "brain damage") encompasses the various types and degrees of nonprogressive brain disorders that develop before, during, or relatively soon after birth. These disorders, which become clinically apparent in early childhood and persist throughout the patient's life, manifest as disturbances of voluntary muscle function and perception. There is often some associated impairment of mental acuity, which is currently referred to as "mental disability."

Because of the effective prevention of musculoskeletal tuberculosis and paralytic poliomyelitis in recent years, cerebral palsy has become one of the foremost causes of musculoskeletal disability in childhood. Furthermore, because of its persistent nature, cerebral palsy presents serious social, psychological, and educational problems.

Incidence

Cerebral palsy is relatively common throughout the world. It has been estimated that every year, for each 100,000 population, six children with cerebral palsy will be born and will survive; a seventh will succumb at birth. Thus, in a country with a population of 100,000,000, there will be 6,000 newborns with cerebral palsy each year.

Etiology

There are many causes of cerebral palsy; indeed any nonprogressive condition that leads to an abnormality of the brain can be responsible. At one time it was thought that the two most common causes were intrapartum cerebral anoxia and actual brain injury during a traumatic delivery. Consequently, the attending obstetrician, family physician, or midwife was often unjustly blamed for a child being born with cerebral palsy. It is now known, as a result of sophisticated diagnostic imaging techniques and other investigations, that such cerebral anoxia (which is currently called cerebral hypoxia/ischemia) and cerebral birth injury are relatively rare causes, accounting for less than 10% of all children with cerebral palsy.

Prenatal causes include genetically determined disorders, congenital cerebral malformations, and prenatal intracranial hemorrhage. Premature birth renders the newborn infant particularly susceptible to cerebral hypoxia/ischemia. Postnatal causes of cerebral palsy include erythroblastosis due to Rh incompatibility and resultant jaundice (icterus) that may affect the basal ganglia (kernicterus)—a less common cause since the development of early treatment by exchange transfusions—cerebral infections (encephalitis), accidental head injury, and nonaccidental injury (child abuse).

Nevertheless, because cerebral palsy is seldom diagnosed until at least several months after birth, the precise cause of the brain lesion in a given child is frequently speculative.

Pathogenesis and Pathology

The underlying brain lesion in cerebral palsy, although irreparable, is not progressive. The loss of function in one neuron system of the brain results in the release of normal control over interdependent systems that, in turn, tend to overact; this is an example of the previously mentioned "release phenomenon."

Manifestations of a brain lesion in an afflicted child are determined by the extent of the lesion and the area of the brain involved: cerebral motor cortex, basal ganglia, or cerebellum. Three main types of cerebral palsy, which comprise 90% of the total are:

1. *Spastic type:* corticospinal system lesion in the cerebral motor cortex, 65%.
2. *Athetoid type:* extrapyramidal system lesion in the basal ganglia, 20%.
3. *Ataxic type:* cerebellar and brain stem lesion, 5%.

Three additional types, tremor, rigidity, and atonia, are rare and make up the remaining 10% of the total.

Clinical Features and Diagnosis

The various types of cerebral palsy are not clinically obvious during the early months of postnatal development because the previously mentioned "release phenomena" tend to appear slowly over several months. Furthermore, during these early months, there is little cerebral activity, even in the normal brain. Cerebral palsy can be suspected, however, when an infant fails to achieve the milestones of motor development at the appropriate ages (an average, normal infant turns over at 5 months, sits up at 7 months, pulls up to a standing position at 10 months, stands alone at 14 months, and walks unaided at 15 months).

In addition to retarded motor development, many children with cerebral palsy exhibit some degree of intellectual disability: 40% are seriously intellectually disabled and considered uneducable, another 40% are less disabled but still below average, and the remaining 20% are average or above. Assessment of intelligence is particularly difficult in children with cerebral palsy because of the associated motor and sensory deficits, as well as their short attention span.

The severity of all types of cerebral palsy varies greatly. In the mildest forms, the patient is capable of leading an almost normal life; in the severe forms the patient is almost completely incapacitated. The clinical manifestations of the three most common types of cerebral palsy are distinctive enough to merit separate consideration.

Spastic Type of Cerebral Palsy: 65%

The characteristic features of spastic paralysis, or paresis, are paralysis of patterns of voluntary movement (rather than of individual muscles) and increased muscle tone (hypertonicity, spasticity, increased deep tendon reflexes, and clonus).

In early life, the disturbance of voluntary movements appears as difficulty in achieving fine, coordinated muscle action. When the infant or child attempts to carry out even simple movements, many muscles contract at the same time, and movement is restricted and laborious. The increased muscle tone can be detected in fairly young infants by the "startle reflex," a mass muscle spasm elicited by any sudden noise (Fig. 12.10). The spastic limbs seem stiff and exhibit an increased stretch reflex (sudden contraction of a muscle when stretched). The deep tendon reflexes in the involved limbs are hyperactive and after the first year, the plantar cutaneous reflex becomes extensor in type (Babinski response).

Depending on the extent of the lesion in the cerebral cortex, the spastic paralysis may involve only one limb, called monoplegia (Fig. 12.11), the upper and lower limbs on one side, or hemiplegia (Fig. 12.12), both lower limbs, known as diplegia or paraplegia (Little's disease) (Fig. 12.13), or all four limbs, called tetraplegia, quadriplegia, or bilateral hemiplegia (Fig. 12.14). The muscles of the throat may also be affected.

Although the paralysis affects movements more than individual muscles, some muscles are more spastic than others and some are weaker than others; consequently, there is serious muscle imbalance in the involved limbs. In general, muscles that cross two joints, such

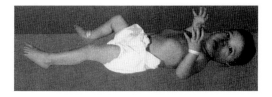

Figure 12.10.   Startle reflex in an infant with cerebral palsy. The infant was startled by a sudden noise immediately before this photograph was taken. Note the mass muscle spasm in the limbs.

as the biceps in the arm and the gastrocnemius in the leg, tend to be more spastic than those that cross only one joint. Furthermore, flexor muscles tend to out-pull extensor muscles, adductors out-pull abductors, and internal rotators out-pull external rotators. Thus, the neurogenic deformities in affected limbs secondary to spastic muscle imbalance are predictable: flexion, adduction, and internal rotation (Figs. 12.11–12.15).

The spastic gait is characteristically stiff, clumsy, and jerky, with the affected limbs held in the position noted above. When the condition is bilateral (diplegia and quadriplegia) these deformities produce a "scissors gait" (Fig. 12.14). Rapid walking or running accentuate the abnormality of the gait, making it more obvious. The child may also exhibit evidence of a central (cortical) type of sensory deficit.

Spastic paralysis of the muscles of speech is reflected in the child's difficulty learning to speak clearly. Spastic paralysis of the muscles of swallowing (dysphagia) interferes with the

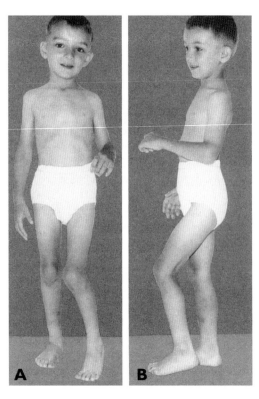

Figure 12.12.   Spastic hemiplegia involving the left upper and lower limbs. This boy is just starting to take a step with his left foot. Note the internal rotation of the arm and the flexion deformities of the elbow and fingers. Note also the flexion, adduction, and internal rotation of the left hip, flexion of the knee and equinus of the ankle.

normally subconscious function of swallowing saliva and accounts for the clinical problem of drooling.

Athetoid Type of Cerebral Palsy: 20%

The characteristic feature of athetosis is the involuntary, uncontrollable movements (mobile spasms) in muscle groups of the face and all four limbs. This purposeless athetotic muscle activity produces twisting, writhing contortions in the limbs and meaningless grimaces in the face (Fig. 12.16). It also causes difficulty with speech and swallowing. The distressing and humiliating phenomenon of athetosis is exaggerated by attempts at voluntary movement as well as by emotional tension; it is absent during sleep. The deep tendon reflexes and the plantar cutaneous reflexes

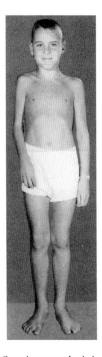

Figure 12.11.   Spastic monoplegia involving the right upper limb. Note the internal rotation of the arm and the flexion deformity of the elbow, wrist, and fingers.

are usually normal. Despite physical appearances to the contrary, the athetoid child's intelligence is usually within normal limits.

Ataxic Type of Cerebral Palsy: 5%

The characteristic features of cerebellar ataxia are disturbed coordination of muscle groups and a relative lack of equilibrium. The gait is unsteady and the child frequently appears about to fall, although this is usually prevented by using the arms to maintain balance (Fig. 12.17). There is neither spasticity nor athetosis and, because the lesion is primarily cerebellar, intelligence is usually unaffected.

Prognosis

Repeated mental and physical assessment of a child with cerebral palsy over many months is necessary to establish a realistic prognosis. Despite the permanent nature of the underlying brain lesion, every cerebral palsied child

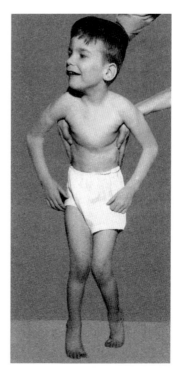

Figure 12.14. Spastic tetraplegia (paraplegia) involving all four limbs. Note the internal rotation of the arms and flexion deformity of the elbows. Note also the flexion, adduction, and internal rotation of the hips, flexion of the knees and equinus of the ankle. When this boy tried to walk, his knees crossed, one in front of the other (scissors gait).

exhibits some improvement in motor skills during the growing years through natural maturation of the part of the brain that remains intact. This improvement, although delayed, is comparable to the improvement of motor skills in a normal child who sits up at 7 months and walks at 15 months.

Cerebral palsy may be so mild that the child is but a few months or a year behind in the milestones of development. It may, however, be so severe that at 5 years of age, the child is unable to sit up and is functioning at the level of a 5-month-old infant, or at 14 years of age is unable to walk and is functioning at the level of a 14-month-old child.

In general, the prognosis of children with cerebral palsy with respect to their intelligence and ability to walk (without treatment) can be stated as follows: of the hemiplegics, 70% have normal intelligence and all will walk; of the

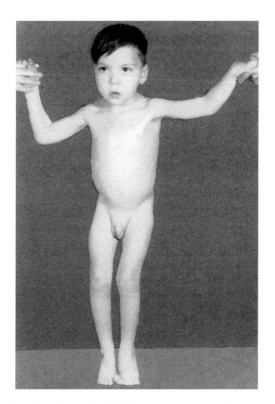

Figure 12.13. Spastic diplegia involving both lower limbs. This boy's upper limbs are normal. Note the flexion, adduction deformities of the hips, and flexion of the knees and equinus of the ankles.

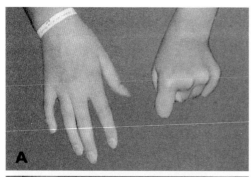

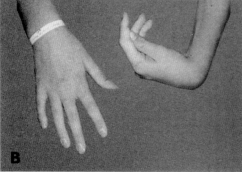

Figure 12.15.   A. Thumb-clutched hand in cerebral palsy due to flexion and adduction of the thumb. **B.** The thumb is released only when the wrist is flexed.

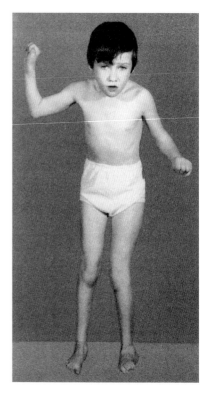

Figure 12.17.   Ataxia and disturbed coordination of muscles in a girl with the ataxic type of cerebral palsy. Note that the child stands with a wide stance and uses her arms to help maintain her balance.

spastic diplegics, 60% have intelligence above 80 and 75% will walk; of the quadriplegics, 90% have an intellectual disability and only 25% will walk. The athetoid children have limited motor skills and problems with verbal

communication even though most of them have a normal intelligence, as do the ataxic children.

Approximately one third of all children with cerebral palsy have a brain lesion so severe that treatment is ineffective and institutional care may be required; one sixth have a lesion so mild that treatment is unnecessary; the remaining half can be helped by realistic treatment.

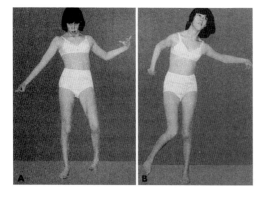

Figure 12.16.   Athetosis in a girl with athetoid-type cerebral palsy. These photographs were taken 2 seconds apart and give some indication of the twisting, writhing contortions in the limbs and the meaningless grimaces in the face.

Treatment of Cerebral Palsy

The overall management of children with cerebral palsy requires the combined skills of the family physician, rehabilitation physician, neurologist, orthopaedic surgeon, neurosurgeon, psychologist, physical, occupational, and speech therapists, medical social worker, and teacher. Ideally, assessment and treatment of these children is carried out in a special treatment center with facilities for both inpatient and outpatient care. Management of the child's physical problem alone, however, is not sufficient. Professional staff who care for children with cerebral palsy require an abundance of compassion, understanding, and patience. The prevailing attitude must be one of kindly realism.

Psychological Considerations

The parents of a child with cerebral palsy need special consideration. Because the diagnosis is seldom made during the early months, the parents have assumed that their child is normal; their disappointment is extreme when they realize that their child will, in fact, never be normal. Indeed, some parents have great difficulty accepting this reality.

The psychological needs of the child depend on the age and the degree of mental development. Many have a labile temperament and a short attention span, both of which render training and teaching difficult. Understandably, most children with cerebral palsy experience psychological problems of adjustment, particularly during adolescence.

Therapeutic Drugs

No type of drug can affect the brain lesion itself and in general, the drugs that have been used to help control the effects of the brain lesion have been disappointing. Epilepsy, which may accompany cerebral palsy, is now being aggressively investigated. It can be controlled to a large extent by drugs and, when necessary, neurosurgical intervention to deal with the offending focus of the epilepsy.

For very young children with spastic diplegia or quadriplegia and dynamic deformities of the lower limbs, but no structural contractures, a relatively new form of treatment is the injection of Botulinum-A toxin into the myoneural junctions of the most spastic muscles (usually calf muscles, hamstrings, and adductors). The toxin blocks the release of acetylcholine, decreasing spasticity. The beneficial effects last from 3 to 4 months, after which the injections can be repeated several times. The long-term results of Botulinum-A injections are yet to be determined.

Physical and Occupational Therapy

The aims are to encourage muscle relaxation, improve muscle coordination, and develop voluntary muscle control so that purposeful patterns of movement can be achieved. Simple activities that a normal child can learn alone, such as standing, walking, eating, and dressing, must be taught the cerebral palsied child by painstaking and repetitive training (Fig. 12.18).

Daily passive stretching of spastic muscles in an attempt to prevent deformity is of limited value in children with marked spasticity and muscle imbalance. Hand skills are difficult to develop, particularly in the presence of a central (cortical) sensory deficit; nevertheless, many cerebral palsied children can become relatively independent through repeated training.

Speech Therapy

With prolonged therapy, the defective speech in many afflicted children can be improved to the point of being reasonably intelligible.

Orthopaedic Appliances

Removable splints are helpful in preventing deformity as well as in preventing recurrence of an already corrected deformity (Fig. 12.1). During the early years, braces for the lower limbs are often necessary to enable a child to stand and walk with the help of crutches (Fig. 12.2). Efforts should be made, however, to correct deformities and improve function by physical therapy and operations, so that the child can be freed from cumbersome bracing as soon as possible.

Surgical Manipulation

Correction of fixed deformities by stretching of muscle contractures under general anesthesia is helpful in milder forms of spastic paralysis; the correction must be maintained by removable splints for many years to prevent recurrence. This method of treatment is of little value, however, for children with severe contractures caused by marked spasticity.

Orthopaedic Operations

The operative treatment of children with cerebral palsy is but one aspect, albeit an important

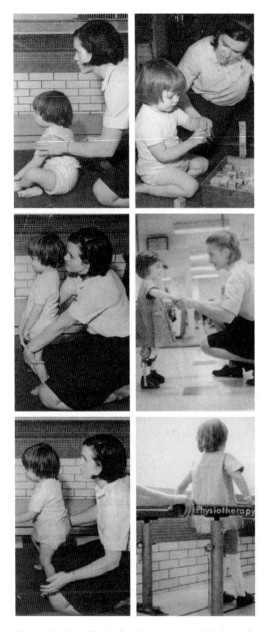

Figure 12.18.   Physical and occupational therapy for children with cerebral palsy involves painstaking and repetitive training by cheerful and dedicated therapists.

one, in the multifaceted approach to management. Operations are based on the first four of the six previously outlined principles of orthopaedic treatment of neurological disorders and injuries. In general, operative treatment is of value primarily in the spastic type of cerebral

palsy but is not indicated until the child has at least developed kneeling balance. Much clinical judgement is required in planning any operations for a cerebral palsied child; after the surgery, the child will still have cerebral palsy and, unless the surgical decision has been sound, he or she will not be any better after operation—just different. Parents must be made aware that well-chosen operations can improve function, but they cannot make spastic limbs function normally.

One or more of the following operations may be required for a child with the spastic type of cerebral palsy: 1) *tendon lengthening* (Fig. 12.4): lengthening of the Achilles' tendon for equinus deformity; of the hamstring tendons for knee flexion deformity; of the iliopsoas tendon for hip flexion deformity; 2) *tendon transfer* (Fig. 12.3): of the tibialis posterior tendon from the medial side of the foot to the dorsum; of the flexor carpi ulnaris from the medial side of the wrist to the dorsum; 3) *arthrodesis* (Fig. 12.7), of the three posterior joints of the foot (triple arthrodesis); of the wrist; of the metacarpophalangeal joint of the thumb.

One of the most serious complications of the complex muscle imbalance around the hip in a child with severe cerebral palsy of the spastic type—especially quadriplegia—is progressive paralytic subluxation of one or both hip joints that eventually become dislocated. Unfortunately, muscle releases designed to prevent this complication often fail to achieve their goal. Once established, such subluxations and dislocations require combined soft tissue releases, capsular repair, and extensive osteotomies of both the femur and the pelvis.

Special seating devices combined with surgical correction of deformities enables children with even the most disabling forms of cerebral palsy to sit comfortably.

A Neurosurgical Operation—Selective Posterior (Dorsal) Rhizotomy

The principle of this neurosurgical operation is to decrease the stimulating inputs from the muscle spindles in the lower limbs that arrive in the spinal cord via afferent fibers in the posterior (dorsal) nerve roots. This is accomplished surgically by cutting from 25% to 50%

of the fascicles of each of the posterior nerve roots from the level of the second lumbar vertebra to the sacrum. The operation, the long-term results of which are still being assessed, is indicated in children from 3 to 8 years of age who have a relatively mild spastic diplegia and are ambulatory. Although the resultant decrease in spasticity would seem to be of long duration, perhaps even permanent, approximately 50% of the children will still require one or more orthopaedic operations.

Very few patients with the athetoid type of cerebral palsy can be helped by orthopaedic surgery; occasionally, a particularly troublesome pattern of athetoid movement can be diminished by selective neurectomy.

The ataxic type of cerebral palsy is not amenable to surgical treatment.

Rehabilitation

For cerebral palsied children who have never been normal and have never "habilitated," the philosophy of *re*-habilitation is, in this sense, one of habilitation. This unfortunate group of children and their anxious parents represent one of the most important challenges to the whole concept of rehabilitation, as described at the end of Chapter 6. No group deserves more compassionate, considerate, and realistic rehabilitation.

Cerebral Palsy in the Adult

The philosophy and principles of treatment described above for children with cerebral palsy must be carried through to meet the continuing needs of adolescents and adults whose cerebral palsy has been with them in their past, is part of their present, and will be with them throughout their future. Although cerebral palsied adults have outgrown the phase of being considered as "a cute little crippled kid," their needs are just as worthy of our consideration. Hopefully, these adults have at least reached their potential, however limited that may be, but they may still not be capable of taking a normal role in society. Under these circumstances, employment in a sheltered workshop or in a modified area within industry is of great importance. If we cannot change the cerebral palsied adult to fit his or her environment, then we must change that environment to fit the cerebral palsied adult.

Cerebrovascular Disease and Hemiplegia

The most common of all neurological disorders is *cerebrovascular disease,* which includes all vascular disorders of the brain. The most catastrophic complication of the various types of cerebrovascular disease is sudden and irreversible ischemia of the brain, which produces the familiar syndrome of stroke (apoplexy, cerebrovascular accident). This complication, which occurs most frequently in the elderly, may be caused by hemorrhage, thrombosis, or embolism; it is particularly serious because brain tissue dies after relatively few minutes of complete ischemia.

The residual effects of a stroke are extremely variable, depending on both the site and extent of the area of cerebral ischemia. Discussions in this textbook, however, will focus on the patient who develops a complete hemiplegia (Fig. 12.19). At the onset the pa-

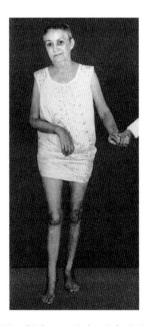

Figure 12.19.   Right spastic hemiplegia in a 63-year-old woman who is recovering from a stroke due to a cerebrovascular accident involving the left cerebral hemisphere. Note the internal rotation of the shoulder, flexion of the elbow and wrist, flexion and adduction of the hip, flexion of the knee and equinus of the ankle. Note also the right facial weakness.

ralysis is flaccid, but within a few weeks it becomes spastic, as evidenced by hypertonicity, increased deep tendon reflexes, and clonus. The plantar cutaneous response becomes extensor in type (Babinski response).

Until recently, most victims of a stroke received only token therapy designed to improve their musculoskeletal function. It is now appreciated, however, that this large group of patients can be rehabilitated much more efficiently if they are vigorously treated in accordance with the previously outlined principles of orthopaedic treatment of neurological disorders and injuries.

The most important aspects of musculoskeletal treatment for stroke victims with residual hemiplegia are psychotherapy, physical and occupational therapy, light braces (Fig. 12.20), selective nerve blocks to relieve spasticity and, occasionally, tendon transfers to restore muscle balance and improve function, such as transfer of the tibialis posterior tendon to the dorsum of the foot (Fig. 12.3) and transfer of the flexor carpi ulnaris tendon to the dorsum of the hand.

Much progress has been made in the rehabilitation of stroke victims through selective electrical stimulation of weak muscles that improves function significantly in both the upper and lower limbs.

Stroke victims often fall at home, sustaining fractures and joint injuries that delay their rehabilitation. Stable devices such as horizontal railings and vertical poles set up in the patient's home provide something for them to hold onto with their normal hand to keep them from falling.

DISORDERS AND INJURIES OF THE SPINAL CORD
Congenital Myelodysplasia

Congenital defects of the spinal cord (myelodysplasia) and nerve roots associated with spina bifida are fully discussed along with other congenital abnormalities in Chapter 8.

Diastematomyelia

The term *diastematomyelia* refers to a rare but important congenital defect of the spinal column in which either the lower part of the spinal cord or the upper part of the cauda equina is split into two vertical components by a spur that passes backward from the posterior surface of a vertebral body and traverses the spinal canal. This congenital spur, which may be fibrous, cartilaginous, or even bony, interferes with the normal upward migration of the conus of the spinal cord during growth; consequently, during childhood the spur produces a progressive neurological deficit, usually of the lower motor neuron type involving the lower limbs, bladder, or bowel.

There is nearly always an associated congenital anomaly, either of the overlying skin, such as a hairy patch, hemangioma, or dermal sinus, or of the regional vertebral bodies. The diagnosis can be suspected on clinical grounds but is confirmed by myelographic evidence of a midline split in the contrast medium (Fig. 12.21) or by either CT or MRI.

Neurosurgical treatment, which involves laminectomy and excision of the congenital spur, prevents further progression of the neurological deficit and may even result in some improvement.

Syringomyelia

This degenerative disorder is characterized by slow but progressive enlargement of an abnormal cavity (i.e., a syrinx) within the spinal cord, most commonly in the cervical region. In more than half of patients, the syringomyelia is associated with prolapse of the cerebellar tonsils through the foramen magnum of the

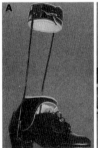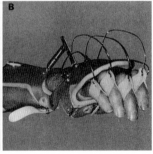

Figure 12.20. **A.** Light spring brace with outside T strap to help overcome a paralytic foot drop and varus deformity for a patient with a spastic hemiplegia from a stroke. **B.** Spring-assisted hand splint to prevent deformities and improve hand function.

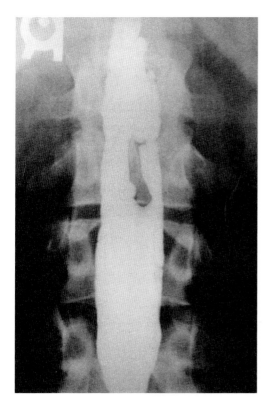

Figure 12.21.   Myelogram in the upper lumbar region showing a midline split in the contrast medium at the level of the second lumbar vertebra due to the spur of a diastematomyelia.

skull (the Chiari malformation). The cavity, or syrinx, is filled with cerebrospinal fluid under pressure. Consequently, the neurological manifestations include a dissociated sensory loss, namely loss of pain and temperature sensation but preservation of light touch, vibration, and position sense. In addition, pressure on the anterior horn cells produces lower motor neuron lesions in the upper limbs, especially in the hands. When the syringomyelia begins in childhood, at least 80% of the children will have developed an atypical scoliosis by adolescence.

The most precise method of diagnostic imaging to demonstrate a syringomyelia is a lateral projection of MRI.

Neurosurgical drainage of the syrinx is required to reduce the fluid pressure on the spinal cord. If the syringomyelia is associated with a Chiari malformation, neurosurgical de-

compression of the foramen magnum is also required. The scoliosis that is secondary to syringomyelia is not responsive to bracing. Consequently if treatment is indicated, it consists of correction and stabilization (fusion) with surgical instrumentation after decompression of the syrinx.

Poliomyelitis

The disease *poliomyelitis* (*"polio," "infantile paralysis"*) is a viral infection that affects the motor cells (anterior horn cells) of the spinal cord and is capable of producing permanent paralysis. It is now an almost completely preventable disease as a result of the development of effective vaccines by both Salk and Sabin. Indeed, by 1991, 85% of children worldwide were receiving three doses of trivalent poliovirus vaccine. Nevertheless, it may be many years before this disease is completely controlled, particularly in the developing countries of the world. Therefore, poliomyelitis still merits consideration in a textbook related to the musculoskeletal system. Also, some patients who had become victims of acute paralytic poliomyelitis 2 to 4 decades earlier, are currently experiencing the onset of increasing weakness and disability, a phenomenon that is called "postpolio syndrome" (described at the end of this section).

Incidence and Etiology

Before the discovery of effective poliomyelitis vaccines, this disease was the most frequent cause of crippling in children and to a lesser extent in adults. In highly developed countries where vaccination programs have been extensive, poliomyelitis is fortunately rare; in some of the developing countries, however, poliomyelitis continues to pose a threat to both life and limb. It affects boys more often than girls and the lower limbs more often than the upper limbs or trunk.

The poliomyelitis virus, of which there are three types, is a member of the enterovirus group. Characteristically, it enters the body via the gastrointestinal tract and spreads through the bloodstream to its target, the anterior horn cells of the spinal cord and brain stem. Usually occurring in epidemics, particularly during late summer, poliomyelitis may also occur sporadically.

Prevention

The development of a killed virus vaccine by Salk, and of an attenuated living virus vaccine by Sabin, are among the most significant medical advances in the present century. Both vaccines are highly effective and safe.

Pathogenesis and Pathology

Poliomyelitis may be *abortive* with no symptoms, *nonparalytic* with systemic symptoms, and *paralytic*. After an incubation period of 2 weeks, the virus attacks anterior horn cells and may destroy them, thereby producing a permanent lower motor neuron type of paralysis of the muscle fibers they innervate. Alternatively, the infection in the cord can produce a temporary inflammatory edema in the anterior horn, or even reversible damage to the cells, with resultant transient paralysis. The remainder of the discussion concerns only paralytic poliomyelitis.

Clinical Features and Diagnosis

During the *prodromal phase*, which lasts 2 days, the patient experiences nonspecific systemic symptoms common to many viral infections: headache, malaise, and generalized muscular aches.

During the *acute phase* of paralytic poliomyelitis, the patient develops a fever, severe headache, neck rigidity (indicating meningeal irritation), painful spasm, and tenderness in affected muscles. At this time the cerebrospinal fluid contains large numbers of lymphocytes. It is during the acute phase, which lasts approximately 2 months, that a flaccid paralysis develops in those muscles innervated by the damaged anterior horn cells. The extent of the paralysis varies from weakness of one muscle or muscle group to complete paralysis of all the muscles of all four limbs and the trunk; if the brain stem is affected as well (bulbar poliomyelitis) the muscles of respiration become paralyzed, and assisted (mechanical) respiration is necessary to preserve life.

During the *recovery phase* (convalescent phase), which lasts up to 2 years, there is gradual recovery of any transient paralysis; most occurs within the first 6 months. Approximately one third of the patients will make a complete recovery during this phase.

The *phase of residual paralysis* persists for the rest of the patient's life and no further recovery can be expected. Approximately half the patients with residual paralysis have only moderate involvement, but the remainder are left with extensive paralysis. The causes of paralytic deformity include muscle imbalance, muscle contracture, muscle atrophy and, during childhood, retarded longitudinal bone growth in an involved limb. A variety of typical postpoliomyelitis deformities develop, depending on the extent and distribution of the paralysis (Figs. 12.22–24).

Treatment

No form of treatment affects the extent of the paralysis or the degree of its recovery. During the acute phase, the patient is kept in bed and treated symptomatically. Removable splints are used to prevent contractures in involved limbs (Fig. 2.1) and, after muscle spasm has subsided, the joints of a paralyzed limb are gently put through a full range of motion for several minutes each day.

Treatment during the recovery phase includes active exercises to strengthen recovering muscles and suitable braces to stabilize weak limbs, prevent contractures, and improve function (Fig. 12.2).

Treatment of patients with residual paralysis is selected in accordance with the six previously outlined principles of orthopaedic treatment of neurological disorders and injuries. Operative treatment is deferred until there is no further hope of muscle recovery. The most efficacious surgical operations for patients with flaccid paralysis in the residual phase of poliomyelitis include: 1) *tendon lengthening* (Fig. 12.4); 2) *tendon transfer* (Fig. 12.3); 3) *tenodesis* (Fig. 12.5); 4) *osteotomy near a joint* (Fig. 12.6); 5) *arthrodesis* (Fig. 12.7); 6) *leg-length equalization* (either epiphyseal arrest or surgical shortening of the longer leg or, alternatively, epiphyseal stimulation or surgical lengthening of the shorter leg). The choice of the many available operations for specific combinations of residual paralysis is not discussed here, but some examples are cited in

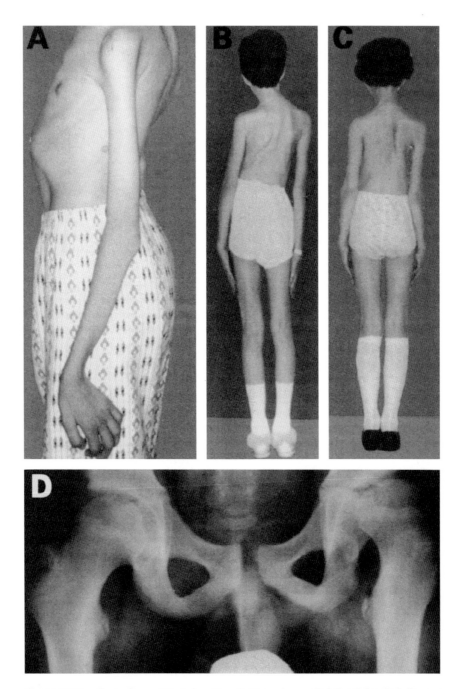

Figure 12.22.   Postpoliomyelitis deformities. **A.** Extensive paralysis involving the left upper limb and spine. Note the paralytic thoracic kyphosis and the marked atrophy of the entire upper limb. This boy's function can be improved by arthrodesis of the wrist, tendon transfers in the hand and elbow, arthrodesis of the shoulder. **B.** Paralytic scoliosis. Note the shift of the trunk to the right (decompensation). **C.** Same child 6 months after correction of the scoliosis by Harrington type of instrumentation and spinal fusion. **D.** Paralytic subluxation of the left hip; the acetabulum has become abnormal secondarily. This problem can be improved by the combination of transfer of the iliopsoas muscle (to make it an abductor instead of a flexor) and innominate osteotomy to redirect the acetabulum.

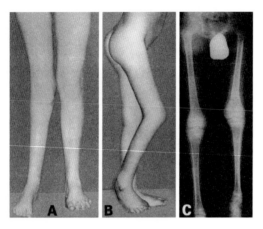

Figure 12.23. Postpoliomyelitis deformities. **A.** Valgus deformity of the right knee, varus deformity of the foot, atrophy, and leg-length discrepancy. This combination of deformities can be improved by supracondylar osteotomy of the femur, triple arthrodesis of the foot, and surgical lengthening of the tibia. **B.** Hip flexion deformity, knee flexion deformity, equinovarus deformity of the foot. This child could be helped by soft tissue release and muscle transfer about the hip, supracondylar osteotomy of the femur, triple arthrodesis of the foot and tendon transfer (tibialis posterior tendon to the dorsum of the foot). **C.** Leg-length discrepancy. This can be improved by surgical lengthening of the shorter femur. Alternatively, the discrepancy could be decreased by epiphyseal arrest of the longer lower limb or surgical shortening of the longer femur.

relation to a group of postpoliomyelitic deformities shown in Figs. 12.22–24.

For some patients, the residual paralysis in a lower limb is so extensive that permanent bracing is required to provide stability for standing and walking (Fig. 12.2). For others with obvious atrophy of a lower limb, the appearance of the limbs can be effectively matched by wearing a cosmetic prosthesis over the atrophied segment of the limb (Fig 12.9).

Patients with extensive residual paralysis, particularly when it involves both upper limbs, require rehabilitation, the philosophy of which is described at the end of Chapter 6.

Postpolio Syndrome

Approximately 50% of patients who had suffered acute paralytic poliomyelitis in the 1940s and 1950s, and who had a long period of stable paralysis, have begun some 2 to 4 decades later to experience increasing muscle weakness, fatigue and discomfort in their involved extremities. There are several hypothetical explanations for this phenomenon that has been termed the "postpolio syndrome." There is no convincing evidence of reactivation of the polio virus. One theory is that there has been gradual degeneration of involved terminal axons over the ensuing decades. Another the-

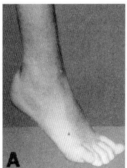
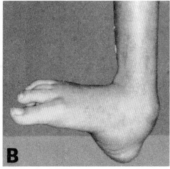
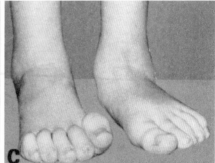

Figure 12.24. Postpoliomyelitis deformities. **A.** Paralytic equinus of the ankle. This can be improved by lengthening the Achilles tendon and tendon transfer (peroneal tendons to the dorsum of the foot). **B.** Paralytic calcaneus deformity of the ankle. Tenodesis of the Achilles tendon and tendon transfer (tibialis anterior to the heel) would improve the function of this child's foot. **C.** Paralytic varus deformity of the right foot and claw toe deformities. Paralytic deformity of the left foot. This child's feet can be improved by triple arthrodesis of both feet and tendon transfer in the right foot (extensor hallucis longus to the first metatarsal).

ory is that as adults become older, there is a gradual decrease in strength even in normal muscles. Thus, if a patient with residual partial paralysis of a given muscle has been able to compensate for that weakness during several decades, such compensation may no longer be possible when the involved muscle becomes even weaker with age. Furthermore, many of these patients develop painful musculoskeletal disorders such as tendinitis, fibrositis, and arthritis that aggravate the syndrome.

The treatment of postpolio syndrome involves reassuring the patients that their poliomyelitis has not recurred, plus gentle exercises to increase strength, light braces when necessary, and an appropriate modification of the patient's lifestyle.

Spinocerebellar Degenerations

A group of genetically related disorders, the *spinocerebellar degenerations*, is characterized by degeneration of ascending and descending tracts in the spinal cord, cerebellum, and even the cerebral cortex. The most common disorder of this group is *Friedreich's ataxia*.

Friedreich's Ataxia

A serious form of spinocerebellar degeneration, Friedreich's ataxia is characterized by degenerative changes in the posterior and lateral tracts of the spinal cord and cerebellum with resultant loss of position sense, poor balance, and ataxia. It may be inherited either as an autosomal dominant or as a recessive, but more often the latter.

The disease becomes manifest in early childhood by the development of bilateral pes cavus with claw toes (Fig. 12.25) and a progressive cerebellar ataxia with a swaying, staggering, irregular gait. Scoliosis develops in approximately 75% of the patients. Nystagmus and dysarthria indicate further cerebellar degeneration. The deep tendon reflexes disappear at the ankle and the plantar cutaneous reflexes become extensor in type (Babinski response). In addition, there is a profound loss of position sense and vibration sense.

Friedreich's ataxia is slowly but relentlessly progressive, rendering most victims wheelchair-bound by the age of 40. Occasionally,

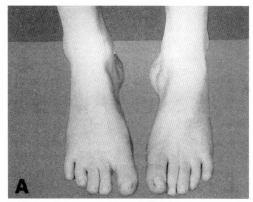

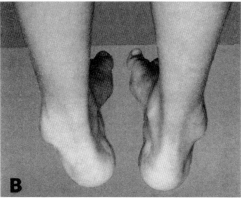

Figure 12.25.   Friedreich's ataxia in a 10-year-old boy showing the bilateral pes cavus deformity and varus of the heels. At a later stage, his toes will become hyperextended at the metatarsophalangeal joints and flexed at the interphalangeal joints (claw toes).

however, the degenerative process becomes arrested. The most common cause of premature death (usually in the third or fourth decade) is progressive cardiomyopathy.

Surgical procedures to correct foot deformities are similar to those described above for paralytic poliomyelitis but are of less permanent value because of the progressive ataxia.

Spinal Paraplegia and Quadriplegia

Disorders and injuries that damage the spinal cord are particularly serious, not only because of the cord's limited power of regeneration but also because of the associated complications. Indeed, before World War II, 80% of all spinal paraplegics were dead within a few years. Fortunately, at present, as a result of better understanding and more vigorous treatment, the mortality figures have been reversed, and 80% of spinal paraplegics are alive even after 10 years.

Incidence and Etiology

The most common cause of spinal paraplegia is acute injury, either indirect in association with fractures or dislocations of the spine (Fig. 12.26) and central herniations of the intervertebral disc, or direct from penetrating injuries such as gunshot and stab wounds. The para-

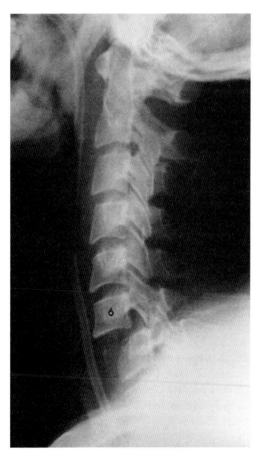

Figure 12.26. Fracture-dislocation of the cervical spine at the C6-7 level in a 34-year-old man as the result of an automobile accident. Note that the inferior facet of C6 has been dislocated to a position in front of the superior facet of C7 and that there is a fracture of the anterosuperior corner of the seventh cervical vertebra. The shadow in front of the vertebral bodies is a gastric suction tube. This man was immediately quadriplegic, complete in the lower limbs and partial in the upper limbs.

plegia is usually immediate. It has been estimated that during each year in Canada and the United States, 12,000 people sustain a spinal cord injury.

Causes of more slowly developing spinal paraplegia include: 1) neoplasms involving the spinal cord (intramedullary and extramedullary, primary and secondary); 2) infection of the vertebral bodies (particularly tuberculosis) with either pressure on the cord or actual invasion by granulation tissue; and 3) diseases of the spinal cord itself, such as multiple sclerosis.

Clinical Features

The clinical picture in the early stages of spinal paraplegia depends on whether the paraplegia is of sudden onset, as with traumatic paraplegia, or of gradual onset.

Complete Paraplegia of Sudden Onset (Traumatic)

Initially, the patient exhibits a state of spinal shock characterized by complete flaccid paralysis of all muscles innervated by that part of the spinal cord below or distal to the level of injury, and a comparable complete loss of sensation. Injuries below the level of the first thoracic vertebra produce a paralysis of both lower limbs (paraplegia), whereas those above this level produce a paralysis of all four limbs (quadriplegia, tetraplegia). In either case, there is also a flaccid paralysis of the urinary bladder and rectal sphincter and absence of deep tendon reflexes in affected muscles.

After a few weeks, the state of flaccid paralysis is superseded by a state of residual spastic paralysis as the cord reflexes below the level of injury take over in the absence of inhibitory impulses from the upper motor neurons. Thus, the muscles in the area of paralysis exhibit hypertonicity, increased deep tendon reflexes, and clonus; the plantar cutaneous reflexes are extensor in type. There is no voluntary power below the injury. Although the loss of sensation remains complete, painful stimuli in the paralyzed areas can cause a massive reflex spasm of muscles that may even cause the bladder to empty.

Incomplete Paraplegia of Sudden Onset (Traumatic)

With incomplete lesions, some tracts have escaped damage at the level of injury; consequently, it is more likely that the damage to the remaining tracts is not severe enough to be permanent and some recovery may be expected.

Paraplegia of Gradual Onset

When the disorder involving the spinal cord is slowly progressive, as with a neoplasm or infection, the phenomenon of spinal shock is not seen. The paralysis progresses slowly and is spastic from the beginning.

Early Treatment of Traumatic Spinal Paraplegia

Scientific investigations by Tator and colleagues have demonstrated that the injured spinal cord, in addition to suffering from the physical effects of trauma, also suffers from secondary pathological processes including ischemia and edema, both of which are amenable to treatment in the first few hours after injury. Consequently the currently recommended immediate treatment includes administration of methylprednisolone to minimize ischemia and edema.

To prevent distension and to keep the skin dry, the bladder is kept empty by means of an indwelling catheter during the flaccid stage of the paraplegia. Surgical decompression is indicated if the paraplegia is incomplete at the onset or if there is evidence of progression in the neurological deficit. If the paraplegia is complete from the beginning, surgical decompression is of no value. In the presence of an unstable fracture-dislocation of the spine, early operative reduction and stabilization of the spine by metal devices and bone grafts may enhance neurologic recovery. Such stabilization facilitates subsequent nursing care and enables the patient to get up with safety and comfort at an early stage during rehabilitation.

The prevention of pressure sores (decubitus ulcers) in the anesthetic areas of skin is of paramount importance from the beginning, because this complication of paraplegia is the greatest single cause of morbidity. Initially, the patient must be turned every 2 hours.

With high spinal cord injuries, the voluntary muscles of respiration are paralyzed and respiratory complications, such as atelectasis, may require bronchoscopic suction even during the first few days after the injury.

Continuing Treatment of Paraplegia

As soon as feasible, paraplegic patients should be transferred to a special paraplegic unit or center for long-term care and rehabilitation. Indeed, the development of paraplegic centers has been one of the most significant factors in the improved results of treatment. The management of paraplegic patients requires the skills and dedication of a large team, including a rehabilitation physician, neurosurgeon, orthopaedic surgeon, urological surgeon, plastic surgeon, nurses, orderlies, physical and occupational therapist, social worker, teacher, and job placement counselor. The most suitable individual to serve as captain of this team is usually the rehabilitation physician, but this individual's ability to be compassionate and understanding is more important than his or her particular specialty.

The following are some of the more important aspects of the long-term care of paraplegic patients:

1. *Care of the urinary tract:* Urological complications account for 40% of deaths in paraplegics; hence, their prevention is of extreme importance. After the early period when continuous drainage of the bladder is necessary, most patients can learn to empty their bladder by suprapubic manual compression. The aim is to establish an "automatic bladder" that empties when the patient initiates a cutaneous reflex.

2. *Care of the skin:* Paraplegics must eventually take the responsibility for preventing decubitus ulcers by turning frequently and by learning to inspect their own skin, with the help of a hand mirror. If a decubitus ulcer does develop, it may necessitate extensive plastic operations.

3. *Musculoskeletal function:* The combination of spasticity with muscle imbalance and dependent edema leads to the development of joint contractures that, in turn, may interfere with the patient's rehabilitation. These contractural deformities are mostly preventable, provided all joints in the area of paralysis are moved through a full range daily. Braces are of little value to the paraplegic who has no control over the pelvic muscles and no sensation in the lower

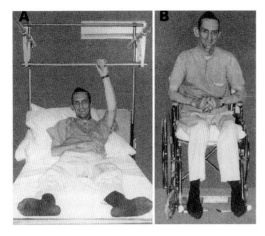

Figure 12.27. This paraplegic man must have a bar over his bed in the hospital and later in his home so that he can pull himself up and swing out of bed to a wheelchair. This young man, who prefers a wheelchair to full control braces and crutches, is well on his way to being rehabilitated.

limbs. Most paraplegics find they have more mobility in a wheelchair to which they can readily transfer from bed or toilet (Fig. 12.27). For quadriplegics, carefully chosen tendon transfers may permit more efficient use of the few remaining muscles controlling the hands.

4. *Rehabilitation:* The philosophy of rehabilitation outlined at the end of Chapter 6 is particularly applicable to spinal paraplegics and quadriplegics. Previous formal education is the most significant factor in employability and many paraplegics require further education before they can become gainfully employed. The improved methods of overall management of spinal paraplegia and quadriplegia have made it possible for the majority of these patients to achieve reasonable independence and to lead useful, as well as rewarding, lives.

DISORDERS AND INJURIES OF THE SPINAL NERVE ROOTS AND PERIPHERAL NERVES
Polyneuropathy
Hereditary Motor and Sensory Neuropathies
Four types of peripheral nerve and nerve root disorders have been classified on the basis of

their specific molecular genetics as the *hereditary motor and sensory neuropathies (HMSNs)*. Types I and II, which together were previously known as Charcot-Marie-Tooth syndrome or peroneal muscular atrophy, are inherited as an autosomal dominant trait.

In type I, the disease becomes manifest in childhood or early adult life by the development of bilateral pes cavus, a paralytic deformity of the feet due to muscle imbalance. As the disease progresses, symmetrical muscular atrophy and weakness become apparent in the peroneal muscles and toe extensors. Subsequently, the disease may advance to involve the tibialis anterior muscles, in which case there is a bilateral drop foot gait. The upper limbs may also become involved, but the muscle atrophy and weakness are primarily peripheral and seldom extend above the knees or the elbows (Fig. 12.28). The disease is characterized by low motor nerve conduction velocities. Sensory changes are slight but there is usually loss of vibration sense below the knee.

This disorder does not shorten the patient's

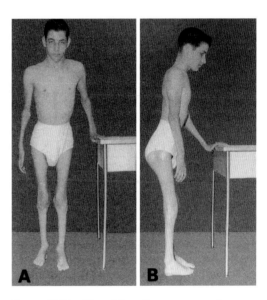

Figure 12.28. Type I hereditary motor and sensory neuropathy (Charcot-Marie-Tooth disease, peroneal muscular atrophy) in a 16-year-old boy. Note the bilateral pes cavus deformities, marked and symmetrical muscular atrophy of the calves, paralytic deformities of the hands, and muscular atrophy of the forearms. The boy walks with a bilateral drop foot gait and requires braces.

life expectancy. Muscular control of the hips and knees is always preserved, so the patient can usually retain his or her ability to walk although braces may become necessary. Surgery, such as lengthening of the Achilles tendon, transfer of the tibialis posterior tendon from the medial side of the foot to the dorsum, and arthrodesis of the posterior joints of the foot (triple arthrodesis), may be required.

In type II HMSN, the disease becomes apparent later in life. Although the signs and symptoms are similar to those of type I, there is usually more muscle atrophy.

Type III HMSN, which presents in infancy, is known as Déjérine-Sottas disease; it is inherited as an autosomal recessive trait. It usually progresses to the point where the patient loses the ability to walk by the third decade.

Type IV HMSN is a rare autosomal recessive disorder that is called Refsum disease. It is characterized by the presence of retinitis pigmentosa and an elevated serum phytanic acid.

Acute Inflammatory Demyelinating Polyneuropathy (Guillain-Barré Syndrome)

This acute form of polyneuropathy is considered to be a T cell-mediated immune disorder. An affliction of young adults and occasionally of children, its clinical features are somewhat similar to those of poliomyelitis except there is no fever and the lower motor neuron paralysis is almost always symmetrical; there may even be sensory changes. The cerebrospinal fluid changes are completely different from those of poliomyelitis in that the cell count is normal and the protein content is increased.

The prognosis of Guillain-Barré syndrome is good in that complete recovery is common. In the more severe forms, both plasma exchange and intravenous infusion of gamma globulin are effective. Nevertheless, there may still be residual paralysis, particularly in the lower limbs. The orthopaedic treatment of such paralysis is similar to that already described in an earlier section of this chapter for poliomyelitis.

Other Forms of Polyneuropathy

Peripheral polyneuropathy is also seen as a manifestation of toxic levels of arsenic, lead, and other heavy metals. A common sign of lead poisoning, for example, is paralytic wrist drop. A nutritional form of polyneuritis may complicate such disorders as alcoholism and beri beri. Diabetic neuritis is seen as a complication in 5% of patients with severe diabetes. In leprosy (Hansen's disease), which is regrettably still common in many of the developing tropical countries, the most significant lesion is a peripheral neuritis with peripheral paralysis and loss of sensation, a combination that often necessitates tendon transfers and always requires precautions to prevent injuries to insensitive hands and feet.

Compression of Spinal Nerve Roots

Disorders of the spine, including the intervertebral discs, may cause either continuous or intermittent compression of associated nerve roots, as discussed in Chapter 11. In the lumbar region, the most common cause is herniation of the intervertebral disc; in the cervical region, it is osteophytic narrowing of the intervertebral foramina. Many other disorders of the spine may produce nerve root compression. These include spinal infections, primary and secondary neoplasms, and spinal injuries.

The cardinal symptom of nerve root compression is pain that radiates in the nerve root distribution (radicular pain). Nerve root pain is increased by the following activities: 1) spinal movements that increase the nerve root compression; 2) coughing or sneezing, which raise the cerebrospinal fluid pressure; 3) straight leg raising, which increases the tension on the compressed nerve root. Paresthesia, such as numbness or tingling in the nerve root distribution may also be experienced.

The motor signs of nerve root compression are those of a lower motor neuron lesion in the muscles innervated by that particular root. In considering nerve root lesions, it is important to appreciate that a given nerve root distributes fibers to more than one peripheral nerve, and a given peripheral nerve receives fibers from more than one nerve root.

Treating nerve root compression means treating the underlying causative condition. In addition to local rest and immobilization of the spine, surgical decompression of the nerve root is sometimes necessary.

Peripheral Nerve Entrapment Syndromes

Theoretically, any peripheral nerve could be subjected to continuous or intermittent compression. Certain nerves course through specific anatomical regions in which they have less room to escape the effects of compression; in these regions, they are more easily "entrapped" by the internal pressure of an adjacent space-occupying lesion, such as edema, or by external pressure; hence the terms *nerve entrapment syndromes* and *entrapment neuropathies*.

The symptoms and signs vary with the degree of compression and whether it is continuous or intermittent. Pain and paresthesia in the sensory distribution of the nerve are common and may be associated with a sensory deficit. Muscle weakness (or even paralysis) and atrophy are commonly seen in the muscles innervated by the involved nerve at a later stage.

The more common nerve entrapment syndromes merit consideration as examples of this phenomenon.

Median Nerve at the Wrist (Carpal Tunnel Syndrome)

At the wrist, the median nerve and flexor tendons pass through a common tunnel whose rigid walls are formed by the carpal bones and joints and the transverse carpal ligament (flexor retinaculum). Any disorder that takes up space in this already crowded tunnel compresses the most vulnerable structure, the median nerve, and produces *carpal tunnel syndrome.*

This fairly common syndrome can be caused by a variety of conditions including: 1) edema of acute and chronic trauma; 2) inflammatory edema associated with rheumatoid tenosynovitis; 3) osteophytes in the carpal joints; 4) ganglion; 5) lipoma.

Occurring most commonly in women of middle age or older, the syndrome produces pain and paresthesia in the sensory distribution of the median nerve in the hand. The patient may notice some clumsiness of finger function. The symptoms are aggravated by

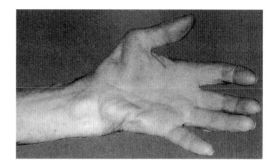

Figure 12.29.   Atrophy of the thenar muscles, especially the abductor pollicis brevis, in a 50-year-old woman due to longstanding compression of the median nerve at the wrist (carpal tunnel syndrome). Note the prominence on the anterior aspect of the wrists; her median nerve compression was caused by a large ganglion in the carpal tunnel. Her condition could have been diagnosed at an earlier stage before muscle atrophy developed.

movements of the wrist. Subsequently, objective findings of sensory loss appear, and eventually there is weakness and atrophy of the thenar muscles, especially the abductor pollicis brevis (Fig. 12.29). Nerve conduction studies are essential for the confirmation of the diagnosis of carpal tunnel syndrome.

In the early stages of carpal tunnel syndrome, temporary immobilization of the wrist and the avoidance of strenuous work for a few weeks may be sufficient to relieve the pressure of edema on the median nerve. If the edema is inflammatory, a local injection of hydrocortisone may bring relief. Frequently, the problem persists and necessitates surgical decompression of the median nerve by longitudinal division of the transverse carpal ligament. During pregnancy, the associated fluid retention and edema can produce an alarmingly rapid onset of carpal tunnel syndrome that requires urgent surgical decompression. In recent years, endoscopic decompression of the median nerve has been performed by some hand and wrist surgeons, but this procedure requires special expertise to avoid complications.

Ulnar Nerve at the Elbow (Delayed or Tardy Ulnar Palsy)

At the elbow, the ulnar nerve passes through a groove behind the medial epicondyle. In the presence of a valgus deformity of the elbow (increased carrying angle), the ulnar nerve is subjected to stretching, intermittent compression, and friction during flexion and extension (Fig. 12.30).

The patient complains of pain and paresthesia in the sensory distribution of the ulnar nerve. Later, objective sensory changes can be detected. Paralysis is usually delayed for many years (tardy paralysis), but eventually weakness and atrophy become apparent in the interosseous muscles of the hand. The only effective treatment is surgical transposition (relocation) of the ulnar nerve to the anterior aspect of the elbow.

Radial Nerve at the Axilla (Crutch Palsy)

Prolonged and faulty use of the axillary type of crutch, taking weight through the axilla rather than through the hands, produces intermittent compression of the radial nerve in the axilla. After several months, the patient experiences pain and paresthesia in the distribution of the radial nerve. Subsequently, paralysis of the finger and wrist extensor muscles becomes apparent. This lesion is completely reversible, provided the cause is eliminated. The patient should be instructed in the proper use of crutches or provided with elbow-length crutches.

Brachial Plexus at the Thoracic Outlet (Scalenus Syndrome)

The lower trunks of the brachial plexus may become entrapped as they cross over the first rib at the site of insertion of the scalenus muscles. Entrapment is more likely to occur if a congenital cervical rib is present. Persons with poor muscle tone and a long, thin thorax are most prone to develop this syndrome, which is manifest by radiating pain and muscular weakness in the upper limb; the precise distribution of the symptoms and signs depend on which trunks of the brachial plexus have become involved. The subclavian artery may also be compressed with resultant cyanosis of the arm and a weak radial pulse.

Exercises to strengthen the muscles that elevate the shoulder may be sufficient to relieve symptoms. Sometimes, however, it is necessary to explore the region surgically, to release the scalenus muscles and, if a cervical rib is present, to excise it.

Digital Nerves in the Foot (Morton's Neuroma and Metatarsalgia)

Women who wear excessively tight shoes run the risk of producing intermittent compression of their digital nerves in the forefoot—the folly of fashionable female footwear (Fig. 12.31). The digital nerve going to the space between the third and fourth toes is most often affected. Because the digital nerves are purely sensory, the only symptoms are pain and paresthesia. The pain may be so severe that the patient must literally stop in her tracks and remove her shoe. As a result of the repeated compression, a painful neuroma develops in the digital nerve. Examination reveals decreased sensation in the adjacent sides of the affected toes; lateral compression of the forefoot reproduces the pain of which the patient complains.

Wearing larger shoes with a metatarsal pad

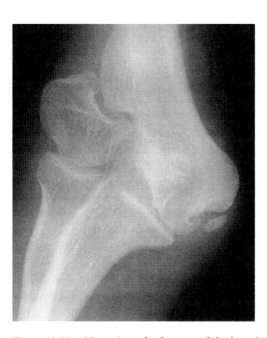

Figure 12.30. Nonunion of a fracture of the lateral condyle of the right humerus in a 21-year-old man. The fracture had occurred at the age of 5 years. The patient had a marked cubitus valgus deformity and a tardy ulnar palsy. Symptoms from the friction neuritis of the ulnar nerve did not develop until 10 years after the original injury.

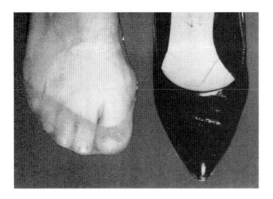

Figure 12.31. Folly of fashionable female footwear. This woman's foot is obviously much wider than her shoe. She had a Morton's neuroma and metatarsalgia from intermittent compression of the digital nerve going to the space between the third and fourth toes.

to elevate the transverse (anterior) arch and separate the metatarsal may relieve the pain, but frequently the only form of treatment that brings permanent relief is surgical excision of a segment of the digital nerve with its neuroma.

Acute Injuries to Nerve Roots and Peripheral Nerves

Nerve roots and peripheral nerves may be injured by a blunt object that causes a *contusion,* by a sharp object that produces a *partial* or *complete laceration,* or by a severe stretch that results in a *traction injury* (a partial or complete tear). In addition, nerves are particularly vulnerable to prolonged ischemia which leads to *necrosis.*

Classification of Nerve Injuries

Seddon has developed the following classification of nerve injuries:

1. Neuropraxia

There is only slight damage to the nerve with transient loss of conductivity, particularly in its motor fibers. Wallerian degeneration (breakdown of the myelin sheaths into lipid material and fragmentation of the neurofibrils) does not ensue and complete recovery may be expected within a few days or weeks.

2. Axonotmesis

The injury damages the axons, which are prolongations of the cells in the spinal cord, but does not damage the structural framework of the nerve itself. The axons distal to the injury undergo Wallerian degeneration. Peripheral regeneration of the axons occurs along the intact neural tubes to the appropriate end organs, but it occurs very slowly, approximately 1 mm each day, or 3 cm each month. Thus, if the axonotmesis in a given nerve occurred 9 cm proximal to its site of entrance into a given muscle, it would take approximately 3 months for the regenerating axons to reinnervate that muscle.

3. Neurotmesis

In this type of injury, the internal structural framework and the enclosed axons are divided, torn, or destroyed. Wallerian degeneration occurs in the distal segment. Because the axons in the proximal segment have lost their neural tubes, natural regeneration is impossible. The neurofibrils and fibrous elements grow out of the divided end of the nerve to produce a bulbous neuroma. The only hope of recovery lies in surgical excision of the damaged section of the nerve and accurate suture of the freshened ends (preferably with the magnification provided by magnifying glasses or a dissecting microscope). Even under ideal circumstances for nerve suture, recovery is less than complete.

Clinical Features and Diagnosis

Immediately after a nerve injury, there is complete loss of conductivity in the motor, sensory, and autonomic fibers. The muscles supplied by the nerve root or peripheral nerve exhibit a flaccid paralysis and subsequently undergo atrophy. A loss of cutaneous sensations, deep sensation, and position sense can be detected. The autonomic deficit is manifest by a lack of sweating (anhydrosis) in the cutaneous distribution of the nerve, as well as a temporary vasodilation and resultant warm skin followed by a vasoconstriction and cold skin.

The precise diagnosis concerning both the type of injury and its location can be helped by appropriate electrical tests (nerve conduction tests, strength duration curves, and electromyography).

Prognosis and Recovery

The prognosis depends on the type of injury (neuropraxia, axonotmesis, or neurotmesis), as described above. If recovery does take place, it is evidenced first by return of muscle power in the most proximally supplied muscle. Return of sensation follows a definite pattern, in that deep sensation returns first, followed by pain and position sense. As regeneration of axons proceeds along the nerve, the regenerated portion is hypersensitive so that finger tapping over it causes a tingling sensation (*Tinel's sign*). Thus, by assessing the distal limit of this phenomenon at intervals, it is possible to determine the progress of regeneration.

A disabling complication of partial nerve lesions during the recovery phase is severe burning pain (*causalgia*) in the sensory distribution of the nerve. The pain is sufficiently incapacitating in some patients that sympathetic denervation of the limb is required.

Treatment of Acute Nerve Injuries
Open Injuries

The open wound is explored and the nerve identified. If the division of the nerve is clean-cut, as by a piece of glass or a knife, immediate suture of the nerve is indicated (*primary repair*). If, however, the divided nerve ends are frayed, it is wiser to simply bring the two ends together with a single suture and defer definitive repair for 2 or 3 weeks (*secondary repair*), at which time it is possible to assess the extent of the damaged portion that must be resected; furthermore, at this time the nerve sheath, having thickened, is more efficiently sutured.

The surgical repair of a divided peripheral nerve (neurorrhaphy) has been tremendously enhanced by the use of the operating microscope. This device enables the surgeon to suture together the cut ends of individual nerve fascicles (perineurial fascicular neurorrhaphy) as well as epineurial neurorrhaphy.

Closed Injuries

In closed injuries that are complicated by loss of nerve function, it can usually, but not invariably, be assumed that the continuity of the injured nerve has not been lost (neuropraxia or axonotmesis). In more than 75% of closed fractures complicated by a nerve injury, the nerve sheath is intact. Accordingly, it is reasonable to wait for the expected time of recovery (as described above for neuropraxia and axonotmesis). In the event that recovery has not occurred in the expected time, it can be assumed that the injury has been a neurotmesis, in which case surgical exploration and repair are indicated. In general, it is unwise to delay repair for longer than 4 months, by which time fibrotic changes in the distal segment of the nerve as well as in the paralyzed muscle militate against a good result.

Residual Paralysis

In some nerve injuries, the damage is irreparable and the paralysis is permanent; in others, even after nerve repair there may be some residual paralysis. Under these circumstances the treatment is based on the principles of orthopaedic treatment of neurological disorders and injuries, as stated earlier in this chapter.

Traction Injuries of the Brachial Plexus

The brachial plexus of nerves is much more vulnerable to traction injuries than is the lumbosacral plexus because the upper limb, being less firmly attached to the trunk than the lower limb, is more easily pulled away by forceful traction. Most traction injuries to the brachial plexus occur when the head and neck are forced laterally while, at the same time, the shoulder on the opposite side is either forced downward or kept from moving with the head and neck. Such injuries may result from a difficult delivery (birth injury) or from a road accident.

Birth Injuries of the Brachial Plexus (Obstetrical Paralysis)

During the difficult delivery of a large baby as a vertex presentation, at the stage when the shoulders are still retained, strong lateral flexion of the head and neck may produce a traction injury of the brachial plexus. The same type of injury may occur during a breech delivery at the stage when the after-coming head is still retained, if strong lateral flexion is applied to the trunk and cervical spine. The resultant brachial plexus injury may range from a mild stretch to complete tearing of one or more trunks, or even avulsion of nerve roots from the spinal cord. The result is a mixed sensory and lower motor neuron lesion.

The precise diagnosis of the site of avulsion of the nerve roots can be improved by CT myelograms or MRI.

Upper Arm Type (Erb's Palsy)

The most common type of obstetrical palsy is a traction injury of upper trunks (C5 and C6) with resultant paralysis of the shoulder and upper arm. The newborn infant exhibits no active movement in the affected arm, which, because of the distribution of muscle paralysis, lies by the side in a position of internal rotation (Fig. 12.32). Any recovery occurs most rapidly during the first 6 months. At 3 months of age, the best predictor of subsequent recovery at 12 months is the combination of active elbow flexion, plus elbow, wrist, thumb, and finger extension. For those children who are deemed at 3 months to have a poor prognosis for recovery, surgical exploration and, when possible, repairs of nerve trunks are indicated. By the end of 1 year, 75% of the children will have made an almost complete recovery. During this year, all joints of the involved limb must be put through a full range of motion in an attempt to prevent contractures; a night splint is of doubtful value. Residual paralysis persists in some children and the residual muscle imbalance produces the typical deformity of adduction and internal rotation at the

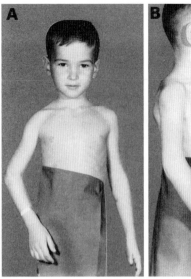
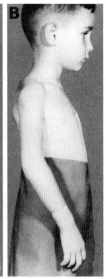

Figure 12.33.   Residual paralysis of Erb's palsy in the right arm of a 6-year-old boy. Note the typical deformity of adduction and internal rotation of the shoulder and flexion of the elbow. This boy's appearance and function could be improved by an external rotation osteotomy of the humerus.

shoulder and flexion at the elbow (Fig. 12.33). For young children, operations such as muscle releases and muscle transfers about the shoulder or, for older children, external rotation osteotomy of the humerus, may be required to permit shoulder abduction and to place the functioning hand in more useful positions.

Lower Arm Type (Klumpke's Paralysis)

In this rare type of obstetrical palsy, the lower trunks of the brachial plexus (C8, T1) are injured and, consequently, the resultant paralysis involves the muscles of the forearm and hand (Fig. 12.34). The prognosis for recovery is unfavorable and operations, such as tendon transfer, may be necessary to improve hand function.

Whole Arm Type

An obstetrical traction injury that involves the entire brachial plexus is usually so severe that no recovery is to be expected. Indeed, it is likely that at least some of the nerve roots are completely avulsed from the spinal cord. There is complete loss of sensation and com-

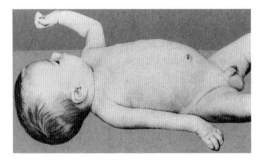

Figure 12.32.   Obstetrical paralysis in an infant due to a traction injury of the brachial plexus at the time of a difficult delivery. From birth, the infant had not moved his right arm but had moved his hand. Note that the arm is adducted and internally rotated at the shoulder. This is the upper arm type of birth injury of the brachial plexus (Erb's palsy).

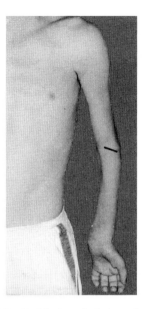

Figure 12.34.   Residual paralysis from the lower arm type of birth injury of the brachial plexus (Klumpke's paralysis) in a 10-year-old child. The hand and wrist are virtually flail and most of the forearm muscles are atrophied. This boy's hand function could be improved by arthrodesis of the wrist and tendon transfer to the fingers and thumb.

plete paralysis of the entire upper limb; in addition there may be a Horner's syndrome on the same side due to injury of the sympathetic fibers of the first thoracic root (Fig. 12.35). The completely flail, insensitive arm is not amenable to surgical treatment.

Psychological Consideration for the Parents

When a child has sustained a birth injury to the brachial plexus, the parents frequently bear some resentment toward the doctor who performed the delivery. This negative attitude, which is understandable but rarely justifiable, may persist for many years. Those who treat the child subsequently have a moral obligation to reassure the parents that, had the doctor not acted as he or she did during the critical stage of the delivery, the child might have suffered irreparable cerebral ischemia/hypoxia with resultant brain damage.

Brachial Plexus Injuries Resulting from Accidents

Major accidents involving a severe fall or blow on the side of the head and simultaneous depression of the shoulder may produce a traction injury of the brachial plexus in both children and adults. Road accidents, particularly motorcycle accidents, are the most frequent cause of such injuries. Neurological examination of the limb reveals the extent and probable site of the injury. The traction force is so severe, however, that in more than half the patients, nerve roots have been avulsed from the spinal cord, in which case there is no hope of nerve regeneration. Avulsion of the roots can be detected by myelogram, which reveals extravasation of the contrast medium along the nerve root sleeves (pseudomeningocele). If there is no radiographic evidence of root avulsion, exploration of the brachial plexus is justifiable in the hope that at least some of the nerves can be repaired.

Brachial plexus surgery including perineurial fascicular nerve grafting with the high power magnification of the operating microscope has improved the results of surgical treatment of these devastating injuries.

Most brachial plexus injuries resulting from severe accidents are extensive and involve the entire plexus (whole arm type). Furthermore,

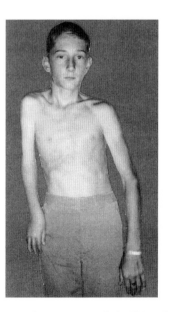

Figure 12.35.   Permanent paralysis of the whole arm type of birth injury of the brachial plexus. The arm is completely paralyzed and completely insensitive. Did you notice the drooping of this boy's right eyelid indicating a Horner's syndrome?

the prognosis for recovery of function, particularly below the elbow, is poor. Persistent pain for a period of 6 months is a bad prognostic sign. Approximately one third of patients recover sufficiently that hand function can be improved by surgery, such as tendon transfer and arthrodesis. When there is no recovery, an alternative to a flail, insensitive arm is amputation above the elbow and arthrodesis of the shoulder, so that the patient can obtain some function by means of a prosthetic limb.

Acute Injuries to Specific Peripheral Nerves

Although any peripheral nerve may be injured, some are injured more frequently than others. Examples of the more common peripheral nerve injuries are given below without discussing details; the previously outlined general features of nerve injuries may be applied to each of these specific injuries.

The *axillary nerve* may be injured in association with a traumatic anterior dislocation of the shoulder, or less commonly, a fracture of the proximal end of the humerus. The *radial nerve,* one of the most frequently injured, is usually involved at the time of a displaced fracture of the humeral shaft. The *ulnar nerve* at the elbow may sustain a mild traction injury at the time of a fracture-separation of the medial epicondyle, whereas the *median nerve* is more likely to be injured in association with a supracondylar fracture of the humerus. The median nerve at the wrist may also be injured by a severely displaced fracture of the distal end of the radius. At the wrist, both the median and ulnar nerves are prone to being divided, as this is a common site of deep lacerations.

The *sciatic nerve* is often injured by a traumatic posterior dislocation of the hip, with or without an associated fracture of the acetabulum. The sciatic nerve may receive a direct injury from an inaccurately placed intramuscular injection of drug into the buttock. The *lateral popliteal (common peroneal) nerve,* as it courses subcutaneously over the neck of the fibula, is particularly vulnerable to laceration as well as to the pressure effects of tight bandages or casts.

DISORDERS OF MUSCLE

The majority of neuromuscular disorders are neurogenic rather than myogenic. Nevertheless, a variety of pure muscle disorders (*myopathies*) cause significant clinical disturbances of the musculoskeletal system and merit consideration.

The *congenital* disorders of muscle, *hypotonia of neuromuscular origin* (formerly known as *amyotonia congenita* or *infantile spinal muscular atrophy*), and *amyoplasia congenita* are discussed in Chapter 8.

The most significant acquired disorders of muscle are the various types of muscular dystrophy.

Muscular Dystrophies

The term *muscular dystrophy* refers to a group of genetically determined disorders of muscle (*primary myopathies*) characterized by progressive muscle degeneration and weakness. In recent years, these tragic disorders have stimulated much interest, particularly in relation to their genetic and biochemical features.

Types of Muscular Dystrophies

Duchenne muscular dystrophy (DMD)
Becker muscular dystrophy (BMD)
Limb girdle muscular dystrophy
Facioscapulohumeral muscular dystrophy

Duchenne Type (Pseudohypertrophic Muscular Dystrophy)

This common, classical form is inherited as a sex-linked recessive trait; consequently, it afflicts males only, although nonafflicted female carriers can transmit the disease to their male offspring.

In 1985, Worton and his associates discovered the gene responsible for both the Duchenne and the Becker types of muscular dystrophy. It is located at the Xp21 region of the X chromosome. Abnormalities of this gene lead to absence of dystrophin (a protein normally present in the sarcolemma of muscle cells) in the Duchenne type and an altered dystrophin in the Becker type. Indeed, these two types of muscular dystrophy are sometimes referred to as "dystrophinopathies." The ultimate goal of the molecular genetics of the muscular dystrophies, of course, is gene therapy. This form of muscular dystrophy becomes apparent in young children of preschool age but may develop in older children or even young adults. The boy is observed to tire easily and cannot keep up with his playmates. Symmetrical weakness of the pelvic muscles, particularly the gluteus maximus, develops early and accounts for the boy's difficulty in climbing stairs and standing up from a sitting or lying position. Getting up from the floor, he must "climb up his legs," which is among the most characteristic signs of muscular dystrophy (Gower's sign) (Fig. 12.36). Pseudohypertrophy develops most characteristically in the calf muscles, the increased bulk

of the muscle being due to excessive fibrous tissue and fat rather than to muscular hypertrophy. Subsequently, the muscles of the trunk and shoulder girdle become weak. Deformities secondary to contractures are common. Nearly all patients with Duchenne muscular dystrophy develop a progressive paralytic scoliosis, especially after they have become consistent wheelchair users.

Progression of the disease is relentless; most boys are physically incapacitated within 10 years of onset and few survive beyond the age of 20; the most common cause of death is cardiac failure due to associated cardiomyopathy.

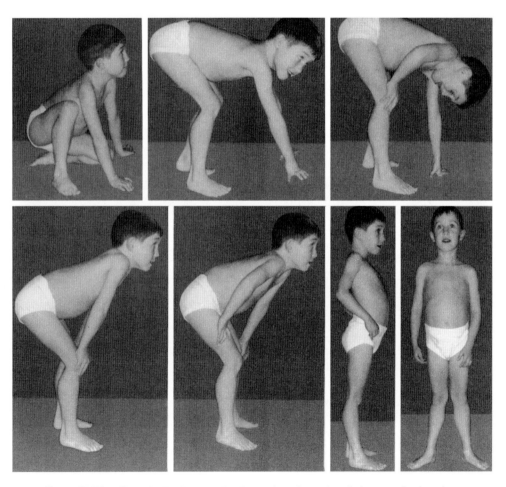

Figure 12.36. Gower's sign in muscular dystrophy. This series of photographs show how a boy with muscular dystrophy must get up from the floor by climbing up his legs with his hands because of weakness in the gluteus maximus and spinal muscles. Note the pseudohypertrophy of his calf muscles and the lumbar lordosis in the standing position.

Laboratory investigation reveals an elevation of certain cellular enzymes that probably arise from affected muscles. These enzymes include creatinine phosphokinase, and aldolase alanine transaminase. Electromyography helps to differentiate neurogenic muscle weakness from myogenic weakness. Muscle biopsy is valuable in determining the exact type of muscular dystrophy.

The aforementioned new genetic knowledge has facilitated the detection of carriers and affected individuals, both before and after birth, and has replaced creatinine phosphokinase assay and muscle biopsy for carrier detection.

Becker Muscular Dystrophy

This uncommon type of muscular dystrophy is also inherited as a sex-linked recessive trait. It appears at a later age, is less severe, and more slowly progressive than the Duchenne type. Otherwise, these two types of muscular dystrophy are similar, as is their treatment.

Limb Girdle-Type Muscular Dystrophy

This rare type of muscular dystrophy, which begins in adult life, is inherited as an autosomal recessive trait. It affects muscles of both the shoulder girdle and the pelvic girdle. Muscle atrophy is characteristic, but pseudohypertrophy is seldom seen. The disease progresses slowly.

Facioscapulohumeral-Type Muscular Dystrophy

Occurring more often in adults than in children, this type of muscular dystrophy is inherited as an autosomal dominant trait that affects the muscles of the face, shoulders, and arms. It may become arrested at any stage and does not shorten the patient's life expectancy.

Treatment of Muscular Dystrophy

In the past, the inevitability of progressive muscular weakness and premature death in this poignant group of children and young adults led to an attitude of apathy in relation to treatment. Although there is no specific cure for the various types of muscular dystrophy, much can be done through overall management to make the remaining years of these patients and their parents more bearable. There is evidence that prednisone can improve strength and function. The procedure of myoblast transfer has not been proven to be beneficial.

Ideally, patients with muscular dystrophy should be seen at regular intervals in combined or multidisciplinary outpatient clinics where their continuing care can be supervised by a team that includes a neurologist, rehabilitation physician, orthopaedic surgeon, physical and occupational therapists, and medical social worker. Active exercises help prevent the otherwise inevitable disuse atrophy of uninvolved muscles, minimize physical disability, and improve the patient's morale. Dietary su-

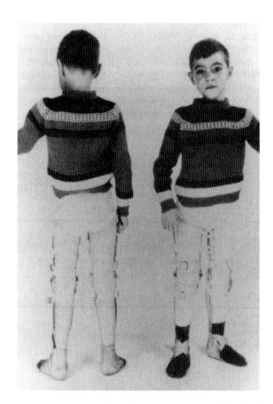

Figure 12.37.   At first glance, you may think this is a composite photograph of a boy taken from the front and back. Actually, it is a photograph of two boys—identical twins—both of whom have inherited the Duchenne type of muscular dystrophy. Note the modern light braces. Their disease had progressed to the point at which they were no longer able to walk unaided. With the help of orthopaedic operations and the support of these braces, they were able to continue walking for 2 more years.

pervision helps to reduce the obesity that accompanies relative inactivity and that accentuates the disability.

When the child can no longer walk unaided, he should be provided with light braces (Fig. 12.37). To overcome disabling contractures of the calf and thigh muscles, minor operations, such as subcutaneous tenotomies of the tendo Achillis and fasciotomies of the fascia lata as well as transfer of the tibialis posterior tendon to the dorsum of the foot, are most helpful. The child can be up and walking the next day, thereby overcoming the ill effects that occur with even a few weeks' confinement to bed.

The combination of light braces and orthopaedic operations will enable children with muscular dystrophy to continue being able to walk for an average of 25 additional months (which represents 10% of their life expectancy).

When a child's paralytic scoliosis is still mild (approximately 20°), it should be treated by surgical correction, instrumentation, and fusion from the upper thoracic spine to the sacrum to enable the child to sit upright in a wheelchair.

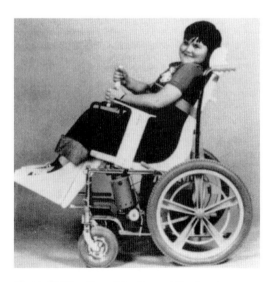

Figure 12.38. Boy with advanced Duchenne muscular dystrophy reclining in a "spinal support system" that fits into his battery-powered wheelchair. Note the electric hand controls for forward and reverse motions, as well as for right and left turns.

Even when these children become wheelchair-bound, the provision of a custom-made "spinal support system" and a battery-powered wheelchair have been very helpful to both the afflicted children and their distressed parents (Fig. 12.38).

SUGGESTED ADDITIONAL READING

Adams R, Victor M. Principles of neurology. 5th ed. New York: McGraw-Hill, 1993.

Albright AL, Cervi A, Singletary J. Intrathecal baclofen for spasticity in cerebral palsy. JAMA 1991;265:1418–1422.

Apley AG, Solomon L. Apley's system of orthopaedics and fractures. 7th ed. Avon: Butterworth-Heinemann, Bath Press, 1993.

Ashbury AK, McKhann GM. Changing views of Guillain-Barré syndrome. (Editorial) Ann Neurol 1997;41(3):287–288.

Birch JD. Neuromuscular disorders in children. In: Kasser JR, ed. Orthopaedic knowledge update 5. Rosemont, IL: American Academy of Orthopaedic Surgeons, 1996;195–202.

Blair E, Stanley FJ. Intrapartum asphyxia: a rare cause of cerebral palsy. J Pediatr 1988;112:515–519.

Bleck EE. Orthopaedic management in cerebral palsy. Philadelphia: Lippincott-Raven, 1987.

Bleck EE. Current concepts review. Management of the lower extremities in children who have cerebral palsy. J Bone Joint Surg Am 1990;72:140–144.

Boscarino LF, Ounpuu S, Davis RB III. Effects of selective dorsal rhizotomy on gait in children with cerebral palsy. J Pediatr Orthop 1993;13:174.

Cashman NR. Polio, including the postpolio syndrome: facts and myths. Curr Opin Orthop 1992;3(3):224–228.

Charry O, Koop S, Winter R. Syringomyelia and scoliosis: a review of 25 pediatric patients. J Pediatr Orthop 1994;14:309–317.

Chow JCV. Carpel tunnel release. In: McGinty JB, Caspari RB, Jackson RW, et al, eds. Operative arthroscopy. 2nd ed. Philadelphia: Lippincott-Raven, 1996.

Clarke HM. An approach to obstetrical brachial plexus injuries. Hand Clin 1995;11(4):563–581.

Cooke PH, Cole WG, Carey RPL. Dislocation of the hip in cerebral palsy. J Bone Joint Surg Br 1989;71(3):441–446.

Cosgrove AP, Corry IS, Graham HK. Botulinum toxin in the management of the lower limb in cerebral palsy. Dev Med Child Neurol 1994;36:386–396.

Cwick VA, Brooke MH. Recent advances in diagnosis and treatment of Duchenne muscular dystrophy. Curr Opin Orthop 1992;3(3):218–223.

DiCesare PE, Young S, Perry J, et al. Perimalleolar tendon transfer to the os calcis for triceps surae insufficiency in patients with postpolio syndrome. Clin Orthop 1995;310:111–119.

Dietz FR. Neuromuscular disorders. In: Weinstein SL, Buckwalter JA, eds. Turek's orthopaedics: principles and their application. 5th ed. Philadelphia: Lippincott-Raven, 1994:213–249.

Dubowitz V. Muscle disorders in children. 2nd ed. Philadelphia: WB Saunders, 1995.

Dürr A, Cossee M, Agid Y, et al. Clinical and genetic abnormalities in patients with Friedreich's ataxia. N Engl J Med 1996;335(16):1169.

Farley FA, Song KM, Birch JG, et al. Syringomyelia and scoliosis in children. J Pediatr Orthop 1995; 15:187–192.

Gelberman RH, ed. Operative nerve repair and reconstruction. Vol I and II. Philadelphia: Lippincott, 1991.

Gilbert A, Brockman R, Carlios H. Surgical treatment of brachial plexus birth palsy. Clin Orthop 1991;264:39–47.

Gilman S. Advances in neurology (review article—Medical Progress). N Engl J Med 1992; 326(24):1608–1616.

Graham HK. The orthopaedic management of cerebral palsy. In: Broughton NS, ed. A textbook of paediatric orthopaedics. London: WB Saunders, 1997;101–113.

Green NE. The orthopaedic care of children with muscular dystrophy. Instructional course lectures. American Academy of Orthopaedic Surgeons 1989;36:267–274.

Griggs RC, Moxley RT III, Mendell JR, et al. Prednisone in Duchenne dystrophy. Arch Neurol 1991;48:383–388.

Jubelt B, Drucker J. Post-polio syndrome: an update. Semin Neurol 1993;13:283–290.

Kalen V, Bleck EE. Prevention of spastic paralytic dislocation of the hip. Dev Med Child Neurol 1985;27:17–24.

Karpati G. Muscle, neuromuscular, and CNS disorders. Editorial overview. Curr Opin Orthop 1992;3(3):213.

Koman LA, Mooney JF III, Smith BP, et al. Management of spasticity in cerebral palsy with Botulinum-A toxin. Report of a preliminary randomized, double-blind trial. J Pediatr Orthop 1995; 14:299–303.

Michelow BJ, Clarke HM, Curtis CG, et al. The natural history of obstetrical brachial plexus palsy. Plast Reconstr Surg 1994;93:675.

Millesi H. Progress in peripheral nerve reconstruction. World J Surg 1990;14:733–747.

Natress GR. Neuromuscular disorders of childhood. In: Broughton NS, ed. A textbook of paediatric orthopaedics. London: WB Saunders, 1997:131–147.

Nonaka I, Kobayashi O, Osari S. Nondystrophinopathic muscular dystrophies including myotonic dystrophy. Semin Pediatr Neurol 1996;3(2): 110–121.

Ouvrier RA. Hereditary neuropathies in children: the contribution of the new genetics. Semin Pediatr Neurol 1996;3(2):140–151.

Park TS, Owen JH. Surgical management of spastic diplegia in cerebral palsy. N Engl J Med 1992; 326(11):745.

Peacock WJ, Arlens L, Berman B. CP spasticity: selective posterior rhizotomy. Pediatr Neurosci 1987;13:61.

Peacock WJ, Standt LA. Spasticity in cerebral palsy and the selective posterior rhizotomy procedure. J Child Neurol 1990;5:179–185.

Perry J. Pathological gait. In: Green WB, ed. Instructional course lectures. American Academy of Orthopaedic Surgeons, vol 39, 1990.

Perry J. Fontaine JD, Mulroy S. Findings in postpoliomyelitis syndrome: weakness of muscles of the calf as a source of late pain and fatigue of muscles of the thigh after poliomyelitis. J Bone Joint Surg Am 1995;77(8):1148–1153.

Pope DF, Bueff HV, De Luca PA. Pelvic osteotomies for subluxation of the hip in cerebral palsy. J Pediatr Orthop 1994;14:724–730.

Rang M. Neuromuscular disease. In: Wenger DR, Rang M, eds. The art and practice of children's orthopaedics. New York: Raven Press, 1993; 534–587.

Ray PM, Belfall B, Duff C, et al. Cloning of the breakpoint on an X:21 translocation associated with Duchenne muscular dystrophy. Nature 1985;318:672–675.

Reiter B, Goebel HH. Dystrophinopathies. Semin Pediatr Neurol 1996;3(2):99–109.

Renshaw TS. Cerebral palsy. In: Morrissy RT, Weinstein SL, eds. Lovell and Winter's pediatric orthopaedics. Philadelphia: Lippincott-Raven, 1996:469–502.

Root L, Laplanza FJ, Brourman SN, et al. The severely unstable hip in cerebral palsy: treatment with open reduction, pelvic osteotomy, and femoral osteotomy with shortening. J Bone Joint Surg Am 1995;77:703–712.

Ropper AH. The Guillain-Barré syndrome (review article). N Engl J Med 1992;326(17):1130–1136.

Roth JH, Richards RS, MacLeod MD. Endoscopic carpel tunnel release. Can J Surg 1994;37(2): 189–193.

Shapiro F, Specht L. Current concepts review. The diagnosis and orthopaedic treatment of inherited muscular diseases of childhood. J Bone Joint Surg 1993;74A:439–441.

Steinbok P, Gustavsson B, Kestle JRW. Relationship of intraoperative electrophysiological criteria to outcome after selective functional posterior rhizotomy. J Neurosurg 1995;83:18–26.

Sutherland DH. Gait analysis in neuromuscular diseases. In: Green WB, ed. Instructional course lectures. American Academy of Orthopaedic Surgeons, vol 39, 1990.

Tachdjian MO. Clinical pediatric orthopedics: the art of diagnosis and principles of treatment. Stamford, CT: Appleton and Lang, 1997.

Tator CH, Rowed DW. Current concepts in the immediate management of acute spinal cord injuries. Can Med Assoc J 1979;121:1453–1464.

Tator CH. Pathophysiology and pathology of spinal cord injury. In: Wilkins RH, Rengachary SS, eds. Neurosurgery. New York: McGraw Hill, 1996;2847–2859.

Thompson GH. Neuromuscular disorders. In: Morrissy RT, Weinstein SL, eds. Lovell and Winter's pediatric orthopaedics. Philadelphia: Lippincott-Raven, 1996;537–577.

Worton R. Muscular dystrophies: diseases of the dystrophin-glycoprotein complex. (Perspectives) Science 1995;270:755–756.

Worton RG, Brooke MH. The X-linked muscular dystrophies. In: Scriver CR, ed. The metabolic and molecular bases of inherited disease. New York: McGraw-Hill, 1995:4195–4226.

Wright PF, Kim-Farley RJ, de Quadros CA, et al. Strategies for the global eradication of poliomyelitis by the year 2000. N Engl J Med 1991; 325(25):1774–1779.

13 Disorders of Epiphyses and Epiphyseal Growth

The epiphyses and their epiphyseal plates (physes) comprise a captivating component of the skeletal system during the growing years of childhood. Because they are unique structural and functional units, it is not surprising that under abnormal circumstances, they react differently from the rest of the skeleton. Consequently, a variety of unique disorders peculiar to epiphyses and epiphyseal growth may be seen in children.

The various *generalized* disorders of epiphyses and epiphyseal plates (physes) of *congenital* origin, such as achondroplasia, are discussed in the latter part of Chapter 8. Those that are *acquired,* such as rickets, are considered in Chapter 9. The present chapter is concerned with a discussion of the *localized* disorders of these unique units and, in particular, with the *pressure* type of epiphyses as opposed to the *traction* type (Fig. 13.1). Injuries involving the epiphyseal plate (physis) are considered in Chapter 16.

Epiphyses appear to be more resistant to many of the disorders seen in other parts of the skeleton. Hematogenous osteomyelitis, for example, never begins in an epiphysis and rarely spreads into it through the epiphyseal plate (physis). Furthermore, during childhood nearly all bone neoplasms, both benign and malignant, avoid the epiphysis. By contrast, the epiphyses are particularly vulnerable to an idiopathic type of avascular necrosis *(osteochondrosis).* In addition, local epiphyseal growth is altered in a variety of childhood disorders such as idiopathic curvature of the spine (scoliosis). Such disorders are likely to be progressive throughout the growing years.

The term "physis" is an accepted synonym for the time-honored term "epiphyseal plate." Consequently, the terms "physis, physes, and physeal" are included (in brackets) throughout this chapter for the sake of clarity.

NUTRITION OF THE EPIPHYSIS AND ITS EPIPHYSEAL PLATE

Knowledge of the unique blood supply to epiphyses and their epiphyseal plates (physes) is pivotal to an understanding of their disorders. Most pressure epiphyses are covered essentially by articular cartilage and receive blood vessels only through their "bare bone areas." Others, such as the femoral head, being completely intra-articular and completely covered by articular cartilage, receive their blood supply precariously from vessels that must penetrate the "cartilage clothing."

In addition to supplying the epiphyses, the epiphyseal blood vessels are also responsible for the nutrition of the growing cells of the epiphyseal plate; therefore, ischemia of the epiphysis is associated with ischemia of the epiphyseal plate and a subsequent disturbance of longitudinal growth of the bone.

Whereas the shaft of a long bone grows in length from the epiphyseal plate (physis), the epiphysis itself grows in three dimensions from the deep zone of the articular cartilage (Fig. 13.2). The same is true of small bones such as the tarsal navicular.

AVASCULAR NECROSIS OF BONE

Death of bone is by no means limited to epiphyses; hence, the general subject of avascular necrosis merits consideration. Variously called avascular necrosis, aseptic necrosis, and ischemic necrosis, this condition represents a series of pathological events from the initial loss of blood supply and resultant death of bone to the gradual replacement of the dead bone by living bone. It is a common phenomenon, inasmuch as after every *fracture,* a minute area of each fracture surface undergoes avascular necrosis. Furthermore, free bone grafts, which initially are both avascular and

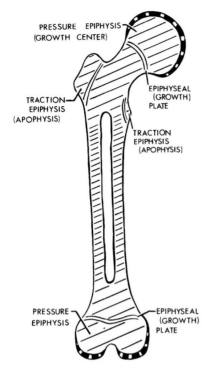

Figure 13.1. Types of epiphyses. A pressure epiphysis, situated at the end of a long bone, is subjected to pressures transmitted to the joint into which it enters. In this sense it may be considered an articular epiphysis. Furthermore, its epiphyseal plate (physis) provides longitudinal growth of the bone. A traction epiphysis, by contrast, is the site of attachment of tendons and muscles; consequently, it is subjected to traction rather than to pressure. Because it does not enter into the formation of a joint, it is nonarticular and does not contribute to the longitudinal growth of the bone.

multiple synonyms (epiphysitis, osteochondritis, aseptic necrosis, ischemic epiphyseal necrosis) may seem confusing. The confusion is not lessened by the multiple eponyms based on the name of the person, or persons, who have described the disorder in a given epiphysis (Kohler's disease, Osgood-Schlatter's disease, Legg-Calvé-Perthes' disease)—the "*osteochondroses eponymous.*" Some semblance of order out of this semantic chaos comes from the realization that the underlying pathogenesis, if not the etiology, is similar in all of these entities, and that the clinical manifestations in any given epiphysis are determined by the stresses and strains to which it is subjected

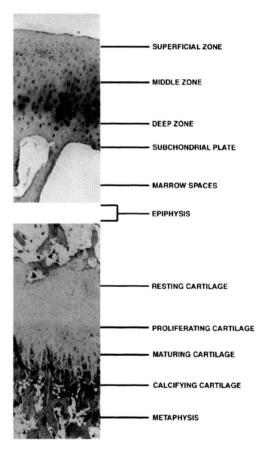

Figure 13.2. Sites of bone growth. The metaphysis grows in length from the epiphyseal plate (physis) (*below*) but the epiphysis itself grows in three dimensions from the deep zone of the articular cartilage (*above*). Small bones, such as the tarsal navicular and lunate, also grow from the deep zone of their articular cartilage.

necrotic, eventually become replaced by living bone.

The present discussion, however, is concerned with avascular necrosis of *subchondral bone* that supports articular cartilage in synovial joints.

IDIOPATHIC AVASCULAR NECROSIS OF EPIPHYSES (THE OSTEOCHONDROSES)

A number of idiopathic clinical disorders of epiphyses in growing children share the common denominator of avascular necrosis and its sequelae. They are therefore considered as a group of disorders, the *osteochondroses*. The with subsequent use. The major concern in any of the osteochondroses is that during the pathological process, the involved epiphysis may become permanently deformed with resultant secondary degenerative arthritis (osteoarthritis) of the joint.

Osteochondrosis usually involves a *secondary* epiphyseal center, or *pressure epiphysis,* at the end of a long bone (such as the femoral head) but may also involve the primary epiphyseal center of a small bone (such as the tarsal navicular). Understandably, the epiphyses that are most susceptible are those that are entirely covered by articular cartilage and therefore have a precarious blood supply. Somewhat similar lesions that affect *traction epiphyses* (such as the tibial tubercle) are sometimes considered as examples of idiopathic osteochondrosis. These are probably traumatic in origin and are discussed separately.

General Features of the Osteochondroses

Many features of the various clinical entities of osteochondrosis are common to all. Hence, to avoid repetition, they are discussed herein as *general features* before proceeding to a consideration of the specific clinical entities.

Incidence and Etiology

The osteochondroses, in general, are most common during the middle years of growth, from the ages of 3 to 10. They affect boys more frequently than girls, and the lower limbs are more often involved than the upper limbs. Osteochondrosis of a given epiphysis is bilateral in approximately 15% of involved children.

As the adjective "idiopathic" implies, the precise *etiology* of the osteochondroses has so far escaped detection and remains an intriguing challenge. Despite the plethora of proposed theories, there have been few proven facts. Although it is generally agreed that the common denominator in the osteochondroses is avascular necrosis of the epiphyseal center, there is less agreement about the mechanism of the initial loss of blood supply.

Certain factors, such as genetically determined vascular configuration, may have a predisposing influence. Because boys sustain

more injuries than girls, and their lower limbs are injured more often than their upper limbs, the sex and site incidence of osteochondroses suggest that trauma may play a role. Trauma of sufficient severity to produce a fracture or a dislocation can definitely produce the well-recognized, posttraumatic type of avascular necrosis. In the idiopathic type, however, less severe trauma may produce a complication, such as a pathological fracture, in already necrotic bone, aggravating the condition sufficiently to bring it to the physician's attention. A tense synovial effusion, either traumatic or inflammatory, may develop enough pressure to obliterate small intra-articular vessels, such as those proceeding to the head of the femur.

Pathogenesis and Pathology

The osteochondroses are self-limiting disorders that eventually heal spontaneously; consequently, relatively little pathological tissue has been available for study. Nevertheless, the pathogenesis and pathology are more clearly understood than the etiology.

The pathological changes in the various phases of this process of events are well correlated with the radiographic changes and are best discussed in relation to a specific epiphysis as an example. Osteochondrosis of the femoral head (Legg-Perthes' disease) is most suitable for this purpose. Its pathogenesis and pathology are presented as being representative of the changes that take place in all the osteochondroses. The description that follows is based partly on clinical and radiographic observations in children and partly on the author's experimental investigations in young pigs.

This fascinating pathological process is best considered in relation to four *phases,* even though the transition from one phase to another is both gradual and subtle. The whole process spans a long period, from 2 to 8 years, depending on the age of onset and the extent of involvement of the epiphysis.

1. Early Phase of Necrosis (the Phase of Avascularity)

After obliteration of the blood vessels to the epiphysis from whatever cause, the osteocytes and the bone marrow cells within the epiphysis die. However, the bone remains unchanged for many months, neither harder nor softer than normal bone. The ossific nucleus of the epiphysis ceases to grow because there is no blood supply for endochondral ossification. The articular cartilage, which is nourished by synovial fluid, remains alive and continues to grow. Over the ensuing months (sometimes up to a year or longer), the ossific nucleus of the involved epiphyseal center is smaller than that on the normal side, whereas the cartilage space is thicker (Fig. 13.3). During the avascular period, the radiographic density of the nucleus remains unchanged, because both bone deposition and bone resorption are biological phenomena that cannot occur without a blood supply. Nevertheless, disuse atrophy (osteoporosis) and hence, decreased radiographic density in the well-vascularized metaphysis may give the appearance of a relative increase in density of the femoral head. This is the "quiet phase" of osteochondrosis, during which the child is usually symptomless and no deformity takes place. Magnetic resonance imaging is (MRI) useful in the earliest diagnosis of avascular necrosis of epiphyses.

2. Phase of Revascularization with Bone Deposition and Resorption

This phase represents the vascular reaction of the surrounding tissues to dead bone. It is

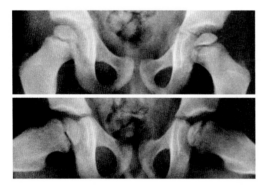

Figure 13.3. Osteochondrosis of the left femoral head (Legg-Perthes' disease) toward the end of the early phase of necrosis. Note that the left epiphyseal center of ossification is significantly smaller than the right, whereas the cartilage space of the left hip is thicker than that of the right. The apparent increase in density at this stage is only relative to the decreased density of the metaphysis.

characterized by revascularization of the dead epiphysis, a process that brings about a series of changes that are detectable radiographically. Beginning peripherally around the rim of the epiphysis, ossification of the thickened preosseous cartilage resumes. At the same time, new bone is laid down on dead trabeculae inside the original ossific nucleus. This *bone deposition,* which is added to the pre-existing bone, renders the original nucleus more dense radiographically and gives the appearance of what the author has termed a "head-within-a-head" (Fig. 13.4). The new bone that forms, however, is primary woven bone comparable to that seen in a fracture callus. It is not soft in a physical sense, but it has the property that the author has termed *biological plasticity* in that, as it grows, it is easily molded into either a normal, or an abnormal, shape, depending on the forces to which it is subjected.

During the phase of revascularization, a *pathological fracture* occurs in the subchondral bone of the original ossific nucleus at the site of greatest stress (in the hip this is the anterosuperior portion of the femoral head) and can be detected radiographically in at least one projection (Fig. 13.5). The fracture, almost certainly the result of superimposed trauma, is associated with pain (heralding the clinical onset of the osteochondrosis). A synovial effusion develops in the joint with synovial thickening and resultant limitation of motion. The overlying joint cartilage remains intact. Continued micromotion at the site of the pathological fracture incites a fibrous and granulation tissue reaction that results in excessive osteoclastic *bone resorption* and interferes with reossification. In the femoral head, this resorption may involve only the anterior part (partial-head type) or the entire head (whole-head type), depending on the extent of the subchondral fracture.

The combination of irregular areas of bone deposition and bone resorption provides the radiographic appearance of apparent "fragmentation" (Fig. 13.6). In the case of the femoral head, the hip may become *subluxated,* with resultant excessive forces being applied to it. During this most vulnerable phase of osteochondrosis, abnormal forces on the already weakened epiphysis may produce a pro-

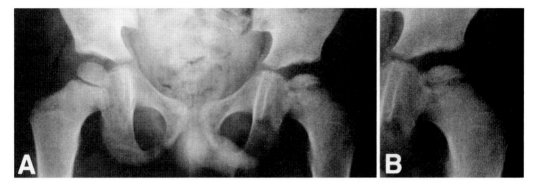

Figure 13.4.   A. Osteochondrosis of the left femoral head (Legg-Perthes' disease) in the phase of revascularization with bone deposition and bone resorption. Note the small, dense head (the size of the head when it stopped growing) and the new bone peripherally on either side of it. This is the "head-within-a-head" phenomenon. This is more clearly seen in the enlarged picture of the left hip (**B**). At this stage, there is an absolute increase in radiographic density because of new bone laid down on dead trabeculae.

gressive *deformity* (in this case, flattening) due to biological plasticity of the new living bone, cartilage, and fibrous tissue (Fig. 13.7). By the same token, suitable molding forces on the epiphysis during this phase can prevent deformity as will be seen later. The epiphyseal plate (physis), also having suffered the effects of ischemia, may cease to grow normally, and the metaphysis may become broadened. The phase of revascularization with bone deposition and bone resorption persists for varying

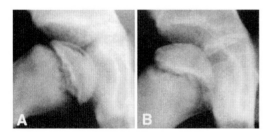

Figure 13.5.   Osteochondrosis of the right femoral head (Legg-Perthes' disease) in the phase of revascularization. **A.** Note the pathological fracture in the subchondral bone of the femoral head in this "frog position" view, which is a lateral projection of the femoral head and neck, but an anteroposterior projection of the pelvis. This fracture is sometimes referred t ɔ as the "crescent sign" or "the radiolucent line." The fracture is pathological in the sense that it occurs through abnormal bone, in this case, dead bone. **B.** The fracture is difficult to see in the anteroposterior projection of the femoral head.

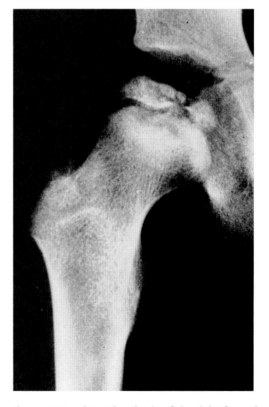

Figure 13.6.   Osteochondrosis of the right femoral head (Legg-Perthes' disease) later in the phase of revascularization with bone deposition and bone resorption going on simultaneously in different areas of the head. Note the radiographic appearance of "fragmentation." (The overlying radiolucent cartilage, however, would still be intact.)

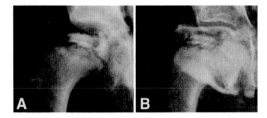

Figure 13.7. Osteochondrosis of the right femoral head (Legg-Perthes' disease) in the phase of revascularization. **A.** Note that the femoral head is subluxated upward and outward in relation to the acetabulum. This complication has produced excessive forces on the femoral head and has resulted in a progressive deformity. **B.** The extent of the deformity in the femoral head at this stage is well appreciated in the arthrogram. Part of the flattened head has extruded beyond the edge of the acetabulum. Such deformity can also be demonstrated well by the noninvasive method of MRI.

periods, from 1 to 4 years. During this phase, the epiphysis continues to be deformable.

3. Phase of Bone Healing

Eventually, bone resorption ceases and bone deposition continues so that the fibrous and granulation tissue are slowly replaced by new bone. The newly formed bone of the healing epiphysis still exhibits "biological plasticity" and can still be molded to some extent, for better or for worse, by forces to which it is subjected. The eventual contour of the epiphysis can be assessed only when reossification of the epiphysis is complete (see Figs. 13.14–13.16).

4. Phase of Residual Deformity

Once bony healing of the epiphysis is complete, its contour remains relatively unchanged. Thus, any residual deformity persists. Because the articular cartilage has remained reasonably normal, function in the joint can continue to be satisfactory for many years. Nevertheless, in weightbearing joints such as the hip, residual deformity, and its associated joint incongruity and limitation of motion eventually lead to the gradual development of degenerative joint disease (osteoarthritis) in later life (Fig. 13.8).

Clinical Features and Diagnosis

The osteochondroses produce neither symptoms nor clinical signs during the quiet, early phase of necrosis. In the phase of revascularization, particularly if a pathological fracture develops in the subchondral bone, the child experiences pain. A synovial effusion develops, which accounts for local tenderness and painful limitation of motion in the joint, especially abduction (Fig. 13.9). If not treated, the symptoms and signs tend to be intermittent, but gradually the muscles controlling the joint exhibit some degree of disuse atrophy (Fig. 13.9). Occasionally, a child goes through all the phases of an osteochondrosis without symptoms, in which case the diagnosis is made fortuitously on the basis of a radiograph taken for some other purpose.

The radiographic features of the various phases of osteochondrosis have been correlated with the pathogenesis and pathology (Figs. 13.3–13.8). The differential diagnosis radiographically includes irregular ossification in a normal epiphysis and generalized disorders, such as hypothyroidism and epiphyseal dysplasia, in which abnormal findings are seen in multiple epiphyses.

Sequelae

The sequelae of osteochondrosis include: subchondral fracture in the epiphysis, subluxation of the involved joint, deformity of the epi-

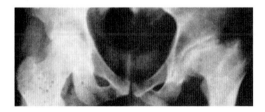

Figure 13.8. Late degenerative joint disease (osteoarthritis) of the left hip in a 36-year-old man secondary to the residual joint deformity and incongruity of Legg-Perthes' disease that he developed at the age of 6 years. Note also the short, broad femoral neck. This man has pain on walking and painful limitation of motion. A reconstructive operation such as femoral osteotomy, prosthetic joint replacement, or even arthrodesis, will eventually be required to relieve his symptoms when they become severe enough to justify surgical treatment.

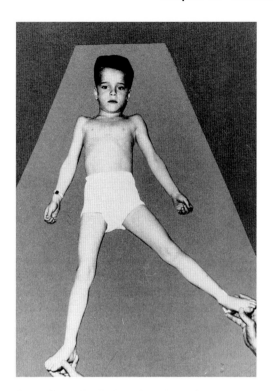

Figure 13.9.   Limitation of passive abduction of the hip and disuse atrophy of the thigh due to Legg-Perthes' disease of the right hip in a 5-year-old boy.

physis with resultant joint incongruity, and late secondary degenerative joint disease (osteoarthritis). A long-term follow-up study by McAndrew and Weinstein revealed that 50% of the patients had disabling osteoarthritis by the age of 50 years.

Aims and Principles of Treatment

Osteochondrosis is a self-limiting disease with or without treatment. Furthermore, the diagnosis is rarely made before the phase of revascularization and neither drugs, nor any other form of treatment, can reverse the process. The aims of treatment must be to prevent deformity of the epiphysis and preserve congruity of the joint to prevent secondary osteoarthritis.

The principles of treatment are concerned with the prevention of abnormal forces on the epiphysis during its vulnerable phases of revascularization and healing. For osteochondrosis involving an epiphysis of the lower limb, this involves preventing subluxation of the joint.

The author's experimental investigations in young pigs have demonstrated that the time-honored practice of prolonged relief of weightbearing over a period of years, either by means of bed rest, or by so-called weight-relieving braces, is neither necessary nor desirable. It also has been demonstrated—in the hip joint for example—that weightbearing can be permitted with impunity, provided the femoral head is kept from subluxating and the hip maintains a good range of movement. Once significant deformity has developed, however, treatment has little effect on the final outcome. The specific methods of treatment are outlined in relation to the various clinical entities.

Specific Osteochondroses of Secondary Centers of Ossification (Pressure Epiphyses)

The foregoing discussion of *general features* of the osteochondroses is applicable to each of the clinical entities to be described and should serve to make a discussion of these *specific* entities both interesting and meaningful.

Osteochondrosis of the Femoral Head (Legg-Perthes' Disease)

Easily the most important of the osteochondroses is Legg-Perthes' disease; it is more common and more serious than the others. Its numerous synonyms include: coxa plana (flat hip); pseudocoxalgia; osteochondritis deformans coxae juvenilis; Legg's disease; Calvé's disease; Perthes' disease; Legg-Calvé-Perthes' syndrome.

Incidence and Etiology

Legg-Perthes' disease occurs most frequently between the ages of 3 and 11 years and is five times more common in boys (particularly physically active boys) than girls. It is bilateral in approximately 15% of affected children and there may be a familial incidence. Of the many proposed theories of etiology, the one that seems most likely, and for which there is some experimental proof, is that the original occlusion of the precarious blood supply to the femoral head is caused by the excessive fluid pressure of a synovial effusion in the hip joint, either inflammatory or traumatic. As mentioned in Chapter 10, approximately 5% of children with transient synovitis of the hip and an associated synovial effusion in the joint develop the complication of Legg-Perthes' disease.

Recently, Gueck and associates have found antithrombotic factor deficiencies and hypofibrinolysis in some children with Legg-Perthes' disease and suggest that the resultant thrombophilia may well be of etiological significance.

Pathogenesis and Pathology

Legg-Perthes' disease was used as an example of all the osteochondroses in discussing pathogenesis and pathology in the preceding general section of this chapter; they need not be repeated here. It is well to emphasize the importance of the pathological subchondral fracture and of secondary subluxation of the hip as harmful factors in the pathogenesis of deformity in Legg-Perthes' disease.

Clinical Features and Diagnosis

The symptoms and signs in the various phases of Legg-Perthes' disease are similar to those described in the general section, but a few points merit further discussion. The absence of clinical manifestations of the disease during the quiet, early phase of necrosis accounts for the fact that the child is seldom brought to a physician until the phase of revascularization, or even later. The pain in this disease may be felt in the region of the hip, but may also be referred to the knee. The specific limitation of hip joint motion involves abduction and internal rotation. The disuse atrophy is most noticeable in the upper part of the thigh (Fig. 13.9). The child walks with a limp of the antalgic, or protective, type (protecting the hip against pain by rapidly taking weight off the foot on the involved side with each step) and exhibits a Trendelenburg sign.

The diagnosis can be suspected clinically but confirmed only by radiographic examination, the findings of which are well correlated with the pathogenesis and pathology (Figs. 13.3–13.8). Magnetic resonance imaging is useful in the early detection of Legg-Perthes' disease.

Complications

Legg-Perthes' disease may be complicated by subchondral fracture in the epiphysis (Fig. 13.5), subluxation of the joint (Fig. 13.7), flattening of the epiphysis (coxa plana) with resultant incongruity (Fig. 13.7), and late degenerative joint disease (osteoarthritis) (Fig. 13.8).

Treatment

The aim of treatment in Legg-Perthes' disease is to prevent deformity of the femoral head, thereby preventing degenerative joint disease in the hip in adult life. The principle of treatment is prevention of excessive forces on the femoral head during its vulnerable phases of revascularization and bony healing. In the hip particularly, this involves prevention of a secondary subluxation.

The methods of treatment of Legg-Perthes' disease in the past (all of which had been based on the avoidance of weightbearing) varied from enforced and continuous confinement to bed in an institution for several years, through various types of so-called weight-relieving braces, to a sling and crutches. At the opposite extreme, some surgeons have adopted the nihilistic attitude that no treatment affects the final outcome of the disease and consequently, no treatment is indicated.

Catterall's radiographic classification of four degrees of involvement of the femoral head is widely used, but the essential point is simply whether less than half or more than half the head is involved (Salter-Thompson classification). Herring's "lateral pillar" classification is also useful. Unless there is subluxation, only those children with more than half the head involved require treatment; this means that approximately half the children with Legg-Perthes' disease require regular observation only.

For those children who do require treatment, the underlying principle (which has been proven in the author's experimental investigations) is *containment* of the femoral head, plus a full range of hip joint motion and full weightbearing so that the involved femoral head may be protected from becoming flattened.

An effective, albeit cumbersome form of

containment is weightbearing in abduction plaster casts (Petrie) (Fig. 13.10) or in some type of removable abduction brace (Fig. 13.11). Both strategies prevent subluxation and enable the acetabulum to mold the "biologically plastic" healing femoral head in such a way that it does not become deformed. The abduction casts are more effective than the various abduction braces.

Surgical procedures, such as varus femoral osteotomy (Fig. 13.12) and innominate (Salter) osteotomy (Fig. 13.13), are designed to prevent or overcome subluxation of the involved hip. They have been used successfully in children older than the age of 5 years with more than half the femoral head involve, who consequently have a bad prognosis. The operation is performed *before* any deformity has developed. After the osteotomy has united (in approximately 6 weeks), the child is allowed to walk and run unhampered by braces or crutches. For children whose onset occurs

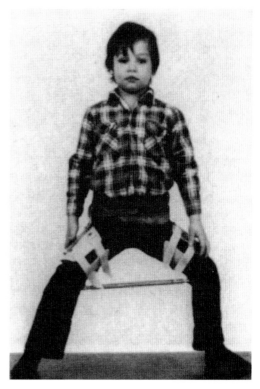

Figure 13.11.   The "Scottish Rite" abduction brace for Legg-Perthes' disease. This brace is less restrictive than the Petrie casts but may not be as effective in keeping the femoral head contained.

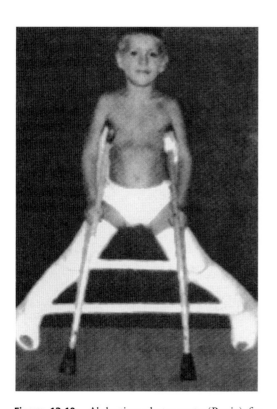

Figure 13.10.   Abduction plaster casts (Petrie) for Legg-Perthes' disease. The abducted position effectively prevents subluxation of the hip.

after the age of 10 years and who have extensive involvement, a combination of femoral and innominate osteotomy may be required.

In the late stages of the disease when deformity of the femoral head has developed, a period of several months in abduction casts after a muscle release may be necessary to improve the shape of the head before the combined osteotomies.

Prognosis

In Legg-Perthes' disease more than in any of the other osteochondroses, the prognosis, even with treatment, is extremely variable. The age of onset is an important factor; in general, the prognosis is good in children whose onset occurs before the age of 5 years (Fig. 13.14). These children seldom require any treatment. The prognosis is fair in children with an onset from 5 to 9 years of age with more than half the head involved (Fig. 13.15)

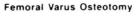

Femoral Varus Osteotomy

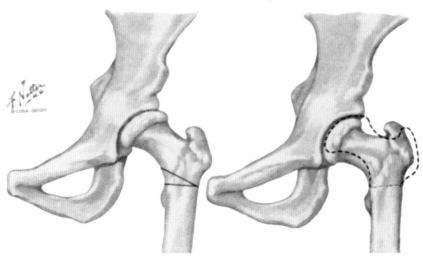

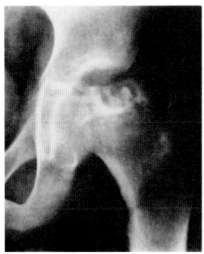

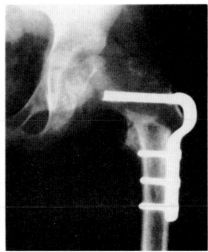

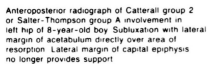

Anteroposterior radiograph of Catterall group 2 or Salter-Thompson group A involvement in left hip of 8-year-old boy Subluxation with lateral margin of acetabulum directly over area of resorption Lateral margin of capital epiphysis no longer provides support

Anteroposterior radiograph. 3 months following varus derotation osteotomy Subluxation corrected: lateral portion of capital femoral epiphysis within acetabulum and again provides support

Figure 13.12. Femoral osteotomy for Legg-Perthes' disease. (Copyright 1986. Novartis. Reprinted with permission Clinical Symposia, illustrated by Frank H. Netter, MD. All rights reserved.)

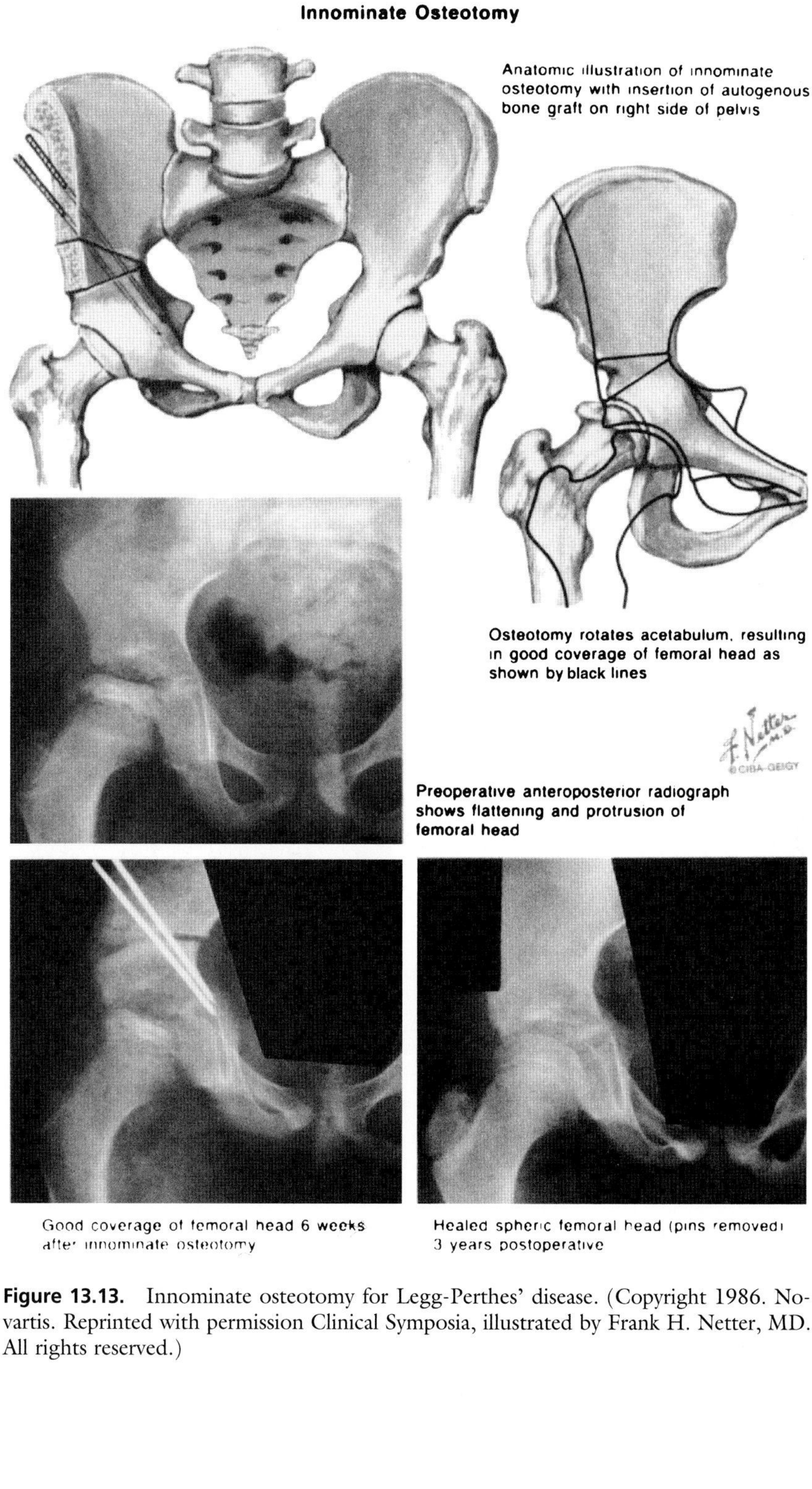
Innominate Osteotomy
Anatomic illustration of innominate osteotomy with insertion of autogenous bone graft on right side of pelvis
Osteotomy rotates acetabulum, resulting in good coverage of femoral head as shown by black lines
F. Netter M.D.
© CIBA-GEIGY
Preoperative anteroposterior radiograph shows flattening and protrusion of femoral head
Good coverage of femoral head 6 weeks after innominate osteotomy
Healed spheric femoral head (pins removed) 3 years postoperative

Figure 13.13. Innominate osteotomy for Legg-Perthes' disease. (Copyright 1986. Novartis. Reprinted with permission Clinical Symposia, illustrated by Frank H. Netter, MD. All rights reserved.)

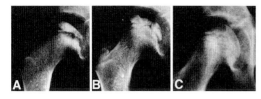

Figure 13.14. Good prognosis. **A.** At the age of 4 years near the end of the early stage of recovery. **B.** Two years later. **C.** Four years later the femoral head is round, a good result.

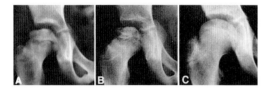

Figure 13.15. Fair prognosis. **A.** At age 6 years, early in the revascularization phase. **B.** One year later. **C.** Five years later the femoral head is large (coxa magna) but reasonably round, a fair result.

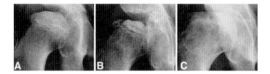

Figure 13.16. Poor prognosis. **A.** At age 8 years early in the revascularization phase. **B.** One year later, there is marked subluxation. **C.** Five years later, the femoral head is not only large but also flat (coxa plana), a poor result.

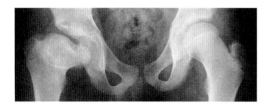

Figure 13.17. Severe residual deformity in the femoral head due to untreated Legg-Perthes' disease in a 14-year-old boy whose parents had refused treatment for him when he first had symptoms at the age of 8 years.

and poor in children when onset occurs after the age of 9 years (Fig. 13.16). The prognosis is definitely worse in the whole head type and in the presence of subluxation as well as persistent loss of hip joint motion. In the older child, failure to treat Legg-Perthes' disease may lead to severe residual deformity (Fig. 13.17). Age for age, the prognosis is somewhat worse for girls than boys.

Osteochondrosis of the Capitellum (Panner's Disease)

The capitellum of the humerus is rarely the site of avascular necrosis. Afflicting children between the ages of 3 and 11 years, its pathogenesis and pathology are those of all osteochondroses (described in an earlier section of this chapter).

Panner's disease is manifest by pain and slight swelling in the elbow, as well as by restriction of joint motion. The radiographic appearance is typical of osteochondrosis in other pressure epiphyses (Fig. 13.18). Because the elbow joint is non-weightbearing, and excessive and abnormal forces are not normally applied to the capitellum, deformity is unlikely and the prognosis is good. Treatment consists of providing the child with a sling during periods of discomfort.

Osteochondrosis of a Metatarsal Head (Freiberg's Disease)

Unlike other osteochondroses, Freiberg's disease begins during adolescence and is more

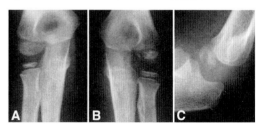

Figure 13.18. Osteochondrosis of the left capitellum (Panner's disease) in a 6-year-old boy. **A.** The normal right elbow for comparison. **B** and **C.** Note the combination of rarefaction due to bone resorption and sclerosis due to bone deposition giving the appearance of "fragmentation." Note also the phenomenon of a "capitellum-within-a-capitellum."

common in girls. Most of those afflicted have a congenitally long second metatarsal, or a short first metatarsal, both of which cause excessive pressures on the head of the second metatarsal, particularly when high-heeled shoes are worn; this may be a predisposing factor. Although the second metatarsal is the common site, Freiberg's disease occasionally affects the third metatarsal.

The pathogenesis and pathology are as for all osteochondroses (described in an early section of this chapter), except that an osteochondral fragment may become loose as occurs in osteochondritis dissecans. The most significant complication is residual deformity with resultant degenerative disease (osteoarthritis) of the metatarsophalangeal joint after the deformity has been present for several years.

The patient complains of pain in the forefoot on standing and walking. Examination reveals local thickening and tenderness as well as painful restriction of motion in the metatarsophalangeal joint. The radiographic appearance is typical of all osteochondroses (Fig. 13.19).

Nonoperative treatment by means of low-heeled shoes and a stiff rocker-bottom sole may relieve the symptoms from the complication of degenerative joint disease. Frequently, excision arthroplasty (accomplished by removal of the distorted metatarsal head or of the base of the phalanx) is necessary for permanent relief.

Osteochondrosis of Secondary Centers of Ossification in the Spine (Scheuermann's Disease)

Each vertebral body increases in height from two epiphyseal plates (physes), one covering the upper surface, the other covering its lower surface. The so-called "ring epiphysis" is, in effect, a traction epiphysis, or apophysis, and does not contribute to the height of the vertebral body. In the thoracic spine a growth disturbance of the epiphyseal plates (physes) anteriorly, with a resultant accentuation of the normal kyphotic curve, is variously known as osteochondrosis of the spine, *Scheuermann's*

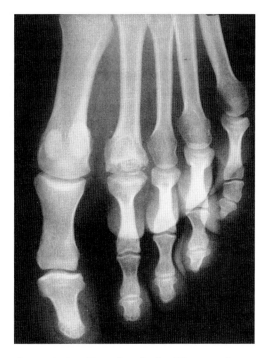

Figure 13.19.   Osteochondrosis of the second metatarsal head (Freiberg's disease) in a 19-year-old girl. The normally dome-shaped head has become flattened, broad, and irregular with resultant joint incongruity and early degenerative joint disease. Originally, this metatarsal would have been longer than the first; the hypertrophy of the shaft suggests that it has been bearing excessive weight for many years.

disease, vertebral epiphysitis, adolescent kyphosis, or adolescent round back (Fig. 13.20).

Incidence and Etiology

This fairly common but poorly understood disorder, which affects both boys and girls, usually begins at puberty and progresses during adolescence until vertebral growth has ceased in the late teens. In at least some of the patients, the disorder is inherited with an autosomal dominant pattern. It commonly involves the epiphyseal plates (physes) of three or four adjoining vertebral bodies in the midthoracic region.

Persistent anterior vascular grooves in the vertebral bodies may be a predisposing factor. Multiple minor injuries to the epiphyses and their epiphyseal plates (physes) have also been incriminated. Whatever the cause, there would seem to be an element of avascular ne-

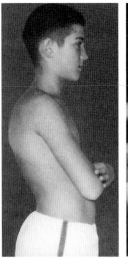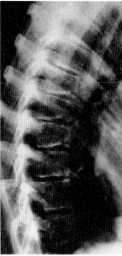

Figure 13.20. **Left.** Osteochondrosis of the secondary centers of ossification in the spine (Scheuermann's disease) in a 14-year-old boy. Note the exaggerated kyphosis in the thoracic region (round back) and the compensatory exaggerated lordosis in the lumbar region.

Figure 13.21. **Right.** The thoracic spine of the same boy as shown at left. The four middle vertebrae are involved. Note the irregular ossification of the anterior portion of the epiphyses of these four vertebrae. The indentations into the bodies of the vertebrae represent Schmorl's nodes. The intervertebral disc spaces are uniformly narrow and the kyphosis is accounted for by the anterior wedging of the involved vertebral bodies.

crosis affecting the anterior portion of the involved epiphyseal plates (physes), but whether this is primary or secondary is not known.

Pathogenesis and Pathology
A consistent finding in the involved vertebral bodies is the presence of herniation of the intervertebral disc through the anterior portion of the epiphyseal plate into the body of the vertebra (Schmorl's node). As a result, there is less disc material between the vertebral bodies, and the intervertebral disc space narrows. Such a herniation may interfere with the epiphyseal plate (physeal) growth directly; or by disturbing the blood supply to the plate (physis), it may interfere with growth indirectly. Ossification in the anterior portion of the vertebral epiphysis becomes irregular and, in this sense, is typical of osteochondrosis. Deficient

growth anteriorly, in the presence of continuing growth posteriorly, inevitably produces a wedge-shaped vertebral body that is shorter in front than behind; a series of three or four such wedge-shaped vertebral bodies accounts for the increased kyphosis.

Clinical Features and Diagnosis
The child is usually noticed by the parents, or by a school physician, to have "poor posture" or "round shoulders" at about the time of puberty. At this stage the disorder is symptomless. During the ensuing few years, however, the round back appearance becomes progressively more noticeable and the patient may complain of moderate back pain, particularly at the end of an active day. Examination reveals an exaggerated kyphosis in the thoracic region and a compensatory exaggerated lordosis in the lumbar region (Fig. 13.20).

There may be local tenderness over the spinous processes of the involved thoracic vertebrae. The hamstring muscles are always tight. The symptoms subside spontaneously when growth ceases, but the spinal deformity persists.

Radiographic examination of the thoracic spine reveals irregular ossification in the anterior portion of the epiphyses of several adjoining vertebrae, as well as indentations through their epiphyseal plates (physes) at the site of the Schmorl's nodes. The intervertebral disc spaces are uniformly narrow but the involved vertebral bodies are wedge-shaped (Fig. 13.21).

Treatment
Because Scheuermann's disease is self limiting and the symptoms are mild, many patients do not require treatment. For those with an anticipated or established unsightly deformity, the aim of treatment during the growing years is to prevent a progressive thoracic kyphosis. An effective method of treatment to help prevent such progression of deformity during growth is the Milwaukee brace (see Fig. 13.48), which is normally used for scoliosis (lateral curvature), but which can be modified for the treatment of kyphosis. Such a brace is used for approximately 1 year.

Once growth is completed, a brace is no

longer effective. Thus in older adolescents and adults—and only those with an unsightly kyphosis (more than 60°) and severe back pain—surgical correction including spinal instrumentation and spinal fusion may be required.

SPECIFIC OSTEOCHONDROSES OF PRIMARY CENTERS OF OSSIFICATION

Short bones, such as the tarsal navicular and the lunate, form as primary centers of ossification and, having no epiphyseal plates (physes), they grow from the deep zone of their articular cartilage. These bones are to a large extent covered by articular cartilage; consequently, they have a precarious blood supply that reaches them only through their "bare areas of bone." Two of the short bones that are prone to develop osteochondrosis are the tarsal navicular and the lunate.

Osteochondrosis of the Tarsal Navicular (Kohler's Disease)

In young children the tarsal navicular bone normally develops from more than one center of ossification, and this should not be confused with true osteochondrosis (which is relatively uncommon).

In children, particularly boys, between the ages of 4 and 8 years, true osteochondrosis may develop in the navicular and initiate the series of events in the pathogenesis and pathology of all osteochondroses outlined early in this chapter. In this particular osteochondrosis, however, healing is usually complete in 2 years and there is seldom a residual deformity. Occasionally the disorder is bilateral.

During the early phase of necrosis, Kohler's disease is symptomless, but in the phase of revascularization, the child usually complains of mild pain in the mid-foot and tends to walk with an antalgic limp. Examination reveals local tenderness and swelling due to a synovial effusion in the region of the navicular. The radiographic findings are comparable to those already described for all osteochondroses earlier in this chapter (Fig. 13.22).

The prognosis of Kohler's disease is excellent in that regardless of the type of treatment, the lesion heals with no significant sequelae.

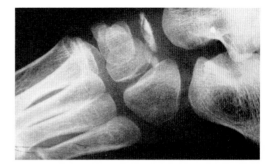

Figure 13.22.   Osteochondrosis of the tarsal navicular (Kohler's disease) in a 5-year-old boy. The process is in the phase of revascularization with areas of bone deposition and bone resorption. The ossific nucleus is thin but the cartilage space is thicker than normal, which means that the overall size of the navicular is not diminished. This explains the eventual normal appearance of the navicular at the end of the healing process.

Treatment is aimed at relief of the transient local symptoms and usually consists of providing the child with a sponge-rubber arch support during the active phases of the osteochondrosis. A walking cast may be required for a few weeks to relieve an episode of acute pain, but this is unusual. However, Williams and Cowell have reported that the short-term use of such a cast reduces the duration of symptoms from more than 1 year to 3 months.

Osteochondrosis of the Lunate (Kienböck's Disease)

The lunate bone is occasionally involved by a process that would seem to represent avascular necrosis. Occurring most frequently in young adults, Kienböck's disease may be secondary to trauma, either major or minor. Workers such as carpenters, as well as pneumatic jackhammer operators and riveters sustain repeated microtrauma to their wrists and are much more often afflicted than others. It may be significant that the right hand is involved more frequently than the left. It is possible that microfractures within the lunate disturb its already precarious blood supply and initiate the necrosis.

The pathogenesis and pathology are similar to those described for all osteochondroses in an earlier section of this chapter, with two exceptions. The healing process is much slower in the adult than in the child and in Kienböck's disease, it is unlikely that the lunate ever reaches complete healing. Furthermore, in the adult, the articular cartilage is likely to be affected as the underlying bone collapses. For these two reasons, degenerative joint disease in the wrist is an almost inevitable complication of Kienböck's disease.

The patient initially complains of mild aching in the wrist, but this tends to become progressive over several years secondary to degenerative joint disease. It may cause considerable disability, particularly in a worker. Examination reveals local tenderness over the lunate but little swelling; wrist motion is restricted by pain and the grip is weaker than on the normal side. The radiographic appearance is characteristic of avascular necrosis, depending on the phase of the process at the time (Fig. 13.23).

Inasmuch as in this disorder the pathological process is irreversible, the aim of treatment is relief of pain. In the early phases, immobilization of the wrist may bring temporary relief,

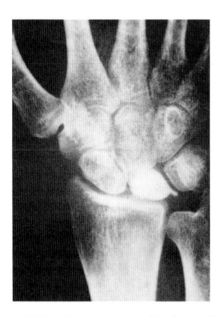

Figure 13.23.   Osteochondrosis of the lunate (Kienböck's disease) in a 30-year-old workman who had complained of pain in his wrist for 2 years. Note the marked sclerosis and irregularity of the lunate as well as the disuse osteoporosis in the surrounding bones.

but the most reasonable treatment is excision of the lunate before degenerative changes develop in the perilunar carpal joints. In the presence of advanced osteoarthritis, the only form of treatment likely to bring permanent relief is arthrodesis of the wrist.

Osteochondrosis of a Primary Center of Ossification in the Spine (Calvé's Disease)

The primary center of ossification of a vertebral body is occasionally the site of osteochondrosis (*Calvé's disease*, vertebral osteochondrosis, vertebra plana) but less commonly than the previously described disorder of Scheuermann's disease which affects the secondary centers. Calvé's disease occurs in children between the ages of 2 and 8 years and is almost always limited to one vertebral body.

Once thought to be an idiopathic type of osteochondrosis, Calvé's disease probably represents avascular necrosis secondary to a local variety of *Langerhans-cell histiocytosis* (formerly known as *eosinophilic granuloma,* discussed in Chapter 9). Because both osteochondrosis and this variety of Langerhans-cell histiocytosis are self-limiting disorders, the prognosis is good.

The child may complain of mild back pain but is otherwise healthy. Examination reveals a slight kyphosis and, occasionally, muscle spasm. Radiographic examination reveals a striking change in the vertebral body, the ossified part of which becomes wafer thin and sclerotic (Fig. 13.24). A radiographic study of other bones (skeletal survey) should be carried out to seek evidence of a widespread variety of Langerhans-cell histiocytosis formerly known as Hand-Schüller-Christian disease. Needle or punch biopsy of the vertebral body may be required to establish the diagnosis. Within 2 or 3 years, reossification of the cartilage model of the vertebral body and the continued growth from its secondary centers of ossification result in an almost complete restoration of the vertebra, which is only slightly thinner than normal.

Because this disorder is self limiting, treatment is aimed at relieving symptoms. A temporary spinal brace usually is sufficient.

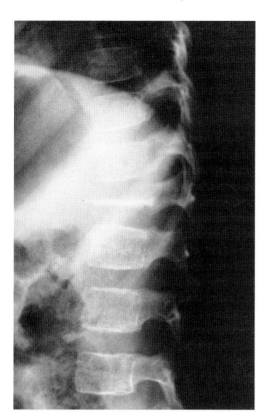

Figure 13.24.   Osteochondrosis of the primary center of ossification of a vertebral body (Calvé's disease) in a 7-year-old boy. The ossified portion of the vertebral body is wafer-thin and sclerotic, but the cartilage spaces above and below are thicker than those in the rest of the spine. This means that the cartilage model of the vertebra has not flattened completely and explains the almost complete restoration in the thickness of the vertebral body after healing of the lesion by ossification of the cartilage model.

TANGENTIAL AVASCULAR NECROSIS OF A PRESSURE EPIPHYSIS (OSTEOCHONDRITIS DISSECANS)

The convex surfaces of certain pressure epiphyses are susceptible to avascular necrosis of a small tangential segment of subchondral bone that may become separated, or "dissected," from the remaining portion of the epiphysis by reactive fibrous and granulation tissue; hence the name, *osteochondritis dissecans.* This relatively uncommon disorder is different from the more common phenomenon of irregular epiphyseal ossification, or a separate center of ossification, both of which are variations of normal.

Incidence and Etiology

Osteochondritis dissecans usually occurs in older children and young adults; boys are afflicted more frequently than girls. The most frequently involved epiphyses are the medial femoral condyle, patella, capitellum, femoral head, and talus.

The etiology of the initial avascular necrosis in osteochondritis dissecans is not known. The observations that this disease is sometimes familial and, in some patients, associated with osteochondrosis elsewhere, suggest that there may be a preexisting abnormality in the epiphysis that plays a predisposing role. In the adult, however, trauma is probably responsible for aggravating the lesion and may even initiate the necrosis.

Pathogenesis and Pathology

The tangential area of avascular necrosis on the convex surface of the epiphysis is usually no larger than 2 cm in diameter and often smaller. Whatever the cause of the necrosis, the osteocytes die, but the overlying articular cartilage, which is nourished by synovial fluid, remains alive. An ingrowth of fibrous and granulation tissue (from the marrow spaces of the remaining healthy part of the epiphysis) dissects in a plane between living and dead bone, thereby isolating the necrotic segment.

As the necrotic segment becomes revascularized, a combination of bone deposition and bone resorption occurs and the convex surface of the epiphysis may flatten. Provided the overlying articular cartilage remains intact, bony healing usually takes place eventually.

Superimposed trauma at this stage may tear the overlying cartilage, in which case the necrotic fragment is forced out of its concave soft tissue bed and becomes an osteocartilaginous loose body (sometimes referred to as a "joint mouse," as it is free to flit elusively from place to place within the synovial cavity).

Clinical Features and Diagnosis

There are usually neither symptoms nor clinical signs during the quiet, early phase of necrosis. During the revascularization phase, the patient may experience intermittent local pain with relatively little disturbance of joint function. Examination reveals a moderate synovial effusion in the joint, slight disuse atrophy of surrounding muscles, but little restriction of joint motion. Should the necrotic segment become partially detached, the symptoms and signs are more marked. Should it become completely detached, the patient complains of intermittent catching, or locking, of the joint due to the presence of the loose body.

Radiographically, the lesion is characterized by a small isolated segment of subchondral bone separated from its bed by a radiolucent line that represents soft tissue (Figs. 13.25 and 13.26). Because the lesion is tangential, its radiographic detection may necessitate special tangential projections.

Arthrography and MRI are helpful in determining whether the overlying cartilage is intact; in the knee joint, arthroscopy is particularly appropriate for this purpose.

Prognosis

Many lesions of osteochondritis dissecans heal spontaneously in 2 or 3 years without leaving any residual joint incongruity, especially in the

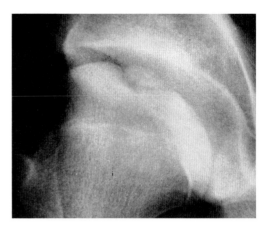

Figure 13.26. Osteochondritis dissecans on the convex surface of the femoral head in a 15-year-old boy. The small subchondral segment of necrotic bone is clearly seen. This segment, however, is unlikely to become separated because it is well protected by the opposing congruous joint surface of the acetabulum.

juvenile type in which the epiphyseal plates (physes) are still open. In the knee and in the elbow, the process is more likely to be complicated by complete separation of the necrotic fragment with its overlying cartilage, thereby forming a loose body and leaving a residual and permanent defect in the joint surface of the epiphysis.

If the defect is small, or is on a nonweightbearing surface of the joint, the consequences are not significant. However, if it is large and involves a weightbearing surface, degenerative disease of the joint may ensue over a period of years.

Treatment

The aims of treatment depend on the phase of the pathological process at the time. If the cartilage overlying the tangential segment of dead bone is still intact, the aim of treatment is to prevent its detachment. This involves restriction of activity and may even necessitate temporary relief of weightbearing from the joint to encourage healing. If the segment is large and involves a weightbearing surface of the joint, particularly in the knee, arthroscopic surgery involving insertion of peg-shaped bone grafts accelerate healing of the fragment to its bed and prevent its separation. Once the overlying cartilage has been torn and the frag-

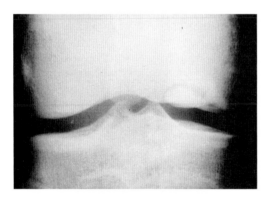

Figure 13.25. Osteochondritis dissecans on the convex surface of the medial femoral condyle in a 19-year-old boy. Note the small subchondral segment of bone separated from the remainder of the epiphysis by a radiolucent line that represents fibrous tissue. In the knee joint, the necrotic segment and its overlying cartilage may become detached and move freely about the joint as a loose body. The same complication is known to occur in the elbow joint when the osteochondritis dissecans involves the capitellum.

ment has become either partially or totally separated, it should be removed unless it is large (more than 2 cm in diameter), in which case it should be replaced and held in its bed either by metal pins or bone pegs. If this is not feasible, autogenous periosteal grafting followed by continuous passive motion (CPM) may be required (as mentioned in Chapter 18).

NONTRAUMATIC OSTEONECROSIS OF THE FEMORAL HEAD IN ADULTS

Nontraumatic osteonecrosis (a form of avascular necrosis) may develop spontaneously in one or both femoral heads in adults. This idiopathic type of femoral head necrosis in adults (also known as Chandler's disease), which seems to have become more prevalent in recent years, is more often seen in middle-aged persons who have a history of some generalized disorder such as alcoholism, or who have received systemic adrenocorticosteroids (as reported by Cruess) for an unrelated condition. It is possible, though unproven, that a pathological fracture in osteoporotic cancellous bone may even initiate the avascular necrosis. The intravascular coagulation within the femoral head may even be the result of fat emboli, as proposed by Jones. As in Legg-Perthes' disease (discussed in an earlier section of this chapter), the thrombophilia secondary to hypofibrinolysis and antithrombotic factor deficiencies may be of etiological significance in nontraumatic osteonecrosis in the adult.

The pathogenesis and pathology of avascular necrosis of the mature femoral head differ significantly from those of osteochondrosis of the immature femoral head (Legg-Perthes' disease). The entire process extends over many years and never heals spontaneously. A large segment of the weightbearing area may collapse. Furthermore, the articular cartilage frequently fails to survive and may even become lifted off the underlying bone. The joint is eventually irreparably destroyed.

The patient complains of severe pain, either in the hip or referred to the knee, and notices a slowly progressive stiffening of the joint. The pain and joint stiffness increase gradually until sudden collapse of a major weightbearing area of the femoral head causes severe pain. Examination reveals painful limitation of hip joint movement that is associated with muscle spasm. Function in the hip deteriorates relentlessly and irreversibly.

The earliest diagnosis is possible with MRI. Later, radiographic changes include marked sclerosis of a major segment of the femoral head that includes the weightbearing area. The sclerotic segment may be demarcated from the rest of the head by irregular areas of rarefaction and sclerosis; it may have collapsed, or become impacted, with resultant incongruity of the joint (Fig. 13.27). Magnetic resonance imaging is also helpful in the diagnosis, particularly in the early stages.

In the early stage of the disease, before any collapse of the femoral head has occurred, surgical core decompression of the femoral head or a vascularized fibular graft inserted into the neck and head of the femur (as recommended by Urbaniak) may prevent such collapse.

The prognosis of advanced nontraumatic osteonecrosis of the adult femoral head is very poor indeed because of the irreparable damage to the joint. Treatment frequently involves surgical operations, such as a varus

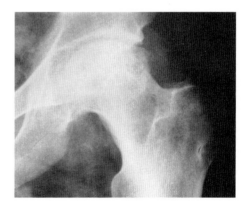

Figure 13.27. Nontraumatic osteonecrosis of the femoral head in a 47-year-old man who had been receiving adrenocorticosteroid therapy for 2 years as treatment for an unrelated disorder. Note the sclerosis of a large segment of the femoral head. The convex weightbearing area has collapsed with resultant incongruity of the joint surfaces. Irregular areas of bone resorption can be seen between the large sclerotic segment and the remainder of the femoral head. This man's hip joint is irreparably damaged.

osteotomy of the femur or a Sugioka-type osteotomy that rotates the femoral head and neck "upside down" so that the uninvolved part of the femoral head comes to bear weight. If, however, the entire femoral head is involved, the patient will require a prosthetic hip joint replacement, either unipolar or bipolar, depending on the state of the acetabulum.

NONTRAUMATIC OSTEONECROSIS OF THE KNEE IN ADULTS

This disorder, a form of avascular necrosis, is also known as *spontaneous osteonecrosis of the knee,* or SONK, and has been recognized only in the past few decades. The medial femoral condyle is usually involved, the average age at onset is older than 60 years, and it occurs more commonly in women than men. Although acute, severe pain in the knee may precede radiographic changes by 6 months, the diagnosis can be made earlier by scintigraphy (a bone scan) because of increased uptake of the radionuclide in the medial femoral condyle, which indicates an attempt at revascularization of the necrotic bone. Eventual collapse of the medial femoral condyle can be managed by either an osteocartilaginous allograft, as advocated by Gross, or a high tibial osteotomy if the area of necrosis is not extensive; otherwise, a prosthetic knee joint replacement is indicated.

POSTTRAUMATIC AVASCULAR NECROSIS OF TRACTION EPIPHYSES (APOPHYSES)

Two disorders that were formerly thought to represent a form of osteochondrosis of traction epiphyses (apophyses) are now thought to be caused by partial avulsion of the apophysis and its related tendon. These disorders, Osgood-Schlatter's disease and Sever's disease, are discussed separately from the osteochondroses of pressure epiphyses.

Partial Avulsion of the Tibial Tubercle (Osgood-Schlatter's Disease)

In very young children, the tibial tubercle is formed by a cartilaginous tongue-shaped downward prolongation of the upper tibial epiphysis. Toward the end of growth, one or more centers of ossification appear in the tibial tubercle. At this stage, it is most vulnerable to the effects of repeated, forceful traction through the attached patellar tendon.

Partial avulsion of the growing tibial tubercle, with subsequent avascular necrosis of the avulsed portion, is probably the explanation for the clinical disorder known as *Osgood-Schlatter's disease.* Boys, particularly active boys, between the ages of 10 and 15 years are most frequently affected. The lesion may be bilateral.

The child complains of local pain aggravated by kneeling on the tibial tubercle, by direct blows, and by running. Clinically, a prominent subcutaneous swelling, some of which is due to reaction in the soft tissues, is apparent in the region of the tibial tubercle (Fig. 13.28). The prominence is tender and

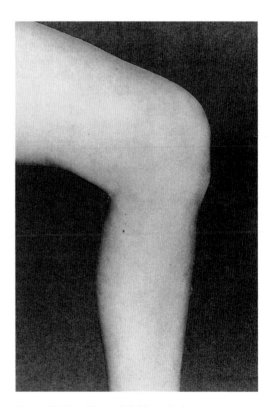

Figure 13.28.   Osgood-Schlatter's disease due to partial avulsion of the tibial apophysis in a 14-year-old boy. Note the prominent subcutaneous swelling over the tibial tubercle. Some of this swelling is due to reaction in the local soft tissues.

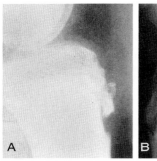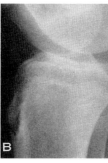

Figure 13.29. Osgood-Schlatter's disease due to partial avulsion of the tibial apophysis in a 14-year-old boy. **A.** Note the irregular areas of bone deposition and bone resorption in the proximal part of the traction epiphysis (apophysis). **B.** The normal tibial tubercle of the opposite knee is perfectly smooth and regular.

the pain can usually be reproduced by having the patient extend the knee against resistance.

Radiographically, the proximal part of the tibial tubercle exhibits irregular areas of bone deposition and bone resorption when compared to the tubercle on the normal side (Fig. 13.29).

Osgood-Schlatter's disease is usually self limiting, in which case the tibial tubercle becomes completely ossified over a period of about 2 years. In some children, a complication develops: a proximal segment fails to unite to the remainder of the tubercle, remains mobile, and persists as a source of local pain and tenderness.

The aim of treatment in uncomplicated Osgood-Schlatter's disease is prevention of further irritation during the healing phase. This is done by avoiding kneeling and jumping. It is not necessary to immobilize the knee nor to restrain the child from running. Residual nonunion of a proximal fragment after the remainder of the tibial tubercle has healed will not improve spontaneously and will continue to cause symptoms. Under these circumstances, excision of the ununited fragment is indicated.

Partial Avulsion of the Calcaneal Apophysis (Sever's Disease)

The traction epiphysis (apophysis), through which the Achilles tendon inserts into the os

calcis, normally ossifies from multiple centers. Being broad and flat, it normally appears radiographically dense in a lateral projection. This combination may lead to an erroneous radiographic diagnosis of osteochondrosis. Nevertheless, a clinical disorder, which may represent chronic strain or even partial avulsion of the calcaneal apophysis, does exist and is seen in children, particularly active boys, between the ages of 8 and 15 years.

The child experiences pain behind the heel and walks with little spring in his step (calcaneus gait) in a subconscious effort to reduce the powerful pull of the Achilles tendon on the apophysis. Local tenderness and slight swelling are usually found over the posterior aspect of the heel. The radiographic findings are within the wide range of normal variations mentioned above.

This self-limiting disorder improves spontaneously in less than a year, but during this time the child's symptoms can be relieved by elevating the heel of the shoe 1 cm, thereby decreasing the pull of the Achilles tendon during walking.

POSTTRAUMATIC AVASCULAR NECROSIS OF SUBCHONDRAL BONE

The main blood vessels to a significant part of a bone may be torn at the time of a severe injury such as a fracture, a dislocation, or a combination of the two (which is referred to as a "fracture-dislocation"). Even if not torn initially, the blood vessels may be compressed by the displaced fragments or by the dislocated bone. In either event, resulting ischemia can lead to the serious complication of avascular necrosis, a complication that occurs most commonly after certain types of fractures and dislocations involving the femoral head and neck, the radial head and neck, the carpal scaphoid, and the talus.

In children, posttraumatic avascular necrosis of a pressure epiphysis is most likely to occur after fracture-separation of the upper femoral epiphysis or after traumatic dislocation of the hip (Fig. 13.30). The course is similar in many ways to that of Legg-Perthes' disease (described in an earlier section of this chapter). The most important sequelae are incongruity of the joint and retardation of growth in the epiphyseal plate (physis).

In adults, fractures of the neck of the femur and traumatic dislocation of the hip are the most common causes of posttraumatic a vascular necrosis. This complication in adults delays, but does not prevent, healing of a fracture. Frequently, it leads to the type of

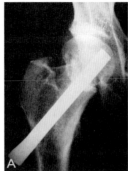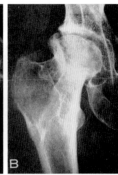

Figure 13.31.   Posttraumatic avascular necrosis of the femoral head in a 65-year-old woman after fracture of the neck of the femur. **A.** The hip 2 months after internal fixation of the fracture with a Smith-Petersen nail (now obsolete) reveals no significant change in the density of the femoral head. **B.** The radiograph 2 years later reveals evidence of extensive avascular necrosis of the femoral head. The fracture of the neck of the femur has healed and the nail has been removed. Proximal to the original fracture site is a large segment of avascular necrosis. This triangular-shaped segment containing the weightbearing surface has collapsed, resulting in significant joint incongruity. Note the evidence of bone deposition and bone resorption in the femoral head demarcating the necrotic fragment from the remainder of the head. Note also that this patient's hip is now adducted due to an adduction contracture. This patient's hip is irreparably destroyed and will require a prosthetic hip replacement.

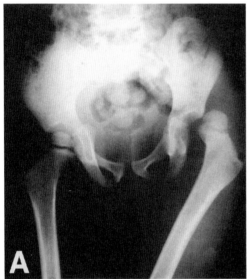

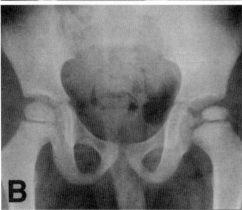

Figure 13.30.   Posttraumatic avascular necrosis of the left femoral head. **A.** Traumatic posterior dislocation of the left hip in a 4-year-old boy. **B.** The radiograph 16 months later reveals definite evidence of avascular necrosis of the femoral head. Note the increased density of the relatively small ossific nucleus of the left femoral head. This ossific nucleus is approximately the same size as it was at the time of the dislocation. Note also the evidence of bone deposition peripherally in the preosseous cartilage of the femoral head. This condition is comparable in many ways to Legg-Perthes' disease.

irreparable joint damage seen in idiopathic avascular necrosis of the femoral head in adults (described in an earlier section of this chapter) (Fig. 13.31).

MISCELLANEOUS CAUSES OF AVASCULAR NECROSIS OF SUBCHONDRAL BONE

The blood supply to bone may be disturbed in a variety of ways, and the subchondral bone at the end of long bones is most susceptible. In certain blood diseases, such as *polycythemia,* the likely cause is thrombosis. In certain metabolic disorders, such as *Gaucher's disease,* accumulation of abnormal cells may obliterate the blood supply (Chapter 9). Nitrogen emboli arising from fatty tissues, such as the fatty marrow, after atmospheric decompression in divers and underground construction workers (*decompression illness, caisson disease, "the bends"*), may cause avascular necrosis of bone

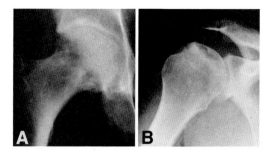

Figure 13.32. Avascular necrosis of **A,** the femoral head, and **B,** the humeral head secondary to caisson disease. The patient is a 42-year-old underground construction worker. The infarcts of bone are due to nitrogen emboli released from the fatty bone marrow during excessively rapid decompression. (The word "caisson" refers to a large underwater watertight chamber, open at the bottom, from which water is kept out by air pressure.)

with subsequent degenerative joint disease (Fig. 13.32). *Burns* and *frostbite* are likely to destroy blood supply to bone, particularly pressure epiphyses in children. Radiation therapy was sometimes complicated by avascular necrosis of bone in the region, particularly the neck of the femur in women who were being radiated for malignant lesions of the uterus. Fortunately, this complication has been reduced in recent years by improved methods of radiotherapy.

DISORDERS OF EPIPHYSEAL GROWTH

A variety of entirely different disorders of childhood share one thing in common: they are related, either directly or indirectly, to epiphyseal growth. Consequently, they begin during the growing years and tend to be progressive as long as the child is still growing. For these reasons they are grouped together in this chapter as "disorders of epiphyseal growth." These disorders include *slipping of the upper femoral epiphysis (adolescent coxa vara), Blount's disease (tibia vara), Madelung's deformity,* and *idiopathic curvature of the spine (idiopathic scoliosis).*

Slipped Upper Femoral Epiphysis (Adolescent Coxa Vara)

The hip joint is probably subjected to greater physical forces than any other joint in the ex-

tremities. Furthermore, the upper femoral epiphyseal plate is set obliquely in relation to the axis of the femoral shaft and is subjected to *shearing* forces. It is not surprising that in the presence of either a generalized or a localized weakness of the epiphyseal plate, the upper femoral epiphysis is particularly prone to slip off the femoral neck through its weakened plate.

In the disorder of slipped upper femoral epiphysis (adolescent coxa vara), the epiphysis either gradually, or suddenly, slips downward and backward in relation to the neck of the femur; or, if you prefer, the femoral neck slips upward and forward in relation to the epiphysis. Another synonym for this disorder is *slipped capital femoral epiphysis (SCFE).*

Incidence and Etiology

Slipping of the upper femoral epiphysis is most likely to develop in older children and adolescents, from the age of 9 years to the end of growth, and is more common in boys than girls. The slip first becomes apparent in one hip, but there is approximately a 30% chance of the second hip becoming involved subsequently. These chances are even greater if the patient is overweight and has 3 or 4 years of anticipated skeletal growth remaining.

Although the upper femoral epiphysis may slip in otherwise normal individuals, it is more likely to do so in the presence of some preexisting endocrine imbalance. Thus, the incidence is high in the very tall, thin, rapidly growing adolescent and is even higher in the obese Fröhlich type of adolescent male with a female distribution of fat and sexual underdevelopment (Fig. 13.33).

The etiology of slipped upper femoral epiphysis is not entirely understood. The experimental investigation of Harris suggests that an imbalance between growth hormone and sex hormones (either excessive growth hormone or deficient sex hormones) weakens the epiphyseal plate and renders it more vulnerable to the shearing forces of both weightbearing and injury. From immunofluorescent staining of the synovial membrane, Morrissy has postulated that, at least in some patients, there is an underlying abnormality of the immune system.

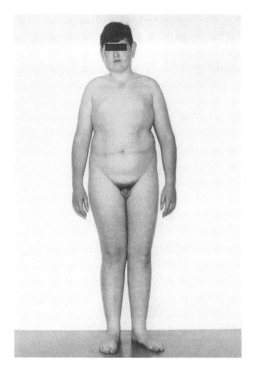

Figure 13.33. Slipped left upper femoral epiphysis of the Fröhlich type in a 14-year-old boy with a female distribution of subcutaneous fat and underdeveloped genitalia. Note that the boy's left lower limb is externally rotated. Radiographic examination confirmed the clinical suspicion of slipping of the left upper femoral epiphysis.

Pathogenesis and Pathology

The femoral epiphysis usually slips slowly and progressively and leads to a progressive coxa vara deformity with secondary remodeling of the femoral neck; the posterior periosteal attachment remains intact. Such a chronic slip is stable. An acute injury superimposed on this pathological process may cause a sudden further slip—an acute-on-chronic slip. Indeed, the epiphysis may become completely separated from the femoral neck, in which case the precarious blood supply of the femoral head may be severely damaged, with resultant avascular necrosis. Understandably, an acute-on-chronic slip is unstable. Once the epiphyseal plate (physis) closes by bony union, no further slip occurs. Nevertheless, residual displacement of the femoral head alters the mechanics of the hip and leads to the development of degenerative disease (osteoarthritis) of the hip in adult life.

Clinical Features and Diagnosis

Early diagnosis is extremely important so that surgical treatment may be instituted in the earliest possible stages of slipping. The most common initial symptom is mild discomfort arising in the hip but referred to the knee. At this stage, the patient's knee may be examined clinically and radiographically, even repeatedly, with negative results. Meanwhile, the underlying slip of the upper femoral epiphysis, having escaped detection, progresses. In the early stages there is usually a slight limp, most noticeable when the patient is tired. As the slip progresses, a Trendelenburg-type gait develops (the patient's trunk leans toward the affected side as weight is borne on the affected lower limb as described in Chapter 5, Fig. 5.13). The lower limb becomes externally rotated (Fig. 13.33). Further examination reveals limitation of internal rotation and abduction of the hip. As the hip is passively flexed, the thigh rotates externally.

The diagnosis can be suspected from the aforementioned symptoms and signs but it can be confirmed only by radiographic examination of the upper end of the femur in two projections. A minimal slip is always more obvious in the lateral projection than in the anteroposterior projection (Fig. 13.34). This is the stage at which the diagnosis should always be made.

If the femoral epiphysis continues to slip gradually, remodeling of the femoral neck becomes apparent (Fig. 13.35). The radiographic appearance of a complete separation of the epiphysis is striking. There is usually evidence of a preceding gradual slip (Fig. 13.36). The slipped upper femoral epiphysis may be classified as acute, chronic, or acute superimposed on chronic.

The most significant complications of slipped upper femoral epiphysis are avascular necrosis (osteonecrosis) of the femoral head and chondrolysis (acute cartilage necrosis) of the hip joint. In unstable slips, a pretreatment technetium bone scan (scintigraphy) that reveals ischemia of the femoral head is a predictor of avascular necrosis and provides evidence that this complication has been caused by the slip rather than by its treatment.

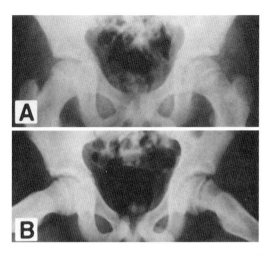

Figure 13.34.   Minimal slip of the left upper femoral epiphysis in a 14-year-old boy. **A.** In the anteroposterior projection there is an abnormal relationship between the femoral head and the neck. The slip is not very obvious. **B.** In the lateral projection of the upper end of the femur ("frog position projection"), the slip of the left upper femoral epiphysis is much more obvious.

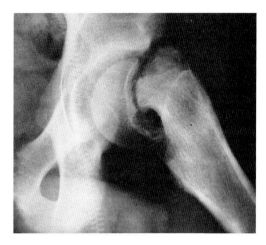

Figure 13.36.   Complete separation of the left upper femoral epiphysis in a 13-year-old boy. The remodeling of the femoral neck provides evidence that the epiphysis had been slipping gradually before the complete separation. This is in keeping with the boy's history of pain in the left hip and a limp during the 4 months preceding the acute injury that caused the complete separation. The risk of avascular necrosis in this femoral head is high.

Treatment

Because the precarious blood supply has already been threatened by the slipping through the epiphyseal plate (physis), forceful manipulation of a slipped upper femoral epiphysis should definitely be avoided to prevent the complication of avascular necrosis (osteonecrosis) of the femoral head.

The aim of treatment in the early stages is to prevent further slip of the epiphysis. If the femoral head has slipped chronically and

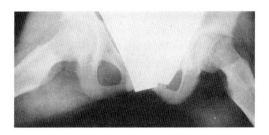

Figure 13.35.   Gradual slipping of the left upper femoral epiphysis in a 15-year-old boy. Note the new bone formation in the angle between slipped femoral head and the posterior aspect of the femoral neck. This type of remodeling always indicates a chronic, slowly progressive slip.

minimally (less than 1 cm in the lateral projection), it should be surgically stabilized *in situ* by means of a centrally placed cannulated threaded screw with the guidance of an image intensifier, after which weightbearing may be resumed (Fig. 13.37). A complete separation of the epiphysis superimposed on a chronic slip can usually be reduced to a satisfactory position by internally rotating the involved hip under general anesthesia (without force and only to the preacute slip position). It then can be stabilized surgically by two centrally placed, cannulated, threaded screws (to provide more secure fixation). After such treatment, weightbearing must be avoided until the epiphysis has healed to the neck, and this may require several months. Even the chronic slip that has progressed well beyond 1 cm, and in which there has not been a superimposed acute slip, should be pinned *in situ*. The subsequent remodeling is often quite satisfactory.

Surgical correction of the residual deformity of the head and neck may become necessary a year or more later, only if there is inadequate remodeling or if the gait remains unsatisfactory. Under these circumstances,

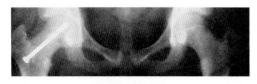

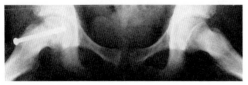

Figure 13.37.   Surgical stabilization of a minimal slip of the right upper femoral epiphysis in situ by means of a single cannulated screw that crosses the epiphyseal plate (physis) and enters the center of the epiphysis as seen in both the anteroposterior projection (*above*) and the frog lateral projection (*below*). Although from the anteroposterior projection, it might seem that the entire screw was buried within the femoral neck and epiphysis, it can be seen in the frog lateral projection that the head of the screw is outside the anterior aspect of the femoral neck. (This is yet another example of the value of two radiographic projections at right angles to each other.)

the associated abnormal relationship between the femoral head and the acetabulum is most safely achieved by a compensatory intertrochanteric or subtrochanteric osteotomy of the femur. Operation in the region of the epiphyseal plate would seem, at least theoretically, to be more logical, but the risk of producing *iatrogenic avascular necrosis* is considerable. Furthermore, the prognosis for future hip function after avascular necrosis of the femoral head in this age group is extremely bad. Such an operation might be called "orthopaedic roulette," because the surgeon never knows which time the operation is going to kill the femoral head!

The follow-up care of patients treated for slipped upper femoral epiphysis must continue at least until the epiphyseal plate (physis) has closed; during this time, the opposite femoral epiphysis must also be assessed at regular intervals because there is a 30% chance that it will begin to slip before growth is complete. The patient and the parents should be informed of this and of the need to seek orthopaedic care immediately should any symptoms or signs develop in the opposite hip.

Tibia Vara (Blount's Disease)

The medial portion of the upper tibial epiphyseal plate may become the site of a localized epiphyseal growth disturbance known as *tibia vara* (*Blount's disease, osteochondrosis deformans tibiae*), which is characterized by a progressive bow leg (varus) deformity.

This disorder is more common in girls than boys. It usually becomes manifest at the age of about 2 years in the infantile type and after the age of 8 years in the adolescent type. The growth disturbance may involve only one tibia or both. Tibia vara is relatively uncommon in most areas of the world but is inexplicably common in two completely different types of country, namely, Finland and Jamaica.

Once considered to be the result of a localized osteochondrosis of the medial portion of the upper tibial epiphysis, tibia vara is now thought to represent a localized form of *epiphyseal dysplasia*. The combination of diminished growth in the medial portion of the epiphyseal plate (physis) and continued normal growth in the lateral portion accounts for the progressive angulatory deformity of varus, that is, bow leg. After a number of years, the medial portion of the epiphyseal plate (physis) closes prematurely.

In the early stages of tibia vara, there are no symptoms. Examination reveals a characteristic varus deformity of the knee, a deformity that is particularly striking when it is unilateral (Fig. 13.38). Radiographically, there is defective ossification of the medial portion of the upper tibial epiphysis, a beaked appearance of the underlying metaphysis, and obvious retardation of longitudinal growth in the medial side of the tibia (Fig. 13.39).

Treatment in the early stages of tibia vara in young children is aimed at preventing progression of the varus deformity. This can sometimes be accomplished by means of a night splint of the type used for physiological bow legs (Chapter 7). In older children, the varus deformity progresses despite splinting. It can be corrected only by osteotomy of the tibia, which may have to be repeated on one or more occasions during the remaining growth period.

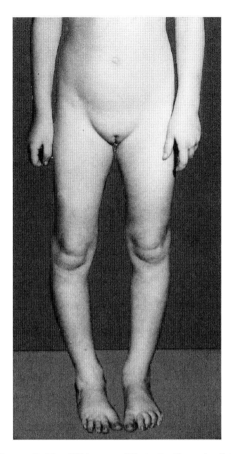

Figure 13.38.   Tibia vara (Blount's disease) of the medial portion of the right upper tibial epiphyseal plate (physis) in a 6-year-old girl. Note the varus deformity as well as the internal tibial torsion in the right lower limb compared to the normal left lower limb.

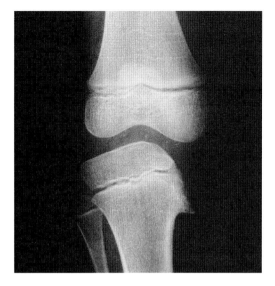

Figure 13.39.   Tibia vara (Blount's disease). This is the radiograph of the girl shown in Figure 13.38. Note the defective ossification of the medial portion of the upper tibial epiphysis, the beaked appearance of the underlying metaphysis, and the evidence of a growth disturbance in the medial portion of the epiphyseal plate (physis).

Madelung's Deformity

An epiphyseal growth disturbance may develop on the medial (ulnar) side of the distal radial epiphysis as the result of a localized form of *epiphyseal dysplasia*. The resultant deformity of the wrist, which does not usually become apparent until adolescence, is known as *Madelung's deformity* and is characterized by prominence of the distal end of the ulna on the dorsum of the wrist and forward displacement of the hand in relation to the forearm. It is more common in girls than boys and is usually bilateral (Fig. 13.40). Further examination reveals limitation of flexion of the wrist and of supination of the forearm.

Treatment is aimed at correction of the

rather ugly deformity as well as improvement of wrist function. This is best accomplished by excision of the distal portion of the ulna and osteotomy of the deformed distal end of the radius.

Scoliosis

Considering the complexity and multiplicity of the intervertebral and apophyseal joints in

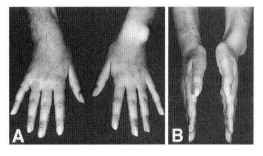

Figure 13.40.   Madelung's deformity in the left wrist of a 14-year-old girl. The distal end of the ulna is prominent on the dorsum of the wrist and the hand appears to be displaced forward in relation to the forearm. In this girl the deformity had been bilateral, but the deformity in the right wrist has been corrected surgically.

the human spinal column, it is remarkable that in the vast majority of people, the spine grows straight during childhood and remains straight throughout adult life. It is not surprising that a variety of disorders are capable of disturbing this normal growth pattern and can lead to a progressive and serious spinal deformity.

The broad term *scoliosis* refers to *a lateral curvature of the spine;* thus, scoliosis is a deformity rather than a specific disease or disorder. As such, it takes many forms, depending on its etiology and the age at which it begins. It is of the utmost importance to learn about the nature of scoliosis, its early diagnosis in childhood, its prognosis and, in a general way at least, what can and should be done for those affected in the way of preventive and corrective treatment.

At the outset a few terms should be defined. A *nonstructural scoliosis* is a reversible lateral curvature of the spine *without rotation.* It can be reversed either voluntarily by the patient, or by correcting the underlying cause (Fig. 13.41). A *structural scoliosis* is an irreversible lateral curvature of the spine *with rotation* of the vertebral bodies in the abnormal area (major curve) (see Fig. 13.46). (The term, major curve, is synonymous with the term primary curve, but the adjective *major* is currently preferred by members of the Scoliosis Research Society of North America). The scoliosis is said to be *compensated* when the shoulders are level and are directly above the pelvis. This is possible because of the development of *compensatory* curves above and below the major curve. When the major curve is greater than the sum of its compensatory curves, however, the scoliosis is said to be *decompensated,* inasmuch as the shoulders are not level and there is a lateral shift or "list" of the trunk to one side. The designations, *right* or *left* scoliosis, refer to the convex side of the major curve.

The following etiological classification should help to put the various types of scoliosis in reasonable perspective.

Etiological Classification of Scoliosis
I. Nonstructural Scoliosis (Reversible)
  1. Habitual poor posture (postural scoliosis)

  2. Pain and muscle spasm
    a) Painful lesion of a spinal nerve root (e.g. sciatic scoliosis, Chapter 11, Fig. 11.39)
    b) Painful lesion of the spine (inflammation, Chapter 10; neoplasm, Chapter 14)
    c) Painful lesion of the abdomen (appendicitis, perinephric abscess)
  3. Lower limb-length discrepancy
    a) Actual shortening of the lower limb (Fig. 13.41)
    b) Apparent shortening of the lower limb (pelvic obliquity)
      i) Adduction contracture of the hip on the shorter side
      ii) Abduction contracture of the hip on the longer side
II. Structural Scoliosis (Irreversible)
  1. Idiopathic Scoliosis (85% of all scoliosis)
    a) Infantile: appears from birth to 3 years
    b) Juvenile: appears from 4 years to 9 years
    c) Adolescent: appears from 10 years to the end of growth (see Fig. 13.45)
  2. Osteopathic Scoliosis
    a) Congenital (discussed in Chapter 8)
      i) Localized: hemivertebrae (failure of formation) (Fig. 8.64); unilateral bony bar (failure of segmentation) (Figs. 8.65 and 13.42)
      ii) Generalized: osteogenesis imperfecta, arachnodactyly (discussed in Chapter 8)
    b) Acquired
      i) Fractures and dislocations of the spine; traumatic and pathological
      ii) Rickets and osteomalacia (discussed in Chapter 9)
      iii) Thoracogenic; unilateral pulmonary disease (emphysema) and unilateral chest operations (thoracoplasty)
  3. Neuropathic Scoliosis

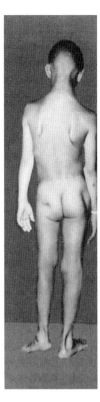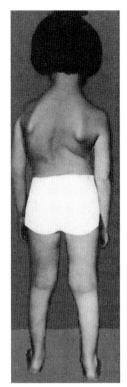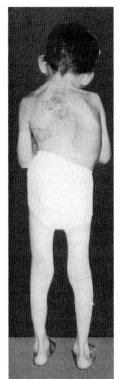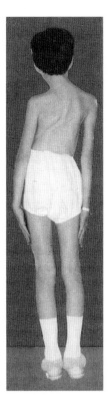

Figure 13.41.   Nonstructural scoliosis (functional scoliosis) secondary to lower limb-length discrepancy in a 6-year-old boy. In the standing position, the left side of this boy's pelvis is lower than the right and consequently, his spine must compensate by curving to the right so that he may remain upright. There is no rotational deformity in the spine. This compensatory type of scoliosis is completely reversible in that the spine straightens when an appropriate lift is put under the short limb and when the individual either sits or lies down.

Figure 13.42.   Congenital scoliosis due to failure of segmentation of the lateral components of the lower thoracic spine in a 5-year-old girl. This girl's deformity is rigid and her scoliosis is decompensated to the left.

Figure 13.43.   Neuropathic scoliosis due to neurofibromatosis (von Recklinghausen's disease) in a 4-year-old boy. Note the large café-au-lait spot on the upper part of his back and the severe right thoracolumbar scoliosis. Scoliosis secondary to neurofibromatosis has an extremely poor prognosis concerning progression of deformity and usually requires operative treatment.

Figure 13.44.   Neuropathic paralytic scoliosis secondary to extensive poliomyelitis involving trunk muscles in a 10-year-old girl. The curve pattern is right thoracic and the scoliosis is decompensated to the right. In the paralytic type of scoliosis, the spine tends to sag, or collapse, in the erect position because of the associated muscle weakness.

a) Congenital (discussed in Chapter 8)
   i) Spina bifida with myelodysplasia
   ii) Neurofibromatosis (von Recklinghausen's disease) (Fig. 13.43)

b) Acquired (paralytic scoliosis) Chapter 12)
   i) Poliomyelitis (Fig. 13.44)
   ii) Paraplegia
   iii) Cerebral Palsy
   iv) Friedreich's ataxia

v) Syringomyelia
4. Myopathic Scoliosis
   a) Congenital (discussed in Chapter 8)
      i) Hypotonia of neuromuscular origin (spinal muscular atrophy)
      ii) Amyoplasia congenita (arthrogryposis)
   b) Acquired
      i) Muscular dystrophy

Idiopathic Scoliosis

All the aforementioned types of structural scoliosis are potentially serious and patients so afflicted merit continuing supervision by an orthopaedic surgeon. For the purpose of this textbook, the major emphasis is placed on the idiopathic type of structural scoliosis, which comprises 85% of the total and which develops in otherwise normal, healthy children and adolescents. The basic clinical problem of the idiopathic type of scoliosis is the unsightly appearance of the deformity. Thus, it is primarily a cosmetic problem, albeit a very significant one.

Incidence and Etiology

Idiopathic scoliosis is a relatively common musculoskeletal deformity in that it is present to some degree in approximately 0.5% of the population; there is a definite familial incidence. The *infantile* type, which appears between birth and 3 years of age, is more common in boys and, for reasons unknown, is seen more frequently in some countries than in others. The *juvenile* type, which appears between the ages of 4 and 9 years, and the more common *adolescent* type, which first becomes apparent between the ages of 10 years and the end of growth, are both much more common in girls.

The pattern of the curve may be *lumbar, thoracolumbar, thoracic,* or *combined lumbar and thoracic* (double major curve), but by far the most common pattern is a right thoracic scoliosis in adolescent girls (Fig. 13.45). Despite much investigation, both clinical and experimental, the precise etiology remains an unsolved and challenging problem; hence, the persistence of the adjective, idiopathic.

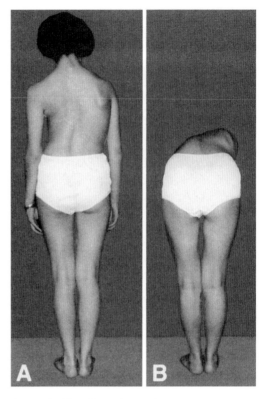

Figure 13.45. Idiopathic scoliosis in a 13-year-old girl. **A.** Note that the right shoulder is higher than the left, the right scapula is more prominent than the left, and the left hip protrudes more than the right. The curvature in the thoracic spine is apparent. This girl's scoliosis is of the right thoracic pattern and is decompensated to the right. **B.** The rotation of the vertebrae and ribs is most readily detected from behind as the girl bends forward.

Pathogenesis and Pathology

The most important aspect of the pathogenesis of the deformity of scoliosis is its *progression,* with skeletal growth that is particularly rapid during adolescence (Fig. 13.47). As the lateral curvature and the coexistent rotation of the spine increase, secondary changes develop in the vertebrae and ribs due to progressive growth disturbance. On the concave side of the curve, increased pressure on one side of the epiphyseal plates of the vertebral bodies produces wedge-shaped vertebrae. Such structural changes help to explain the irreversibility of structural scoliosis (Fig. 13.46). Persistent malalignment of the spinal joints may become worse very slowly (1° per year) even

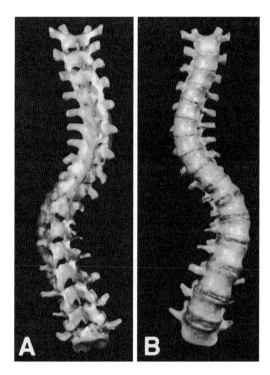

Figure 13.46. Idiopathic scoliosis as seen in the postmortem specimen of a spine from an adolescent (who died of an unrelated cause). The curve pattern is a combined left lumbar and right thoracic scoliosis (double major curve). **A.** In this view from behind, note the rotation of the spine in both major curves. **B.** In this view from the front, note the secondary changes, particularly wedging in the vertebral bodies, due to a growth disturbance.

after growth is over, especially when the curve is more than 40°. Such malalignment eventually leads to painful degenerative joint disease of the spine in adult life.

Clinical Features and Diagnosis

Idiopathic scoliosis begins slowly, insidiously, and painlessly. Thus, in the early stage of its development, the patient is not aware of the curvature, and because it is well concealed by clothing at this stage, the parents are not aware of it either. Later, the parents may observe that one shoulder is higher than the other, one shoulder blade is more prominent than the other, or one hip protrudes more than the other. By the time a spinal curvature has progressed sufficiently to be readily detected clinically, it has usually reached 30°.

Examination of the otherwise healthy child or adolescent from behind reveals a *lateral curvature* of the spine and *rotation* in the area of the major curve. The rotation of the spine is most noticeable from behind when the patient is asked to bend forward (Fig. 13.45). Complete physical examination, including lower limb-length measurement and neurological assessment, is necessary to exclude other causes of scoliosis.

Radiographic examination, which should include an anteroposterior and lateral projection of the full length of the spine in the *standing* position, reveals a curvature that is always more marked than would be expected from the external physical appearance (Fig. 13.51).

Assessment of the scoliosis by MRI is indicated in the presence of any neurological deficit, neck stiffness, or headache.

During the past decade, widespread school screening programs to detect scoliosis in girls from 12 to 14 years of age have detected a curvature of 10° or more in 2% of such girls (a radiographic curve of less than 10° is considered to be a variation of normal). Of all girls screened in these programs, approximately 0.3% require treatment and the majority are mild curves that can be managed by bracing. Happily, scoliosis is being detected early so that the incidence of severe curvatures (more than 40°), and hence the need for major spinal operations, is decreasing. An alternative to radiographic diagnosis of minimal scoliosis is moiré fringe photography by which ordinary light is projected through special grids. Its major advantage is the avoidance of exposure to radiation. Although these massive school screening programs have been found not to be "cost effective" they have provided useful information concerning the natural history of scoliosis in its earliest stages.

Prognosis

Because the deformity of scoliosis increases with growth, it is obvious that an important factor in assessing the prognosis for a given child is the amount of growth that remains. In addition, the more severe the degree of curvature is at the time of assessment, the more likely it is to increase. For example, a mild curvature (less than 30°) first noticed in a 14-

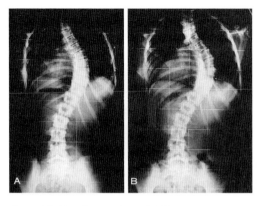

Figure 13.47. Progression of deformity with growth (viewed from behind). **A.** Idiopathic scoliosis of the right thoracic type in a 12-year-old girl. The curve is relatively mild. The girl's parents declined treatment at this time. **B.** The same girl just 1 year later shows a considerable progression in the severity of the curve. The scoliosis has become decompensated and the curve has become relatively rigid. These radiographs emphasize how much progression of the curvature can take place in just 1 year of rapid growth.

epidemiological outcome study, Nachemson has proven that the proper use of bracing does have a significantly beneficial effect on the natural history of progression of mild adolescent scoliosis. For many years, the Milwaukee brace has been the standard orthosis for this form of nonoperative management (Fig. 13.48). A more recent modification, proven to be effective for lumbar and thoracolumbar curves, is the Boston brace (as developed by Emans and his associates, including Hall) that eliminates the metal superstructure and is consequently hidden by ordinary clothes, a feature that is particularly appreciated by adolescent girls. In the 1990s, the prefabricated Boston brace and the custom-made variation of it are the most commonly used types of thoracolumbosacral orthosis (TLSO) (Fig. 13.49 and 13.50).

Another option is the night-time use of the lateral bending Charleston splint, especially for relatively mild thoracolumbar curves.

year-old girl may not increase significantly, whereas the same degree of curvature, first noticed in a 10-year-old girl, is almost certain to increase, particularly during a period of rapid growth (Fig. 13.47).

Treatment

The patient with idiopathic scoliosis should be seen by an orthopaedic surgeon to determine the need for correction of the deformity, and thereafter should be assessed at regular intervals throughout the growing period.

The aims of treatment are to prevent progression of a mild scoliosis and to correct and stabilize a more severe deformity. The indications for treatment and the methods of treatment require the judgment and skills of an experienced orthopaedic surgeon.

Nonoperative Methods. Exercises designed to prevent the progression of idiopathic scoliosis have been proven ineffectual, as have body casts.

For children with curves of 20° to 40° and with 2 years or more of anticipated skeletal growth, spinal braces can usually prevent increasing curvature and may even provide some permanent correction. From a very extensive

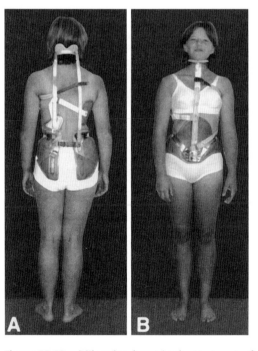

Figure 13.48. Milwaukee brace in the treatment of idiopathic scoliosis. This brace combines the forces of longitudinal traction and lateral pressure. It must be "custom-made" to fit very accurately and requires careful continuing supervision to be effective. The head and chin extension of this brace is used only for the treatment of high thoracic curves.

Operative Treatment. Idiopathic scoliosis with a curve of more than 40° that is already producing an obvious clinical deformity, or that can be predicted to do so in the future (because of predicted growth), is best treated by the combined operation of mechanical correction of the curvature by internal *spinal instrumentation. and spinal fusion*. The original system was designed by Harrington and reported by him in 1962 (Fig. 13.51). More recent designs include the Cotrel-Dubousset (CD) system and the Texas Scottish Rite Hospital (TSRH) system (Fig. 13.52). After the operation of spinal fusion for scoliosis, the patient's spine must be protected by a body cast for at least 3 months, and sometimes longer, to allow the fusion area in the spine to become consolidated.

Operative treatment is usually deferred

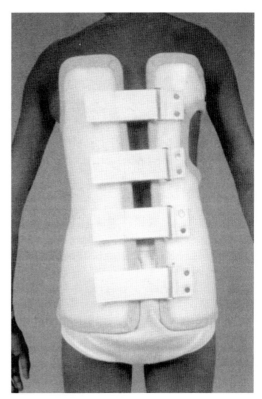

Figure 13.50. A custom-made thoracolumbar (TLSO) brace that applies corrective forces on the scoliotic spine.

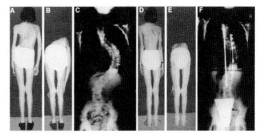

Figure 13.51. Severe idiopathic scoliosis of the right thoracic pattern in a 15-year-old girl. **A, B,** and **C.** Before treatment; note the decompensation of this girl's scoliosis and the severe rotational rib deformity. Her scoliosis could have, and ideally should have, been treated earlier. **D, E,** and **F.** One year after mechanical correction of the scoliosis by means of Harrington-type internal spinal instrumentation (distraction rod on the concave side, compression rod on the convex side). The operation included spinal fusion of the curved portion of the spine. This girl's spine is better compensated and the rib deformity has been well corrected. A completely different type of spinal instrumentation (involving staples, screws, and a cable) applied to vertebral bodies—after excision of intervertebral discs—has been developed in Australia by Dwyer.

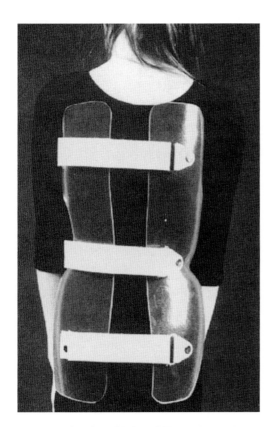

Figure 13.49. A prefabricated Boston brace. Appropriately placed pads attached to the inner surface of the brace provide the desired pressures that exert corrective forces on the scoliotic spine. This is the original type of thoracolumbosacral (TLSO) brace.

until the child is at least 10 years old. Under certain circumstances, it may be performed at an earlier age.

For adolescents with severe lumbar and thoracolumbar curves, especially those of paralytic origin and those in which the posterior elements are deficient, the Dwyer method of anterior correction and interbody fusion using staples and cables has been useful. Subsequently, other methods of anterior interbody fusion (which involve plates and screws) have been developed.

For children with paralytic forms of scoliosis, the method of "segmental spinal instrumentation," developed by Luque, provides good correction and an effective internal splint for the spine.

Very young children with progressive idiopathic scoliosis present a challenging problem.

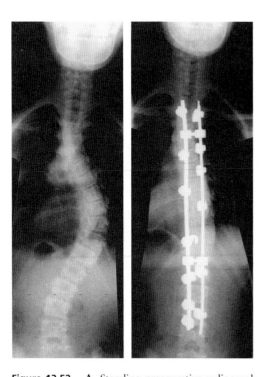

Figure 13.52.   A. Standing preoperative radiograph of severe idiopathic thoracic scoliosis in a 12-year-old girl. The curve in the thoracic region measured 60°. **B.** Standing postoperative radiograph of the same patient. The operation consisted of correction of the curvature by means of the Texas Scottish Rite Hospital (TSRH) type of spinal instrumentation and posterior spinal fusion. Note the excellent correction of the deformity.

In such instances, bracing is usually inadequate to control their curves and spinal fusion is contraindicated because it stops vertical growth of the fused part of the spine. For these children, Gillespie has placed the end hooks of a Harrington rod in bone but has passed the rod subcutaneously and has avoided a fusion. Vertical growth continues, necessitating exchange of the rod for a longer one from time to time but the system (which is combined with bracing) has allowed these children to grow relatively straight and reach an age when definitive spinal fusion can be performed.

The development of more physiological methods of treatment must await the discovery of the precise etiology of idiopathic scoliosis, which conceivably might even be of a metabolic nature. In the meantime, early diagnosis and early, effective orthopaedic treatment can do much to prevent the dreadfully severe spinal curvatures and rib deformities that have been allowed to develop all too often in the past.

SPONDYLOLYSIS

A mysterious defect occasionally develops in one or both sides of the neural arch of a lower lumbar vertebra for no apparent reason. Approximately 85% of such defects occur in the fifth lumbar vertebra and most of the remaining 15% occur in the fourth lumbar vertebra.

The defect, which consists of fibrous tissue, is known as *spondylolysis*. It always develops in the weakest part of the neural arch—the narrow isthmus (pars interarticularis) between the superior articular process and the inferior articular process. Being in the posterolateral part of the neural arch, the defect of spondylolysis is not readily detected in either anteroposterior or lateral radiographic projections. It is clearly seen, however, in an oblique projection (Fig. 13.53).

Incidence and Etiology

Once thought to be a congenital defect, spondylolysis is now known to develop during postnatal life. Moreover, the incidence of spondylolysis has been discovered to increase with age—not only during the growing years but also during adult life. Indeed, the defect can be demonstrated radiographically in ap-

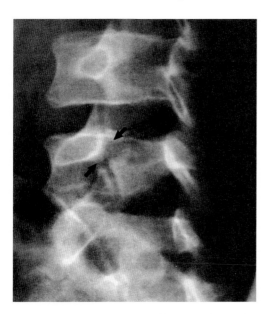

Figure 13.53. Spondylolysis of the pars interarticularis of the neural arch of the fifth lumbar vertebra as seen in an oblique radiograph (*arrows*). Note the intact pars interarticularis of the fourth lumbar vertebra above. The pars interarticularis in this projection may be likened to the narrow knot of an obliquely placed bow tie or to the neck collar on a Scotty dog (the head of which is to the left in this radiograph). The defect of spondylolysis is at the site of the knot.

proximately 10% of adults. Because the lower lumbar region of the human spine is subjected to much stress in the erect position, it is possible that spondylolysis represents either a stress fracture (fatigue fracture) from frequently repeated stresses or an ordinary fracture from a single injury. Nevertheless, the precise etiology remains obscure.

Clinical Features and Treatment

In the majority of individuals with spondylolysis, the defect produces neither symptoms nor signs. After an injury or chronic strain, however, the fibrous tissue in the defect may be stretched. The resultant pain may persist for many months and necessitate the use of a lumbosacral-type brace. As a practitioner you must always rule out other causes of low back pain in a patient who has spondylolysis, because the spondylolysis may be an incidental

finding that is unrelated to the source of the patient's pain.

Complication

When spondylolysis is bilateral, the vertebra is in a sense separated into two parts: the vertebral body, pedicles, and superior articular processes anteriorly, and the lamina and inferior articular processes posteriorly. Under these circumstances, the anterior part may slip forward in relation to the posterior part and produce one form of spondylolisthesis.

SPONDYLOLISTHESIS

Forward slipping of one vertebral body (and the remainder of the spinal column above it) in relation to the vertebral segment immediately below is referred to as *spondylolisthesis*. It usually occurs in the lower lumbar spine, particularly between the fifth lumbar vertebra and the sacrum. A normal lumbar vertebral body is prevented from slipping forward by an intact neural arch and the almost vertically inclined posterior facet joints on each side through which it articulates with the vertebral segment below. With loss of continuity of the pars interarticularis or an abnormality of the posterior facet joints, the intervertebral disc is not sufficiently strong to prevent forward displacement of the body of the involved vertebra.

Incidence and Etiology

Some degree of spondylolisthesis of a lower lumbar vertebra is detectable in approximately 2% of adults. The most common type is secondary to the aforementioned bilateral defect in the pars interarticularis of the neural arch (spondylolysis). Consequently, the usual site is the fifth lumbar vertebra. In this type (*spondylolytic spondylolisthesis*) the vertebral body, its pedicles and superior articular processes—and the spinal column above—become progressively displaced forward, leaving the inferior articular processes, the lamina, and the spinous process behind as a separated neural arch (Fig. 13.54). Forward displacement is most likely to be progressive during the rapid growth spurt of early adolescence and is almost never progressive during adult life.

Less common is the type of spondylolisth-

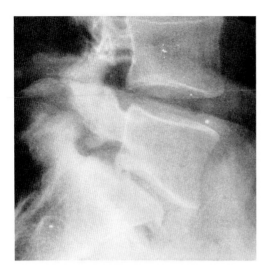

Figure 13.54. Spondylolisthesis of the fifth lumbar vertebra in relation to the sacrum. The body of the fifth lumbar vertebra, its pedicles and superior articular processes—and the spinal column above—have become displaced forward leaving the inferior articular processes, the lamina, and the spinous process behind. There is a bilateral defect in the pars interarticularis through which the spondylolisthesis has occurred; hence, this is the spondylolytic type of spondylolisthesis.

esis secondary to degenerative disc disease and subluxation of the posterior facet joints. In this type (*degenerative spondylolisthesis*), the displacement may be either forward or backward; the usual site is the fourth lumbar vertebra.

In a third type (*congenital spondylolisthesis*), which is associated with either a congenital abnormality of the posterior facet joints or congenital elongation of the pars interarticularis, the anterior displacement of the fifth lumbar vertebra is severe.

Two rare types are *traumatic spondylolisthesis* secondary to a single injury and *pathological spondylolisthesis* secondary to a pathological weakness of bone.

Clinical Features and Diagnosis

Spondylolytic spondylolisthesis usually becomes manifest during childhood by the gradual onset of low back pain that is aggravated by standing, walking, and running and relieved by lying down. The associated clinical

deformity, which is related to the degree of forward slip, is characterized by a "step" in the lumbosacral region at the level of the spondylolisthesis and an increased lumbar lordosis above (Fig. 13.55). The hamstring muscles are tight, with resultant limitation of straight leg raising. Significant involvement of

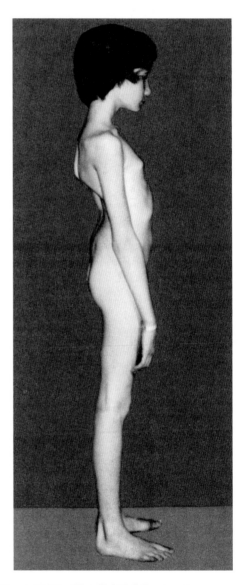

Figure 13.55. The clinical deformity of severe spondylolisthesis of the fifth lumbar vertebra in an 11-year-old girl. Note the vertical inclination of the sacrum, the step in the lumbosacral region, and the increased lumbar lordosis above. Chronic low back pain and a progressive anterior displacement of the fifth lumbar vertebra necessitated a local spinal fusion.

the nerve roots is not common in this type of spondylolisthesis, although nerve root irritation may produce sciatica. Radiographic examination reveals forward displacement of the affected vertebral body in the lateral projection (Fig. 13.54). Oblique radiographic projections are required to detect the underlying spondylolysis (Fig. 13.53).

In degenerative spondylolisthesis, the displacement—either forward or backward (retrospondylolisthesis)—is relatively slight. Osteophyte formation in relation to the subluxated and degenerated posterior facet joints may produce compression of the related nerve roots. The predominant symptom is chronic low back pain due to instability of the abnormal segment.

In congenital spondylolisthesis, the forward displacement of the fifth lumbar vertebra in relation to the sacrum is severe. Consequently there may be pressure on the cauda equina as well as on the nerve roots. Such pressure may be increased during a period of rapid growth, as in early adolescence and may produce acute low back pain with or without sciatica.

Treatment

Spondylolisthesis may cause no symptoms, in which case the patient should be examined clinically and radiographically at regular intervals to detect any progression of the forward slip of the affected vertebral body. Progressive forward slip is an indication for stabilization of the unstable segment by means of a local spinal fusion, which may be achieved posteriorly, anteriorly (interbody fusion), or laterally (intertransverse process fusion). The latter is the most effective type of fusion for spondylolisthesis. Surgical reduction of this slip is controversial because of potential neurological complications.

Mild low back pain in the absence of a progressive slip can usually be relieved by wearing a lumbosacral-type brace. Severe back pain and nerve root irritation in children and adolescents do not usually necessitate surgical decompression of the nerve roots, but the development of a cauda equina syndrome is an absolute indication for such decompression. In a patient with spondylolisthesis who has

either back pain or nerve root irritation, you, as a practitioner, must look for other causes of the symptoms, because their source may be at a level other than that of the spondylolisthesis.

Complications

Severe forward displacement of the fifth lumbar vertebra (which was first described by an obstetrician) may narrow the pelvic inlet sufficiently in the female that normal delivery is impossible and Caesarean section becomes necessary. This is particularly true of the congenital type of spondylolisthesis.

SUGGESTED ADDITIONAL READING

Al-Rowaih A, Lindstrand JA, Bjorkengren A, et al. Osteonecrosis of the knee: diagnosis and outcome in 40 patients. Acta Orthop Scand 1991; 62(1):19–23.

Axer A. Subtrochanteric osteotomy in the treatment of Perthes' disease. J Bone Joint Surg 1965;47B:489–499.

Barrie HJ. A diagram of the form and origin of loose bodies in osteochondritis dissecans. J Rheumatol 1984;11(4):512–513.

Bell DF, Armstrong P, et al. The use of Ilizarov technique in the correction of limb deformities associated with skeletal dysplasias. J Pediatr Orthop 1992;12:283–290.

Bradway JK, Klassen RA, Peterson HA. Blount's disease: a review of the English literature. J Pediatr Orthop 1987;7:472–480.

Brotherton BJ, McKibbin B. Perthes' disease treated by prolonged recumbency and femoral head containment: a long-term appraisal. J Bone Joint Surg 1977;59B:8–14.

Broughton NS, ed. A textbook of paediatric orthopaedics (from the Royal Children's Hospital, Melbourne). London: WB Saunders, 1997.

Bunnell WP. Outcome of spinal screening. Spine 1993;18(12):1572–1580.

Cahill BR. Osteochondritis dissecans of the knee: treatment of juvenile and adult forms. Journal of the American Academy of Orthopedic Surgeons 1995;3(4):237–247.

Carney BT, Weinstein SL. Long-term follow-up of slipped capital femoral epiphysis. J Bone Joint Surg 1991;73A(5):667–674.

Catterall A. The natural history of Perthes' disease. J Bone Joint Surg 1971;53B:37–53.

Catterall A. The place of femoral osteotomy in the management of Legg-Calvé-Perthes' disease. The Hip 1985:24–27. Proceedings Hip Society.

Cohen J, Bonfiglio M, Campbell CJ. Orthopedic pathophysiology in diagnosis and treatment. New York: Churchill Livingstone, 1990.

Emans JB, Kaelin A, Bancell P, et al. The Boston

bracing system for idiopathic scoliosis: follow-up results in 295 patients. Spine 1986;11(8):792–801.

Fernandez-Feliberti R, Flynn J, Ramirez N, et al. Effectiveness of TLSO bracing in the conservative treatment of idiopathic scoliosis. J Pediatr Orthop 1995;15:176–181.

Ferriter P, Shapiro F. Infantile tibia vara: factors affecting outcome following proximal tibial osteotomy. J Pediatr Orthop 1987;7:1–7.

Fredrickson BE, Baker D, McHolick WK, et al. The natural history of spondylolysis and spondylolisthesis. J Bone Joint Surg 1984;66A(5):699–707.

Garino J, Steinberg ME. Etiology, diagnosis and treatment of avascular necrosis of the femoral head. Current Opin Orthop 1994;5(1):3–10.

Glueck CJ, Crawford A, Roy D, et al. Association of antithrombotic factor deficiencies and hypofibrinolysis with Legg Perthes' disease. J Bone Joint Surg 1996;78A:3–13.

Golding JSR, McNeil-Smith JDG. Observations on the etiology of tibia vara. J Bone Joint Surg 1963;45B:320–325.

Hall JE. Anterior surgery in the treatment of idiopathic scoliosis. J Bone Joint Surg 1994;76B(Suppl 1):3.

Hall JE. Spinal deformities (Editorial). Current Orthopaedics 1989;3:69–71.

Harrington PR. Treatment of scoliosis—correction and internal fixation by spinal instrumentation. J Bone Joint Surg 1962;44A(4):591–610.

Harris IE, Weinstein SL. Long-term follow-up of patients with Grade III and Grade IV spondylolisthesis: treatment with and without spinal fusion. J Bone Joint Surg 1992;69A(7):960–704.

Harris WR. The endocrine basis for slipping of the upper femoral epiphysis: an experimental study. J Bone Joint Surg 1950;32B:5–11.

Haupt JB, Pritzker KPH, Alpert B, et al. Natural history of spontaneous osteonecrosis of the knee (SONK). A review. Semin Arthritis Rheum 1983;13(2):212–227.

Herring AH. Legg-Calvé-Perthes' disease. Monograph series. Rosemont: American Academy of Orthopaedic Surgeons, 1996.

Herring JA, Neustadt JB, Williams JJ, et al. The lateral pillar classification of Legg-Calvé-Perthes' disease. J Pediatr Orthop 1992;12:143–150.

Herring JA. Current concepts review: the treatment of Legg-Calvé-Perthes' disease: a critical review of the literature. J Bone Joint Surg 1994;76-A(3):448–458.

Jerre R, Billing L, Hansson G. The contralateral hip in patients primarily treated for unilateral slipped upper femoral epiphysis. J Bone Joint Surg 1994;76B(4):563–567.

Jones JP Jr. Concepts of etiology and early pathogenesis of osteonecrosis. In: Schafer M, ed. Instructional course lectures. Chicago: American Academy of Orthopaedic Surgeons, 1994;499–512.

Jones JR, Paterson DC, Hillier TM, et al. Remodelling after pinning for slipped capital femoral epiphysis. J Bone Joint Surg 1990;72B(4):568–573.

Kostuik JP. Operative treatment of idiopathic scoliosis. Current concepts review. J Bone Joint Surg 1990;72A(7):1108–1113.

Logue E, Sarwark JF. Idiopathic scoliosis: new instrumentation for surgical management. Journal of the American Academy of Orthopaedic Surgeons 1994;2(1):67–77.

Lonstein JE, Winter RB. The Milwaukee brace for the treatment of adolescent idiopathic scoliosis: a review of one thousand and twenty patients. J Bone Joint Surg 1994;76A(8):1207–1221.

Lowe TG. Scheuermann disease. Current concepts review. J Bone Joint Surg 1990;72A(6):940–945.

Luque ER. Segmental spinal instrumentation for reduction of scoliosis. Clin Orthop 1982;163:192–198.

Mankin HJ. Nontraumatic necrosis of bone (osteonecrosis). Current concepts review article. N Engl J Med 1992;326(22):1473–1479.

Martinez AG, Weinstein SL, Dietz FR. The weight-bearing abduction brace for the treatment of Legg-Perthes' disease. J Bone Joint Surg 1992;74-A(1):12–21.

McAndrew MP, Weinstein SL. A long-term follow-up of Legg-Calvé-Perthes' disease. J Bone Joint Surg 1984;66-A(6):860–869.

Meechan PL, Angel D, Nelson JM. The Scottish Rite abduction orthosis for the treatment of Legg-Perthes' disease: a radiographic analysis. J Bone Joint Surg 1992;74A(1):2–12.

Moberg A. Legg-Calvé-Perthes' Disease: an epidemiological, clinical and radiological study. Acta Universitatis Upsaliensis. Comprehensive summaries of Uppsala dissertations from the faculty of medicine 583. Uppsala, 1996.

Mont MA, Hungerford DS. Non-traumatic avascular necrosis of the femoral head. J Bone Joint Surg 1995;77A(3):459–474.

Morrissy RT, Kalderson AE, Gerdes MH. Synovial immunofluorescence in patients with slipped capital femoral epiphysis. J Pediatr Orthop 1981;1:55–60.

Morrissy RT, Weinstein SL. Lovell and Winter's pediatric orthopaedics. 4th ed. Volume II. Philadelphia: Lippincott-Raven, 1996.

Mubarak SJ, Carroll NC. Juvenile osteochondritis dissecans of the knee: etiology. Clin Orthop 1981;157:200–211.

Nachemson AL, Peterson L-E, and Members of the Brace Study Group of the Scoliosis Research Society. Effectiveness of treatment with a brace in girls who have adolescent idiopathic scoliosis: a prospective controlled study based on data from the Brace Study of the Scoliosis Research

Society. J Bone Joint Surg 1995;77-A(6): 815–822.

O'Brien ET, Fahey JJ. Remodelling of the femoral neck after in-situ pin for slipped capital femoral epiphysis. J Bone Joint Surg 1977;59A:62–68.

Paley D. Deformity planning for frontal and sagittal plane corrective osteotomies. Orthop Clin North Am 1994;3:425–465.

Petrie JG, Bitenc I. The abduction weight-bearing treatment in Legg-Perthes Disease. J Bone Joint Surg 1971;53B:54–62.

Rattey T, Piehl F, Wright JG. Acute slipped capital femoral epiphysis: review of outcomes and rates of avascular necrosis. J Bone Joint Surg 1996; 78A(3):398–402.

Sachs B, Bradford D, Winter RB, et al. Scheuermann kyphosis: follow-up of Milwaukee brace treatment. J Bone Joint Surg 1987;69A(1): 50–57.

Salter RB. The present status of surgical treatment for Legg-Perthes' disease. J Bone Joint Surg 1984;66A:961–966.

Salter RB, Bell M. The pathogenesis of deformity in Legg-Calvé-Perthes' disease: an experimental investigation. J Bone Joint Surg 1968;50B:436.

Salter RB, Thompson GH. Legg-Calvé-Perthes' disease: the prognostic significance of the subchondral fractures and a two-group classification of the femoral head involvement. J Bone Joint Surg 1984;66A:479–489.

Salter RB. Legg-Perthes' Disease. The scientific basis for the methods of treatment and their indications. Clin Orthop 1980;150:8–11.

Salter RB. Legg-Perthes' disease: relevant research and its application to treatment. In: Leach RE, Hoagland FT, Riseborough EJ, eds. Controversies in orthopaedic surgery. Philadelphia: WB Saunders, 1982:287–325.

Schenck RC Jr, Goodnight JN. Current concepts review. Osteochondritis dissecans. J Bone Joint Surg 1996;78A(3):439–456.

Schoenecker PW, Meade WC, Pierron RL, Sheridan JJ, Capelli RN. Blount's disease: a retrospective review and recommendations for treatment. J Paediatr Orthop 1985;5(2):181–186.

Schwend RM, Hennrikus W, Hall JE, et al. Childhood scoliosis: clinical indications for magnetic resonance imaging. J Bone Joint Surg 1995; 77A(1):46–53.

Sponseller PD, Desai SS, Millis MB. Comparison of femoral and innominate osteotomies for the treatment of Legg-Calvé-Perthes' disease. J Bone Joint Surg 1996;70A:1131–1139.

Stevens DB, Short BA, Burch JM. In situ fixation of the slipped capital femoral epiphysis with a single screw. J Pediatr Orthop 1996;(5):85–89.

Stulberg SD, Cooperman DR, Wallensten R. The natural history of Legg-Calvé-Perthes' disease. J Bone Joint Surg 1981;63A:1095–1100.

Stulberg SD, Salter RB. The natural course of Legg-Perthes' disease and its relationship to degenerative arthritis of the hip: a long-term follow-up study. Orthop Trans 1997;1:105.

Sugioka Y, Hotokebuchi T, Tsutsui H. Transtrochanteric anterior rotational osteotomy for idiopathic and steroid induced necrosis of the femoral head: indications and long-term results. Clin Orthop 1992;277:112–120.

Tachdjian MO. Clinical pediatric orthopedics: the art of diagnosis and principles of management. Stamford, CT: Appleton & Lange, 1997.

Thompson GH, Salter RB. Legg-Calvé-Perthes' disease: current concepts and controversies. Orthop Clin North Am 1987;18:617.

Twyman RS, Desai K, Aichroth PM. Osteochondritis dissecans of the knee. A long-term study. J Bone Joint Surg 1991;73B(3):461–464.

Urbaniak JR, Coogan PG, Gunneson EB, et al. Treatment of osteonecrosis of the femoral head with free vascularized fibular grafting: a long-term follow-up study of one hundred and three hips. J Bone Joint Surg 1995;77A(5):681–694.

Warner WC Jr, Beaty JH, Canale ST. Chondrolysis after slipped capital femoral epiphysis. J Pediatr Orthop 1996;(5):168–172.

Weiner D. Pathogenesis of slipped capital femoral epiphysis: current concepts. J Pediatr Orthop 1996;(5):67–73.

Weinstein SL, ed. The pediatric spine: principles and practice. New York: Raven Press, 1994.

Weinstein SL, Buckwalter JA. Turek's orthopaedics: principles and their application. Philadelphia: JB Lippincott, 1994.

Wenger DR, Rang M. The art and practice of paediatric orthopaedics. New York: Raven Press, 1993.

Wenger DR, Ward WT, Herring JA. Current concepts review: Legg-Calvé-Perthes' disease. J Bone Joint Surg 1991;73A:778.

Williams GA, Cowell HR. Köhler's disease of the tarsal navicular. Clin Orthop 1981;158:53–58.

Winter RB. The pendulum has swung too far: bracing for adolescent idiopathic scoliosis in the 1990s. Orthop Clin North Am 1994;25(2): 195–204.

14 Neoplasms of Musculoskeletal Tissues

As practitioners of the future, it is most important that you learn about the *general features* of this wide variety of lesions, the *incidence,* the *diagnosis,* the *prognosis* as well as the available *principles and methods of treatment* for patients so afflicted. Less important at this stage for you as students are the minute details of the microscopic characteristics of these lesions, let alone the interpretation of these changes. Even the most experienced bone pathologists may cavil about the interpretation of the microscopic minutiae of these perplexing lesions.

NEOPLASM-LIKE LESIONS AND TRUE NEOPLASMS OF BONE
Definition of Terms

The term *tumor* (often loosely used to describe any localized swelling or lump) seems less precise than the term *neoplasm,* or new growth, which refers to a new and abnormal formation of cells, a process that progresses throughout the life of the patient unless some type of therapy intervenes. The hereditary mechanism of the neoplastic cells has been irreversibly altered so that they and their "offspring cells" *do not reach maturity.* Thus, succeeding generations of neoplastic cells continue to divide by mitosis more rapidly than do normal cells of that particular tissue, consequently producing a *progressive* lesion. This explains the presence of excessive numbers of mitotic figures in rapidly growing neoplasms.

If, in addition, neoplastic cells demonstrate the ability to initiate independent growth in distant sites (*metastases*), the neoplasm is *malignant* and is referred to as *cancer.* Primary neoplasms of a given structure arise from cells that are normally "local inhabitants" of that structure, whereas metastatic, or *secondary* neoplasms arise from cells that are "outside invaders" from the primary neoplasm. Thus, one might speak of a primary neoplasm *of* bone and of a secondary neoplasm *in* bone, or in other tissues such as lung.

It is more difficult to define a *benign* neoplasm, one that remains localized in its primary site. Indeed, many so-called benign neoplasms may not be truly neoplastic. They may be more reasonably considered either as *reactive lesions* (constituting a self-limiting reaction to some other phenomenon) or as *hamartomas* (lesions in which cells normally present in a local area grow faster than others but do reach maturity, just as do normal cells. They exist as a useless but relatively harmless cell mass). On the basis of these definitions, neither reactive lesions nor hamartomas are progressive, as true neoplasms are progressive and thus have a much better prognosis. Still other lesions of bone, such as *fibrous dysplasia* and *simple bone cysts,* do not fit any of these categories, but in some ways simulate neoplasms. They are also considered in the present chapter. The various forms of *Langerhans' cell histiocytosis*—particularly *eosinophilic granuloma*—may also simulate neoplasms. They are discussed in Chapter 9.

CLASSIFICATIONS

Our limited understanding of neoplasms in general, and of neoplasms of bone in particular, makes it difficult to arrive at a universally acceptable classification.

The cells of the musculoskeletal tissues all share a common *mesodermal* origin but have differentiated along a variety of lines to become *osteoblasts, osteoclasts, chondroblasts, fibroblasts* (*collagenoblasts*), *pericytes,* and *myeloblasts* (of the bone marrow). It seems reasonable to use a classification based (insofar as is known at present) on the cell origin or *genesis* of the lesion. Thus, both the neoplasm-like lesions and the true neoplasms of bone can be subdivided into the following groups: osteogenic, chondrogenic, fibrogenic, angiogenic, and myelogenic. The neoplastic-like lesions and the true neoplasms are most appropriately classified separately.

Classification of Neoplasm-like Lesions of Bone

A. Osteogenic
  1. Osteoma (ivory exostosis)
  2. Single osteochondroma (osteocartilaginous exostosis)
  3. Multiple osteochondromata (multiple hereditary exostoses)
  4. Osteoid osteoma
  5. Benign osteoblastoma (giant osteoid osteoma)
B. Chondrogenic
  1. Enchondroma
  2. Multiple enchondromata (Ollier's dyschondroplasia)
C. Fibrogenic
  1. Subperiosteal cortical defect (metaphyseal fibrous defect)
  2. Nonosteogenic fibroma (nonossifying fibroma)
  3. Monostotic fibrous dysplasia
  4. Polyostotic fibrous dysplasia
  5. Osteofibrous dysplasia (Campanacci syndrome)
  6. "Brown tumor" (hyperparathyroidism; see Chapter 9)
D. Angiogenic
  1. Angioma of bone (hemangioma and lymphangioma)
  2. Aneurysmal bone cyst (ABC)
E. Uncertain origin
  1. Simple bone cyst (unicameral bone cyst) (UBC)

Classification of True Primary Neoplasms of Bone

A. Osteogenic
  1. Osteosarcoma (osteogenic sarcoma)
  2. Surface osteosarcoma (parosteal sarcoma; periosteal sarcoma)
B. Chondrogenic
  1. Benign chondroblastoma
  2. Chondromyxoid fibroma
  3. Chondrosarcoma
C. Fibrogenic
  1. Fibrosarcoma of bone

  2. Malignant fibrous histiocytoma of bone
D. Angiogenic
  1. Angiosarcoma of bone
E. Myelogenic
  1. Myeloma of bone (multiple myeloma)
  2. Ewing's sarcoma (Ewing's tumor)
  3. Hodgkin's lymphoma of bone
  4. Non-Hodgkin's lymphoma (reticulum cell sarcoma)
  5. Skeletal reticuloses (Langerhans' cell histiocytoses; see Chapter 9)
  6. Leukemia
F. Uncertain origin
  1. Giant cell tumor of bone (osteoclastoma)

GENERAL CONSIDERATIONS

Although much remains to be discovered about the nature and the etiology of neoplasms and neoplasm-like lesions of bone, much knowledge has been accumulated concerning their incidence, pathogenesis, clinical features, diagnosis, and the principles as well as the methods of their treatment. Some of this knowledge is best considered in a general way before discussing the various specific clinical entities.

Incidence

In the experience of a primary care physician in medical practice, malignant neoplasms, or new growths, that develop as primary lesions in the musculoskeletal tissues are relatively rare. They represent only 1% of malignant disease in all age groups and 5% in childhood. Less rare are benign neoplasms and neoplasm-like lesions that simulate neoplasms. Secondary neoplasms that develop in bone as metastases from a primary neoplasm (especially metastatic carcinoma) are common.

In the experience of certain types of specialists—orthopaedic surgeons, diagnostic imagers, pathologists, radiotherapists, and medical oncologists—musculoskeletal neoplasms and lesions that simulate them are less rare and constitute an extremely important, although incompletely understood, group of disorders.

The *age incidence* of some of these lesions is quite distinctive. For example, osteosarcoma occurs principally during childhood and adolescence. Ewing's sarcoma is seen mostly in adolescents and young adults, whereas osteoclastoma (giant cell tumor), chondrosarcoma, and fibrosarcoma occur almost exclusively during middle adult life. Multiple myeloma primarily afflicts older adults, whereas metastatic neoplasms are most common in the elderly. The differences in *sex incidence* of the various lesions are less striking. The *site incidence* is of particular value inasmuch as some of these lesions are common in certain bones but almost unknown in others. Even the *anatomical* site within a given bone is of significance. For example, many of the lesions that develop during childhood seem to be related to the rate of "bone turnover" or cellular activity. This is greatest in the flared-out metaphyseal regions of long bones at the most rapidly growing end (lower end of femur, upper end of tibia, upper end of humerus). The epiphyses, by contrast, are usually spared.

A knowledge of the incidence of the various lesions may be useful in the differential diagnosis of a lesion in a certain area of a certain bone in a patient of a certain age.

Diagnosis

Because primary true neoplasms of bone, especially those that are malignant, are rare, the primary care family physician should be constantly alert to the possibility of such a neoplasm in the differential diagnosis of unexplained pain, swelling, a lump, or decrease in function. Thus, the initial suspicion or even the provisional diagnosis of a true neoplasm is likely to be raised either by the primary care physician or the secondary care (community) orthopaedic surgeon. However, the evaluation and treatment of patients with malignant neoplasms of bone are highly specialized. Consequently, patients in whom such a diagnosis is suspected should be referred for further evaluation (including a biopsy) and definitive treatment to a tertiary care musculoskeletal oncology unit. This should be staffed by a multidisciplinary team of experts, including oncological orthopaedic surgeons, diagnostic imagers (radiologists), oncological pathologists, radiation oncologists, medical oncologists, and rehabilitation physicians (physiatrists). By far the most accurate evalua-

tion and best results of treatment are achieved in such tertiary care oncology units.

The diagnostic and evaluation methods for possible malignant neoplasms of bone include a complete history and physical examination, diagnostic imaging, laboratory investigation, staging of the neoplasm, and biopsy.

Clinical Features

A history of recent local trauma is often given by patients with a neoplasm of the musculoskeletal tissues; such trauma usually only brings the preexisting neoplasm to the attention of the patient.

Slowly growing neoplasms and neoplasm-like lesions of bone seldom cause symptoms unless, because of their location, their physical presence interferes with function in surrounding tissues, or they have been complicated by a pathological fracture, that is, a fracture through abnormal bone.

Pain is the most significant symptom of rapidly growing malignant neoplasms. Initially mild and intermittent, the pain becomes progressively more severe and constant, to the point of interfering with the patient's sleep. It is caused either by tension or pressure on the sensitive periosteum and endosteum. A history of sudden onset of severe pain usually indicates the complication of a pathological fracture, and this may be the first manifestation of a weakened area of bone from an underlying neoplasm-like lesion or true neoplasm.

Local swelling or a lump can be detected by inspection when the lesion protrudes beyond the normal confines of the bone (Fig. 14.1). Otherwise, it can be detected by palpation. The swelling of a benign lesion is usually firm and nontender. In the presence of a rapidly growing malignant neoplasm, however, the swelling is more diffuse and frequently is tender (Fig. 14.2). When the lesion is vascular, the overlying skin may be warm and the superficial veins dilated. The latter are best seen under infrared light (Fig. 14.3).

If the lesion is close to a joint, function in that joint may be disturbed and there may also be painful restriction of joint motion.

Diagnostic Imaging and Correlation with Pathology

For the diagnosis and evaluation of neoplasm-like lesions and true neoplasms of bone, the methods of diagnostic imaging include plain radiography (x-rays), plain (conventional) tomography, CT, MRI, and scintigraphy (bone scan).

Plain Radiography

High quality, well-centered plain radiographs in at least two planes continue to be the initial method of diagnostic imaging for suspected neoplasm-like lesions and true neoplasms of bone. Such radiographs reveal the location and size of the lesion, the resorption of bone, the margins of the lesion (either a clear or a fuzzy margin), the reaction of the bone to the

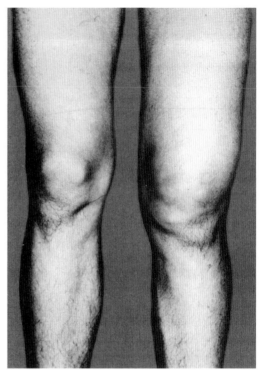

Figure 14.2. Diffuse swelling in the region of the left knee of a 16-year-old boy. This swelling, which was warm and tender, was due to an underlying osteosarcoma.

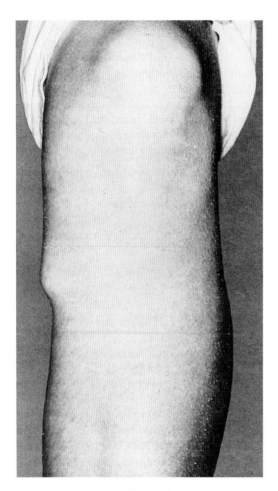

Figure 14.1. Local swelling, or lump, on the medial aspect of the left leg just below the knee in a 10-year-old boy. This local swelling, which was firm and nontender, was due to an underlying osteochondroma (osteocartilaginous exostosis) arising from the medial aspect of the metaphysis of the tibia.

lesion, and the effect of the lesion on the cortex (none, expansion, penetration). Occasionally an asymptomatic, unsuspected lesion, especially a neoplasm-like lesion or a benign neoplasm, is discovered by chance as an incidental finding in a radiograph taken for an entirely different purpose such as an injury.

Because the pathology of neoplasm-like lesions and true neoplasms of bone is well reflected by changes in density in the radiographic appearance of the bone and soft tissues, a correlation of the two will make the study of each aspect more interesting and more meaningful.

Neoplastic cells do not themselves destroy bone, but their presence incites local *osteoclastic resorption of bone*. The cells of certain neoplasms also incite local *osteoblastic* deposition of normal bone, referred to as *reactive bone*. The neoplastic cells of the osteogenic group of neoplasms are capable of producing osteoid

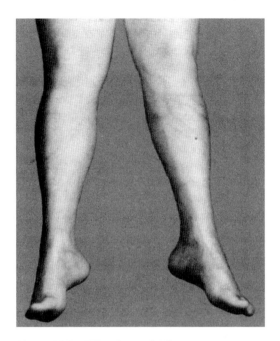

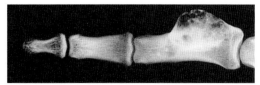

Figure 14.5.   Expansion of a bone by a slowly growing lesion. The enchondroma in this proximal phalanx is slowly eroding the cortex from the inside. Simultaneously, periosteal new bone is being deposited from the outside. When the rate of erosion exceeds that of periosteal bone formation, the bone expands.

Figure 14.3.   Dilated superficial veins in the left leg just below the knee in a 10-year-old boy. This photograph was taken under infrared light. The skin in the area of dilated veins was warm. The underlying lesion was a vascular, rapidly growing osteosarcoma.

teolysis) and bone deposition (osteosclerosis), some of the latter being reactive bone and some being neoplastic bone.

Some slowly growing lesions incite a marked reaction in the surrounding bone; indeed, the reactive bone may almost obscure the underlying neoplasm (Fig. 14.4).

In a slowly growing lesion within the bone,

and bone, which are then referred to as *tumor bone* or *neoplastic bone*. Thus, in a lesion affecting bone, the radiographic appearance reflects varying proportions of bone resorption (os-

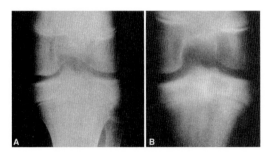

Figure 14.4.   Reactive bone surrounding a slowly growing benign neoplasm, in this case, a chondroblastoma of the upper tibial epiphysis in a 13-year-old boy. **A.** In the plain radiograph, the reactive bone almost obscures the neoplasm. **B.** In this tomogram, the radiolucent neoplasm is seen clearly in the center of the reactive bone. By means of this special technique (tomography, laminography), many films are taken, each of which shows a different layer, or slice, of the tissue in focus. Plain tomography has been replaced to a large extent by CT.

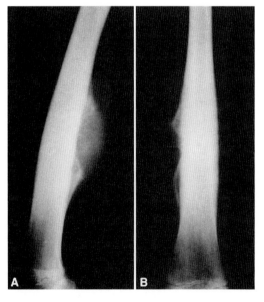

Figure 14.6.   Triangular-shaped areas of reactive bone (Codman's triangles) that have been deposited by the elevated periosteum. In these radiographs of the femur, a malignant neoplasm, an osteosarcoma, has eroded the cortex and elevated the periosteum. The reactive new bone is laid down around the periphery of the neoplasm in the angle between the elevated periosteum and the cortex. Codman's triangle is not always so apparent. It is not pathognomonic of any one bone lesion.

the deep surface of the cortex is gradually eroded from the inside; at the same time, the periosteum reacts by depositing bone on the outside. These combined phenomena explain expansion of a bone (Fig. 14.5).

When the periosteum is elevated by a neoplasm that has eroded the cortex, it produces reactive bone in the angle where it is still attached. This triangular-shaped area of reactive bone is often called *Codman's triangle* (Fig. 14.6).

Elevation of the periosteum in "stages" stimulates the formation of successive layers of periosteal reactive bone, and this phenomenon explains the radiographic "onion-skin" appearance (Fig. 14.7).

As a malignant neoplasm grows rapidly beyond the confines of the cortex, its blood vessels keep pace and grow in a radial fashion from the cortex. Both neoplastic bone and reactive bone form along these radiating vessels,

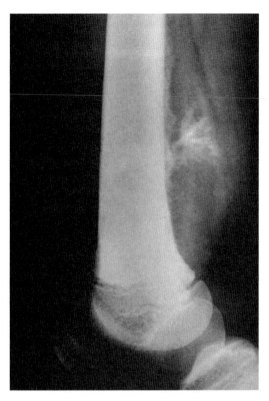

Figure 14.8. Neoplastic and reactive bone radiating out from the cortex into the radiolucent tumor mass. The bone is deposited along the course of blood vessels that radiate out from the cortex; this accounts for the radiographic "sunburst" appearance. In the lower end of this femur, the neoplasm is an osteosarcoma. The radiographic sunburst appearance may also be seen in other malignant neoplasms and is not invariably present in osteosarcoma.

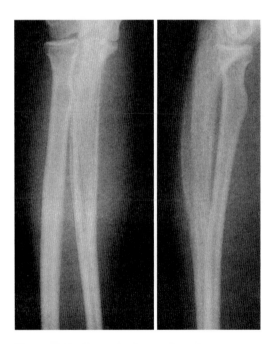

Figure 14.7. Successive layers of reactive bone that have been deposited by the periosteum as it has been elevated in "stages." In these radiographs of the radius and ulna, the underlying neoplasm is a Ewing's sarcoma of the ulna. This radiographic "onionskin" appearance is not pathognomonic of any one bone lesion.

which explains the radiographic "sunburst" appearance (Fig. 14.8).

Bone that has been weakened by local destruction (osteoclastic resorption) from any cause is more readily fractured than normal bone. This complication is referred to as a *pathological fracture* because it occurs through an area of abnormal or pathological bone (Fig. 14.9). If the regenerative process of fracture healing is more rapid than the destructive process of the neoplasm, the pathological fracture will eventually unite. If the reverse is true, however, the pathological fracture will never unite.

In the presence of rapidly growing malignant neoplasms, there may be little or no reac-

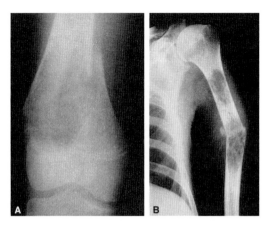

Figure 14.9. Pathological fractures through an abnormal area of bone that has been weakened by the local destruction (osteoclastic resorption) of a neoplasm. **A.** Pathological fracture through an osteosarcoma of the lower end of the femur in a 14-year-old girl. **B.** Pathological fracture through one of the two lesions of myeloma (multiple myeloma) in the humerus of a 43-year-old man.

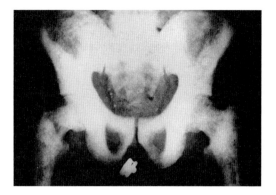

Figure 14.11. Osteosclerotic, or osteoblastic, type of secondary (metastatic) neoplasms in the pelvis and femora of a 75-year-old man. The primary neoplasm was carcinoma of the prostate. The metallic clamp is on an indwelling catheter.

tive bone, in which case the radiographic appearance is that of an osteolytic defect. This is particularly true of the osteolytic type of metastases in bone (Fig. 14.10). Certain primary neoplasms, particularly carcinoma of the prostate, incite a brisk osteoblastic reaction when

they metastasize to bone and produce the osteoblastic, or osteosclerotic type of metastases (Fig. 14.11).

The only true cyst (a cavity containing gas or fluid) in bone is the *simple bone cyst*, which is a neoplasm-like lesion (Fig. 14.12). Other osteolytic lesions may appear to be cystic radiographically, but because they contain tumor tissue, they are in fact solid lesions (Fig. 14.13).

Certain of these radiographic signs are sometimes considered by the inexperienced to be pathognomonic of a given type of neoplasm ("sunburst appearance indicates osteosarcoma," "onion-skin appearance indicates Ewing's tumor"). These signs, however, are by no means either specific or constant. Consequently, a "spot diagnosis" on the basis of a single radiograph is an example more of cleverness than of wisdom. Indeed, all available data from the various diagnostic methods must be correlated to reach a high standard of diagnostic accuracy.

Plain (Conventional) Tomography

This radiographic method provides images of a series of "sections" or "slices" of the tissues at varying depths from the skin surface. Such sections, each of which is focused at a specific level, are particularly helpful in evaluating abnormalities within high-contrast tissues such as bone (Fig. 14.4). Although plain tomogra-

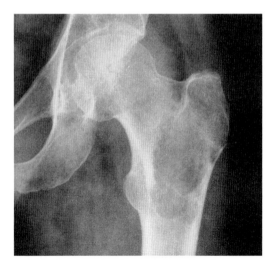

Figure 14.10. Osteolytic type of secondary (metastatic) neoplasm in the intertrochanteric region of the femur of a 62-year-old woman. The primary neoplasm was carcinoma of the breast.

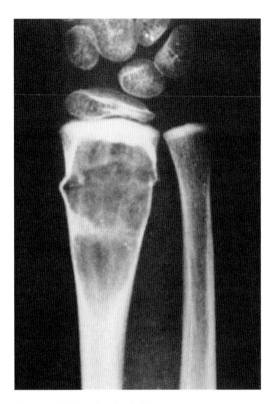

Figure 14.12. Simple (solitary) bone cyst of the lower end of the radius of a 10-year-old boy. This is a true cyst in that it is a lined cavity that contains fluid. Note also the transverse pathological fracture through the cyst.

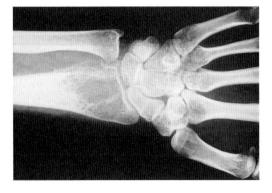

Figure 14.13. Osteolytic neoplasm that, radiographically, has a "cystic" appearance, but is a solid lesion filled with neoplastic tissue. Hence, it is not a true cyst. This neoplasm in the lower end of the radius in a 32-year-old man is a giant cell tumor (osteoclastoma).

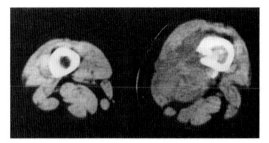

Figure 14.14. Computed tomogram of the cross-section of both thighs. Note the destructive lesion within femur on your right (the left femur viewed from below) and the large extension of the lesion into the soft tissues. The diagnosis is a far-advanced osteosarcoma.

phy has been replaced to a large extent by CT and MRI, it still has a place in centers where these much more expensive modalities are not available.

Computed Tomography (CT)

This sophisticated method of diagnostic imaging through which accurate images of "sections" or "slices" of the body are generated provides a degree of diagnostic imaging not previously possible. By means of CT scans, tissues of varying radiographic densities are more clearly differentiated with less radiation to the patient than with plain (conventional) tomograms.

In the musculoskeletal system, CT is preferred for accurately depicting the site and extent of a lesion, as well as "skip" lesions and soft tissue extension within bone (Fig. 14.14). Computed tomography also provides better bone detail in deep regions such as the pelvis and the spine (Fig. 14.15). It is more useful in detecting areas of ossification and calcification and subtle pathological fractures. In addition, CT scans of the chest reveal very small pulmonary metastases that would not be revealed by plain radiographs (Fig. 14.16).

Magnetic Resonance Imaging

The development of the highly complex diagnostic modality of MRI in the 1980s has been another major breakthrough in the rapidly changing field of diagnostic imaging. The most significant advantages of MRI over CT

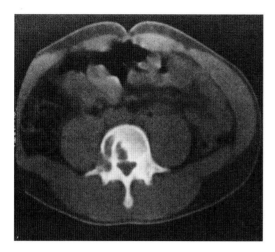

Figure 14.15. Computed tomogram of the cross-section of the trunk at the level of the fourth lumbar vertebra (viewed from below). Note the extensive osteolytic lesions of the vertebral body and pedicle. The diagnosis is an aneurysmal bone cyst.

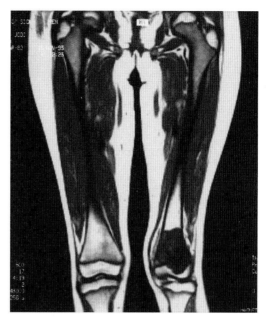

Figure 14.17. Magnetic resonance imaging of both femora of a 13-year-old boy. In this T1-weighted image, there is a large, low-density (dark) lesion in the distal end of the left femur. The diagnosis is an osteosarcoma that has extended from the metaphysis into the epiphysis.

are that it uses non-ionizing radiofrequency radiation rather than ionizing radiation. It provides better images of soft tissues, including bone marrow, as well as of major nerves and blood vessels and the relationship of neoplasms to those structures. It can also provide physiological as well as anatomical data (especially when combined with contrast agents and spectroscopy).

Bone marrow lesions have low signal-intensity in T1-weighted images (appear dark), whereas soft tissue extensions and soft tissue

neoplasms have high signal intensity (appear bright) in T2-weighted images (Figs. 14.17 and 14.18). As exceptions to this generalization, fat (as in a lipoma) has a high signal intensity in both T1- and T2-weighted images, and predominantly fibrous lesions have a low signal intensity in both T1- and T2-weighted images.

Magnetic resonance imaging is especially useful in the staging of malignant neoplasms (as described below).

Scintigraphy (Bone Scan)
Since the 1970s, the specialty of nuclear medicine has made great strides in the detection of a variety of lesions of bone through the use of bone-seeking radionuclides such as technetium-99-labeled polyphosphate. The resultant "bone scans" reflect changes in the local blood flow in bone, as well as the degree of local metabolic activity, especially increased bone formation. Areas of increased radionuclide uptake are referred to as "hot spots."

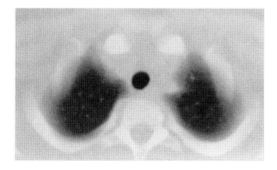

Figure 14.16. Computed tomogram of the cross-section of the chest. Note the multiple tiny radiographic densities throughout both lungs. These are metastases that were not detectable in plain radiographs of the chest.

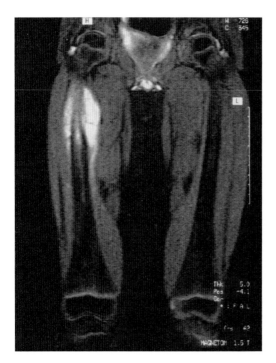

Figure 14.18. Magnetic resonance imaging of both femora of a 7-year-old boy. In this T2-weighted image, note the extensive high density (bright) lesion both inside and outside the proximal area of the diaphysis (shaft) of the right femur. The diagnosis is a Ewing's sarcoma of the femur with soft tissue extension.

Thus, scintigraphy is very helpful in revealing lesions, either benign or malignant, that are highly vascular (Fig. 14.19). The total body bone scan has largely replaced radiographic "skeletal surveys" in the detection of multiple lesions in other bones, as with polystotic fibrous dysplasia and skeletal metastases.

Laboratory Investigations
The following laboratory investigations, most of which are relevant in a given patient, can be helpful in distinguishing between various differential diagnoses.

Complete blood count (CBC), including a white blood cell differential.
Erythrocyte sedimentation rate (ESR)—often elevated in Ewing's sarcoma.
Serum calcium—elevated in multiple myeloma and metastatic bone disease.
Serum phosphorus—lowered in hyperparathyroidism (with "brown tumors").

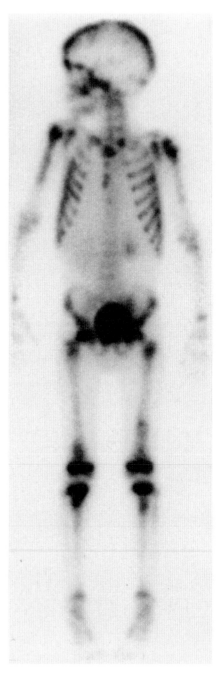

Figure 14.19. Scintigraphy. In this technetium-99-labeled polyphosphate total body bone scan of a 5-year-old girl, there are multiple dark ("hot") spots—both proximal tibiae, both distal femora, both proximal humeri, and the thoracic spine. The diagnosis is metastatic neuroblastoma.

Serum alkaline phosphatase—elevated in osteosarcoma and Paget's disease.

Serum acid phosphatase—elevated in carcinoma of the prostate (spread beyond the capsule).

Prostatic specific antigen (PSA)—elevated in carcinoma of the prostate.

Serum protein electrophoresis—abnormal pattern in multiple myeloma and metastatic bone disease.

Urinary Bence-Jones protein—elevated in multiple myeloma.

Staging of Benign, Potentially Malignant, and Malignant Neoplasms of Bone

Enneking in 1980, and subsequently in 1983 and 1986, reported his widely accepted system of "staging" benign, potentially malignant, and malignant neoplasms of bone. The required methods of assessment for the staging of a suspected malignant neoplasm include plain radiography, CT scan (local and chest) MRI, and scintigraphy (bone scan). The factors involved in assessing the staging of a given lesion include:

1. The histological grade of the lesion: benign (such as a nonosteogenic fibroma), potentially malignant (as a giant cell tumor of bone), low-grade malignancy (locally aggressive but metastasizes late, as a parosteal sarcoma, or a chondrosarcoma), high grade malignancy (locally very aggressive and metastasizes early, as an osteosarcoma and fibrosarcoma).
2. The size of the lesion and whether it is limited to one compartment, such as bone (intracompartmental), or has extended into one or more soft tissue compartments (extracompartmental).
3. Whether the lesion has already metastasized.

Thus, for a malignant neoplasm, the staging can be determined as follows:
  I. Low grade malignancy
    A. Intracompartmental
    B. Extracompartmental
  II. High grade malignancy
    A. Intracompartmental
    B. Extracompartmental
  III. Metastases

The staging of suspected neoplasms of bone is an essential part of the evaluation of the lesion, especially when the lesion is suspected of being malignant. The purpose of the staging system is to determine the prognosis of the lesion, both without and with treatment, and to plan the ideal method of treatment (chemotherapy, radiation therapy, surgical resection). Furthermore, the staging system is helpful in standardizing nationwide and international clinical outcomes of various forms of treatment.

The staging of a given lesion should be carried out *before* a biopsy is performed because the biopsy will alter the diagnostic images that are essential to the staging evaluation.

Biopsy

In the diagnosis of neoplasms and neoplasm-like lesions of the musculoskeletal tissues, a biopsy is essential to avoid two serious errors in relation to treatment: 1) failure to recognize a malignant neoplasm (*underdiagnosis*), which results in inadequate treatment; 2) diagnosis of a nonmalignant lesion as a malignant neoplasm (*overdiagnosis*), which results in excessive treatment.

Multicenter investigations by Mankin (1982, 1985, 1987, 1996) have revealed that one quarter of the surgical biopsies of musculoskeletal neoplasms are either improperly performed or misinterpreted (or both). In addition, they are associated with preventable complications two to twelve times more often when the biopsy is performed in a secondary referring hospital rather than a tertiary referral center. Indeed, the biopsy should be performed by the oncological orthopaedic surgeon who is going to carry out the patient's definitive treatment. Frozen sections ("quick sections") are helpful in determining that the biopsy specimen is representative, but definitive radical treatment should await the interpretation of paraffin sections. The surgical incision for biopsy in an extremity should be longitudinal rather than transverse and should transgress the minimum number of compartments to avoid contamination of uninvolved tissues with malignant cells.

The biopsy samples must be adequate in size and must also be representative of the lesion. In general, open surgical biopsy is more accurate than aspiration biopsy (needle or punch biopsy), although in relatively inaccessible sites, such as vertebral bodies for which open biopsy would require an extensive operation, punch biopsy with radiographic control is often of value. In patients suspected of having a widespread neoplasm of the bone marrow, such as myeloma (multiple myeloma), aspiration biopsy of the marrow in the sternum or the iliac crest is usually adequate.

Transmission electron microscopy has supplemented routine histology and histochemistry in the differentiation of neoplasms containing small round cells, for example, Ewing's sarcoma and metastatic neuroblastoma. By using surface-marker antigens, it is now possible to differentiate Hodgkin's lymphoma from other lymphomas.

The percentage of the resected neoplasm that is necrotic as the result of neoadjuvant (preoperative) chemotherapy is an indication of the appropriateness of the chosen chemotherapeutic agents and hence, of the patient's prognosis.

All the available data are required to make an accurate diagnosis of a given lesion before definitive treatment is instituted. The final decision concerning both diagnosis and the optimal method of treatment is reached ideally from the combined opinions of the oncological orthopaedic surgeon, diagnostic imager, radiation oncologist, medical oncologist, and pathologist.

Principles and Methods of Treatment

Principles

The following well-established principles of treatment are relevant to all patients with neoplasm-like and true neoplasms of bone:

1. The final evaluation of the patient, including the aforementioned staging and biopsy (especially when a malignant neoplasm is suspected) should be carried out by the oncological orthopaedic surgeon who ac-

cepts the responsibility for that patient's definitive treatment in a tertiary care orthopaedic oncological unit.

2. Compassionate communication with the patient and the appropriate relatives (or the parents or guardians if the patient is a child) by the responsible oncological orthopaedic surgeon is a pivotal part of the patient's total care during evaluation, treatment, and follow-up assessments. Unpleasant though it is to be the messenger of bad news, realize that the adult patient and relatives (and the parents or guardians if the patient is a child) want, need, and deserve the truth. The attitude must always be one of *kindly realism* and both patient and relatives deserve the assurance that everything possible will be done to help. Even when, from a scientific point of view, the situation is deemed hopeless, the patient must never be left to feel bereft of compassionate care.

3. A most important principle in the treatment of patients with neoplasms and neoplasm-like lesions of the musculoskeletal tissues is that the treatment must be based on an accurate diagnosis. This is of particular importance when the contemplated treatment involves such major and irreversible operations as limb-sparing surgery or amputation. The prognosis of malignant musculoskeletal neoplasms, although improving, is still relatively poor with currently available methods of treatment. Therefore, failure to treat a patient early for a malignant lesion is serious—yet needless radical surgery of a limb on the basis of a mistaken diagnosis is also serious.

4. The prognosis for each patient, with and without treatment, and the choice of treatment method, should include consideration of both the anticipated duration, or *quantity* of the patient's remaining life and, as important, the *quality* of that life. The prognosis is most accurately assessed by data obtained from the staging of the lesion.

5. The advantages and disadvantages of the various treatment options should be presented to the patient, relatives, or both in a comprehensible manner that will allow

them to become involved in the decision-making process.

6. Ideally, the diagnosis and the proposed treatment plan should be discussed in a conference with all members of the interdisciplinary oncological unit.

7. Surgical methods of treatment must be planned meticulously based on all the available data, especially the staging.

Methods of Treatment
Surgical Procedures

The most effective treatment for most musculoskeletal neoplasms is surgical resection (excision, ablation) either alone or, in the case of malignant neoplasms, combined with adjuvant chemotherapy or radiation therapy (radiotherapy). The types of surgical procedures include the following degrees of resection: intracapsular (intralesional) resection, such as curettage; marginal resection (narrow margins beyond the capsule); wide local resection (wide margins); and radical resection (all, or a large part of the involved bone plus all involved soft tissue compartment[s]). The residual defect after intracapsular resection or marginal resection may require bone grafts (Fig.14.20), whereas the defect after wide local resection always requires such grafts.

The two main types of radical resection are limb-sparing (limb-salvage) procedures and

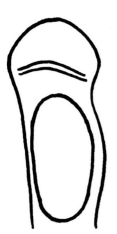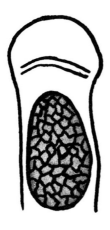

Figure 14.20.   Bone grafting with fragments of cancellous bone to fill a defect after curettage (curettement) of a nonmalignant lesion of bone.

amputation (or disarticulation). In recent decades, limb-sparing procedures have become more widely performed than either amputation or disarticulation. The long-term survival rates are much the same for these two types of radical resection, but the criteria required and the number of complications differ. For a limb-sparing procedure to be indicated, the criteria are: that there are no "skip" lesions (that is, additional lesions in the proximal part of the involved bone); the lesions in the bone and the involved soft tissue compartments are resectable without jeopardizing the subsequent function of the limb; and reconstruction of the residual defect is feasible. When these criteria cannot be met, the only recourse is amputation (or disarticulation). Reconstruction of the major residual defect created by limb-sparing procedures may be accomplished by large bone allografts (with or without supplemental vascularized autogenous bone grafts), arthrodesis (fusion of the bones across the site of the previous joint) or a custom-made endoprosthesis (artificial metallic device). The complications of massive allografts include a significant infection rate, delayed union (or even nonunion) of the graft bone to the host bone, and late pathological fracture of the incompletely revascularized allograft. For the custom-made endoprosthesis, the complications include late loosening and mechanical failure. An alternative method of reconstruction of the defect created by limb-sparing procedures, and one that is appropriate for the lower limb in children—especially boys—is the "rotationplasty" Van Nes procedure. This involves major shortening of the lower limb through the defect, so that the foot is then at the level of the opposite knee joint and rotating the tibia and foot through 180° so that it faces backward. The new position of the proximal femur and the distal femur is maintained by internal skeletal fixation. The child can then use the ankle joint as a knee joint, which provides much better function in a specially designed prosthesis (artifical limb) than an above-knee amputation or a knee disarticulation.

Pathological fractures that occur through a nonmalignant lesion of bone will usually heal, but the risk of repeated pathological fractures may necessitate bone grafting to reinforce the weakened area of bone. Pathological fractures that occur through a malignant neoplasm, however, will not heal spontaneously if the destructive process of the neoplasm exceeds the reparative process of fracture healing. Under these circumstances, *rigid intramedullary metallic fixation* of a fractured long bone may be required as palliative treatment to relieve persistent pain.

When the destruction of bone is extensive, it may be necessary to use bone cement (methylmethacrylate) as an adjunct to the internal fixation so that the patient may regain some effective use of the involved limb during the remaining months of life.

Chemotherapy

The dramatic improvement in the percentages of long-term survival of children and adults with malignant neoplasms of bone is due to the introduction of effective chemotherapeutic agents targeted at the rapidly dividing malignant cells in the primary neoplasm and in any subclinical micrometastases. The success of these chemotherapeutic agents depends on several factors, including the antineoplasm activity of the agent, its mechanism of action, and the biology of the neoplasm. Regimens of chemotherapy that combine agents with differing mechanisms of action are often more effective in maximizing the numbers of susceptible neoplastic cells killed.

Neoadjuvant chemotherapy is given preoperatively, whereas adjuvant chemotherapy is administered postoperatively. The percentage of necrotic cells in a resected neoplasm after a course of neoadjuvant therapy provides useful data concerning both the effectiveness of the chemotherapeutic agent(s) and the prognosis for that particular patient.

The toxic effects of both neoadjuvant and adjuvant chemotherapy include neutropenia, thrombocytopenia, wound complications, infection, nausea, alopecia, and delayed healing (of bone allografts). These effects are reversible after the chemotherapy has been discontinued.

Malignant neoplasms vary in their sensitivity, or response, to chemotherapy. The most sensitive are osteosarcoma, Ewing's sarcoma, malignant fibrous histiocytoma of bone, and childhood rhabdomyosarcoma. Chondrosarcoma, fibrosarcoma of bone, and soft tissue sarcomas are relatively resistant, or unresponsive, to chemotherapy.

The wide variety of currently prescribed chemotherapeutic agents can be categorized into four groups according to their mode of action:

Alkylating agents (cyclophosphamide, cisplatin)
Antineoplasm antibodies (doxorubicin, actinomycin D)
Folate antagonists (methotrexate with citrovorum "rescue")
Antimetabolites (mercaptopurine, 5-flurouracil, i.e. 5-FU)

Much basic research is being conducted to find the ideal chemotherapeutic agents, the effectiveness of which must be assessed by meticulous double-blind, randomized clinical outcome investigations.

Radiation Therapy (Radiotherapy)

This method of treatment, which is often combined with a surgical procedure, adjuvant chemotherapy, or both is described as the ninth General Form of Treatment in Chapter 6, which may be useful for you to review in the context of the present chapter.

SPECIFIC NEOPLASM-LIKE LESIONS OF BONE
Osteoma (Ivory Exostosis)

This relatively rare lesion may develop on the surface of cortical bone of the skull or the tibia. It can be seen on a plain radiograph as a well-demarcated area of increased density. No treatment is required unless the lesion presses on significant soft tissues.

Single Osteochondroma (Osteocartilaginous Exostosis)

Although often considered to be a benign neoplasm, an osteochondroma is probably an abnormality of growth direction and remodeling in the metaphyseal region of long bones in growing children. As indicated by the synonym (osteocartilaginous exostosis), this lesion consists of an outgrowth of both bone and cartilage that forms a prominent "tumor," in the sense of a local swelling, or lump.

A single osteochondroma usually is seen in young persons, although if untreated, it persists into adult life. The lesion always arises from the metaphyseal region; the most common sites are the lower end of femur, upper end of tibia, and upper end of humerus, that is, the most actively growing ends of long bones.

An osteochondroma is comparable pathologically to each of the osteochondromata seen in the congenital condition of *diaphyseal aclasis* (multiple osteocartilaginous exostoses, Chapter 8). The protruding lesion, which always points away from the nearest epiphyseal plate, consists of normal bone and is capped by normal cartilage. Indeed, during the growing years, an osteochondroma has its own epiphyseal plate from which it grows, but growth ceases about the same time as in the neighboring epiphyseal plates (physes). A synovial bursa of the friction type develops between the protruding part of the osteochondroma and the surrounding soft tissues. Osteochondromata may be long with a narrow base (pedunculated or stalked type), or they may be short with a broad base (sessile type) (Fig. 14.21). Malignant change (usually chondrosarcomatous) occurs in approximately 1% of a single osteochondroma in adult life, although the incidence is higher in the multiple form. Such transformation should be suspected if an osteochondroma becomes symptomatic or if it begins to enlarge in adult life.

Osteochondromata are not painful lesions in themselves, but they may interfere with the function of surrounding soft tissues such as tendons and nerves. If sufficiently large, they may even limit joint motion.

Usually the patient happens to become aware of the firm, localized swelling incidentally; understandably, the parents are often concerned about the possibility of "bone cancer" (Fig.14.1). Radiographic examination reveals only the bony part of the osteochondroma, which explains why the lesion is always

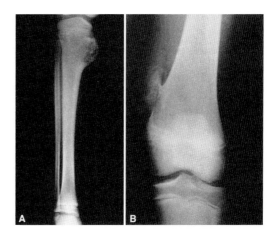

Figure 14.21. Osteochondroma (osteocartilaginous exostosis). **A.** Sessile type of osteochondroma arising from the metaphyseal region of the tibia in a 7-year-old boy. The radiolucent cartilage cap accounts for the lesion being larger clinically than is apparent radiographically. **B.** Pedunculated, or stalked, type of osteochondroma arising from the metaphyseal region of the femur in a 13-year-old girl. Note that the osteochondroma points away from the epiphyseal plate. It will continue to grow slowly from its cartilage cap until the distal femoral epiphyseal plate (physis) stops growing.

larger clinically than it appears radiographically.

Not all osteochondromata require treatment. If the osteochondroma is producing an ugly lump, or if it is interfering with normal function of the limb in any way, it should be surgically excised.

Multiple Osteochondromata (Multiple Hereditary Exostoses) (Diaphyseal Aclasis)

Please see Chapter 8.

Osteoid Osteoma

Osteoid osteoma, which is probably a "reactive" bone lesion rather than a true neoplasm, is a relatively uncommon but distinctive clinical entity characterized by persistent pain. It usually develops in children and adolescents, particularly boys, but occasionally in young adults. Although an osteoid osteoma may occur in almost any bone except the skull, it has a predilection for bones of the lower limb, especially the femur and tibia. Its etiology remains a puzzle.

This curious lesion, which consists of a small, round nidus (a nest) of osteoid tissue surrounded by reactive bone, does not continue to grow and is seldom larger than 1 cm in diameter. When the nidus of osteoid (which is uncalcified and therefore radiolucent) develops in cancellous bone, it incites very little reactive bone (Fig. 14.22). When it develops in cortical bone, the amount of reactive bone is strikingly out of proportion to the size of the central lesion (Fig. 14.23).

The predominant symptom of an osteoid osteoma is mild and nagging pain, more noticeable at night and characteristically relieved by mild analgesics such as aspirin or nonsteroidal anti-inflammatory drugs (NSAIDS). When the lesion is located near a joint, a synovial effusion develops and interferes slightly with joint function. Local muscle atrophy may ensue. An osteoid osteoma in the spine may produce a painful type of scoliosis. The radiographic features, which are well correlated with the pathology of the lesion, are almost pathognomonic (Figs. 14.22 and 14.23). The

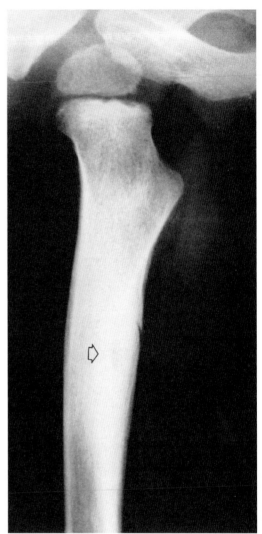

Figure 14.23. Osteoid osteoma in the cortical bone of the femoral shaft in a 5-year-old boy. The radiolucent lesion, which is less than 1 cm in diameter, is almost obscured by remarkably extensive reactive bone that is out of proportion to the size of the lesion (*arrow*).

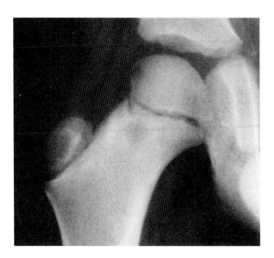

Figure 14.22. Osteoid osteoma in the cancellous bone of the right femoral neck in a 7-year-old boy. The round, radiolucent lesion, which is approximately 1 cm in diameter, has incited relatively little reactive bone formation. This boy complained of pain in the right knee (referred pain), but examination revealed painful limitation of motion in the right hip and atrophy of the muscles in the upper part of the right thigh.

lesion must be differentiated from a local area of chronic osteomyelitis. Scintigraphy (bone scan) is of special value in the diagnosis of an osteoid osteoma as discussed in Chapter 5.

Although osteoid osteomas are not progressive and may even be self-limiting over many years, the persistent pain usually necessitates their surgical excision. The central nidus of osteoid and a narrow margin of surrounding bone should be completely removed to prevent a recurrence. To avoid a large incision and excision of a block of bone including the osteoid osteoma, various less invasive techniques have been developed. These involve percutaneous CT-guided insertion of a guide wire directly into the nidus and ablating it by overdrilling, cauterization, laser coagulation, or cryotherapy.

After complete excision or ablation of an osteoid osteoma in cortical bone, the residual reactive bone gradually disappears. The instant relief of pain and the rapid return of normal function after adequate excision or ablation of an osteoid osteoma are gratifying to both the patient and the orthopaedic surgeon.

Osteoblastoma (Giant Osteoid Osteoma)

Another reactive bone lesion, which is similar in some ways to an osteoid osteoma, but much larger, is benign osteoblastoma (giant osteoid osteoma). This rare lesion, which tends to develop in vertebrae and flat bones with relatively little sclerosis, consists of osteoid. It is usually painful and is best treated by surgical excision followed by bone grafting of the resultant surgical defect.

Single Enchondroma

Enchondroma is a lesion comprising a mass of relatively normal cartilage cells within the interior of a single bone. Although sometimes considered to be a benign neoplasm, it probably develops as a local abnormality of growth from cartilage cells of the epiphyseal plate during childhood. The patient may not become aware of the lesion until adolescence or early adult life. The most frequent sites are the tubular bones of the hands and feet (phalanges, metacarpals, metatarsals), usually near one end; a less common site is one of the larger long bones.

The cartilage cells of an enchondroma divide only slowly. As the lesion grows, bone is slowly absorbed from the inner cortex; at the same time, periosteal reactive bone is deposited on the outer surface. Because resorption exceeds deposition, the involved bone slowly becomes expanded with a thinned-out overlying cortex. Histologically, an enchondroma may be difficult to differentiate from a slowly

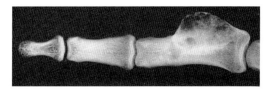

Figure 14.24. Single enchondroma in the proximal phalanx of the finger of a 25-year-old man. Note the expanded cortex.

growing chondrosarcoma. In 2% of patients, a single enchondroma in a large, long bone does undergo malignant change to become a chondrosarcoma.

Because enchondromata are not painful lesions in themselves, the patient is usually unaware of the lesion until a firm swelling is noticed or a local injury causes a pathological fracture in the thin cortex. The radiographic features are quite characteristic (Figs. 14.24 and 14.25). In long-standing enchondromata, particularly in large bones, irregular calcification may appear within the radiolucent cartilage.

Enchondromata are best treated by thorough curettage and packing of the residual cavity with cancellous bone grafts (Fig. 14.20).

Multiple Enchondromata (Ollier's Dyschondroplasia)

The multiple or disseminated form of enchondroma, namely multiple enchondromata, is

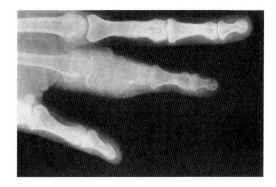

Figure 14.25. Enchondroma in the proximal phalanx of the index finger of a 21-year-old man. Note the central radiolucent lesion that has expanded the phalanx. There is a small pathological fracture through the thinned-out cortex on both sides of the lesion.

also known as Ollier's dyschondroplasia. The lesions in this condition tend to be predominantly in the extremities of one side of the body. The pathology of each individual enchondroma is similar to a single enchondra as is the treatment.

Subperiosteal Cortical Defect (Metaphyseal Fibrous Defect)

By far the most common radiographic lesion in bone is the *subperiosteal cortical defect,* a small, eccentrically placed, superficial crater filled with fibrous tissue that seems to arise from the periosteum. It is estimated that these lesions can be detected in 10% to 20% of all children at some stage of skeletal growth. They are usually seen in the metaphyseal region of the lower end of the femur and often represent an incidental finding (Fig. 14.26).

Subperiosteal cortical defects, which probably constitute a local area of defective endochondral ossification, tend to fill in with bone spontaneously after a number of years, having caused neither symptoms nor clinical signs.

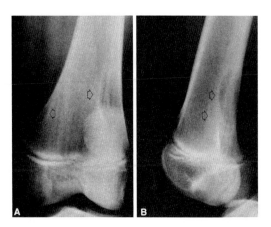

Figure 14.26. Subperiosteal cortical defects (metaphyseal fibrous defects) in the metaphysis of the lower end of the left femur in a 13-year-old boy. Both of these two small defects are just under the periosteum when viewed tangentially (*arrows*). This boy complained of pain in the left knee, which prompted his physician to obtain these radiographs. These lesions, however, could not account for the boy's pain. Examination revealed limitation of internal rotation and abduction of the left hip. Radiographs of the hips revealed a minimal slip of the left upper femoral epiphysis, which was the cause of the referred pain in the knee.

The clinical significance of these lesions lies in the fact that they may be overdiagnosed as a more serious lesion that requires treatment. Furthermore, their presence in a child who is complaining of local pain cannot explain such pain, the cause of which must be sought elsewhere. No treatment is required for subperiosteal cortical defects.

Nonosteogenic Fibroma (Nonossifying Fibroma)

Nonosteogenic fibroma is a relatively common fibrous lesion that is somewhat similar to the aforementioned subperiosteal cortical defect. Whether it is a reactive bone lesion or simply a local developmental disorder is not clear but being self-limiting, it is not a true neoplasm. Although it may persist into early adult life, nonosteogenic fibroma is seen primarily in children and adolescents. The most common sites are the long bones of the lower limbs.

Nonosteogenic fibromata do not cause symptoms and are therefore usually incidental findings. The fibrous lesion arises in the cortex and gradually replaces it from within. It grows slowly to about 4 cm and incites a thin zone of reactive bone around it, thereby producing a characteristic radiographic appearance (Fig. 14.27). Pathological fractures may occur, but only after a fairly severe injury. Furthermore, in this condition, such fractures heal well.

The clinical significance of nonosteogenic fibroma, like that of a subperiosteal defect, is that it may be overdiagnosed as a more serious lesion and overtreated, or it may be considered the explanation for local pain. Because most nonosteogenic fibromata fill in with bone spontaneously over a few years, no treatment is required.

Monostotic Fibrous Dysplasia

Although fibrous dysplasia of bone is not a neoplasm, it is included in this chapter because it simulates a neoplasm radiographically (Fig. 14.28). *Monostotic fibrous dysplasia* consists of a local lesion of fibrous tissue proliferation in the cancellous area of a single bone. It occurs in children, adolescents, and young adults. Radiographically, the osteolytic lesion has a "ground glass" appearance. As a progressively

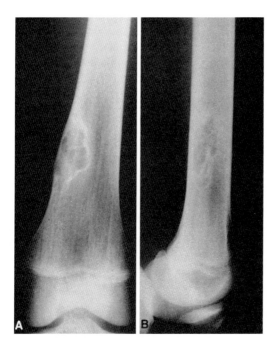

Figure 14.27. Nonosteogenic fibroma in the metaphyseal region of the femur in a 16-year-old boy. **A.** In the anteroposterior projection, which is tangential to the lesion, it can be seen to be eccentrically placed just under the periosteum. **B.** The lateral projection gives the impression that the lesion is centrally placed. Note the clearly defined edges and the zone of reactive bone around this slowly growing lesion. The nonosteogenic fibroma was an incidental finding in these radiographs, which were taken because of a recent mild injury.

larger area of bone is replaced by fibrous tissue, a pathological fracture may ensue.

The prognosis of monostotic fibrous dysplasia is excellent and malignant transformation is rare. Treatment consists of curettage of the lesion and reinforcement of the weakened area by bone grafts to prevent repeated pathological fractures.

Polyostotic Fibrous Dysplasia

This is a widely disseminated polyostotic form of fibrous dysplasia. The pathology of each of the individual lesions is the same as noted above for the monostotic form and is described in Chapter 9.

Osteofibrous Dysplasia (Campanacci Syndrome)

The tibia is the characteristic site of this rare and unusual lesion that in some ways resem-

bles fibrous dysplasia. Usually, there is a bony, hard swelling on the anterior surface of the tibia, which is already bowed anteriorly. Radiographically, the lesions have a bubble-like appearance. If the area of involvement is large, it may have to be resected, after which the residual defect requires bone grafting.

"Brown Tumor" (Hyperparathyroidism)

The disseminated osteolytic lesions of bone known as "brown tumors" are associated with hyperparathyroidism and are described in Chapter 9.

Angioma of Bone

Hemangioma, a vascular type of hamartoma, is relatively common in many tissues. Occasionally, in adults, a hemangioma develops in

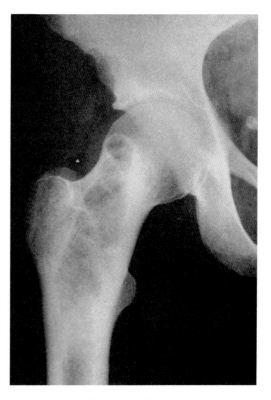

Figure 14.28. Monostotic fibrous dysplasia in the upper end of the femur of a 25-year-old woman. This lesion, which is not a neoplasm but merely fibrous tissue proliferation in cancellous bone, simulates a neoplasm radiographically. Note the clearly defined margins and the surrounding zone of reactive bone.

bone, usually the vertebral bodies or the skull, but these lesions seldom cause symptoms and consequently may remain undiagnosed. In the vertebral body, a hemangioma causes a radiographic appearance of coarse vertical trabeculation. If the lesion does become painful and surgical resection is contemplated, preoperative radiographically controlled embolization may be required to minimize bleeding at operation.

Rarely, a rapidly growing *lymphangioma* in bone causes alarming destruction ("massive osteolysis") in one or more bones and leads to the bizarre condition of "disappearing bone" or "phantom bone."

Aneurysmal Bone Cyst

The curious lesion called *aneurysmal bone cyst (ABC)* is not a true neoplasm, but its pathogenesis is not understood. It is a solitary vascular abnormality that begins within the marrow tissue of cancellous bone.

Aneurysmal bone cysts develop most frequently in adolescents and young adults, usually in the spine, less often in the metaphyseal region of a long bone such as the humerus. Locally destructive, it rapidly erodes cortical bone from the inner surface. At the same time, periosteal reactive bone deposition on the outer surface contains the lesion but allows it to expand to such a degree that it resembles an aneurysmal dilatation—hence the term, *aneurysmal* bone cyst. Because the lesion contains vascular tissue rather than mere fluid, it is not a true cyst. If left untreated, an aneurysmal bone cyst may reach an alarming size and may even rupture into the surrounding tissue, producing a hematoma. Histologically, aneurysmal bone cysts contain a spongelike network of large vascular channels that carry circulating blood and may represent some type of arteriovenous malformation.

Because aneurysmal bone cysts expand rapidly, they are usually painful and tender; pathological fracture of the thinned-out cortex is not uncommon. Radiographic examination reveals a large, expanded osteolytic lesion that looks like an aneurysm (Fig. 14.29).

With the help of arteriography, the main "feeder" vessels can be identified and embolized, after which curettage and bone grafting

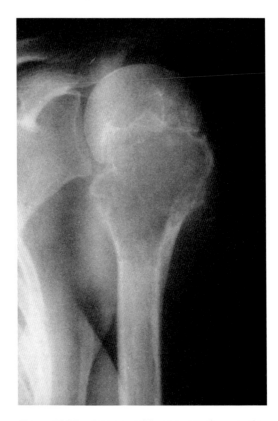

Figure 14.29.   Aneurysmal bone cyst in the metaphyseal region of the upper end of the humerus in a 15-year-old girl. Note the large osteolytic lesion and the thin cortex that has been expanded from within, thereby resembling an aneurysmal dilatation. There is a healed pathological fracture on the lateral aspect of the lesion. At operation, this lesion was found to be exceedingly vascular, and hemorrhage was difficult to control.

may be required. In the past, radiation treatment (radiotherapy) had been recommended but is no longer preferred because of the inherent risk of late radiation-induced sarcoma.

Simple Bone Cyst (Solitary Bone Cyst; Unicameral Bone Cyst)

Simple, solitary bone cyst, or *unicameral bone cyst (UBC),* is not a neoplasm but it can simulate a neoplasm. The only true cyst of bone, it develops most commonly in children and adolescents. The most frequent sites are the upper end of humerus, upper end of femur, upper end of tibia and lower end of radius, in that order.

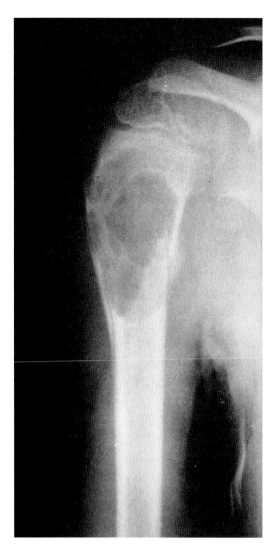

Figure 14.30.   Simple (solitary) bone cyst in the metaphyseal region of the upper end of the humerus in a 10-year-old boy. Note the healing pathological fracture through the weakened cortex on the medial side. This boy had sustained a minor injury 3 weeks previously.

For reasons unknown, the cyst develops subjacent to the epiphyseal plate and gradually expands to fill the entire metaphysis and even part of the diaphysis. Cortical bone is resorbed from the inner surface, but periosteal reactive bone on the outer surface contains the lesion. The cavity is lined by non-neoplastic connective tissue cells and is filled with serous or serosanguinous fluid (reminiscent of the lining and contents of a chronic subdural hema-

toma). The overlying cortex becomes markedly thinned, making pathological fractures common (Fig. 14.30).

Simple bone cysts expand slowly and are painless. The event that usually brings them to the attention of a physician is a pathological fracture resulting from a minor injury. The radiographic features of simple bone cysts are characteristic (Figs. 14.30 and 14.31).

As the cyst becomes more mature and less active, it stops enlarging, in which case the epiphyseal plate grows away from it. Because simple bone cysts are almost never seen in adults, they are obviously due to a self-limiting process. In the meantime, repeated pathological fractures are not only painful and inconvenient for the child, but may lead to progressive deformity, particularly when the cyst is in

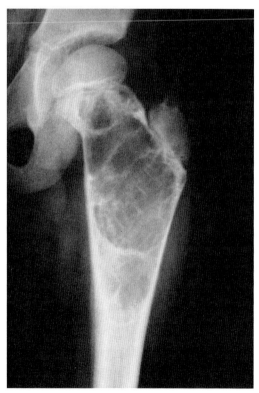

Figure 14.31.   Simple (solitary) bone cyst in the upper end of the femur in an 8-year-old boy. There is only one cavity (unicameral). The radiographic appearance of several cavities (multilocular) is due to ridges of bone on the deep surface of the thin cortex. The proximal end of this cyst extends to the upper femoral epiphyseal plate.

the upper end of the femur, in which case bone grafting and even internal fixation may be required. Although pathological fractures through a simple bone cyst heal readily, the cyst usually persists. Until recently, the most appropriate treatment of simple bone cysts in any site was thorough curettage of the cystic cavity and filling it with bone grafts (Fig. 14.20).

In the early 1970s, however, Scaglietti initiated the transcutaneous injection of corticosteroid (in the form of methylprednisolone acetate) into simple bone cysts as a means of arresting the osteolytic process and reversing it so that the cyst could heal by bone deposition. Theoretically, the corticosteroid inhibits the growth of the connective tissue cells in the lining of the cyst, and hence favors progressive healing by new bone formation. The injection may have to be repeated on several occasions, but in growing children the reported results have been moderately satisfactory: 45% of the cysts disappeared over a period of 3 years; in most of those remaining, the wall of the cyst became sufficiently thick and strong that there have been no further pathological fractures. Long-term outcome studies have revealed less satisfactory results. Recently, encouraging results have been reported by Lokiec et al. from the percutaneous injection of autologous bone marrow in the treatment of simple bone cysts. A number of bone graft substitutes for this purpose are also being investigated.

Thus, for many children with an immature, "active" bone cyst, it may now possible to avoid the open surgical procedure of curettage with its attendant risk of damage to the adjacent epiphyseal plate.

SPECIFIC TRUE NEOPLASMS OF BONE

Osteosarcoma (Osteogenic Sarcoma)

Osteosarcoma is an extremely malignant neoplasm that arises from primitive (poorly differentiated) cells in the metaphyseal region of a long bone in young individuals. It is frequently referred to as osteogenic sarcoma, not because it produces osteoid and bone (although it often does) but because of its genesis from the osteoblastic series of primitive mesenchymal cells.

All primary malignant neoplasms of bone are relatively rare but, of these, osteosarcoma is the second most common (being exceeded only by myeloma). The majority of its victims are children, adolescents, and young adults, which makes it all the more distressing. The most common sites are those of most active epiphyseal growth—the lower end of femur, upper end of tibia or fibula, upper end of humerus, and pelvis. In older persons osteosarcoma may also develop as a complication of Paget's disease in which case the prognosis is extremely grave (Chapter 9).

Osteosarcoma grows rapidly and is locally destructive. Some of these neoplasms produce considerable neoplastic bone (tumor bone) and in this sense are *osteosclerotic,* whereas others, which arise from more primitive cells, are predominantly *osteolytic.* This aggressive neoplasm soon erodes the cortex of the metaphyseal region and predisposes it to pathological fracture (Fig. 14.32). As it continues to grow wildly beyond the confines of the bone, it lifts the periosteum. Reactive bone forms in the angle between elevated periosteum and bone, which accounts for the radiographic phenomenon of Codman's triangle (Figs. 14.6 and 14.33). A combination of reactive bone and neoplastic bone deposited along blood vessels that radiate through the neoplasm from the cortex to the elevated periosteum accounts for the radiographic "sunburst" appearance seen in approximately 50% of osteosarcomas (Fig. 14.8). Osteosarcoma metastasizes to the lungs very early in the course of its development.

The most consistent symptom of rapidly growing osteosarcoma is pain, which is initially mild and intermittent but becomes progressively more severe and constant. Because this neoplasm nearly always arises in the metaphysis, close to a joint, it may interfere with joint function. A diffuse tumor mass develops rapidly and is usually tender (Fig. 14.2). This aggressive neoplasm is very vascular and the overlying skin is usually warm. The superficial veins become dilated and are best seen under infrared light (Fig. 14.3). The serum alkaline phosphatase is usually elevated.

The radiographic features of osteosarcoma,

which have been described above in relation to its pathogenesis, are often, but by no means always, characteristic.

The most accurate form of diagnostic imaging to determine the intraosseous and extraosseous extent of the sarcoma is MRI. Scintigraphy is useful in detecting "skip" lesions and CT scans of the chest are the best way to depict minute pulmonary metastases (Fig. 14.16). Thus, all three modalities of imaging are required to complete the staging of a given osteosarcoma.

Until a few decades ago, the prognosis of osteosarcoma was extremely grave because of its early spread to the lungs via the bloodstream; indeed, more than 90% of patients with osteosarcoma succumbed from pulmonary metastases within 3 years of the time of diagnosis despite treatment (Fig. 14.34).

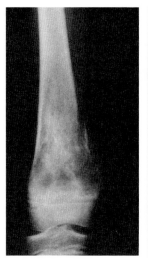
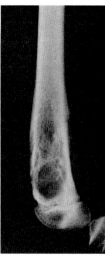

Figure 14.33. Osteosarcoma in the metaphyseal region of the lower end of the femur in a 10-year-old girl. Note the combination of bone resorption and bone deposition. This particular osteosarcoma is predominantly osteolytic, but some neoplastic bone is beginning to form beyond the confines of the metaphysis. A Codman's triangle can be seen in the lateral projection. (Other examples of osteosarcoma are shown in Figures 14.2, 14.3, 14.6, 14.8, 14.9A, 14.14, 14.17, and 14.32).

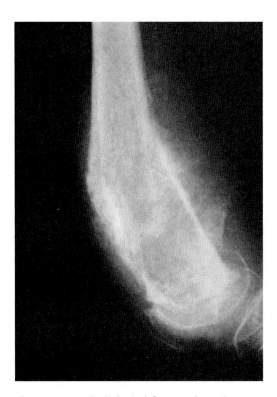

Figure 14.32. Pathological fracture through an osteosarcoma in the lower end of the femur of a 9-year-old girl. The angulated fracture is beginning to unite by subperiosteal callus despite the presence of the rapidly growing malignant neoplasm. Note the soft tissue mass containing neoplastic bone and the Codman's triangle of reactive bone posteriorly.

During the past few decades, the combination of neoadjuvant (preoperative) and adjuvant (postoperative) chemotherapy and more effective surgical procedures have resulted in a dramatic increase in the 5-year disease-free survival to more than 70%.

The chemotherapeutic agents being used include high-dose methotrexate (with citrovorum "rescue") adriamycin, doxorubicin, cisplatin, and ifosphamide.

Based on the staging of the osteosarcoma, limb-sparing procedures (as described in an earlier section of this chapter) are performed much more frequently than the previous method of radical resection, namely amputation (or disarticulation). The long-term survival rates from limb-sparing procedures and amputations (or disarticulation) are virtually the same, but the complication rate is considerably higher with the limb-sparing operations.

In recent years, there has been—and continues to be—exciting basic research on the

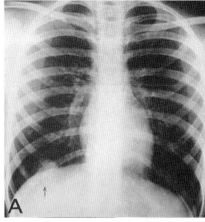

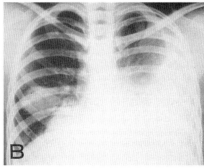

Figure 14.34. Pulmonary metastases secondary to osteosarcoma of the femur in a 9-year-old girl. **A.** Note the round metastasis at the base of the right lung (*arrow*). **B.** The radiograph only 2 months later reveals a massive pleural effusion on the left side, a small pneumothorax on the right side, and multiple metastases in both lungs.

molecular genetics of osteosarcoma. For example, Gallie and her associates found that children with hereditary retinoblastoma who have structural alterations in one allele of the retinoblastoma (RB1) gene are 400 times more likely to develop an osteosarcoma than are normal children. This retinoblastoma gene has been identified as a tumor-suppressive gene, the absence of which leads to the development of the retinoblastoma as well as osteosarcoma. This type of research may lead eventually to effective gene therapy for both retinoblastoma and osteosarcoma.

Molecular biologists have produced sophisticated tumor "markers" to identify specific variations of osteosarcoma and other malignant neoplasms of bone.

Surface Osteosarcoma

Parosteal Osteosarcoma

In recent decades, *parosteal sarcoma* has been considered separately from osteosarcoma because of significant differences. Less common than osteosarcoma, it tends to afflict adolescents and young adults. The most frequent site is the distal end of the femur. This lesion appears to arise from the osteoblastic cells of the periosteum. It grows mostly beside the intact cortex of the bone (parosteal) as a radiographically dense, osteoblastic lesion (Fig.14.35). It may even be mistaken for the sessile type of osteochondroma.

Because parosteal sarcoma is a low-grade malignancy that grows relatively slowly, at least in comparison with osteosarcoma, pain is not an early clinical feature. Also, the cortex

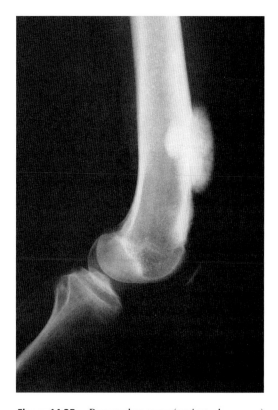

Figure 14.35. Parosteal sarcoma (periosteal sarcoma) arising from the anterior surface of the lower end of the femur in an 18-year-old girl. The major portion of the neoplasm is outside the confines of the bone. It is predominantly osteoblastic (osteosclerotic) and consequently is very dense radiographically.

is seldom eroded, making pathological fracture rare. Parosteal sarcoma metastasizes relatively late to the lungs; consequently, its prognosis is much better than that of osteosarcoma. Early total resection, either by limb-sparing procedures or by amputation, results in a permanent cure in 80% of patients.

Periosteal Osteosarcoma

This type of surface osteosarcoma is somewhat more aggressive than the parosteal variation. It tends to erode the cortex from the outside and may also invade the soft tissues. The treatment is similar to parosteal osteosarcoma's, but if the histological studies of the resected lesion reveal areas of higher grade malignancy, adjuvant chemotherapy should also be used.

Benign Chondroblastoma

A rare, benign neoplasm, *chondroblastoma* develops within the epiphysis of older children and adolescents, particularly at the upper end of tibia, lower end of femur, and upper end of humerus. In this last site, it is known as a Codman's tumor. Indeed, it is one of the few neoplasms to arise in the epiphysis. Because the lesion is subjacent to the articular cartilage, the patient complains of pain and experiences disturbed function in the nearby joint. A synovial effusion may develop.

Chondroblastoma grows slowly and becomes surrounded by sclerotic reactive bone that may even obscure the underlying cartilaginous neoplasm radiographically (Fig. 14.36). Computed tomography and MRI are useful in revealing this neoplasm. Histologically, this lesion may be difficult to differentiate from a chondrosarcoma. Chondroblastomas are benign neoplasms, however, and respond well to local curettage and bone grafting.

Chondromyxoid Fibroma

Chondromyxoid fibroma is actually more of a chondroma than a fibroma inasmuch as it is a mucin-containing neoplasm of chondroblastic origin. It develops eccentrically in the metaphyseal region of long bones and in the small bones of adolescents and young adults. Although usually benign, chondromyxoid fi-

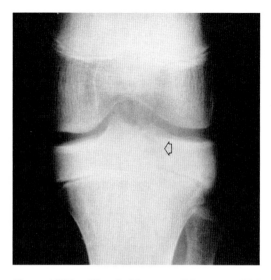

Figure 14.36.   Chondroblastoma of the upper tibial epiphysis in a 13-year-old boy (*arrow*). The small benign neoplasm is almost obscured by the surrounding sclerosis that is due to reactive bone. A tomogram of this boy's lesion (shown in Figure 14.4B) reveals the radiolucent neoplasm much more clearly.

broma is considered to be potentially malignant neoplasms.

Chondromyxoid fibroma grows relatively slowly and tends to maintain an eccentric location in the bone. The overlying cortex is often expanded, and the neoplasm is surrounded by a sclerotic zone of reactive bone (Fig. 14.37). Because chondromyxoid fibromas are poten-

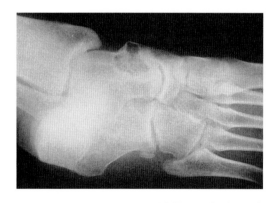

Figure 14.37.   Chondromyxoid fibroma in the neck of the talus in a 25-year-old man. Note the eccentric location of the neoplasm in the bone, the expanded and thin overlying cortex, and the surrounding sclerotic zone of reactive bone.

tially malignant, they are more effectively treated by local excision that includes a margin of normal bone rather than by simple curettage.

Chondrosarcoma

Chondrosarcoma is usually a relatively slow-growing malignant neoplasm that arises either spontaneously in previously normal bone, or as the result of malignant change in a preexisting, nonmalignant lesion, such as an osteochondroma or an enchondroma. Occurring mostly in adults older than age 30, it is the third most common malignant neoplasm of bone (after myeloma and osteosarcoma) and tends to develop in the pelvic and shoulder girdles and proximal long bones. There is often radiographic evidence of patchy calcification within this cartilaginous neoplasm. Such calcification is best seen with CT imaging. Histologically, the lesion consists of poorly differentiated cartilage cells but relatively few mitotic figures. Nevertheless, varying grades of malignancy exist within this category.

Chondrosarcoma grows relatively slowly, so pain is not a prominent clinical feature. A large cartilaginous mass slowly develops. Metastases tend to develop late, making the prognosis of chondrosarcoma considerably better than that of osteosarcoma. Because chondrosarcomas are radioresistant and exhibit only a limited response to chemotherapy, the optimum form of treatment is complete removal of the neoplasm. This usually necessitates either limb-sparing procedures or amputation. After such treatment, the patient has at least a 35% chance of cure with a high-grade chondrosarcoma and an 80% chance of cure with a chondrosarcoma that is of low-grade malignancy.

Fibrosarcoma

Fibrosarcoma is an uncommon malignant neoplasm that may arise in a long bone in young adults either as primary neoplasm or secondary to radiation. The principal sites are the femur, tibia, and radius. Because it grows relatively slowly, it is seldom painful. Radiographically, fibrosarcoma produces a fairly well de-

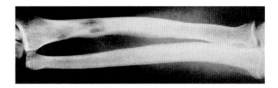

Figure 14.38.   Fibrosarcoma in the radius of a 28-year-old woman. Note that there are several well-demarcated osteolytic defects, all of which are part of the same neoplasm.

marcated osteolytic defect with little reaction in the surrounding bone (Fig.14.38).

The prognosis of fibrosarcoma is only slightly better than that of osteosarcoma because it metastasizes later. Its treatment, which involves complete resection of the lesion with wide margins, may necessitate either a limb-sparing procedure or amputation.

Malignant Fibrous Histiocytoma

This neoplasm, which resembles fibrosarcoma somewhat, usually develops in middle-aged adults. It produces an ill-defined osteolytic lesion that spreads early into the soft tissues, as revealed by CT and MRI.

Treatment involves wide resection either by a limb-sparing procedure or amputation, depending on the staging of the neoplasm. In either case, neoadjuvant and adjuvant chemotherapy are indicated with the same protocol as for osteosarcoma. For deep-seated, inaccessible neoplasms, radiation therapy remains an option.

Myeloma (Multiple Myeloma)

Myeloma is a widespread, multicentric neoplasm that arises from plasma cells in the hemopoietic tissue of the bone marrow in older persons, usually over the age of 50. It may occasionally remain localized as a solitary myeloma for many years, but even then it usually becomes multicentric. Pain is a prominent clinical feature. This neoplasm is particularly fascinating; recent electrophoretic studies of the associated changes in specific fractions of the serum proteins suggest that the initial neoplastic change may start in a *single* cell, as opposed to a *group* of cells. Myeloma is the most common of all primary malignant neoplasms of bone, constituting 50% of such neoplasms. In older individuals, hemopoietic (red) marrow is most prevalent in the spine, pelvis, ribs, sternum, and skull, and these are the most frequently involved sites. However, multiple bones may become riddled with rapidly destructive lesions that are painful (Fig. 14.39). The rapid destruction of bone with little reactive bone formation accounts for the high incidence of pathological fractures (Fig. 14.39A). Open reduction, internal fixation, and the addition of methylmethacrylate may be required to relieve the associated pain. A spinal brace provides comfort for patients with vertebral fractures.

Because plasma cells of the bone marrow normally produce γ-globulin, the concentration of this protein in the serum is markedly elevated in patients with myeloma. The excessive γ-globulin is excreted in the urine and may interfere with renal function. A specific protein—Bence-Jones protein—can be detected in the urine of approximately 50% of the patients. Anemia and an elevated erythrocyte sedimentation rate (ESR) are common, as is a decreased resistance to infection.

Because this neoplasm is so widespread, the diagnosis of myeloma can often be confirmed by needle aspiration biopsy of the marrow from either the iliac crest or the sternum. Until recently, the prognosis was extremely grave in that most patients succumbed within 2 years of diagnosis. In recent years, encouraging results are being obtained with intensive chemotherapy that may include cyclophosphamide, melphalan, with prednisone. Bisphosphonates, which inhibit bone resorption, help to control the patient's hypercalcemia. Bone marrow transplantation may improve the long-term results.

Ewing's Tumor (Ewing's Sarcoma)

Ewing's tumor is a rapidly growing malignant neoplasm that arises from primitive cells of the bone marrow in young persons, usually in the medullary cavity of long bones. It accounts for 5% of malignant neoplasms of bone. Like osteosarcoma, it develops in children, adolescents, and young adults, most commonly in the femur, tibia, ulna, and metatarsals.

Beginning within the medullary cavity, Ewing's tumor soon perforates the cortex of the shaft and elevates the periosteum. The repeated elevation of the periosteum and consequent reactive bone formation account for the laminated, or "onionskin" appearance seen radiographically (Figs. 14.7 and 14.40). Computed tomography, MRI, and scintigra-

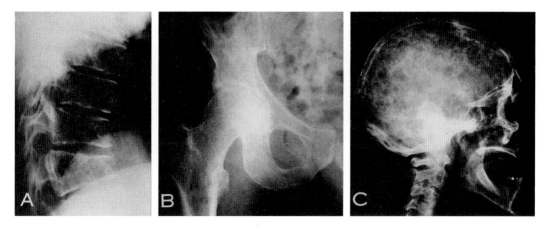

Figure 14.39.   Myeloma (multiple myeloma) in the spine, pelvis, and skull of a 58-year-old man. **A.** Note the pathological compression fracture through an osteolytic lesion in a thoracic vertebra. **B.** There are multiple lesions in the innominate bone of the pelvis as well as in the femur. **C.** The skull is riddled with multiple, small, clearly defined osteolytic defects.

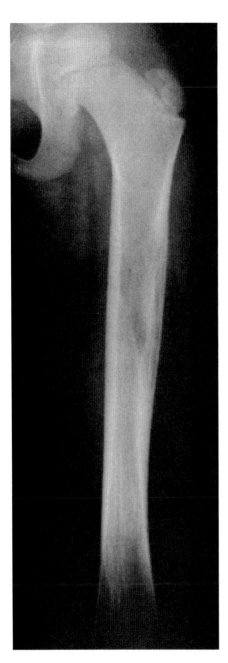

Figure 14.40.   Ewing's tumor (Ewing's sarcoma) in the shaft of the femur in a 6-year-old girl. This neoplasm is in an early stage of its development and is only moderately destructive. Note the radiographic "onionskin" appearance of periosteal reactive bone on the lateral aspect of the lesion. More advanced stages of Ewing's tumor are shown in Figures 14.7 and 14.18.

phy are all required for staging of the neoplasm. Ewing's tumor metastasizes early to the lungs and to other bones. Microscopically, this neoplasm is characterized by poorly differentiated round cells of marrow origin that contain intracellular glycogen as detected by means of a periodic acid-Schiff stain.

Ewing's tumor grows so rapidly that it often outgrows its blood supply; consequently, central areas of the neoplasm become necrotic. The products of this enter the bloodstream and produce systemic manifestations that include slight fever, moderate leukocytosis, and an elevated sedimentation rate. Also, the blood supply to local areas of bone may be compromised, with resultant avascular osteonecrosis.

As with other rapidly growing malignant neoplasms, the principal symptom is pain of progressive severity. A diffuse soft tissue mass is usually palpable and is moderately tender. Initially, the neoplasm exhibits relatively little bone destruction but subsequently, there is considerable reactive bone from the periosteum (Fig. 14.40).

The pain, local tenderness, systemic manifestations and radiographic features raise the differential diagnoses of chronic osteomyelitis and eosinophilic granuloma. The only certain method of diagnosis of Ewing's tumor is surgical biopsy and histological examination of representative samples of the lesion.

The prognosis of Ewing's tumor, like that of osteosarcoma, is extremely grave. Until recently, regardless of whether the patient was treated surgically or by radiation, the mortality rate within the first few years after diagnosis was approximately 95%.

Because the primary lesion is relatively radiosensitive and may "melt away" after intensive radiotherapy, this was the initial treatment of choice for many years. Nevertheless, metastases were still very common. Consequently, in recent decades, increasing emphasis has been placed on the combination of neoadjuvant chemotherapy and radical surgical resection (either a limb-sparing procedure, when feasible, or amputation) followed by adjuvant chemotherapy with or without radiation therapy. The chemotherapy may include vincristine, actinomycin D, doxorubicin, or cyclophosphamide. This combination of treatments has already increased the 5-year disease-free rate from 5% to more than 50%.

Hodgkin's Lymphoma

Most of the *Hodgkin's lymphomas* that involve bone are secondaries, that is, metastases rather than primary neoplasms. Middle-aged adults are usually inflicted, usually in the spine, ribs, and pelvis. Pain from the osteolytic lesions is a prominent feature. Scintigraphy may reveal multiple neoplasms, and CT as well as MRI are necessary for staging of the neoplasm. The most appropriate treatment is a combination of chemotherapy and radiation therapy.

Non-Hodgkin's Lymphoma (Reticulum Cell Sarcoma)

This variation of a lymphoma in bone arises in cells of the reticuloendothelial system. It was previously called "reticulum cell sarcoma" or "reticulosarcoma" (Fig. 14.41). The usual age incidence is middle-age and the most common sites are femur, tibia, humerus, pelvis, and vertebrae. The neoplasm may be secondary rather than primary; the distinction is important because the prognosis is better for the latter. Examination of the bone marrow is required to determine the presence or absence of disseminated disease. Scintigraphy is used to detect multiple lesions.

Pathological fractures through the osteolytic defect are common and may require open reduction and internal fixation to relieve the pain.

Solitary (primary and secondary) non-Hodgkin's lymphomas of bone are radiosensitive, and the combination of radiation therapy and chemotherapy renders surgical resection unnecessary.

Skeletal Reticuloses (Langerhans' Cell Histiocytosis)

The three forms of skeletal reticuloses (formerly called histiocytosis X, and now called Langerhans' histiocytoses) are Letterer-Siwe disease, Hand-Schüller-Christian disease, and eosinophilic granuloma. They are discussed in Chapter 9 under the heading of "The Histiocytoses."

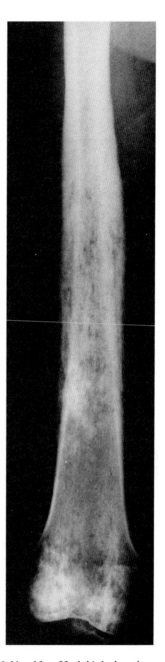

Figure 14.41. Non-Hodgkin's lymphoma (reticulum cell sarcoma) of the femur in a 29-year-old woman. Note the mottled appearance due to a combination of osteoclastic bone resorption (osteolysis) and osteoblastic bone deposition (osteosclerosis). The layers of subperiosteal reactive bone are somewhat similar to those seen in Ewing's sarcoma.

Leukemia

The various leukemias, which are malignant neoplasms arising from the hemopoietic stem cells, may be lymphocytic or myelogenous, and either acute or chronic. The leukemic deposits in the bone marrow may be painful, especially in children. Radiographically, these deposits are depicted as multiple ill-defined areas of rarefaction in long bones (Fig. 14.42). The diagnosis can usually be made by a complete blood count and differential, plus a bone marrow aspirate.

For these widespread leukemic deposits, the treatment is the same as for the underlying leukemia, that is, chemotherapy.

Giant Cell Tumor of Bone (Osteoclastoma)

A variable lesion, *giant cell tumor of bone* or *osteoclastoma* is a potentially malignant, and

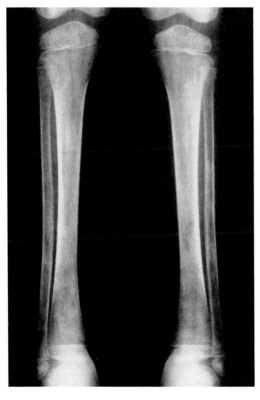

Figure 14.42.   Acute leukemia in a 7-year-old boy. The multiple, ill-defined areas of rarefaction in the long bones represent leukemic infiltrations. This boy complained of deep pain in his legs and examination revealed bone tenderness.

sometimes frankly malignant, neoplasm that arises in the cancellous end of long bones in young adults.

Much confusion and divergence of opinion surround this neoplasm. The origin of the osteoclast is not known; there is not even general agreement that the osteoclast is the principal neoplastic cell of an osteoclastoma. Formerly, several benign neoplasms, and even non-neoplastic lesions that contained osteoclasts, or giant cells, were considered to be giant cell tumors. Now that these less serious "giant cell variants" have been excluded, what remains as a true giant cell tumor is a formidable neoplasm.

These neoplasms develop in the region of the former epiphysis of long bones after the epiphyseal plate has closed. Therefore, it is rare before the age of 20 years. The most common sites are the lower end of radius, upper end of tibia, lower end of femur, and upper end of humerus. The neoplasm usually extends to the articular cartilage.

Giant cell tumors are locally destructive neoplasms. The cancellous and cortical bone are resorbed from the inside and simultaneously, the periosteum deposits bone on the outside so that the end of the bone eventually becomes expanded. Growth may be slow or relatively rapid, depending on the aggressiveness of the particular lesion. Two-thirds of these neoplasms are benign in their behavior, one sixth are locally aggressive, and one sixth become frankly malignant. Areas of hemorrhage within the lesion are common, and a phenomenon comparable to aneurysmal bone cyst may be superimposed on the original lesion, causing it to expand at an alarming rate. Even those giant cell tumors that are frankly malignant tend to metastasize late. Microscopically, osteoclastomas consist of a vascular network of stromal cells and large numbers of multinucleated giant cells.

The patient complains of local pain, the severity of which is related to the rate of growth of the neoplasm. Because the lesion abuts the articular cartilage, there is nearly always some disturbance of joint function. The radiographic appearance is variable but reveals local

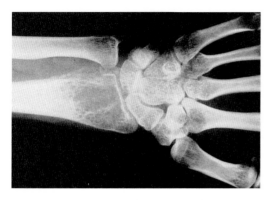

Figure 14.43. Giant cell tumor of bone (osteoclastoma) in the lower end of the radius of a 32-year-old man. Note that the destructive (osteolytic) neoplasm includes the site of the former epiphysis and extends to the subchondral bone. In this relatively early stage, the radius is just beginning to expand on the medial (ulnar) side.

bone destruction and eventually expansion of the end of the bone (Fig. 14.43).

Giant cell tumors have a disturbing tendency to recur after local surgical treatment such as simple curettage. Therefore, the original operation should be as aggressive as necessary to remove all neoplastic tissue without being so extensive that it disturbs function in the limb unnecessarily. A local recurrence after curettage is an indication for radical excision of the entire lesion in a limb-sparing procedure, with replacement of the resected part of the bone by methylmethacrylate, an autogenous bone graft, an osteocartilaginous allograft, or a custom-made endoprosthesis as a joint replacement. For the most aggressive giant cell tumors, or for local recurrence, radiotherapy is one option that can be used in an attempt to avoid amputation.

METASTATIC (SECONDARY) NEOPLASMS IN BONE

By far the most common malignant neoplasms *in* bone (rather than *of* bone) are *metastatic neoplasms,* or "bone secondaries," that have invaded bone from a primary malignant neoplasm elsewhere. In adults, particularly the elderly, these "outside invaders" almost always originate from *carcinoma,* whereas in children their usual source is *neuroblastoma.*

Metastatic Carcinoma

Metastatic carcinoma is common, as evidenced by the postmortem evidence that at least 25% of all patients who have died from carcinoma have one or more metastases in bone. Viable neoplastic cells from a primary carcinoma may reach bone by the bloodstream, by the lymphatics, or by direct extension. Hemopoietic (red) bone marrow seems to provide the most fertile "soil" for the "seeding" of carcinoma cells, making the vertebrae, pelvis, ribs, and proximal long bones of the limbs the most common sites for metastatic carcinoma, that is, the sites of persistent hemopoietic bone marrow in the elderly.

The most frequent *primary* sources for metastatic carcinoma in bone are breast, prostate, lung, kidney, thyroid, bladder, and colon (in that order). Most of the metastatic neoplasms in bone are locally destructive and produce *osteolytic metastases* (Fig. 14.44). Others, particularly those from carcinoma of the prostate, incite a marked osteoblastic reaction in their metastatic site and produce *osteosclerotic metastases* (Fig. 14.45). Total body scintigraphy is useful in detecting asymptomatic lesions. The primary organ from which the metastases have originated is usually known, but if it is unknown or not obvious, it should be found by further investigation.

The most prominent and distressing symp-

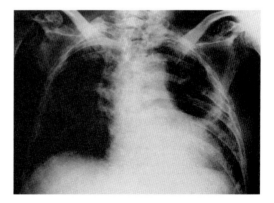

Figure 14.44. Widespread osteolytic metastases in the vertebrae, scapulae, and ribs of a 49-year-old woman. The primary neoplasm was carcinoma of the breast. Another example of the osteolytic type of metastatic carcinoma in bone is shown in Figure 14.10.

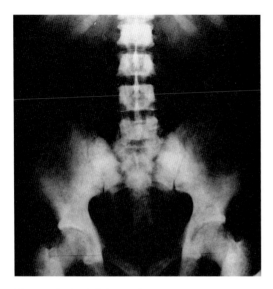

Figure 14.45.   Widespread osteosclerotic (osteoblastic) metastases in the femora, pelvis, and vertebrae of a 60-year-old man. The primary neoplasm was carcinoma of the prostate. Another example of the osteosclerotic type of metastatic carcinoma in bone is shown in Figure 14.11.

onstrated by CT that a given pulmonary metastasis is, in fact, solitary and when the resection is combined with adjuvant chemotherapy.

Various forms of hormone therapy and even endocrine operations such as castration, adrenalectomy, and hyophysectomy, depending on the source of the primary neoplasm, may help to retard the rate of progression of the metastases and relieve pain, as well as prolong life somewhat.

Whenever feasible, pathological fractures in limb bones are stabilized by metallic internal fixation, with or without bone cement (methylmethacrylate), to relieve the associated pain. Even for impending pathological fractures through large metastases in long bones, prophylactic internal fixation is appropriate. Pathological fractures of the spine can be immobi-

tom of metastatic carcinoma in bone is severe and unrelenting pain, some of which is due to the complication of pathological fracture (Fig. 14.46). Indeed, metastatic neoplasms in bone are the most frequent cause of a pathetically painful demise of a patient dying of cancer.

Osteoclastic resorption in multiple bones releases excessive amounts of calcium into the bloodstream. In patients with multiple metastases, the resultant hypercalcemia may cause anorexia, nausea, general weakness, and depression. These symptoms may be relieved by the use of bisphosphonates. The reactive bone formation stimulated by these lesions accounts for the elevation of serum alkaline phosphatase. A raised serum acid phosphatase and prostatic-specific antigen (PSA) are an indication of advanced carcinoma of the prostate as the primary site.

The treatment of patients with metastatic carcinoma is palliative. Local radiation therapy and appropriate chemotherapy may retard the rate of growth of a metastasis and help to relieve pain.

Resection of solitary lung metastases has shown promising results when it can be dem-

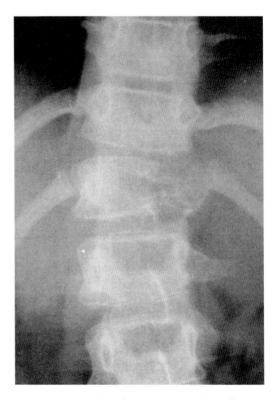

Figure 14.46.   Pathological compression fracture through an osteolytic metastasis in the body of the 12th thoracic vertebrae in a 54-year-old man. Note the asymmetrical collapse of the vertebral body. The primary neoplasm was bronchogenic carcinoma of the lung.

lized in an appropriate spinal brace, but a progressive neurological deficit is an indication for urgent decompression.

The total care of a patient with metastatic carcinoma requires unending understanding and kindly compassion, with palliative care and hospice management, either in hospital or at home. The comfort, composure, companionship, counseling, and dignity of the dying must always be a priority.

Metastatic Neuroblastoma

In infants and young children, *neuroblastoma*, an extremely malignant neoplasm of the adrenal medulla, is the most common primary source of multiple metastases in bone, usually developing in the vertebrae, skull, and metaphysis of long bones (Fig. 14.47). There is often a high urinary excretion of catecholamines. Chemotherapy and local radiation therapy tend to retard the growth of these me-

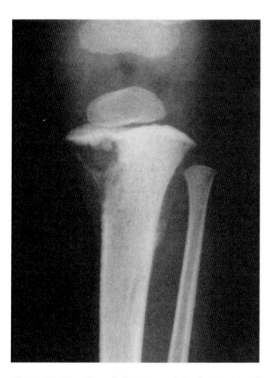

Figure 14.47. Osteolytic metastasis in the upper end of the tibia in a 2-year-old child. Note the marked bone destruction in the medial part of the metaphyseal, as well as the subperiosteal reactive bone on the lateral aspect. The primary neoplasm was a neuroblastoma of the adrenal medulla.

tastases and relieve pain. A bone marrow allograft may actually prolong the child's life.

NEOPLASM-LIKE LESIONS AND TRUE NEOPLASMS OF SOFT TISSUES

In the extremities and the trunk, soft tissue lesions that appear as visible "bumps" or "swellings" or palpable "lumps" are relatively common, but at least 95% are either neoplasm-like lesions or benign neoplasms. The Definition of Terms and General Considerations, including the diagnosis, principles, and methods of treatment, described at the beginning of this chapter for neoplasm-like lesions and true neoplasms of *bone* are applicable to those of *soft tissues*.

CLASSIFICATIONS

As with the neoplasm-like lesions and true neoplasms of bone, so also with those of soft tissues, the following classifications are based (insofar as is known at present) on the cell origin or *genesis* of the lesion.

Classification of Neoplasm-like Lesions and Benign Neoplasms of Soft Tissues

A. Myogenic
   1. Rhabdomyoma
B. Lipogenic
   1. Lipoma
C. Fibrogenic
   1. Fibroma
   2. Aggressive fibromatosis
D. Neurogenic
   1. Neuroma
   2. Neurilemmoma (benign schwannoma)
   3. Neurofibroma
E. Angiogenic
   1. Hemangioma of soft tissue
   2. Lymphangioma of soft tissue
   3. Glomus tumor
F. Synoviogenic
   1. Synovial chondrometaplasia (synovial chondromatosis)
   2. Pigmented villonodular synovitis (PVNS)
   3. Giant cell tumor of tendon sheath

Classification of Malignant Neoplasms of Soft Tissues

A. Myogenic
1. Rhabdomyosarcoma
B. Lipogenic
1. Liposarcoma
C. Fibrogenic
1. Fibrosarcoma of soft tissue
2. Malignant fibrous histiocytoma
D. Neurogenic
1. Neurosarcoma
E. Synoviogenic
1. Synovial sarcoma
F. Uncertain histiogenesis
1. Epithelioid sarcoma

SPECIFIC NEOPLASM-LIKE AND BENIGN NEOPLASMS OF SOFT TISSUES

Lipoma

The most common soft tissue neoplasm of the musculoskeletal system, *lipomas* are benign collections of mature fat cells. They usually develop in middle-aged and elderly adults and are neither painful nor tender. Lipomas are soft, mobile, and almost fluctuant. On plain radiographs, they appear as a clearly demarcated radiolucent lesion and they have a high signal density on both T1-weighted and T2-weighted MR images. Only those lipomas that are either a cosmetic problem or symptomatic require surgical resection, which can be accomplished using narrow (marginal) margins, with very little chance of recurrence. Even without surgical treatment, lipomas are unlikely to ever undergo malignant transformations.

Fibroma

A solitary *fibroma* usually presents as an asymptomatic nodule or lump in the subcutaneous tissues. No treatment is required.

Aggressive Fibromatosis

This rare lesion is more aggressive than a solitary fibroma. It requires complete resection with a wide margin and has a tendency to recur locally even after complete resection.

Neuroma

After either partial or complete division of a peripheral nerve, a combination of nerve tissue and fibrous tissue grows from the cut end of the nerve, producing a *neuroma* (a post-traumatic neuroma), which is not a true neoplasm.

Neurilemmoma (Benign Schwannoma)

A benign nerve sheath neoplasm, a *neurilemmoma*, also known as a benign schwannoma, develops in middle-aged adults as an asymptomatic mass attached to a peripheral nerve. Treatment consists of surgical resection of the neoplasm with narrow (marginal) margins, leaving the underlying nerve intact.

Neurofibroma

This is a benign neoplasm of neural and fibrous tissue arising in a peripheral nerve. It usually causes pain and paresthesias. When symptomatic, a *neurofibroma* should be resected intracapsularly to preserve the associated nerve. Multiple neurofibromas (neurofibromatosis) are associated with other manifestations of von Recklinghausen's disease, a condition that is described in Chapter 8.

Hemangioma

This relatively common benign neoplasm can occur in either superficial or deep tissues. These lesions tend to "fill" more completely when the patient is erect rather than supine, in which case they may cause a dull, aching discomfort. When they involve a synovial joint, they may result in recurrent hemarthroses. Their treatment involves wide resection, but hemangiomas tend to recur locally.

Glomus Tumor

This relatively uncommon neoplasm-like lesion is tiny (only a few millimeters in diameter) and usually develops in the nail bed of a finger or toe. Consisting of neurovascular tissues, a *glomus tumor* causes episodes of excruciating pain in association with exquisite local tenderness. These symptoms, which are completely out of proportion with the minute size of the lesion, justify surgical excision.

Synovial Chondrometaplasia (Synovial Chondromatosis)

Metaplasia is a change in adult cells of a given tissue in which they produce a different type of cell and consequently, a different type of tissue. On rare occasions in adults, and for reasons unknown, the cells of the synovial membrane may undergo metaplasia (*synovial chondrometaplasia*), whereby they come to resemble chondroblasts and produce deposits of cartilage tissue within the membrane. These cartilaginous deposits may become vascularized, develop centers of ossification, and become radiopaque. As these osteochondral masses grow, they become pedunculated and may be torn loose from the synovial membrane to become free bodies in the synovial cavity (osteochondral loose bodies or "joint mice"). The ossific nucleus, having lost its blood supply, dies but remains in its coffin of cartilage. The cartilaginous portion, being nourished by synovial fluid, survives and may even continue to grow. Arthroscopic examination is helpful in establishing the diagnosis.

Adults older than 40 years of age are most likely to develop this unusual type of metaplasia. The typical sites are the knee, hip, and elbow. The patient complains of "grinding" in the joint and the sensation of something moving about inside the joint. The radiographic appearance of synovial chondrometaplasia, or synovial chondromatosis is characteristic (Fig. 14.48).

Simple removal of the multiple osteochondral loose bodies is inadequate, because more will form. Therefore, to deal definitively with this condition, surgical synovectomy is required. This can be achieved either through an open arthrotomy or through an arthroscope.

Pigmented Villonodular Synovitis

Definitely not a neoplasm, *pigmented villonodular synovitis* (PVNS) is probably a proliferative reaction to some type of inflammatory agent. This reaction, characterized by large numbers of giant cells, produces villous and nodular masses that fuse together in the synovial membrane to form a single mass. Arthroscopy and biopsy through the arthroscope are of value in making the diagnosis. The pigment of PVNS is hemosiderin, which gives the lesion a yellowish color. Microscopically, these lesions contain lipid-filled histiocytes and giant cells.

Pigmented villonodular synovitis, which is relatively rare, occurs in adults and the knee is the usual synovial joint affected. The lesion produces a bulky mass in the synovial membrane and may even erode bone. Involvement of the synovial sheath of tendons is most common in the flexor tendon sheaths of the hand where the lesion forms a solitary, firm nodule.

This lesion in synovial joints responds well to surgical excision of the involved area of synovial membrane. For diffuse and widespread intra-articular disease, extensive synovectomy (either open or arthroscopic) is required.

Giant Cell Tumor of Tendon Sheath

This benign lesion, which some pathologists consider a manifestation of villonodular synovitis in the synovial tendon sheath of the hand or the foot, is not a true neoplasm. It is characterized by a firm nodule that consists of giant cells and xanthoma cells (hence the synonym *xanthoma* (Fig. 14.49). Treatment consists of surgical resection of the lesion without disturbing the underlying tendon.

SPECIFIC MALIGNANT NEOPLASMS OF SOFT TISSUES

The various malignant neoplasms of soft tissues are *sarcomas* and, in general, are best

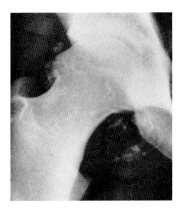

Figure 14.48. Synovial chondrometaplasia (synovial chondromatosis) in the hip joint of a 54-year-old man. Note the multiple radiopaque loose bodies in the joint. Each of these ossified bodies is encased in cartilage.

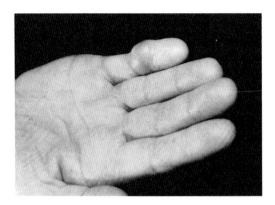

Figure 14.49. Pigmented villonodular synovitis in the flexor tendon sheath of the fifth finger in a 42-year-old woman. The nodular swelling was firm. This lesion, which is not a neoplasm, is sometimes referred to as a xanthoma, or giant cell tumor, of the tendon sheath.

treated by radical surgical resection. With the exception of rhabdomyosarcoma, they tend to be resistant to both chemotherapy and radiation therapy.

Rhabdomyosarcoma

A high-grade malignancy and the most common of the soft tissue sarcomas in children and young adults, it occurs especially around the shoulder or hip. In very young children, the embryonic type of *rhabdomyosarcoma* may involve the genitourinary muscles. It is best treated by radical surgical excision. In addition, because it is relatively sensitive to chemotherapy and radiation, these methods of treatment should be combined with surgical resection. Current chemotherapeutic agents in use for rhabdomyosarcoma are vincristine, actinomycin D, and cyclophosphamide.

Liposarcoma

The most frequently occurring soft tissue sarcoma in middle-aged and elderly adults, *liposarcomas* usually arise in the deeper tissues, especially within muscles. They present as a mass that is firmer than a lipoma and they vary from low-grade to high-grade malignancy. All grades are best treated by wide surgical resection. For liposarcomas in inaccessible sites, radiation therapy is indicated.

Fibrosarcoma and Malignant Fibrous Histiocytoma

These two malignant neoplasms of fibrous tissue origin usually become apparent because of a progressively enlarging but painless mass in the soft tissues. They can be distinguished from one another by immunohistochemical markers but their treatment is the same, namely wide local resection including either a limb-sparing procedure or, if not feasible, amputation.

Neurosarcoma

This rare malignant soft tissue sarcoma, also known as malignant schwannoma, arises in peripheral nerves in young adults. The clinical features of pain, paresthesias, and paralysis are due to pressure on the involved nerve. Treatment consists of wide surgical resection.

Synovial Sarcoma (Synovioma)

Synovial sarcoma is a high-grade malignant neoplasm that arises from cells of synovial potential, often in tendon sheaths near, but not actually within, a major joint in young adults. More common in the lower limbs than elsewhere, synovial sarcoma usually becomes manifest by the development of a painful, tender soft tissue swelling near a joint, typically the knee. Because the bone is not involved, radiographic examination reveals only a soft tissue mass that may show calcification within it. Histologically, tissue spaces or clefts may be seen within the neoplasm.

The treatment of synovial sarcoma is radical surgical incision, preferably a limb-sparing procedure but if that is not feasible, then amputation. Even with such surgical treatment, synovial sarcoma may recur locally. Furthermore, metastases may appear as late as 5 years after the surgical resection or amputation, and the long-term disease-free survival rate is only 50%.

Epithelioid Sarcoma

This relatively rare high-grade malignant neoplasm of soft tissues tends to occur in the hands or feet of young adults. When an *epithelioid sarcoma* arises in the subcutaneous tissues, it may ulcerate through the skin and yet, the histological characteristics may look misleadingly benign. This particular sarcoma spreads rapidly, both locally and to the lungs. Treatment consists of early radical-surgical resection, either a limb-sparing procedure or amputation and chemotherapy as well as radiation therapy.

SUGGESTED ADDITIONAL READING

Alman BA, de Bari A, Krajbich JI. Massive allografts in the treatment of osteosarcoma in children and adolescents. J Bone Joint Surg 1995;77-A(1): 54–64.

Apley AG, Solomon L. Apley's system of orthopaedics and fractures. 7th edition. Oxford: Butterworth-Heinemann Ltd., 1993.

Bacci G, Toni A, Avella M, et al. Long-term results in 144 localized Ewing's sarcoma patients treated with combined therapy. Cancer 1989; 63:1477–1486.

Bataille R, Harousseau, J-L. Multiple myeloma. (Medical Progress). N Engl J Med 1997; 336(23):1657–1664.

Bell RS, Davis A. Diagnosis, survival and options for surgical care in osteosarcoma. Current Opinions in Orthopaedics 1992;3(6):792–797.

Bell RS, Davis A, Allan DG, et al. Fresh osteochondral allografts for advanced giant cell tumors at the knee. J Arthroplasty 1994;9(6):603–609.

Bennett CJ Jr, Marcus RB, Million RR, et al. Radiation therapy for giant cell tumor of bone. Int J Radiat Oncol Biol Phys 1993;26:299–304.

Biermann JS. Musculoskeletal neoplasms. In: Richards S, ed. Orthopaedic knowledge update—paediatrics. Rosemont, IL: The American Academy of Orthopaedic Surgeons, 1996; 55–64.

Bonfiglio M, Buckwalter JB. Musculoskeletal tumors. In: Clark CR, Bonfiglio M, eds. Orthopaedics, essentials of diagnosis and treatment. New York: Churchill Livingstone, 1994;351–372.

Brien EW, Terek RM, Healey JH, et al. Allograft reconstruction after proximal tibial resection for bone tumors: an analysis of function and outcome comparing allografts and prosthetic reconstruction. Clin Orthop Rel Res 1994;303: 116–127.

Bruchner JD, Conrad EV III: Musculoskeletal neoplasms. In: Kasser JR, ed. Orthopaedic knowledge update 5. Rosemont, IL: The American Academy of Orthopaedic Surgeons, 1996; 133–148.

Buckwalter JA. Musculoskeletal neoplasms and disorders that resemble neoplasms. In: Weinstein SL, Buckwalter JA, eds. Turek's orthopaedics: principles and their application. 5th ed. Philadelphia: J.B. Lippincott, 1994.

Cammisa FP Jr., Glasser DB, Otis JC, et al. The van Nes tibial rotationplasty: a functionally viable reconstruction procedure for children who have a tumor of the distal end of the femur. J Bone Joint Surg 1990;72A:1541–1547.

Campanacci M, Capanna R, Picci P. Unicameral and aneurysmal bone cysts. Clin Orthop Rel Res 1986;204:25–36.

Clohisy DR, Mankin HJ. Osteoarticular allografts for reconstruction after resection of a musculoskeletal tumor in the proximal end of the tibia. J Bone Joint Surg 1994;76-A:549–554.

Cohen J, Bonfiglio M, Campbell CJ. Orthopaedic pathophysiology in diagnosis and treatment. New York: Churchill Livingstone, 1990.

Davis AM, Goodwin P, Bell RS. Prognostic factors in osteosarcoma. J Clin Oncol 1994;12(2): 423–431.

Enneking WF, Spanier SS, Goodman MA. A system for the surgical grading of musculoskeletal sarcoma. Clin Orthop 1980;153:106–120.

Enneking WF. Musculoskeletal tumor surgery. New York: Livingstone, 1983.

Enneking WF. A system of staging musculoskeletal neoplasms. Clin Orthop Rel Res 1986;204: 9–24.

Finn HA, Simon MA. Musculoskeletal neoplasms. In: Goldberg V, ed. Orthopaedic knowledge update 3. Rosemont, IL: The American Academy of Orthopaedic Surgeons, 1990;115–144.

Frassica FJ, Thompson RC. Evaluation, diagnosis, and classification of benign soft-tissue tumors. An instructional course lecture. The American Academy of Orthopaedic Surgeons. J Bone Joint Surg 1996;78-A(1):126–140.

Gallie BL, Dunn JM, Chan HSL, et al. The genetics of retinoblastoma: relevance to the patient. Pediatr Clin North Am 1991;38:2:299–315.

Gitelis S, Wilkins R, Conrad EV III. Benign bone tumors. An instructional course lecture. The American Academy of Orthopaedic Surgeons. J Bone Joint Surg 1995;77-A(11):1756–1782.

Gottsauner-Wolf F, Kotz R, Knahr K, et al. Rotationplasty for limb salvage in the treatment of malignant tumors at the knee: a follow-up study of seventy patients. J Bone Joint Surg 1991;73-A(9):1365–1375.

Green JA, Bellemore MC, Marsden FW. Embolization in the treatment of aneurysmal bone cysts. J Pediatr Orthop 1997;17:440–443.

Hashemi-Nejad A, Cole WG. Incomplete healing of simple bone cysts after steroid injections. J Bone Joint Surg 1997;79-B(5):727–730.

Horowitz S. Musculoskeletal neoplasms. In: Frymoyer JW, ed. Orthopaedic knowledge update 4. Rosemont, IL: The American Academy of Orthopaedic Surgeons, 1993;169–178.

Levesque J, Marx RG, Wunder JS, et al. A clinical guide to bone tumors. Baltimore: Williams and Wilkins, 1998.

Lokiec F, Ezra E, Khermosh O, Weintroub S. Simple bone cysts treated by percutaneous autologous marrow grafting. J. Bone Joint Surg (Br) 1996;78B:934–937.

Mankin HJ, Lange TA, Spanier SS. The hazards of biopsy with malignant primary bone and soft tissue tumors. J Bone Joint Surg 1982;64-A: 1121.

Mankin HJ, Gehardt MC. Advances in the management of bone tumors. Clin Orthop Rel Res 1985;200:73–84.

Mankin HJ, Gebhardt MC, Tomford WW. The use of frozen cadaveric allografts in the management of patients with bone tumors of the extremities. Orthop Clin North Am 1987; 18:275–289.

Mankin HJ, Mankin CJ, Simon MA. The hazards of biopsy, revisited. J Bone Joint Surg 1996;78-A(5):656–663.

Nelson TE, Enneking WF. Staging of bone and soft-tissue sarcomas revisited. In: Stauffer RN, ed. Advances in operative orthopaedics. Vol. 2. St. Louis: Mosby-Year Book, 1994;379–391.

O'Sullivan MD, Saxton VJ. Bone and soft tissue tumors. In: Broughton NS, ed. A textbook of pediatric orthopaedics. London: W.B. Saunders, 1997.

Ogilvie-Harris DJ, Saleh K. Generalized synovial chondromatosis of the knee: a comparison of removal of the loose bodies alone with arthroscopic synovectomy. Arthroscopy 1994;10(2): 166–170.

Pettersson H, Gillespy T, Hamlin DJ et al. Primary musculoskeletal tumors: examination with MR imaging compared with conventional modalities. Radiology 1987;164:237–241.

Roberts P, Chan D, Grimer RJ, et al. Prosthetic replacement of the distal femur for primary bone tumors. J Bone Joint Surg 1991;73-B(5):762.

Rosen G, Capparow B, Huvos AG, et al. Preoperative chemotherapy for osteogenic sarcoma: selection of post-operative chemotherapy based on the response of the primary tumor to pre-operative chemotherapy. Cancer 1982;49:1221–1230.

Rosen G. Neoadjuvant chemotherapy for osteogenic sarcoma. In: Enneking WF, ed. Limb salvage in musculoskeletal oncology. New York: Churchill Livingstone, 1987.

Rosenthal OI, Springfield DS, Gebhardt MC, et al. Osteoid osteoma: percutaneous radiofrequency ablation. Radiology 1995;197:451–454.

Rougroff BT, Kneisl JS, Simon MA. Skeletal metastases of unknown origin. J Bone Joint Surg 1993;75-A:1276–1281.

Ruggieri P, De Cristofaro R, Picci P, et al. Complications and surgical indications in 144 cases of nonmetastatic osteosarcoma of the extremities treated with neoadjuvant chemotherapy. Clin Orthop Rel Res 1993;295:226–238.

Scaglietti O, Marchetti PG, Bartolozzi P. Final re-

sults obtained in the treatment of bone cysts with methylprednisolone acetate (depo-medrol) and a discussion of results obtained in other bone lesions. Clin Orthop 1982;165:34–42.

Schmale GA, Conrad EV III, Raskind WH. The natural history of hereditary multiple exostoses. J Bone Joint Surg 1994;76-A:986–992.

Sim FH, ed. Diagnosis and management of metastatic bone disease: a multidisciplinary approach. New York: Raven Press, 1988.

Simon MA, Aschliman MA, Thomas N, et al. Limb-salvage treatment versus amputation for osteosarcoma of the distal femur. J Bone Joint Surg 1986;68A:1331–1337.

Sjostrom L, Jonsson H, Karlstrom G, et al. Surgical treatment of vertebral metastases. Contemporary Orthopaedics 1993;26:3:247–254.

Springfield DS, Gebhardt MC, McGuire MH. Chondrosarcoma: a review. An instructional course lecture. The American Academy of Orthopaedic Surgeons. J Bone Joint Surg 1996; 78-A(1):141–149.

Springfield DS. Bone and soft tissue tumours. In: Morrissy RT, Weinstein S, eds. Lovell and Winter's pediatric orthopaedics. Vol 1.4th ed. Philadelphia, New York: Lippincoth-Raven, 1996.

Springfield DS. Orthopaedic oncology. In: Sledge CB, ed. Year Book of Orthopaedics, 1996; 225–250.

Stark A, Kreicbergs A, Nilsonne U, et al. The age of osteosarcoma patients is increasing. J Bone Joint Surg 1990;72B:89–93.

Sweetnam R. Tumors of bone and soft tissues. In: Hughes S, Sweetnam R, eds. The basis and practice of orthopaedics. London: William Heinemann Medical Books Ltd., 1980.

Tachdjian MO. Clinical pediatric orthopaedics. The art of diagnosis and principles of treatment. Stamford, CT: Appleton and Lange, 1997.

Tolo V. Tumor management (editorial). J Pediatr Orthop 1997;17:421–423.

Vander Griend RA, Funderburk CH. The treatment of giant-cell tumors of the distal part of the radius. J Bone Joint Surg 1983;75-A:899–908.

Wenger DR, Rang M. The art and practice of children's orthopaedics. New York: Raven Press, 1993.

Wold LE, McLeod RA, Sim FH, et al. Atlas of orthopaedic pathology. Philadelphia: W.B. Saunders, 1990.

Womer RB. The cellular biology of bone tumors. Clin Orthop Rel Res 1991;262:12–21.

Yasko JW, Lane JM. Current concepts review: chemotherapy for bone and soft-tissue sarcomas of the extremities. J Bone Joint Surg 1991;73-A:1263–1271.

Zatsepin ST, Burdygin VN. Replacement of the distal femur and proximal tibia with frozen allografts. Clin Orthop Rel Res 1994;303:95–102.

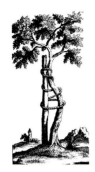

Section 3

Musculoskeletal Injuries

15 Fractures and Joint Injuries—General Features

*"He who loves practice without theory is like
a seafarer who boards a ship without wheel or
compass and knows not whither he travels."*
—Leonardo da Vinci (1495)

GENERAL INCIDENCE AND SIGNIFICANCE

The present age, which is characterized by increasing individual participation in high-speed travel by land, sea, and air, complex industry, and competitive and recreational sports, might well be called the *age of injury*, or the *age of trauma*. The present incidence of injuries is disturbingly high, and continues to rise. Indeed, trauma remains the number one killer of young people in North America. This epidemic of fatal injuries merits more research concerning both prevention and treatment, even though advances in traumatology during the past three decades have significantly reduced the morbidity and mortality from trauma.

The estimated annual cost of trauma in North America alone is over $160 billion. Approximately 10% of all hospital beds are occupied at any given time by the victims of trauma. Of all the significant injuries that befall humans, at least two-thirds involve the musculoskeletal system, including fractures, dislocations, and associated soft tissue injuries. Thus, musculoskeletal injuries have become

increasingly common and important and will continue to be so throughout your life.

Although isolated musculoskeletal injuries in healthy individuals are seldom fatal, they are serious in that they cause much physical suffering, mental distress, and loss of time for the victim; that is to say, they have a low mortality but a high morbidity. Multiple injuries involving other body systems are, in a given individual, even more serious in that they endanger life as well as limb; they have a high mortality and a high morbidity. As a result of our increasing life span, more people are now reaching "old age," when decreasing coordination causes more frequent falls. In addition, senile weakening of the bones from osteoporosis renders older individuals more susceptible to even minor injury. In this elderly age group, musculoskeletal injuries, particularly if treated by prolonged bed rest, may initiate a series of pathological processes that lead to the patient's progressive deterioration and even to his or her death.

The important *general features* of fractures, dislocations, and soft tissue injuries are dis-

417

cussed in the present chapter so that you may be better prepared to understand and appreciate the significance of the more common *specific* injuries in children and adults, as discussed in the subsequent two chapters. Indeed, your knowledge and understanding of the general features of musculoskeletal injuries, combined with good common sense, will enable you to deduce and to anticipate the appropriate methods of treatment for specific injuries under specific circumstances. As a student, there is much you must learn about musculoskeletal injuries, including their *production, complications, diagnosis,* and *healing process,* and the *general principles,* as well as the *specific methods of their treatment.* Later, during intensive postgraduate hospital training, clinical teachers will instruct you on the *special techniques* of the various methods of treatment through "live demonstrations," the most effective way to teach the *technical details* of treatment.

FRACTURES AND ASSOCIATED INJURIES

A *fracture,* whether of a bone, an epiphyseal plate, or a cartilaginous joint surface, is simply a *structural break in continuity.* Because bones are surrounded by soft tissue, the physical forces that produce a fracture, as well as the physical forces that result from sudden displacement of the fracture fragments, always produce some degree of soft tissue injury as well. When you imagine a fracture, it is natural to visualize a radiographic picture of a broken bone, because radiographs provide such graphic evidence of a fracture. However, they seldom provide evidence of the extent of the associated soft tissue injury. Therefore, you must constantly think in terms of the fracture and of what has happened to the surrounding soft tissues. Sometimes, the associated soft tissue injury, particularly if it involves brain, spinal cord, thoracic or abdominal viscera, a major artery, or a peripheral nerve, may assume much greater clinical significance than the fracture itself.

Physical Factors in the Production of Fractures

To understand why and how a bone breaks, the physical nature of bone itself must be ap-

preciated, as well as the nature of the physical forces required to break it. Normal living bone, rather than being absolutely rigid, has a degree of elasticity or flexibility, and is capable of being bent slightly; it is more like wood in a living tree than it is like a nonliving material such as a stick of chalk.

Cortical bone as a structure can withstand compression and shearing forces better than it can withstand tension forces; in fact the majority of fractures represent *tension failure* of bone, in that bone is actually pulled apart or torn apart by the tension forces of bending, twisting, and straight pull. Thus, a bending (angulatory) force causes a long bone to bend slightly and, if the force is great enough, it suddenly causes an almost explosive tension failure of the bone on the *convex* side of the bend. The failure usually then extends across the entire bone and produces either a *transverse* fracture or an *oblique* fracture (Fig. 15.1). In young children, cortical bone is like green wood in a living young tree. Consequently, an angulatory force may produce tension fail-

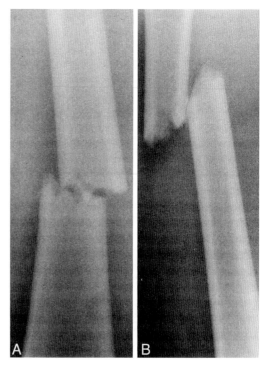

Figure 15.1.   A. Transverse fracture of the femoral shaft. **B.** Oblique fracture of the femoral shaft.

ure on the convex side of the bend and only bending on the concave side of the *greenstick* fracture (Fig. 15.2). A twisting (torsional, rotational) force causes a spiraling type of tension failure in a long bone and produces a *spiral* fracture (Fig. 15.3). A sudden, straight, pulling (traction) force exerted on a small bone (such as the patella) or part of a bone (such as the medial malleolus of the tibia) through attached ligaments or muscle attachments may also result in tension failure of bone and produce an *avulsion* fracture (Fig. 15.4). A fracture that involves the articular cartilage of a joint is referred to as an *intra-articular fracture*.

Cancellous bone, having a sponge-like structure (spongiosa), is more susceptible to crushing (compression) forces than is cortical bone. Sudden compression may produce a *crush* fracture (*compression* fracture) in which one fracture surface is driven, or *impacted*, into its opposing fracture surface (Fig. 15.5). In young children a compression fracture may

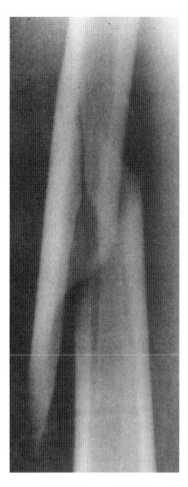

Figure 15.3.   Spiral fracture of the femoral shaft.

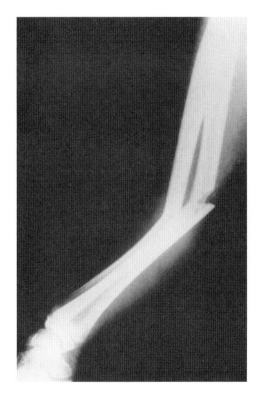

Figure 15.2.   Greenstick fracture of the radius and ulna in a child.

merely "buckle" the thin cortex surrounding the cancellous bone of the metaphysis, producing a *buckle fracture*, sometimes referred to as a "torus fracture" (Fig. 15.6).

The causative force that produces a fracture may be a *direct injury* or blow to the bone by either a sharp or dull object which fractures the bone at the site of impact. More frequently the causative force is an *indirect injury*, in which the initial force is transmitted indirectly through one or more joints to the involved bone, which fractures at some distance from the site of impact.

Descriptive Terms Pertaining to Fractures

The infinite variety and significance of individual fractures necessitates the use of qualifying

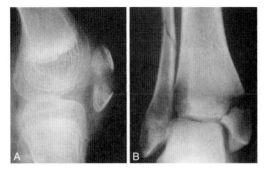

Figure 15.4.   Avulsion fractures. **A.** Avulsion fracture of the patella, which is a sesamoid bone in the quadriceps tendon. The fragments remain distracted because of quadriceps muscle pull. **B.** Avulsion fracture of the medial malleolus that has been pulled off by the intact medial collateral ligament of the ankle at the time of a severe abduction, external rotation injury of the right ankle. Note also the slightly angulated fracture of the fibula and the lateral position of the talus. The attachment of normal ligaments to bone via Sharpey's fibers is so secure that the tendon does not pull out of bone. Tension failure occurs either through the bone or through the ligament first.

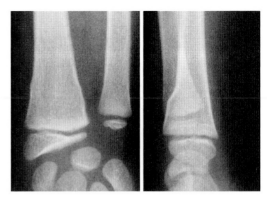

Figure 15.6.   Buckle fracture in the metaphysis of the radius of a 7-year-old boy. The thin cortex has buckled but has not completely broken. In this child, the buckle fracture is more obvious in the lateral projection than in the anteroposterior projection.

terms so that a given fracture may be accurately described. These terms are of great clinical importance because they indicate the nature of the clinical problem and the type of

treatment that will be required. Thus, a fracture is described according to its *site, extent, configuration, the relationship of the fracture fragments to each other, the relationship of the fracture to the external environment* and finally, *the presence or absence of complications.*

1. **Site.** A fracture may be *diaphyseal, metaphyseal, epiphyseal,* or *intra-articular;* if associated with a dislocation of the adjacent joint it is a *fracture-dislocation* (Fig. 15.7).
2. **Extent.** A fracture may be *complete* or *incomplete.* Incomplete fractures include

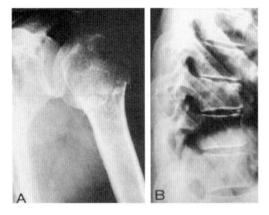

Figure 15.5.   Compression fractures of cancellous bone. **A.** Compression fracture of the surgical neck of the humerus in an elderly adult. Note the impaction of the fracture on the medial side. **B.** Compression fracture of a vertebral body in the midthoracic region of an adult. The vertebral body has lost height anteriorly and has become wedge-shaped as a result of being compressed.

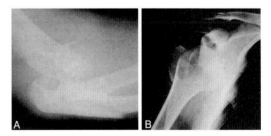

Figure 15.7.   Fracture-dislocations. **A.** Fracture-dislocation of the elbow in an adult. Note the fracture of the shaft of the ulna and the neck of the radius as well as the dislocation of the elbow joint. **B.** Fracture-dislocation of the right shoulder in an adult. Note the fracture of the greater tuberosity of the humerus and the dislocation of the humeral head in relation to the glenoid cavity.

crack or *hairline* fractures (Fig. 15.8), *buckle* fractures (Fig. 15.6) and *greenstick* fractures (Fig. 15.2).

3. **Configuration.** A fracture may be *transverse, oblique* (Fig. 15.1), or *spiral* (Fig. 15.3). With more than one fracture line, and therefore more than two fragments, it is a *comminuted* fracture (Fig. 15.9).

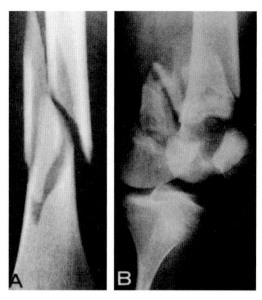

Figure 15.9.   Comminuted fractures. **A.** Comminuted fracture of the shaft of the femur in a child. There are two fracture lines and hence three fragments. Because of its shape, the third fragment in this type of comminuted fracture is referred to as a "butterfly fragment." **B.** Severely comminuted fracture of the distal end of the femur in a young adult who had fallen from a fifth story window. The tremendous force of the impact has shattered the bone into many fragments.

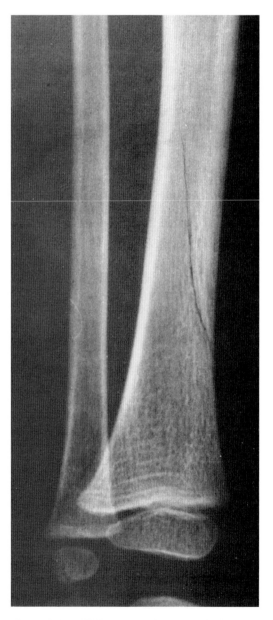

Figure 15.8.   Hairline or crack fracture in the distal third of the tibia in a child. Because there is no displacement, the fracture line is apparent in only one projection.

4. **Relationship of the fracture fragments to each other.** A fracture may be *undisplaced*, or it may be *displaced*, in which case the fracture fragments may be displaced in one or more of the following six ways: 1) *translated (shifted sideways);* 2) *angulated;* 3) *rotated;* 4) *distracted;* 5) *overriding;* 6) *impacted.* At the time the bone is fractured, the causative force usually "follows through," and the degree of displacement of the fragments is maximal at that precise moment. An immediate elastic recoil of the surrounding soft tissues, including periosteum, reduces the displacement to some extent, and the efforts of attendants at the scene of injury to straighten the crooked limb may further reduce the displacement at the fracture site before the patient is seen by an orthopedic surgeon. The relationship of the fracture fragments depends on the effects of gravity, as well as on the ef-

fects of muscle pull on the fragments. These are important factors in the treatment of fractures, as you will see.

5. **Relationship of the fracture to the external environment.** A *closed* fracture is one in which the covering skin is intact. By contrast, an *open* fracture is one that has communicated with the external environment, either because a fracture fragment has penetrated the skin from within or because a sharp object has penetrated the skin to fracture the bone from without (Fig. 15.10). Open fractures, of course, carry the serious risk of becoming complicated by infection. Closed fractures used to be called "simple" and open fractures were "compound"; the terms, *closed* and *open,* however, are more accurate descriptions.

6. **Complications.** A fracture may be *uncomplicated* and remain uncomplicated. It also may be *complicated* or become complicated. The complication may be local or systemic, and it may be caused either by the original injury or by its treatment. A complication that is caused by the treatment is referred to as *iatrogenic* (literally, "caused by the doctor").

Associated Injury to the Periosteum

Because the periosteum is an *osteogenic* sleeve surrounding bone, it is an important structure in relation to fracture healing. The periosteum is thicker, stronger, and more osteogenic during the growing years of childhood than in adult life. In all ages, it is thicker over portions of bone surrounded by muscle (such as the diaphysis, or shaft of the femur) than it is over portions of bone that lie subcutaneously (such as the anteromedial surface of the tibia, or portions of bone that lie within synovial joints, such as the neck of the femur).

The periosteum, being a close-fitting sleeve, is certain to be injured at the moment a bone fractures. In young children the thick periosteum is easily separated from the underlying bone and is not readily torn across; whereas in adults the thin periosteum is more firmly adherent to bone, is less easily separated and is more readily torn across. Except in severely displaced fractures in older children and adults, the periosteal sleeve usually remains intact on at least one side. This portion is referred to as the *intact periosteal hinge* (Fig. 15.11). If the periosteal sleeve is intact around most of its circumference, it can be used to advantage in reducing the fracture and in maintaining the reduction. It also serves as a relatively intact osteogenic sleeve across the fracture site and aids fracture healing. By contrast, a periosteal sleeve that is torn around most of its circumference is of little help in reducing the fracture and in maintaining the reduction, and is ineffective as an aid to fracture healing.

These facts concerning the periosteum help to explain why fractures heal more rapidly and certainly in childhood; why relatively undisplaced fractures heal more rapidly than severely displaced fractures; and why fractures of some bones heal more rapidly than fractures of other bones at any age.

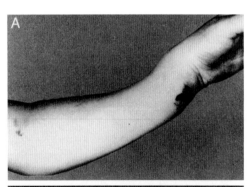
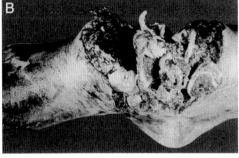

Figure 15.10. Open fractures. **A.** Open fracture of the distal metaphysis of the ulna. A sharp fracture fragment has penetrated the skin from within. **B.** Open fractures of the foot. The blades of a hay mower have penetrated the skin from without and have produced multiple fractures.

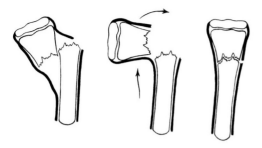

Figure 15.11. The intact periosteal hinge. In the left drawing, the periosteum is intact on the concave side of the angulatory fracture deformity but is torn on the convex side. The middle drawing demonstrates how this type of fracture should be reduced. The fracture deformity is first increased, after which the distal fragment is moved distally. Only then is it possible to engage the fracture surfaces and correct the angulation. The right drawing shows how the intact periosteal hinge helps to prevent overcorrection of the deformity and to maintain the reduction of the fracture. (The role of the intact periosteal hinge is also depicted in Figure 15.36.)

Diagnosis of Fractures and Associated Injuries

Usually when a patient sustains a fracture, both the patient and those who do the transporting are well aware that "a bone has been broken." Under certain circumstances, however, the diagnosis is not at all apparent and careful investigation is necessary lest the serious error of allowing a fracture to go unrecognized is made. This is particularly true when the patient is unable to communicate clearly because of infancy, language barrier, unconsciousness, or mental confusion. Likewise, the fracture may not be obvious when it is undisplaced, or if it is impacted and stable, especially in patients who have sustained multiple serious injuries. Even when the diagnosis of a fracture is obvious, you must be diligent in diagnosis lest you overlook an associated soft tissue injury, a visceral injury, a coexistent dislocation, or even a second fracture (Fig. 15.12). Thus, the methods of obtaining data—the investigation—as outlined in Chapter 5 are as important in the precise diagnosis of musculoskeletal injuries as in the diagnosis of other musculoskeletal conditions.

PATIENT'S HISTORY

The history of a fall, a twisting injury, a direct blow, or a road accident may be given but often the exact details of the *mechanism* of injury are lacking because, as patients sometimes say, "it all happened so suddenly." In addition, one patient may suffer a severe injury without a fracture, whereas another may suffer a seemingly minor injury and sustain a significant fracture. The common symptoms of a fracture are *localized pain*, which is aggravated by movement, and *decreased function* of the involved part. The patient may even have "heard the bone break" or may "feel the ends of the bone grating" (*crepitus*).

Not all fractures are equally painful or interfere equally with function. These manifesta-

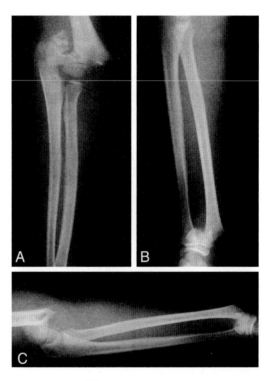

Figure 15.12. The danger of overlooking a second fracture. **A.** If the physical examination revealed an obvious fracture of the elbow and the wrist was not examined also, a radiograph like this might be obtained, which demonstrates a displaced supracondylar fracture of the humerus. **B.** If the physical examination revealed an obvious fracture of the wrist and the elbow was not examined also, a radiograph similar to this might be requested, which demonstrates a displaced fracture of the radius and an undisplaced fracture of the ulna. **C.** Careful physical examination would have led a practitioner to obtain this radiograph, which provides clear evidence of all three fractures.

tions are most severe when the fracture is unstable. Thus, when a patient has sustained a stable fracture of one bone in addition to an unstable fracture of another, the severe pain of the unstable fracture may mask the mild pain of the stable fracture initially until the more severe pain subsides as a result of treatment.

PHYSICAL EXAMINATION

On inspection, you will observe evidence of pain in the patient's facial expression and in the way the patient is protecting the injured part. Local inspection may reveal *swelling* (unless the fractured bone is deep in the tissues, as in the neck of the femur or a vertebral body), *deformity* (angulation, rotation, shortening), or *abnormal movement* (occurring at the fracture site) (Fig. 15.13). Discoloration of the

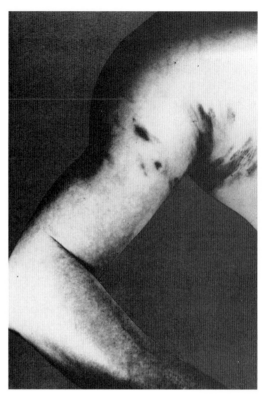

Figure 15.14.   Ecchymosis in the skin of the axilla and upper arm of an adult 3 days after he had sustained a fracture-dislocation of the right shoulder. The hematoma in the deep tissues has gradually spread into the subcutaneous tissues.

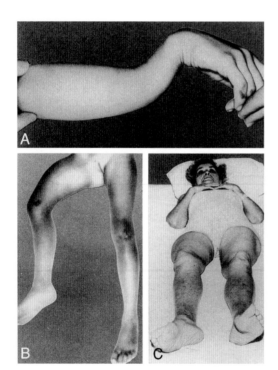

Figure 15.13.   Examples of clinical fracture deformities. **A.** Angulation deformity in the right forearm of a child with a greenstick fracture of the radius and ulna. **B.** Angulation, external rotation and shortening deformities in the right thigh of a child with a completely displaced and overriding fracture of the femoral shaft. **C.** External rotation deformity of the entire right lower limb of an elderly lady with a displaced fracture of the femoral neck.

skin by subcutaneous extravasation of blood (*ecchymosis*) usually is apparent after a few days (Fig. 15.14). By *feeling* (palpation), the examiner can detect *sharply localized tenderness* at the site of fracture as well as *aggravation of pain* and *muscle spasm* during even the slightest passive movement of the injured part. Consequently, feeling or listening for the crepitus of moving bone ends is neither necessary nor kind. You should always look and feel for other less apparent injuries in the same limb and elsewhere, bearing in mind that there may be more than one injury. Many fractures escape detection because of an inadequate physical examination. This, in turn, results in failure to obtain the appropriate diagnostic imaging (Fig. 15.12).

Physical examination must always include a careful assessment of the patient's general condition as well as a diligent search for any associated injuries to brain, spinal cord, peripheral nerves, major vessels, skin, thoracic and abdominal viscera.

DIAGNOSTIC IMAGING

The presence of a fracture can usually be suspected and often established by physical examination alone, but diagnostic imaging is required to determine the exact nature and extent of the fracture.

To avoid causing unnecessary pain or further soft tissue injury, the patient should be provided with some type of radiolucent splint for immobilization before being subjected to radiographic examination (one form of diagnostic imaging). The radiograph should include the entire length of the injured bone and the joints at each end (Fig. 15.15). At least two projections at right angles to each other (*anteroposterior* and *lateral*) are essential for accurate diagnosis (Fig. 15.16). For certain fractures, particularly those of small bones, the ankle, the pelvis, and the vertebrae, special *oblique* projections are often required (Fig. 15.17).

For fractures of the spine and pelvis that may be difficult to visualize by conventional radiography, CT and MRI scans can provide useful additional data (Fig. 15.18).

The radiographic features of a given fracture should provide you with a three-dimensional concept of where the fragments lie in relation to each other and how they came to be in that position (the mechanism of injury). As mentioned previously, however, because of the immediate elastic recoil of the soft tissues, the bone fragments, at the precise moment that the fracture occurred, would have been more widely displaced than at the time of the radiographic examination.

When definite physical signs of a fracture are not confirmed even by additional radiographic projections, you would be wise to treat the patient as though a fracture were present because an undisplaced fracture, which may not be radiographically apparent at first, may become so after 1 or 2 weeks as a result of the healing process (Fig. 15.19).

Normal Healing of Fractures

The normal healing of a fracture is a fascinating biological process, especially because a *fractured bone,* unlike any other tissue that has been torn or divided, is capable of healing *without a scar,* that is, of healing by *bone* rather than by fibrous tissue. An understanding of the response of living bone and periosteum during the healing of a fracture is pivotal in the appreciation of how fractures should be treated. Although mechanical factors of treatment (such as physical immobilization of the fracture fragments) are very important for healing in certain types of fractures, the biological factors are absolutely essential to healing. They must always be respected, to avoid the error of treating fractures as a mechanic or a carpenter would, or of "treating the x-ray picture" at the risk of interfering seriously with the normal biological phenomenon of healing. Fractures are wounds of bone and as with all wounds, treatment must be designed to cooperate with the "laws of nature" concerning biological healing (described as the fourth general principle of fracture treatment in a later section of this chapter).

A number of growth factors secreted by local cells at the fracture site are involved in the fracture healing. These are members of the transforming growth factor beta (TGF-β) superfamily, including insulin-like growth factor (IGF), platelet-derived growth factor (PDGF), and at least seven individual bone

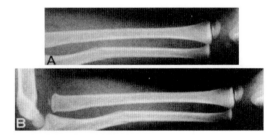

Figure 15.15. The importance of including the entire length of the fractured bone and the joints at each end in the radiographic examination. **A.** This inadequate radiographic examination reveals only an angulated fracture of the ulna. **B.** This radiograph reveals, in addition to the fracture of the ulna, a complete anterior dislocation of the proximal end of the radius in relation to the capitellum. (The combination is known as a Monteggia fracture-dislocation.)

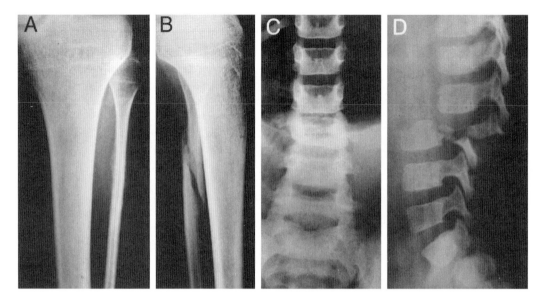

Figure 15.16.   The importance of at least two radiographic projections at right angles to each other (anteroposterior and lateral). **A.** The anteroposterior projection reveals little evidence of disturbance of the tibia or fibula. **B.** The oblique fracture of the fibula is obvious in the lateral projection. **C.** The anteroposterior projection of this severely injured boy reveals relatively little evidence of disturbance of the spine. The radiolucent area across the top half of this radiograph represents gas in a dilated stomach (acute gastric dilatation). **D.** The lateral projection reveals a severe fracture-dislocation of the lumbar spine.

morphogenetic proteins (BMPs). Urist is the discoverer of the osteoinductive BMPs that induce perivascular mesenchymal cells to produce bone at the fracture site. Recombinant human BMP-2 (rh BMP-2) is especially osteoinductive. The interleukins (IL) belong to a group of cell-regulating molecules known as cytokines that also enhance fracture repair.

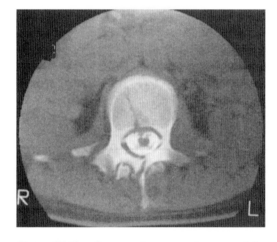

Figure 15.18.   Computed tomography scan of the first lumbar vertebra of a young adult who had sustained a spinal injury from an automobile accident (a cross-sectional "slice" of the spine at this level as viewed from below). Note the fractures of the vertebral body, the lamina (in the midline), and the right transverse process (on the left of the computed tomograph). The fractures of the vertebral body and lamina were not readily detectable in the conventional anteroposterior and lateral radiographs.

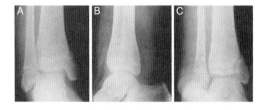

Figure 15.17.   The importance of oblique radiographic projections. **A.** In the anteroposterior projection, there is only slight evidence of a fracture of the medial malleolus. **B.** The lateral projection reveals no evidence of a fracture. **C.** This oblique projection clearly demonstrates a displaced intra-articular fracture of the medial malleolus and disruption of the joint surface as well as of the epiphyseal plate (the physis).

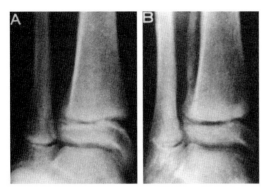

Figure 15.19. Late evidence of a fracture. **A.** Ankle of a 10-year-old boy on the day of injury. He was thought to have a sprained ankle and there is no radiographic evidence of a fracture. **B.** The same boy's ankle 2 weeks later reveals subperiosteal new bone formation along the lateral aspect of the tibia and this provides late evidence that the original injury was a fracture-separation of the distal tibial epiphysis with spontaneous reduction rather than a mere sprain.

The process of fracture healing is different in the dense cortical bone of the shaft of a long bone than in the spongy cancellous bone of the metaphysis of a long bone or the body of a short bone, as you might expect from looking at a cross-section of these two types of bony architecture (Fig. 15.20). These two types of fracture healing, therefore, will be considered separately.

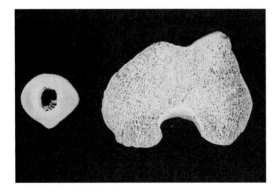

Figure 15.20. Cross-section of the dense cortical bone of the mid-shaft of an adult femur (left) and of the trabeculated sponge-like cancellous bone of the distal metaphyseal region of the same femur. You would expect that fracture healing would differ in these 2 completely different types of bony architecture.

HEALING OF A FRACTURE IN CORTICAL BONE (DIAPHYSEAL BONE; TUBULAR BONE)
Initial Effects of the Fracture

At the moment of fracture in the shaft of a long bone, the tiny blood vessels coursing through the canaliculi in the haversian systems are torn across at the fracture site. After a brief period of local internal bleeding, normal clotting occurs in these tiny vessels and extends for a short distance from the fracture site (to intact anastomosing vessels within bone). Thus the osteocytes in their lacunae for a distance of a few millimeters from the fracture site lose their blood supply and die; consequently there is always a ring of avascular, dead bone at each fracture surface shortly after the injury. These segments of dead bone are eventually replaced by living bone through the simultaneous process of bone resorption and new bone deposition, but it is obvious that initially, the two surfaces of dead bone cannot contribute to the early stages of fracture healing.

In a relatively undisplaced fracture of a long bone, most of the internal bleeding in and around the fresh fracture site comes from the torn nutrient artery or its branches and from the vessels of the periosteal sleeve so that the resultant *fracture hematoma* is well localized around the bone ends. When the fracture site has been severely displaced and the periosteal sleeve severely disrupted, larger arteries in the surrounding muscle and fat are also torn, resulting in a massive hematoma that spreads throughout the surrounding soft tissues.

Early Stages of Healing from Soft Tissues

The fracture hematoma is the medium in which the early stages of healing take place through the reactions of the *soft tissues around the fracture*. The repair cells of fracture healing are osteogenic cells that proliferate from the deep, or cambium, layer of the periosteum to form an *external callus*, and to a lesser extent from endosteum to form an *internal callus*. When the periosteum is severely torn, the healing cells must differentiate from the ingrowth of undifferentiated mesenchymal cells in the surrounding soft tissues. During the early stages of fracture healing, a population explosion of osteogenic cells results in an extremely rapid growth of osteogenic tissue, more rapid than the rate of growth of the most malignant bone neoplasm. Indeed, by the end of the first few weeks, the *fracture callus* consists of a thick enveloping mass of osteogenic tissue.

At this stage the callus does not contain bone and is radiolucent, that is, not apparent radiographically. The fracture callus, initially soft and almost fluid in consistency, becomes progressively firmer like a slowly setting glue, and the fracture site becomes "stickier" and less mobile. Histologically, this stage of callus maturation is characterized by new bone formation in the osteogenic callus, first at a site away from the fracture (where the periosteum still has a good blood supply and where there is least movement). Chapter 2 noted that whenever new bone is formed rapidly, it is the *primary woven type of bone*—early fracture healing is a good example of this phenomenon. Thus, the osteogenic cells differentiate into osteoblasts, and primary woven bone is formed. Closer to the fracture site, where the blood supply is less adequate and more movement is taking place, the osteogenic cells differentiate into chondroblasts and cartilage is formed initially.

Stage of Clinical Union

A temporary external and internal callus, consisting of a mixture of primary woven bone and cartilage, comes to surround the fracture site, forming a "biological glue" that gradually hardens as the cartilaginous components of the callus are replaced by bone through a process of endochondral ossification. When fracture callus becomes sufficiently firm that movement no longer occurs at the fracture site, the fracture is said to be clinically united (*clinical union*), but it has by no means been restored to its original strength. Radiographic examination reveals evidence of bone in the callus but the fracture line is still apparent. Histological examination reveals varying amounts of primary woven bone, as well as cartilage undergoing endochondral ossification.

Stage of Consolidation (Radiographic Union)

As time goes on, the primary, or temporary callus, is gradually replaced by mature lamellar bone, and the excess callus is gradually resorbed. Many months after the fracture, when all the immature bone and cartilage of the temporary callus have been replaced by mature lamellar bone, the fracture is said to be *consolidated* by sound bony union (*radiographic union*). Once bony union has been established, the now redundant mass of callus is gradually resorbed, and the bone eventually returns to almost its normal diameter. Sharp corners of residual angulation, displacement, or overriding become smoothed off or remodeled by the process of simultaneous bone deposition and bone resorption—another example of *Wolff's law* (previously described in Chapter 2). Although the corners of a residual angulation deformity become rounded off, the actual change in alignment tends to persist, except under certain circumstances during childhood when subsequent epiphyseal growth may partially correct such malalignment spontaneously.

The various stages of fracture healing in cortical bone are illustrated in a series of radiographs of a diaphyseal (shaft) fracture in a child (Fig. 15.21).

HEALING OF A FRACTURE IN CORTICAL BONE WITH RIGID INTERNAL FIXATION

When a fracture in cortical bone has been accurately reduced at open operation, and the fracture fragments have been compressed and then held by rigid internal fixation by metallic devices (osteosynthesis), the fracture site is stress protected and indeed the bone hardly knows it has been fractured. The Association for Osteosynthesis/Association for the Study of Internal Fixation (AO/ASIF) system of fracture treatment (which originated in Switzerland in 1958 and is described in a subsequent section of this chapter) achieves such reduction and fixation. Under these circumstances, there is no stimulus for the production of either external callus from the periosteum or internal callus from the endosteum

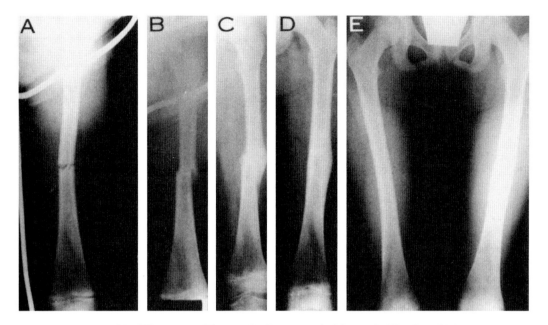

Figure 15.21. The stages of fracture healing in cortical bone. **A.** The day of injury, a transverse fracture is seen in the midshaft of the left femur of this 8-year-old girl. The fracture has been aligned by means of continuous traction and a Thomas splint (part of which is seen in this radiograph). **B.** Two weeks after injury, callus is evident on the lateral aspect of the fracture and has "glued" the fragments together. At this stage the fracture was clinically "sticky" and, consequently, continuous traction was replaced by a hip spica cast. **C.** Eight weeks after injury, callus is abundant and the fracture line is barely apparent. Clinical examination at this stage revealed no movement at the fracture site and no pain on attempting to move it. Thus the fracture had healed to the stage of clinical union. The cast was removed and full weightbearing was allowed. **D.** Six months after injury, the excess callus has been resorbed, the medullary cavity has been re-established and fracture healing has reached the stage of radiographic consolidation. **E.** Eighteen months after injury, the fractured femur has returned almost to its normal shape through the process of remodeling, which is an example of Wolff's law.

and consequently, the fracture healing occurs directly between the cortex of one fracture fragment and the cortex of the other fracture fragment. This process is referred to by the AO/ASIF fracture surgeons as primary bone healing, as opposed to the secondary bone healing involving external and internal fracture callus. In the areas of precise contact (that are under compression), osteoclastic "cutter heads" cross the microscopic fracture site and are followed by new bridging osteons. Even when there is a tiny gap, the healing is direct by the formation of new osteons that become oriented through haversian remodeling to the axis of the bone.

As long as the metallic device, such as a rigid plate, remains in place, the bone underlying the plate continues to be stress protected, because the normal stresses bypass the bone through the plate. Thus the bone in this region tends to develop disuse osteoporosis, which is sometimes referred to as "stress-relief osteoporosis." For this reason, when the fracture has united, the plate and screws may have to be removed to allow reversal of this osteoporosis. Nevertheless, the removal of fixation devices from healed bones is no longer "routine." During the ensuing few months, the healed bone must be protected from excessive stress until it regains its normal strength. In recent years, the AO/ASIF surgeons have become less rigid in their thinking about the need for rigidity in their internal fixation devices.

HEALING OF A FRACTURE IN CANCELLOUS BONE (METAPHYSEAL BONE AND CUBOIDAL BONES)

Cancellous bone (sponge bone) in the flared out metaphysis of long bones and in the bodies of short bones, (cuboidal bones) as well as in the flat bones such as the pelvis and ribs, consists of a spongelike lattice of delicate interconnected trabeculae. The surrounding cortex, which is a relatively thin shell of cortical bone, represents only a small fraction of the cross-sectional area of these bones in contrast to the shafts of long bones, which may be considered as hollow tubes with thick walls of dense cortical bone (Fig. 15.20). Just as the structural arrangement of these two types of bone differs, so also does the process of healing after a fracture.

The healing of a fracture in cancellous bone occurs principally through the formation of an *internal* or *endosteal* callus, although the external or periosteal callus surrounding the thin shell of cortex does play an important role, particularly in children. Because of the rich blood supply to the thin trabeculae of cancellous bone, little necrosis of bone occurs at the fracture surfaces, and there is a large area of bony contact at the fracture site. Therefore, in relatively undisplaced fractures and in well-reduced fractures through cancellous bone, union of the fragments proceeds more rapidly than in dense cortical bone. The osteogenic repair cells of the endosteal covering of trabeculae proliferate to form primary woven bone in the internal fracture hematoma. The resultant *internal callus* fills the open spaces of the spongy cancellous fracture surfaces and spreads across the fracture site wherever there is good contact.

Thus, early fracture healing in cancellous

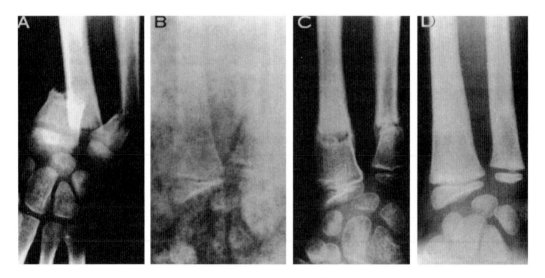

Figure 15.22.   The stages of fracture healing in cancellous bone. **A.** The day of injury a transverse, angulated overriding fracture of the metaphyseal region of the distal end of the radius and an angulated fracture of the same region of the ulna are seen in this radiograph of the wrist of a 10-year-old boy. **B.** The same day, the post reduction radiograph (taken through the plaster cast) reveals satisfactory reduction of both fractures. **C.** Six weeks after injury, endosteal callus and periosteal callus are adequate, although the fracture lines are still apparent. At this stage there was no movement at the fracture site and no pain on attempts to move it. This is the stage of clinical union and immobilization was discontinued. **D.** Six months after injury, radiographic examination reveals obliteration of the fracture line. The fracture healing has reached the stage of radiographic consolidation. Internal and external remodeling of bone at the fracture sites is also apparent. Note the amount of longitudinal bone growth that has taken place from the epiphyseal plates since the injury (the distance between the epiphyseal plate and the fine radiopaque line (Harris line) just proximal to it).

bone occurs at sites of direct contact between the cancellous fracture surfaces by means of endosteal callus. Once union is established at a point of contact, the fracture is clinically united and union spreads across the entire width of the bone. Then, the woven bone is replaced by lamellar bone as the fracture becomes *consolidated*. Eventually the trabecular pattern is re-established by internal remodeling of bone. You will recall that cancellous bone, unlike cortical bone, is particularly susceptible to forces that result in a compression, or crush-type, fracture. Impaction of cancellous fragments provides a broad surface contact for fracture healing. If the crushed surfaces are pulled apart (during reduction of the fracture), a space, or gap, is created, healing is delayed, and there may be subsequent collapse at the fracture site before bony union is consolidated.

The various stages of fracture healing in cancellous bone are illustrated in a series of radiographs of a metaphyseal fracture (Fig. 15.22).

HEALING OF A FRACTURE IN ARTICULAR CARTILAGE

In contrast to bone, the hyaline cartilage of joint surfaces is extremely limited in its ability to either heal or regenerate. Whereas a fracture through bone normally heals by bone, a fracture through articular cartilage either heals by fibrous scar tissue or fails to heal at all. If the fracture surfaces of the cartilage are perfectly reduced, the thin scar leads to local degenerative arthritis. If there is a gap, the fibrous tissue that comes to fill this gap will not withstand the normal wear and tear of joint function and more widespread degenerative changes ensue. Furthermore, any irregularity, such as a "step" in the fractured joint surface, that produces joint incongruity leads inevitably to degenerative arthritis (Fig. 15.23).

In my laboratory, we have investigated the biological effects of immobilization (cast), intermittent active motion (cage activity), and continuous passive motion (CPM) on the healing of the articular cartilage in an experimental model of an intra-articular fracture in the rabbit. The accurate reduction of the fracture was maintained by a metal screw. At 4 weeks postoperatively, we found that in the immobilized casted knees, the fracture in the cartilage had not healed by cartilage. It had healed by cartilage in only 20% of the cage activity group, compared to 80% of the CPM group (Fig. 15.24). We then conducted a

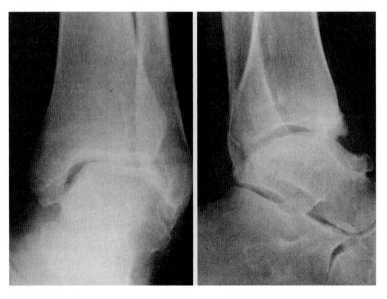

Figure 15.23.   Posttraumatic degenerative arthritis in the ankle of a 57-year-old man whose original intra-articular fracture had occurred 25 years previously. Note the incongruity of the joint surfaces, subchondral sclerosis, and osteophyte formation.

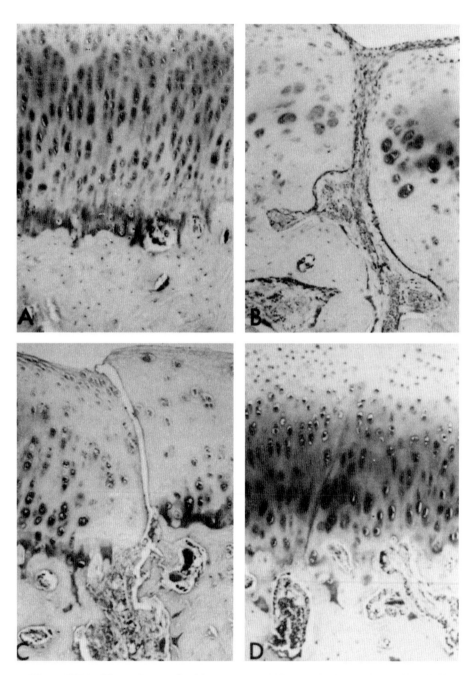

Figure 15.24.   Photomicrograph of the experimental fracture site in articular cartilage (safranin O stain). **A.** Normal intact articular cartilage of the femoral condyle of a rabbit. **B.** After 4 weeks of cast immobilization, the fracture in the cartilage has healed by fibrous scar tissue. **C.** After 4 weeks of cage activity, the fracture has failed to heal. **D.** After 4 weeks of CPM, the fracture in the cartilage has healed well.

long-term study at 6 months in another series of rabbits in which, after a 1- or 3-week period of postoperative management by one of the three aforementioned methods, the animals were allowed to run freely for the remaining 6 months. From this investigation we found that degenerative arthritis had developed in 90% of the knees managed postoperatively by immobilization for 1 or 3 weeks, in 76% of the knees managed by cage activity throughout the 6 months, compared to only 20% of the knees managed postoperatively by either 1 or 3 weeks of CPM. These experimental investigations are relevant to the immediate postoperative management of patients with intra-articular fractures after open reduction and internal fixation.

HEALING OF A FRACTURE INVOLVING THE EPIPHYSEAL PLATE (THE PHYSIS)

The inclusion of an epiphyseal plate (physis) in a fracture alters the picture of fracture healing considerably and adds the risk of local growth disturbance. The normal healing of fractures that involve the epiphyseal plate is discussed, along with other important aspects of these special injuries of childhood, in Chapter 16.

TIME REQUIRED FOR UNCOMPLICATED FRACTURE HEALING

The healing time of fractures is extremely varied, but it is possible to estimate healing time by considering the following important factors: age of the patient, site and configuration of the fracture, initial displacement, and the blood supply to the fracture fragments.

Age of the Patient

The rate of healing in bone varies much more with age than it does in any other tissue in the body, particularly during childhood. At birth, fracture healing is remarkably rapid, but it becomes less rapid with each year of childhood. From early adult life to old age, the rate of fracture healing remains relatively constant. It would seem that the rate of healing in bone is closely related to the osteogenic activity of periosteum and endosteum, which, in turn, is

related to the normal process of remodeling of bone. This process, remarkably active at birth, becomes progressively less active with each year of childhood and remains relatively constant from early adult life to old age. Fractures of the shaft of the femur serve as an example of this phenomenon: a fracture occurring at birth will be united in 3 weeks; a comparable fracture at the age of 8 years will be united in 8 weeks; at the age of 12 years, it will be united in 12 weeks; and from the age of 20 years to old age it will be united in approximately 20 weeks.

Site and Configuration of the Fracture

Fractures through bones that are surrounded by muscle heal more rapidly than fractures through portions of bones that lie subcutaneously or within joints. Fractures through cancellous bone heal more rapidly than fractures through cortical bone; epiphyseal separations heal approximately twice as quickly as cancellous metaphyseal fractures of the same bone in the same age group. Long oblique fractures and spiral fractures of the shaft, having a large fracture surface, heal more readily than transverse fractures having a small fracture surface.

Initial Displacement of the Fracture

Undisplaced fractures, having an intact periosteal sleeve, heal approximately twice as fast as displaced fractures. The greater the initial displacement, the more extensive is the tearing of the periosteal sleeve, and the more prolonged is the healing time of the fracture.

Blood Supply to the Fragments

If both fracture fragments have a good blood supply and are alive, the fracture will heal provided there are no other complications. If, however, one fragment has lost its blood supply and is dead, the living fragment must become united, or fused, to the dead fragment in the same manner as living bone in a host site becomes united to a dead bone graft. Union will be slow and rigid immobilization of the fracture will be required. If both fragments are avascular, bony union cannot occur until they are revascularized, despite rigid immobilization of the fracture.

ASSESSMENT OF FRACTURE HEALING IN PATIENTS

The state of union of a fracture is assessed by both clinical and radiographic examination. The clinical examination for union consists of applying bending, twisting, and compression forces to the fracture to determine the presence, or absence, of movement (Fig. 15.25A). If there is considerable movement at the fracture site, it can be seen as well as felt by both patient and examiner. If there is only minimal movement, the patient alone will feel it because it is painful. Thus, if neither you nor the patient is able to detect movement at the fracture site, the fracture is *clinically united* (Fig. 15.25B).

At the time of *clinical union,* radiographic examination reveals evidence of bony callus, but the fracture line is still apparent because clinical union precedes radiographic consolidation (Figs. 15.21 and 15.22). At this stage

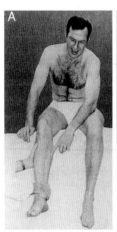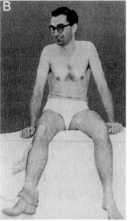

Figure 15.25. Clinical assessment of fracture healing in patients. **A.** Bending and twisting forces applied to this man's leg produce only minimal movement at the fracture site but cause the patient local pain as he is indicating. Note his facial expression of pain. His fracture is not yet clinically united. **B.** Bending and twisting forces applied to this man's leg produce neither movement nor pain at the fracture site. Note his painless facial expression. Therefore, his fracture is clinically united.

immobilization is no longer required, but the healing bone has not regained its normal strength; consequently, it must still be protected from undue stress until *radiographic consolidation* has been achieved, as evidenced by a bony callus that completely bridges the fracture and obliterates the fracture line (Figs. 15.21 and 15.22). The reestablishment of the medullary cavity in shaft fractures and of the trabeculae across fractures in cancellous bone are radiographic evidence of the *remodeling phase* of united fractures.

Abnormal Healing of Fractures

The healing of a given fracture may be abnormal in one of three ways:

1. The fracture may heal in the normally expected time but in an unsatisfactory position with residual bony deformity (*malunion*).
2. The fracture may heal eventually but it takes considerably longer than the normally expected time to do so (*delayed union*).
3. The fracture may fail completely to heal by bone (*nonunion*) with resultant formation of either a *fibrous union* or a false joint (*pseudarthrosis*).

Malunion, delayed union, and nonunion are discussed further in this chapter in the section that deals with the recognition and treatment of the complications of fractures.

Complications of Fractures

Fortunately the majority of fractures are uncomplicated by any serious associated injury or serious reaction to injury. With reasonable treatment the injured patient may be expected to make a full recovery without any significant disability. However, some fractures are either accompanied by or followed by *complications,* some of which have serious local consequences, whereas others endanger not only limb but life itself.

Before proceeding to a discussion of the general principles of fracture treatment, be aware of the possible complications of fractures to avoid the error of focusing only on the fractured bone and overlooking an associated complication. A fracture may be complicated initially by an associated injury, or it may become complicated subsequently, either *early* or *late*. The complication may be *local* at the fracture site or *remote* in other organs. It may be caused by the original injury or it may be iatrogenic, that is, resulting from the doctor's treatment of the injury.

Those complications of fractures that are the result of the injury itself are classified below; those that are iatrogenic are classified after a discussion of fracture treatment. The recognition and treatment of all complications of fractures are discussed together in a subsequent section of this chapter.

CLASSIFICATION OF THE COMPLICATIONS OF THE ORIGINAL INJURY

I. Initial (immediate) complications
   A. Local complications (associated injuries)
      1. Skin injuries
         a) From without: abrasions, laceration, puncture wound, penetrating missile wound, avulsion, loss of skin
         b) From within: penetration of the skin by a fracture fragment
      2. Vascular injuries
         a) Injury to a major artery: division, contusion, arterial spasm
         b) Injury to a major vein: division, contusion
         c) Local hemorrhage
            External
            Internal
            Into soft tissues—hematoma
            Into body cavities—intracranial hemorrhage, hemothorax, hemoperitoneum, hemarthrosis
      3. Neurological injuries
         a) Brain
         b) Spinal cord
         c) Peripheral nerves
      4. Muscular injuries
         a) Division (usually incomplete)
      5. Visceral injuries
         a) Thoracic—heart and great vessels, trachea, bronchi and lungs
         b) Intra-abdominal gastrointestinal tract, liver, spleen, urinary tract
   B. Remote complications
      1. Multiple injuries
         Simultaneous injuries to other parts of the body (unrelated to a fracture)
      2. Hemorrhagic shock
II. Early complications
   A. Local complications
      1. Sequelae of immediate complications
         Skin necrosis, gangrene, Volkmann's ischemia (compartment syndromes), gas gangrene, venous thrombosis, visceral complications
      2. Joint complications
         Infection (septic arthritis)—from an open injury
      3. Bony complications
         Infection (osteomyelitis) at fracture site—from an open injury
         Avascular necrosis of bone—usually of one fragment
   B. Remote complications
      1. Fat embolism
      2. Pulmonary embolism
      3. Pneumonia
      4. Tetanus
      5. Delirium tremens
III. Late complications
   A. Local complications
      1. Joint complications
         a) Persistent joint stiffness
         b) Posttraumatic degenerative arthritis
      2. Bony complications
         a) Abnormal fracture healing: malunion, delayed union, nonunion
         b) Growth disturbance—from epiphyseal plate (physeal) injury
         c) Persistent infection (chronic osteomyelitis)
         d) Posttraumatic osteoporosis

      e) Sudeck's posttraumatic painful osteoporosis (reflex sympathetic dystrophy, sympathetically mediated pain syndrome)

      f) Refracture

   3. Muscular complications

      a) Posttraumatic myositis ossificans

      b) Late rupture of tendons

   4. Neurological complications

     Tardy nerve palsy

 B. Remote complications

   1. Renal calculi

   2. Accident neurosis

General Principles of Fracture Treatment

The six general principles of treatment for all musculoskeletal conditions discussed in Chapter 6 are as applicable to traumatic musculoskeletal conditions (fractures, dislocations, associated soft tissue injuries) as they are to non-traumatic musculoskeletal disorders. A review of these general principles is necessary before you proceed to learn about their application to the treatment of fractures and associated injuries.

1. First, Do No Harm

Whereas some of the problems and complications of fractures are caused by the original injury, others are caused by the treatment of the injury and are iatrogenic (from the Greek iatros, meaning *physician* or *surgeon,* and genic, meaning *produced by*). The incidence and significance of such iatrogenic complications are evidenced by the increasing frequency and magnitude of lawsuits initiated by dissatisfied patients or their relatives against their physician or surgeon. Many of these lawsuits are preventable, at least those that result from a combination of unrealistic expectations by the patient or relatives and inadequate communication between the treating physician or surgeon and the patient and relatives. In addition, many of the iatrogenic complications themselves are preventable; their prevention is one of the important general principles of fracture treatment. The recognition, prevention, and treatment of such complications are discussed in a subsequent section of this chapter, but a few examples are listed here: a) further damage to important soft tissues by careless first aid treatment and reckless transportation of the patient to the hospital as well as within it; b) damage to soft tissues such as skin, blood vessels, and nerves by incorrectly applied plaster casts as well as by excessive traction; c) opening the path to infection of the fracture site by the careless and injudicious application of open reduction with internal skeletal fixation.

2. Base Treatment on an Accurate Diagnosis and Prognosis

The necessity for accurate clinical and radiographic diagnosis of fractures and associated injuries has already been stressed. In addition to diagnosing a fracture and any associated soft tissue injury, the necessary information must be gathered to make a reasonable estimate of the prognosis of the injury. The choice of the specific method of treatment of a fracture must be based on its prognosis.

The following factors are of particular importance in relation to the healing of uncomplicated fractures: age of the patient, site and configuration of the fracture, amount of initial displacement, and the blood supply to the fracture fragments. The significance of these factors has already been discussed in a previous section of this chapter. In general, when good external (periosteal) callus can be expected, as in a shaft fracture without excessive periosteal disruption, or when a combination of periosteal and internal (endosteal) callus can be expected, as in an impacted metaphyseal fracture, perfect reduction and rigid fixation (rigid immobilization) are not essential. By contrast, when healing can be expected to occur from endosteal callus *alone,* as in a fracture of the neck of the femur where the periosteum is exceedingly thin or in an intra-articular fracture of a small bone such as the carpal scaphoid, perfect reduction and rigid fixation are essential.

The first decision is whether the fracture requires reduction and if so, what type is best—closed or open. The second decision concerns the type of immobilization, if any, required—external or internal.

3. Select Treatment with Specific Aims

The specific aims of fracture treatment are: a) to relieve pain; b) to obtain and maintain satisfactory position of the fracture fragments; c) to allow or encourage bony union; d) to restore optimum function in the fractured limb or spine and in the patient as a whole person.

a) *To relieve pain.* Because bone is relatively insensitive, the pain from a fracture arises from the associated injury to the soft tissues, including periosteum and endosteum. The pain is aggravated by movement of the fracture fragments, associated muscle spasm, and progressive swelling in a closed space. Thus, the pain from a fracture can usually be relieved by immobilizing the fracture site and by avoiding a too tight encircling bandage or cast. During the first few days after a fracture, analgesics may be required, provided there is no compromise of circulation in the involved limb.

b) *To obtain and maintain satisfactory position of the fracture fragments.* Some fractures are either undisplaced, or displaced so little that no reduction is indicated. Reduction of a fracture to obtain a satisfactory position is indicated only when it will be necessary to obtain good function, to prevent subsequent degenerative arthritis, or to obtain an acceptable clinical appearance of the injured part. It is not necessary to obtain a perfect radiographic appearance of the bone; remember that it is a patient and his or her fracture being treated, not a radiograph. Maintenance of satisfactory position of the fracture fragments usually requires some degree of immobilization, which may be achieved by a variety of methods, including continuous traction, a plaster-of-Paris cast, external skeletal fixation, and internal skeletal fixation, depending on the degree of stability or instability of the reduction.

c) *To allow and, if necessary, to encourage bony union.* In most fractures, union will occur provided that the natural healing processes are allowed to occur. In certain fractures, however, such as those with severe tearing of the periosteum and surrounding soft tissues or those with avascular necrosis of one or both fragments, union must be encouraged by the judicious use of autogenous bone grafts, either early or late in the healing process.

d) *To restore optimum function.* During the period of immobilization of the healing fracture, disuse atrophy of regional muscles must be prevented by active static (isometric) exercises of those muscles that control the immobilized joints and active dynamic (isotonic) exercises of all other muscles in the limb or trunk. The preservation of good muscle power and tone throughout this period improves local circulation and facilitates subsequent restoration of normal joint motion and optimum function in the fractured limb or spine and in the patient as a whole person. After the period of immobilization, active exercises should be continued even more vigorously. Rehabilitation of the whole person, as discussed in Chapter 6, is always important but usually presents problems only when the fracture has involved a particularly long period of treatment or is associated with serious complications.

4. Cooperate with the "Laws of Nature"

The musculoskeletal tissues react to a fracture in accordance with "laws of nature," as described in a previous section of this chapter dealing with the normal healing of uncomplicated fractures. Treatment must respect and cooperate with these natural laws of tissue behavior to avoid preventing or even delaying normal healing. For example, inadequate protection and immobilization, excessive traction with resultant distraction at the fracture site, operative destruction of blood supply to fragments, and postoperative infection all delay fracture healing and may prevent it. Treatment of a fracture should be planned to create the ideal setting and circumstances so that the patient's natural restorative powers and tissues can reach their full potential. In addition, a knowledge of the natural laws of late remodeling of a healed fracture at various sites and at various ages is important in determining how much deformity at the site of a fracture can be accepted.

5. Make Treatment Realistic and Practical

When considering a specific method of treatment for a fracture, common sense and sound judgement will lead you to ask yourself three important questions concerning the proposed method.

a) *Precisely what am I aiming to accomplish by this method; what is its specific aim or goal?* The specific aims of fracture treatment have been discussed above.

b) *Am I likely to accomplish this aim or goal by this method of treatment?* This question can be answered in part as a result of your knowledge of the previously discussed factors in the prognosis of fractures. In addition, as will be discussed later, certain fractures, such as displaced fractures of the lateral condyle of the humerus in children and displaced fractures of the neck of the femur in adults, cannot be adequately treated by means of external immobilization alone. Such fractures require accurate reduction and internal fixation.

c) *Will the anticipated end result justify the means or method; will it be worth it to your patient in terms of what he or she will have to endure—the risks, the discomfort, the period away from home, work, or school?* This question is of particular importance in fracture treatment. For example, intertrochanteric fractures of the femur in the elderly will nearly always unite whether treated by continuous traction and prolonged immobilization of the patient (bed rest) and the limb, or by operative reduction with internal skeletal fixation and early mobilization of both patient and limb. For an elderly patient, however, the risk of prolonged bed rest is too great, in that it may initiate a series of pathological events that lead to progressive deterioration and even to death. Under such circumstances, operative treatment is preferable because it carries less risk for the elderly person than prolonged bed rest.

6. Select Treatment for Your Patient as an Individual

A given fracture may present an entirely different problem for one individual than for another, particularly in relation to age, sex, occupation, and any coexistent disease. For example, residual deformity of a healed fracture (malunion) of the clavicle presents little problem for a young child (because it will remodel over the growing years) or for a laboring man (because he is not concerned about its appearance), but it may be quite distressing for a female model or an actress. Likewise, malunion of a finger fracture may not interfere

significantly with hand function for a taxi driver but it may be catastrophic for a concert pianist. Therefore, the choice of fracture treatment must be tailored to fit the needs of your patient.

Emergency Life Support Systems

As an undergraduate student you should avail yourself of courses in Basic Life Support (BLS) and Advanced Trauma Life Support (ATLS).

Basic life support (BLS) includes a series of emergency life-saving procedures designed to treat acute failure of the respiratory system, the cardiovascular system, or both without the use of complex mechanical devices. These procedures, which constitute cardiopulmonary resuscitation (CPR) must be started as soon as possible after the emergency has occurred. They are indicated for the following life-threatening emergencies of the ABCs System:

A—Airway (obstruction)
B—Breathing (respiratory arrest)
C—Circulation (cardiac arrest or severe bleeding)

Advanced trauma life support (ATLS) includes more advanced hospital procedures, such as cardiac monitoring, defibrillation, and administering intravenous fluids, medications, and airway devices (such as an endotracheal tube). These procedures may be performed by highly trained emergency medical technicians (EMTs), or paramedics. The ABC system used for basic life support is also used for advanced trauma life support.

Preliminary Care For Patients with Fractures

The interval between the time an individual is injured and the time definitive treatment in a hospital is received may vary from less than 1 hour to several hours or more (and it always seems longer to the injured person and the relatives). During this interval, much can be done to deal with life-threatening injuries, to prevent further injury, and to make the patient more comfortable. This preliminary care for patients with fractures is best considered in three phases: 1) immediate care outside a hospital (resuscitation and first aid); 2) care during transportation to hospital; 3) emergency care in a hospital.

Immediate Care Outside a Hospital (First Aid)

As a healthcare professional who happens on the scene of an accident, you should always accept the moral obligation to stop and render help to the injured. The summoning of emergency services—police, firemen, ambulance—can usually be delegated to someone else while you create order out of disorder, make a rapid assessment of the situation, and initiate immediate care of the injured, relying on the following basic life support system. The ABC priorities are discussed in their order of urgency.

Airway (Obstruction)

If the injured person is unconscious (from fainting, shock, or head injury), the airway may become obstructed by the tongue having dropped back into the pharynx or by aspiration of mucus, blood, vomitus, or a foreign body. This life-threatening complication can usually be relieved by gently rolling the person to the prone position, pulling the jaw and tongue forward, and clearing the pharynx with a finger. During this maneuver, the patient's neck should not be moved just in case there is a coexistent cervical fracture.

Breathing (Respiratory Arrest)

Once the airway has been cleared, mouth-to-mouth resuscitation is required if the patient is not breathing.

Circulation (Cardiac Arrest or Severe Bleeding)

For cardiac arrest, CPR is required. For severe external bleeding, the most effective method of control is firm manual pressure applied to the open wound through a temporary dressing improvised from the cleanest material available. Local pressure on an extremity wound is not only more effective than a tourniquet but also much safer. A tourniquet that is applied too loosely occludes only the venous

return, which increases the bleeding, whereas a tourniquet that is too tight or left on too long causes permanent damage to blood vessels, nerves, and other soft tissues. Firefighters play an extremely important part, using varieties of the "Jaws of Life" in extricating injured individuals who are trapped within a crushed vehicle (Fig. 15.26D).

The most severe bleeding may be hidden because it is internal, (intra-abdominal, intra-thoracic, or within the soft tissues of an extremity).

Shock

At the scene of an accident, you can at least help to prevent shock or an increase in severity of existing shock by controlling hemorrhage and minimizing pain. Pallor combined with cold, moist skin and a weak, rapid pulse are the most obvious manifestations of shock. Careless and rough handling of an injured person aggravates both pain and shock and must be avoided. Neither food nor fluids should be given by mouth during the preliminary treatment of an injured person who may require a general anesthetic shortly after admission to hospital.

Fractures and Dislocations

Obvious fractures and dislocations of the limbs should be splinted before the person is moved to minimize pain and to prevent further injury to the soft tissues. Traction applied slowly and steadily is the most effective and least painful way of straightening a gross deformity and of holding an injured limb while it is being splinted. An injured upper limb is best splinted by being bound to the person's trunk; an injured lower limb can be bound to the opposite lower limb. Temporary limb splints can also be improvised from many available objects (Fig. 15.26A, B, C). Spinal injury may be less obvious. Its presence or absence should be determined by testing for local tenderness along the spine before the injured person is moved, because movement, particularly flexion, of an injured spinal column endangers the spinal cord and nerve roots.

Pertinent information concerning the circumstances of the accident, injuries sustained,

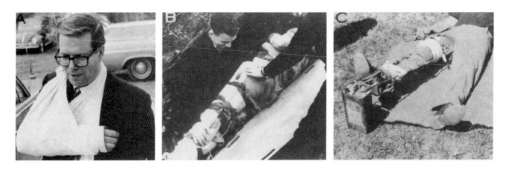

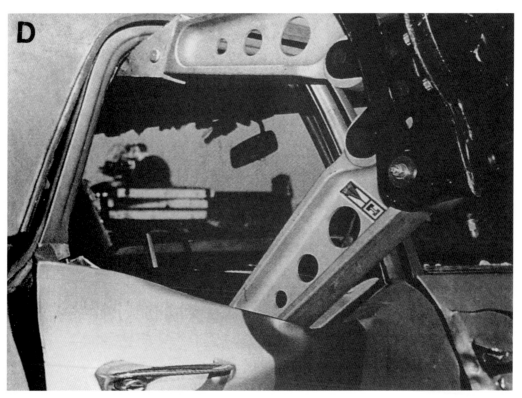

Figure 15.26. Temporary limb splints at the scene of an accident. **A.** Upper limb splint. A short board has been bandaged to this man's fractured forearm before the sling is applied. For an injury above the elbow, a second sling or bandage can be used to bind the upper limb to the trunk. **B.** Lower limb splint. A long board has been bandaged to this man's injured lower limb and then the two lower limbs have been bound together. He was also thought to have a spinal injury and so is being gently rolled onto a long spinal board. **C.** Temporary Thomas splint that has been applied by an ambulance attendant for a man with an open fracture of the femur. The pressure dressing over the open wound and the splint were applied before the accident victim was transported to hospital. **D.** The "jaws of life" being used by a firefighter to spread open a jammed car door to extricate a trapped occupant.

and their emergency treatment should be transmitted to ambulance attendants so that it will be available to hospital attendants.

Transportation

Individuals with major injuries deserve gentle care while being placed in an ambulance or other suitable vehicle. Unless there is no alternative, they should not be squeezed into the narrow confines of a car seat. Those who may have sustained a spinal injury require extremely careful handling. They should be lifted onto a stretcher or suitable alternative, such as a door, by at least two, and preferably four, individuals so that the spine is kept straight while the person is lifted as "an immobilized unit." When possible, a short spinal board should be strapped to the injured person's back before he or she is moved (Fig. 15.27). Likewise, a cervical collar should be applied in case there is a cervical spine injury. Motorcycle or football helmets should not be removed at this time. During the trip to hospital in an ambulance, good care and comfort are much more important to the injured person than careless speed. There is seldom justification for an ambulance driver to break local traffic laws; furthermore, a jolting, swinging ride is painful and dangerous for the injured person and dangerous to others. The modern well-equipped ambulance should be a mobile minor emergency room complete with suction and an oxygen inhalator (Fig. 15.28A). The attendants are well-trained paramedics (Fig. 15.28B). Emergency medical technicians or paramedics merit and appreciate commendation when they have effectively carried out their essential part of the preliminary care of the injured. Their expertise and dedication have saved vast numbers of lives. The use of helicopters or even fixed-wing aircrafts as air ambulances (MEDEVAC) has become very common, particularly in situations where ground travel is impractical or unsatisfactory, such as rough terrain or dense highway traffic. (Figs.15.28C, D).

Emergency Care in a Hospital

On the patient's arrival at the hospital, all essential information should be gathered from the patient, if possible, as well as from rela-

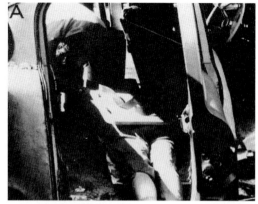
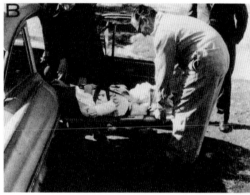

Figure 15.27. Moving an accident victim who has a suspected spinal injury. **A.** A short spinal board is being strapped to the victim's back even before he is extracted from the wrecked automobile. **B.** The victim is then extracted as an immobilized unit.

tives, friends, EMTs or paramedics, ambulance attendants, and police. Such a history, which can be obtained quickly, should be adequate, or "ample," and has been referred to in the ATLS Guidelines of the American College of Surgeons as being AMPLE, an acronym for the following items of information:

A—Allergies of any kind, including antibiotics
M—Medication being taken prior to the accident
P—Past history of relevant diseases
L—Last meal before the accident
E—Events related to the accident: nature and velocity of the injury, others injured, what actually happened?

This information is helpful in the initial *triage* of the injured patient immediately on arrival at the hospital.

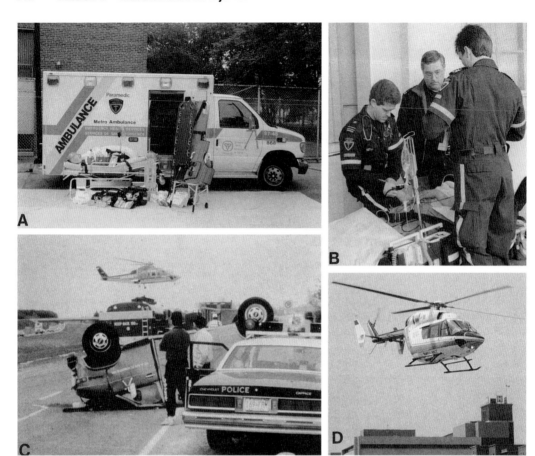

Figure 15.28.   A. A modern, well-equipped ambulance. The displayed equipment includes stretchers, spinal boards, air splints, oxygen tanks, positive pressure face mask, suction apparatus, gloves, and simple surgical instruments. **B.** Paramedics (emergency medical technicians) attending an injured patient. **C.** Helicopter air ambulance leaving the scene of a serious traffic accident and **D,** arriving at a major trauma center.

The emergency or accident room of a hospital will have the facilities necessary to provide continuation of preliminary care for the injured patient at a more sophisticated level (Fig. 15.29). Using the procedures of advanced trauma life support, pertinent data concerning the nature of the accident and the patient's subsequent condition, including some indication of the amount of blood loss, should be obtained from those who have brought him or her to hospital. Emergency treatment is based on the same ABC system as in basic life support.

Airway (Obstruction)
Persistent obstruction of the patient's airway may be relieved by suction and the insertion of a pharyngeal airway but may require tracheal intubation or even an emergency tracheostomy. Supportive oxygen therapy is frequently necessary.

Breathing (Respiratory Arrest)
If, after the airway has been restored and any tension pneumothorax has been decompressed, the patient is still not breathing spontaneously, mechanically assisted respiration is indicated.

Circulation (Cardiac Arrest, or Severe Bleeding)
For cardiac arrest that has not responded to CPR, electrical defibrillation should be con-

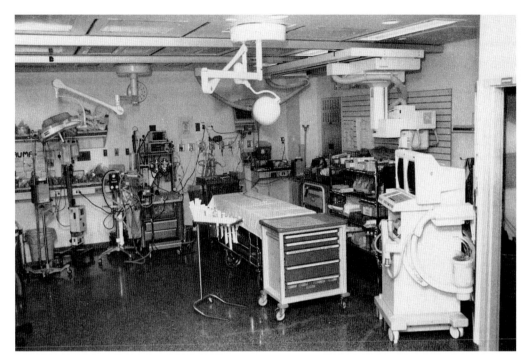

Figure 15.29.   An emergency or accident room equipped to treat patients who have sustained critical injuries. The equipment shown includes the following: anesthetic instruments to provide an airway (pharyngeal airways, laryngoscopes, endotracheal tubes), ceiling source of oxygen, nitrous oxide, suction and diagnostic imaging, anesthetic machine, electrocardiograph with oscilloscope, defibrillator, firm surface under the patient's thorax in the event that closed cardiac massage is required), auxiliary suction machine, blood pump for rapid transfusion, drugs for cardiac arrest ready for immediate injection, and cut-down tray for cannulation of veins.

sidered. If local pressure has not arrested external severe bleeding from an open wound, it may be necessary to clamp one or more vessels, after which the wound is covered with a temporary sterile dressing. Internal hemorrhage secondary to closed fractures is usually underestimated; for example, an adult with a closed fracture of the femoral shaft may lose from 1000 to 2000 ml of blood into tissues, and with a fracture of the pelvis, the patient may lose even more.

Shock

Prevention of shock and urgent treatment of either impending or established shock are imperative before definitive treatment of any fracture is instituted. Vital signs, including pulse rate, respiratory rate, blood pressure, and level of consciousness, are monitored and recorded. Blood is obtained for typing and cross-matching. At the same time, an intravenous infusion is started using two large bone cannulas and large tubing. In severe shock, the central venous pressure should also be monitored via a catheter inserted into a peripheral vein and passed proximally into the vena cava. While waiting for compatible blood, intravenous administration of fluids such as Ringer's lactate or plasma help to control shock temporarily, but hemorrhagic shock is best treated by transfusion of packed homologous red blood cells. Provided there is no head injury or significant abdominal injury, severe pain should be relieved by morphine or a comparable narcotic, which may have to be given intravenously if the peripheral circulation is inadequate.

The detailed complex treatment of shock in patients with multiple injuries (polytrauma) is constantly changing and is best learned in major trauma units in hospitals.

Responsibilities for the Care of the Critically Injured

Although several physicians and surgeons representing various specialties are involved as a trauma team in the total care of the patient who has sustained multiple critical injuries (polytrauma), one surgeon must serve as the team captain. This surgeon must assume the role of leadership and accept the coexistent responsibility for the total welfare of the patient. The captain should seek immediately the help of colleagues in other specialties as necessary and coordinate the efforts of all, but a critically injured patient is in dangerous jeopardy when the final responsibility for lifesaving care is uncoordinated among a number of specialists.

Fractures and Dislocations

Once treatment for the first three priorities has been initiated, a rapid but systematic physical examination is conducted. Vascular impairment and nerve injury should be assessed and their presence or absence recorded before definitive fracture treatment is initiated; otherwise there may be doubt subsequently whether the lesion was caused by the original injury or by the treatment of the injury.

After a rapid assessment of the patient's obvious injury or injuries, the whole patient (including all body systems) must be carefully examined for other fractures as well as for soft tissue injuries and visceral lesions. More injuries escape early detection because of an inadequate physical examination in the emergency assessment of the patient and consequent failure to proceed with further investigation than from incorrect interpretation of radiographs.

Before a patient's fractured extremity is subjected to radiographic examination, it should be splinted to minimize pain and to protect the related soft tissues from further injury (Fig. 15.30). For the same reasons the patient and the injured part should be moved as little as possible during the radiographic examination. It is important to move the tube and film of the radiographic equipment to obtain various projections rather than to move

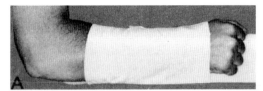
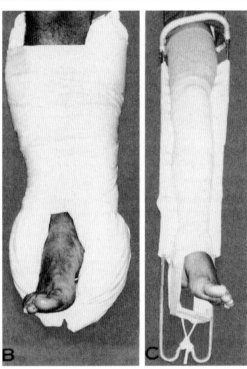

Figure 15.30. Temporary splints for fractured limbs prior to radiographic examination. **A.** Arm splint for a forearm fracture—a simple covered board and bandages. **B.** Pillow splint for a fractured leg or ankle. There is less risk of circulatory disturbance and skin maceration with this type of splint than with an air splint. **C.** Thomas splint for a fractured femur.

the patient or the fractured extremity (Fig. 15.31). The projections and extent of the radiographic examination required for accurate diagnosis are discussed in an earlier section of this chapter.

Throughout the emergency treatment for an injured patient, compassionate care for the patient and the injured tissues and kindly communication with the relatives are essential, deserved, and appreciated. As much information as possible should be obtained about the patient, particularly concerning any pre-existing disorder and its treatment, before definitive treatment of the fracture is undertaken.

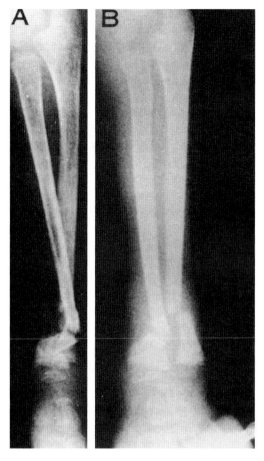

Figure 15.31. This child had an unstable fracture of the distal end of his radius and ulna. Radiographs requested: anteroposterior and lateral projections (the child's forearm should have been splinted before radiographic examination). **A.** A lateral projection of both proximal and distal fracture fragments. **B.** A lateral projection of the proximal fragments and an anteroposterior projection of both distal fragments. Obviously, between two radiographic projections, the child's forearm has been rotated through the unstable fracture sites by the technician. The child would have experienced much pain at this time and might even have sustained further injury to the related soft tissues.

SPECIFIC METHODS OF DEFINITIVE FRACTURE TREATMENT

Having learned the broad general principles of treatment as applied to fractures, you will now wish to learn the various *specific methods* of definitive fracture treatment. In the subsequent two chapters, these methods are discussed in relation to fractures in children and in adults. In this chapter, all of these methods are discussed as a group so that they may be considered in perspective and discussion of treatment for specific fractures in the subsequent two chapters may be more meaningful.

For each method of fracture treatment, there are favorable circumstances in which the method *should* be used (*indications*), as well as unfavorable circumstances in which it should *not* be used (*contraindications*). A knowledge of the indications and contraindications is of great importance in selecting a method or combination of methods of treatment for a particular patient. There is not always unanimity of opinion, even among "fracture experts," about indications and contraindications in relation to the treatment of various fractures. Opinions are based on general principles and on individual experience and preference. They are based as well on our present state of knowledge. With continuing advances in knowledge and improvement in methods and techniques, indications and contraindications become modified. There may be more than one pathway by which a desired goal in fracture treatment may be reached, but some pathways are smoother, easier, and safer for your patient than others.

The specific methods of treatment are discussed, together with their indications and risks. Contraindications for the various methods of treatment can be considered in a more general way now. The absence of an indication for a specific method represents a contraindication in itself. In addition there are three main situations that represent a contraindication for a specific method of treatment: 1) the fracture is not sufficiently serious to require the method; 2) the fracture cannot be adequately treated by the method; 3) either the patient or the fracture is likely to be made worse by the method.

While studying the specific methods of fracture treatment outlined below, bear in mind the four basic goals of all fracture treatment: 1) to relieve pain; 2) to obtain and maintain satisfactory position of the fracture fragments; 3) to allow, and if necessary encourage, bony union; 4) to restore optimum function, not only in the fractured limb or spine but also in the patient as a person. The fourth goal is discussed further in a subsequent section in relation to after-care and rehabilitation for patients with fractures.

In the broad spectrum of fracture treatment, two completely divergent schools of thought have emerged and both have gained much support. One is the Swiss AO/ASIF system of precise open reduction and rigid internal fixation (AO—in German, Arbeitsgemeinshaft-für Osteosynthesefragen; in English—Association for Osteosynthesis; and ASIF—Association for the Study of Internal Fixation). The other is the American "functional fracture-bracing" system (each of which is described in a subsequent section of this chapter). Although seemingly on the surface the exact antithesis of one another, these two well-established methods of fracture management have one important common denominator, namely the preservation of function in the injured limb and the prevention of iatrogenic joint stiffness (fracture disease). As stated in the previous section, "Healing of a Fracture in Cortical Bone with Rigid Internal Fixation," in recent years, the AO/ASIF surgeons have become less rigid in their thinking about the need for rigidity in their internal fixation devices.

Specific Methods of Treatment for Closed Fractures

1. Protection Alone (without Reduction or Immobilization)

Protection of a fracture from the usual forces applied to the particular bone as well as from further injury can be accomplished in the upper limb by means of a simple sling and in the lower limb by relief of weightbearing with crutches, at least for older children and adults (Fig. 15.32).

Indications (Fig. 15.33). Protection alone is indicated for undisplaced or relatively undisplaced, stable fractures of the ribs, phalanges, metacarpals—and in children, of the clavicle. A second indication is that group of fractures, such as mild compression fractures of the spine and impacted fractures of the upper end of the humerus, in which the total result will be better without either reduction or immobilization. Protection alone is also indicated after clinical union has been obtained by other

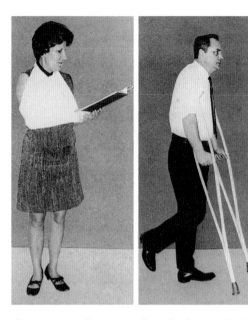

Figure 15.32. Protection alone (without reduction or immobilization). Simple sling for an upper limb injury and crutches with non-weightbearing on an injured lower limb.

means, but before complete radiological consolidation has been established.

Risks. The protection provided may not be adequate for the particular patient (especially a very young child or an uncooperative adult), in which case the fracture may become displaced; hence, the need for radiographic examinations of the fracture site at regular intervals during the healing process.

2. Immobilization by External Splinting (without Reduction)

Immobilization of a fracture by external splinting is only *relative* immobilization, as opposed to rigid fixation, inasmuch as some motion can still occur inside the limb or trunk at the fracture site during the early phases of healing. Relative immobilization is usually achieved by the use of plaster-of-Paris casts of varying design (Fig. 15.34) and occasionally by metallic or plastic splints.

Indications (Fig. 15.35). Immobilization by external splinting without reduction is indicated for fractures that are relatively undisplaced, yet unstable. Such fractures merely require maintenance of the existing position of

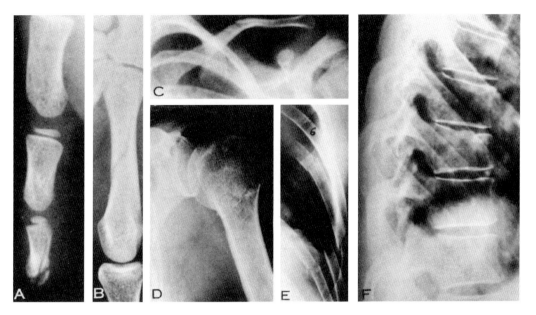

Figure 15.33.   Fractures that can be treated by protection alone. **A.** Crush fracture of the distal phalanx. **B.** Undisplaced fracture of a metacarpal. **C.** Greenstick fracture of the clavicle in a young child. **D.** Impacted compression fracture of the surgical neck of the humerus in an elderly adult. **E.** Undisplaced fractures of ribs (seventh, eighth and ninth). **F.** Mild compression fracture of the thoracic spine.

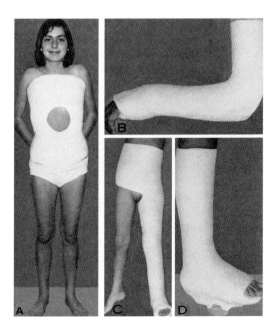

Figure 15.34.   Immobilization by external splinting (without reduction)—plaster-of-Paris casts of varying design. **A.** Body cast (used more for children than for adults); **B.** Above-elbow cast; **C.** Hip spica cast; **D.** Below-knee walking cast.

the fracture fragments during the healing process. A long bone fracture in which there is only sideways shift of the fragments in relation to one another but good contact and no significant angulation or rotation does not require reduction; it does, however, require relative immobilization. The immobilizing splint or cast must be carefully applied and molded to prevent further displacement.

Risks. Despite the fact that the fracture is relatively undisplaced at the time it is immobilized by a cast or splint, subsequent muscle pull and gravitational forces may cause further displacement such as angulation, rotation, or overriding that is unacceptable; hence the need for repeated radiographic examinations during the early stages of healing. Improperly applied casts or splints may cause local pressure sores over bony prominences, or constriction of a limb with resultant impairment of venous or arterial circulation, or both.

3. Closed Reduction by Manipulation Followed by Immobilization

Closed reduction of a fracture, which is a form of surgical manipulation, is by far the most

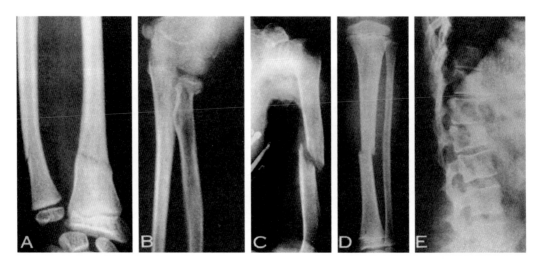

Figure 15.35.   Fractures that can be treated by external splinting (without reduction). **A.** Undisplaced fracture of the radius and ulna of a child. **B.** Undisplaced fracture of the neck of the radius in a child. **C.** Oblique fracture of the shaft of the humerus in an elderly lady. Notice the metallic corset stays. Did you notice the second fracture? There is a coexistent impacted compression fracture of the surgical neck of the humerus. **D.** Stable transverse fracture of the tibial shaft. **E.** Compression fracture of the second lumbar vertebra. The lumbar spine is more mobile and less stable than the thoracic spine.

common method of treatment for the majority of displaced fractures in both children and adults. Immobilization of the fracture by means of a plaster-of-Paris cast is the most common method of *maintaining* the reduction.

The precise technique of manipulative reduction, which is usually performed under anesthesia (general, regional, or local), varies with each fracture, but in general it involves placing the fracture fragments where they were at the time of maximal displacement and then reversing the path of displacement. This requires some knowledge of the likely mechanism of the fracture as well as a three-dimensional appreciation of the relationship of the fragments to one another and to the surrounding soft tissues. The forces involved in reduction are the opposite of those that produced the fracture (Fig. 15.36). The "feel" of stability of a reduced fracture comes only with clinical experience. The completeness of reduction is assessed by radiographs taken at right angles to each other, without moving the limb. The various techniques of closed reduction of fractures by manipulation depend on many factors and must be seen to be appre-

ciated. These can be learned by "live demonstrations" from your surgical teachers.

Plaster casts for immobilization of the fracture and maintenance of the reduction must be carefully and thoughtfully applied and molded or the reduction can be subsequently lost within the cast. The cast should hold the fracture fragments in the same manner as the surgeon's hands were holding them in their most stable position at the completion of the reduction.

Indications (Fig. 15.37). Closed reduction by manipulation followed by immobilization is indicated for displaced fractures that require reduction and when it is predicted that sufficiently accurate reduction can be both *obtained* and *maintained* by closed means.

Risks. Closed reduction that is ineptly and inaptly applied with more force than skill may cause further damage to soft tissues including blood vessels, nerves and even the periosteum. Excessive traction in the longitudinal axis of the limb during reduction may even produce arterial spasm, particularly at the elbow and knee, with resultant Volkmann's ischemia (compartment syndrome, which is discussed in a subsequent section of this chapter). Like-

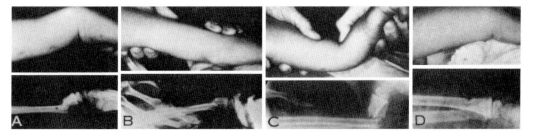

Figure 15.36.   Closed reduction of a fracture by manipulation. **A.** Fractures of the distal end of radius and ulna with angulation and overriding in a child. **B.** Longitudinal traction corrects the angulation but does not reduce the fractures because the intact periosteal hinge will not allow the fracture fragments to be distracted sufficiently to obtain reduction. (These radiographs were taken for teaching purposes. Normally, the surgeon's hands would not be exposed to radiation.) **C.** The fracture deformity must first be increased (to the extent that it was with the maximum displacement at the very moment of the fracture occurring). Then the distal fragment can be moved distally so that the fracture surfaces can be engaged. Only after this manipulation to correct the overriding is angulation corrected. The intact periosteal hinge on the concave side of the angulation then prevents overcorrection of the fracture deformity. (The role of the intact periosteal hinge is also depicted by line drawings in Fig. 15.11.) **D.** The reduced fracture is ready to be immobilized in a well-molded plaster cast that will maintain the reduction.

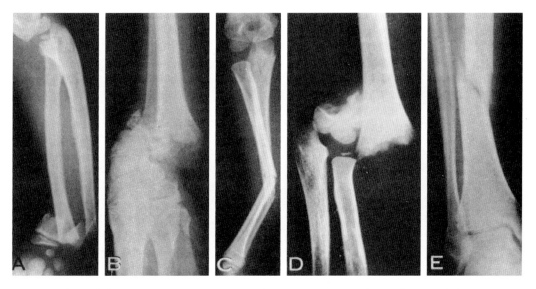

Figure 15.37.   Fractures that can be treated by closed reduction followed by immobilization. **A.** Displaced fractures of the distal end of the radius and ulna of a child. **B.** Colles' fracture of the distal end of the radius of an adult. **C.** Greenstick fracture of the shaft of the radius and ulna of a child. **D.** Displaced supracondylar fracture of the humerus in a child (in whom percutaneous pinning is added). **E.** Angulated spiral fracture of the tibial shaft in an adult.

wise, progressive swelling of a limb within the confines of a tight and rigid cast may also seriously impair circulation. Pressure sores over bony prominences and pressure injuries to peripheral nerves over bony prominences (especially the lateral popliteal nerve where it crosses the neck of the fibula) may also occur as a result of incorrectly applied casts.

Fractures in which the reduction is not sufficiently stable, especially oblique, spiral, and comminuted fractures, may become displaced subsequently within the cast and repeated radiographic assessments of the position of the fragments are essential during the early stages of healing. These risks are minimal when the appropriate technique of manipulative reduction is applied to an appropriate type of fracture by an appropriately experienced surgeon, and the signs of circulatory impairment and pressure are recognized after reduction.

4. Closed Reduction by Continuous Traction Followed by Immobilization

Closed reduction of a fracture by means of continuous traction can be achieved in several ways. For fractures in young children, continuous traction can be applied through the skin by means of extension tape (*skin traction*) (Fig. 15.38). For older children and adults in whom greater traction force is required, it is best applied through bone by means of a transverse rigid wire or pin (*skeletal traction*) (Fig. 15.39). Furthermore, the traction device may be fixed to the end of the bed (*fixed traction*), or it may be balanced by cords with pulleys and weights (*balanced traction*).

Traction in the long axis of the limb is effective in realigning fracture fragments only because the remaining intact soft tissues surrounding the fracture are put on the stretch and thereby guide the fragments into alignment. Continuous traction on the distal fragment is designed to overcome the previously mentioned effects of muscle pull and gravity on the fracture fragments and should be arranged to bring the distal fragment in line with the proximal fragment. For example, in a subtrochanteric fracture of the femur, the proximal fragment is pulled into flexion, abduction, and external rotation by the muscles attached to the lesser and greater trochanters; thus,

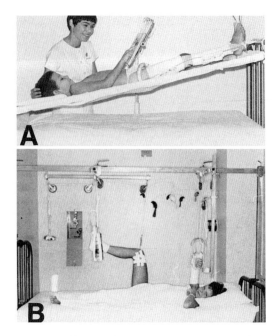

Figure 15.38. Continuous skin traction. **A.** Continuous fixed skin traction combined with a Thomas splint for a boy with an unstable fracture of the femur. **B.** Continuous balanced skin traction on the arm for a boy with an unstable fracture of the humerus. Note also the skeletal traction on the femur for an unstable subtrochanteric fracture of the femur in the same boy. Although these traction methods are both safe and sound, they have been replaced to a large extent in an era of cost constraint by operative methods that enable the child to be discharged from the hospital within days rather than weeks.

traction should be applied to the distal fragment in flexion, abduction, and external rotation to align it with the proximal fragment. Under certain circumstances, manipulative reduction is required to reduce the fracture and continuous traction is used to maintain the reduction. When the fracture has healed to the point of becoming "sticky" and nontender so that traction is no longer required to prevent redisplacement, continuous traction can be replaced by immobilization of the limb or trunk in an appropriate cast, after which the patient may be able to return home while awaiting clinical union of the fracture.

Indications (Fig. 15.40). Closed reduction by continuous traction is indicated for unstable oblique, spiral, or comminuted fractures of major long bones, and unstable spinal

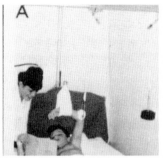
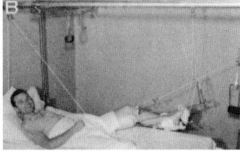
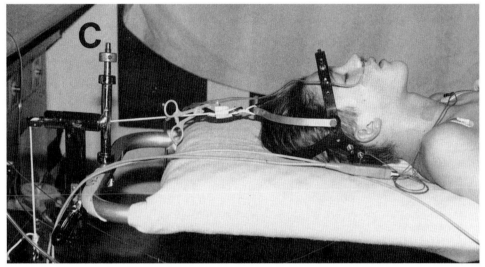

Figure 15.39. Continuous skeletal traction. **A.** Continuous skeletal traction through the olecranon for an unstable supracondylar fracture of the humerus in a child. An alternative that has become popular for such a fracture is closed reduction combined with percutaneous pinning. **B** Continuous balanced skeletal traction through the upper end of the tibia for an unstable fracture of the femur in an adult. For fractures of the femur in adults, continuous traction may be used temporarily but has to a large extent been replaced by either external or internal skeletal fixation. **C.** Continuous skeletal traction through a "halo" attached to screws in the outer table of the skull for an unstable fracture-dislocation of the cervical spine.

fractures. Skeletal traction is also applicable to the treatment of fractures complicated by vascular injuries, excessive swelling, or skin loss in which an encircling bandage or cast would be dangerous.

Risks. Excessive longitudinal traction, particularly if applied several hours or longer after the fracture occurred, may produce arterial spasm with resultant Volkmann's ischemia (compartment syndrome). Ineptly applied skin traction, excessive traction, or both may result in superficial skin loss, whereas skeletal traction may become complicated by pin track infection that reaches the bone. Furthermore,

continuous traction, if inaccurately applied and monitored, may fail to achieve and maintain adequate reduction of the fracture. Excessive traction may also distract the fracture fragments with resultant delayed union or even nonunion; osteoblasts can creep but cannot leap. These risks, like those of closed reduction, are largely preventable, but their prevention requires clinical vigilance by an experienced surgeon.

In many countries, for economic reasons and the resultant policy of short hospital stays, this method of treatment involving prolonged traction has, to a large extent, been replaced

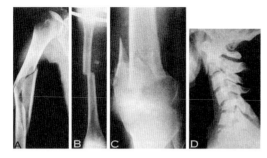

Figure 15.40. Fractures that can be treated by continuous traction. **A.** Unstable comminuted fracture of the shaft of the humerus. **B.** Unstable fracture of the shaft of the femur. **C.** Unstable comminuted supracondylar fracture of the femur. **D.** Unstable fracture-dislocation of the cervical spine (which would be followed by a local spinal fusion after reduction of the dislocation).

by early external or internal skeletal fixation with or without open reduction. These alternative methods of treatment enable the patient to be discharged from the hospital in a few days rather than weeks.

5. Closed Reduction Followed by Functional Fracture-Bracing

In 1961, Dehne advocated the early use of weightbearing plaster casts in the treatment of fractures of the tibia. Two years later, Sarmiento expanded on this concept by conceiving the principle of early function combined with allowing motion at the joints above and below the fractured bone. This method of fracture treatment is variously known as "closed functional treatment," "cast-bracing," or "functional fracture-bracing." Adapting the principles involved in fitting prostheses to amputation stumps (for example, patella tendon-bearing for below-knee prostheses), Sarmiento first used plaster casts and more recently plastic (Orthoplast) splints, both of which are hinged at the level of joints.

The principle of functional fracture-bracing is based on the following concepts: 1) that rigid immobilization of fracture fragments is not only unnecessary but also undesirable for fracture healing; 2) that function and the resultant controlled motion at the fracture site actually stimulate healing through abundant callus formation; 3) that such function prevents iatrogenic joint stiffness; 4) that some-

what less than perfect (anatomical) reduction of a fracture of the shaft of a long bone does not create significant problems concerning either function or appearance (cosmesis). A beneficial socioeconomic spin-off of this method of fracture treatment is the combination of a shorter period of hospitalization, no risk of infection, and a more rapid return of the patient to normal activities, including work.

The initial treatment consists of either closed reduction of the fracture, or continuous traction for a few days followed by immobilization in a plaster cast for a period of 3 to 4 weeks (that is, until the acute pain and swelling have subsided and the soft tissues have begun to heal). At the end of this preliminary period, the hinged cast-brace or plastic brace is applied to splint the fracture while allowing motion in the joints above and below the fractured bone (Figs. 15.41 and 15.42). The encircling external splint combined with the viscoelastic nature of the soft tissues creates a "hydraulic effect" that prevents any initial shortening of the limb from increasing. In large series of patients with fractures of long bones treated by this method, the incidence

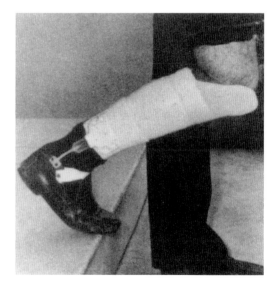

Figure 15.41. Functional fracture-brace for a fracture of the shaft of the tibia in an adult. Note that the well-molded and close-fitting plastic (Orthoplast) brace allows full motion of both the ankle and the knee and in this sense is much more "functional" than a plaster cast that immobilizes both joints.

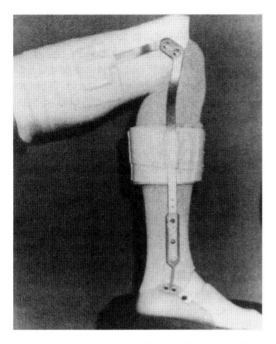

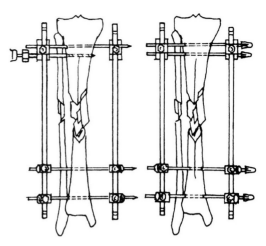

Figure 15.43.   Simplest form of external skeletal fixation to provide fixation of a comminuted fracture of the tibia "at a distance."

Figure 15.42.   Functional fracture-brace for a fracture of the distal third of the femur in an adult. Note that the brace, which has a metal hinge at the knee and a plastic hinge at the ankle allows motion at the hip, knee, and ankle.

of nonunion has been only 1%, which is remarkable.

Indications.   Closed reduction followed by functional fracture-bracing is indicated for fractures of the shaft of the tibia, the distal third of the femur, the humerus, and the ulna in adults. The method is contraindicated for fractures that can be more effectively treated by open reduction and internal skeletal fixation, including intertrochanteric fractures of the femur, subtrochanteric and mid-shaft fractures of the femur, and shaft of the radius and intra-articular fractures.

Risks.   Although functional fracture-bracing is relatively risk free, there is a possibility that the method will fail to maintain an acceptable position of the fracture fragments, in which case alternative methods such as open reduction and internal fixation may still be applied.

6. Closed Reduction by Manipulation Followed by External Skeletal Fixation

External skeletal fixation of fractures, first devised by Stader, a veterinary surgeon, to avoid

the use of plaster casts in animals, was modified for humans over 5 decades ago by Roger Anderson. After a long period of relatively little use, external skeletal fixation is currently undergoing a rebirth of clinical interest and application.

In its simplest form, two or three metal pins are inserted percutaneously through the bone above and below the fracture site and held together by external bars to provide firm (but not rigid) fixation of the fracture "at a distance" (Fig. 15.43). In recent years, devices such as the Hoffman type of external fixation have become increasingly sophisticated to provide more rigid fixation in three dimensions (Fig. 15.44). Circular metal frames that

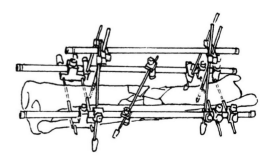

Figure 15.44.   More sophisticated form of external skeletal fixation to provide more rigid fixation in three dimensions.

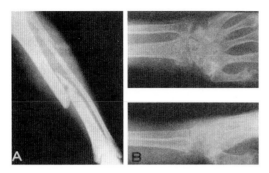

Figure 15.45. Fractures that can be treated by closed reduction and external skeletal fixation. **A.** Unstable comminuted fracture of the tibia in an adult. **B.** Unstable comminuted Colles' fracture of the distal end of the radius in an adult.

encircle the fractured limb and to which the pins are attached are known as "circular external fixation" of which the Ilizarov frame is an example, as described in Chapter 6 (see Fig. 6.26). At an early stage of fracture healing, the external fixator can be "dynamized" to allow axial micromotion at the fracture site, either active (from weightbearing), or passive from a mechanical device, both of which have a stimulating effect on fracture healing as shown by Goodship and Kenright.

Indications (Fig. 15.45). Closed reduction by manipulation followed by external skeletal fixation is primarily indicated for severely comminuted (and unstable) fractures of the shaft of the tibia or femur, especially type 3 open fractures with extensive injuries to soft tissues including arteries and nerves, the repair of which necessitates immobilization of the fracture site. For such fractures, this method offers the distinct advantage of allowing changes of the wound dressing as well as the application of skin grafts. External skeletal fixation may also be indicated for unstable fractures of the pelvis, humerus, radius, and metacarpals.

Risks. The main risk of external skeletal fixation is pin track infection with or without osteomyelitis. If the pins are inserted by means of a high-speed power drill, the surrounding bone may be "burnt to death" by the heat of friction, in which case superimposed infection will produce a *ring sequestrum* (see Fig. 15.68).

7. Closed Reduction by Manipulation Followed by Internal Skeletal Fixation

After accurate manipulative reduction of an unstable fracture, the reduction can be maintained by the percutaneous insertion of metallic nails or intramedullary rods across the fracture site for the purpose of providing internal skeletal fixation of the fracture (Fig. 15.46). Both the closed manipulative reduction of the fracture and the "blind" insertion of the internal skeletal fixation are performed using radiographic control, either by means of repeated single radiographs or short periods of fluoroscopy with an image intensifier. Fractures should never be reduced under ordinary fluoroscopy because of the radiation hazard to the patient as well as to the surgeon.

Indications. Manipulative reduction followed by internal skeletal fixation is indicated for certain fractures in which accurate reduction can be obtained by closed means but cannot or should not be maintained by external immobilization. The most common indica-

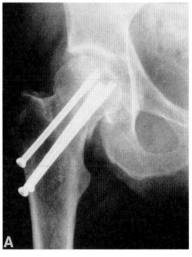
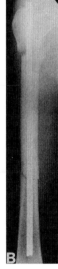

Figure 15.46. Closed reduction followed by internal skeletal fixation. **A.** Three cannulated screws that have been inserted blindly and percutaneously across a fracture of the neck of the femur after closed reduction. This so-called blind pinning of a fracture is not really blind; it is performed under radiographic control. **B.** Intra-medullary rod that has been inserted percutaneously across a segmental fracture of the shaft of the femur after closed reduction.

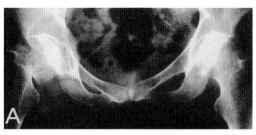

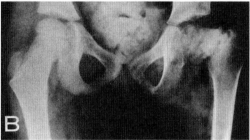

Figure 15.47. Fractures that can be treated by closed reduction and internal skeletal fixation. **A.** Fracture of the neck of the right femur in an adult. **B.** Fracture of the neck of the left femur in a child.

tion for manipulative reduction followed by internal skeletal fixation is the unstable fracture of the neck of the femur in both children and adults (Fig. 15.47). After accurate reduction, the internal fixation device is driven across the fracture site through a small skin incision using radiographic control. Certain fractures in the midshaft of the long bones that can be reduced by closed means also lend themselves to blind intramedullary nailing under radiographic control.

Risks. The closed manipulative reduction may fail to obtain a satisfactory position of the fracture fragments and the skeletal fixation may fail to achieve sufficiently rigid fixation of the fracture. Because with internal skeletal fixation the skin is traversed, the risk of infection is ever present.

8. Open Reduction Followed by Internal Skeletal Fixation

Open reduction has an important place in the treatment of uncomplicated closed fractures but should never be undertaken lightly. When the results are good they are very good, but when they are bad they are horrid—and may even be catastrophic! The fracture site is ex-

posed surgically so that the fracture fragments may be reduced perfectly *under direct vision*. A fracture that is open to inspection, however, is also open to infection. The operative reduction of fractures should be performed (or at least supervised) only by an experienced surgeon and only in a favorable setting such as an operating theater that has a consistently low infection rate and is properly equipped with adequate instruments. To convert a closed fracture to an infected fracture is a terrible tragedy!

Once the fracture has been reduced at open operation, the reduction must be maintained by internal fixation, which is achieved by using some type of metallic device, a technique that is sometimes referred to as *osteosynthesis*. Surgical skill is required to avoid unnecessary further damage to the surrounding soft tissues and in particular to the blood supply of the fracture fragments. The surgeon must constantly think as a biologist with reverence for living tissues rather than merely as a carpenter of cortical bone, even though the technical application of internal fixation must of course be structurally sound.

A variety of mechanical devices has been developed to provide rigid internal fixation of fractures. These metallic devices, each of which has its special uses and advantages, include various types of transfixation screws, onlay plates held by screws, intramedullary nails and rods, smooth and threaded pins, encircling bands, and wire sutures (Fig. 15.48). In the past, it was thought that all internal metallic fracture fixation devices should be removed after they had served their purpose. The current thinking, however, is that many such devices should not be removed because the risks of doing so are greater than the risks of leaving them in place.

Biodegradable screws made of polyglycolic acid maintain their strength for up to 6 months and are gradually resorbed in 2 to 5 years. They are useful for the internal fixation of fractures involving cancellous bone, especially in children, and have a distinct advantage over metallic pins and screws in that they do not need to be removed after the fracture has united.

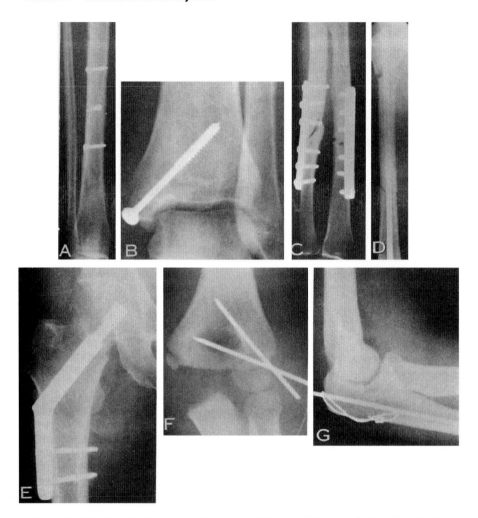

Figure 15.48.   Metallic devices used for internal fixation of fractures. **A.** Interfragmentary transfixion screws for a long oblique fracture of the tibia. (This fracture could have been more effectively treated by an intramedullary rod.) **B.** Lag screw (compression screw) for an avulsion fracture of the medial malleolus. **C.** Heavy onlay compression plate and screws (AO compression device) for fractures of the radius and ulna. (One screw in the ulna is incorrectly placed in that it traverses the fracture line.) **D** Intramedullary rod for a segmented fracture of the femur. **E.** Nail-plate combination for a fracture of the neck of the femur. **F.** Kirschner wires for a fracture of the lateral condyle of the humerus in a child. **G.** Intramedullary Kirschner wire and a "tension-relieving" figure-eight wire loop (AO device) for a fracture of the olecranon.

The AO/ASIF System of Internal Fixation. In 1958 a small group of Swiss surgeons including Müller, Allgower, and Willeneger, who were dissatisfied with the existing systems and techniques of internal fixation of fractures, formed a study group called AO, which was subsequently called ASIF. These innovative surgeons and their research colleagues, who are concerned with biomechanical improvements of the internal fixation for fractures, have developed the best system, techniques, and equipment available for this purpose. More recently, this group of fracture surgeons has become less fixed in their thinking about the need for rigidity of their internal fixation devices.

The principle of the AO/ASIF system is to achieve internal fixation of fracture fragments rigid enough that external immobilization is not necessary and full, active function of muscles and joints is possible very soon after operation. The underlying reason for this system is the avoidance of what this group refers to as "fracture disease," or what might also be considered as "immobilization disease," that is, the iatrogenic sequelae of prolonged immobilization of extremities, joint stiffness, muscle atrophy, disuse osteoporosis, and chronic edema. In essence, the aim of the AO/ASIF system is the rapid recovery of function in the injured limb. As mentioned in an earlier section of this chapter, fracture healing in the presence of rigid, stable internal fixation (applied under compression) is of the "direct" or "primary" type.

The surgeon who treats fractures must be skilled in all methods of fracture treatment and not just in a system of internal fixation, lest that surgeon exemplify the phenomenon stated by Abraham Maslow, namely that "if the only tool you have is a hammer, you tend to see every problem as a nail."

Indications (Fig. 15.49). Open reduction and internal skeletal fixation of a closed fracture should be undertaken only for definite and justifiable indications, which may be either absolute (a matter of necessity) or relative (a matter of judgment). Open operation is indicated to *obtain* reduction, when closed reduction by manipulation would clearly be impossible or has already been proven to be so. Examples are displaced avulsion fractures, intra-articular fractures in which reduction of the joint surface must be perfect, displaced fractures in children that cross the epiphyseal plate (physis), and fractures in which soft tissues have become interposed and trapped between the fragments. With grossly unstable fractures, it may be possible to *obtain* reduction by closed means, but impossible to *maintain* the reduction. Therefore, for these fractures operative treatment is indicated, not so much for the reduction of the fracture as for the maintenance of reduction by internal fixation. Examples are intertrochanteric fractures of the femur, fractures of both bones of the forearm in adults, and displaced fractures of phalanges.

Open reduction and internal fixation of a fracture are also indicated where there is a coexistent vascular injury that requires exploration and repair. Operative treatment of a fracture may be indicated to *facilitate nursing care* of the patient and prevent serious complications as occur with unstable intertrochanteric fractures of the femur in the elderly, extremity fractures associated with severe head injury, and fracture-dislocations of the spine complicated by paraplegia. Under certain circumstances, a *pathological fracture* through a metastatic neoplasm merits internal fixation (with or without methylmethacrylate) to relieve pain and make the remaining months of the patient's life more bearable.

In general, combined open reduction and internal fixation is contraindicated in fractures of the shaft of the tibia and shaft of the humerus (both of which can usually be adequately managed either by closed nailing or by functional fracture bracing).

Risks. The most serious risk of open operative reduction of fractures is *infection*. Even in the best of operating rooms, every operative wound becomes *contaminated* by bacteria from the air. The longer the wound is open, the more bacteria enter it. Furthermore, the torn and bruised muscles, as well as the fracture hematoma itself, serve as an ideal culture medium for bacteria. The fact that contamination does not invariably lead to infection attests to the local and general resistance of the host. Nevertheless, the risk is real and an infected fracture is a catastrophe. Operative reduction of a fracture also carries the risk of further *damage to the blood supply* of the fracture fragments which, in turn, may lead to delayed union and even nonunion. Unless the device used for internal fixation provides rigid immobilization of the fracture fragments in a suitable position of reduction, there is a possibility of continued movement at the fracture site, of *metal failure*, and of delayed union or nonunion. In addition, *postoperative adhesions* between muscle groups may lead to persistent restriction of joint motion.

The controversial concept of using less rigid or semiflexible plates to diminish the "stress protection" of bone offers some theoretical advantages but is still in the investigative stage, both experimentally and clinically.

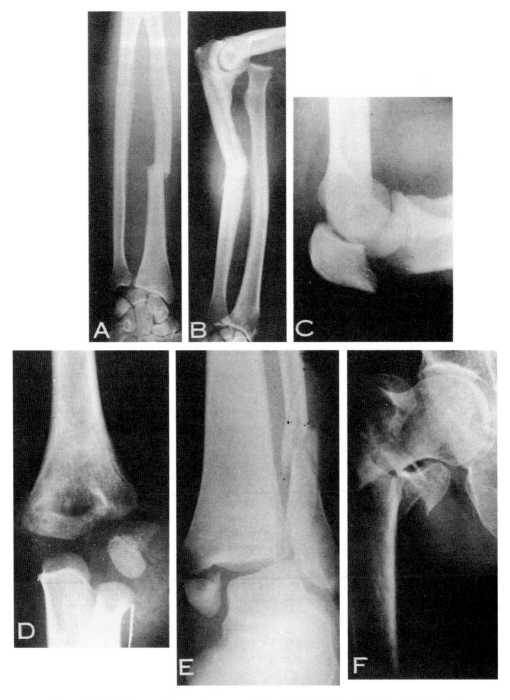

Figure 15.49.   Fractures that are best treated by open reduction and internal fixation. **A.** Fracture of the shaft of the radius and subluxation of the inferior radioulnar joint in an adult. **B.** Fracture of the shaft of the ulna and anterior dislocation of the proximal end of the radius (Monteggia fracture-dislocation) in an adult. **C.** Widely separated intra-articular fracture of the olecranon. **D.** Displaced fracture of the lateral condyle of the humerus in a child. **E.** Fracture-subluxation of the ankle with an avulsion fracture of the medial malleolus and a comminuted fracture of the shaft of the fibula. **F.** Comminuted intertrochanteric fracture of the femur.

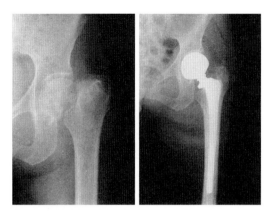

Figure 15.50. Excision of a fracture fragment and replacement by a prosthesis. In this elderly patient who had a femoral neck fracture, the proximal fragment (femoral head and neck) has been excised and replaced by an endoprosthesis (in this case, a cemented hip prosthesis), the stem of which penetrates the distal fragment.

9. Excision of a Fracture Fragment and Replacement by an Endoprosthesis

For certain fractures of the hip and elbow, the results of internal fixation are relatively unsatisfactory because of the high incidence of avascular necrosis of the articular fragment, nonunion of the fracture, and posttraumatic degenerative joint disease. Under these circumstances, the articular fragment may be excised and replaced by a suitable endoprosth-

esis to provide a prosthetic joint replacement (Fig. 15.50).

Indications (Fig. 15.51). Because of the high incidence of avascular necrosis of the femoral head and nonunion of the fracture, displaced intracapsular fractures of the neck of the femur in the elderly cannot always be managed satisfactorily by internal fixation. Excision of the proximal fragment (femoral head) combined with replacement with an endoprosthesis overcomes both of these problems and permits earlier mobilization of the patient as well as of the hip. Comminuted fractures of the radial head in adults are not amenable to internal fixation and, because residual incongruity of the joint leads to posttraumatic degenerative joint disease, it is preferable to excise the radial head. If the elbow joint is grossly unstable as a result of coexistent ligamentous injury, the radial head may be replaced by an endoprosthesis. If the elbow joint is not unstable, no endoprosthesis is required and the patient is left with an excision arthroplasty. Excision of the radial head is contraindicated in children because of the resultant loss of the epiphyseal (physeal) growth at this site. For severely comminuted and grossly unstable supracondylar fractures of the humerus in adults, an elbow prosthesis may be required. Severely comminuted fractures of the patella are best treated by excision of the

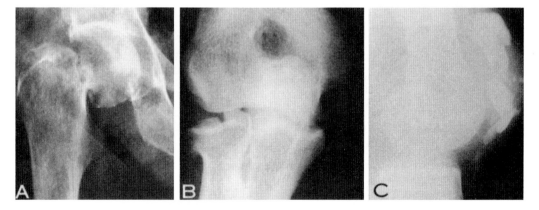

Figure 15.51. Fractures that may require excision of a fragment. **A.** Fracture of the femoral neck in an elderly adult. The femoral head fragment should be replaced by an endoprosthesis. **B.** Severely comminuted, intra-articular fracture of the radial head in an adult. **C.** Severely comminuted (shattered) patella.

entire patella and reconstruction of the quadriceps mechanism. Comminuted fractures of the humeral head can be treated by excision and replacement with a hemiarthroplasty.

Risks. As with other methods of operative treatment of fractures, the most serious risk is infection, a complication that is particularly serious in the presence of an endoprosthesis. Indeed, severe infection may necessitate removal of the endoprosthesis, with a resultant false joint (excision arthroplasty). There is also a risk, particularly in the elderly hip, that the endoprosthesis will gradually migrate through osteoporotic bone of the pelvis or femur.

Treatment for Open Fractures

Because open (compound) fractures have communicated with the external environment through the skin and have already been complicated by *bacterial contamination*, they carry the serious risk of becoming further complicated by *infection*. Thus, they merit special consideration, with particular emphasis on the *prevention of infection* and *obtaining union of the fracture*. Because of the extensive soft tissue injury associated with open fractures, they usually take much longer to unite than closed fractures.

The extent of the skin wound of an open fracture varies considerably. It may be a small puncture wound caused by penetration of the skin from within by a sharp, jagged spike of bone (Fig. 15.10), or by penetration of the skin from without by a missile such as a bullet. The wound may be a sizeable tear in the skin through which bare bone is still protruding (Fig. 15.52). Alternatively, the wound may

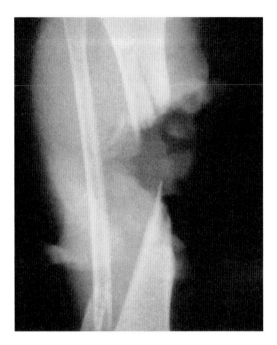

Figure 15.53. Open fracture of the shaft of the tibia. The blades of a power lawn mower penetrated the skin from without and fractured the tibia. There is extensive soft tissue loss as well as loss of a large segment of bone. Notice also the associated closed fracture of the fibula.

consist of extensive lacerations from without (Fig. 15.53) or even *avulsion* of a large area of skin and subcutaneous fat (Fig. 15.54). The soft tissue injury associated with an open fracture is usually even more extensive than is immediately apparent. The external blood loss through the open wound before hospital admission is also frequently underestimated.

An instant ("polaroid") photograph should be taken of every open fracture in the emergency room before a sterile dressing has been applied, or in the operating room, to provide an important item for the hospital record and to avoid the risk of additional contamination from repeated preoperative inspections of the open wound by consulting surgeons.

Classification of Open Fractures

From the experience of more than 1000 open fractures of long bones, Gustilo and Anderson were able to distinguish three distinct categories of such injuries and to develop the follow-

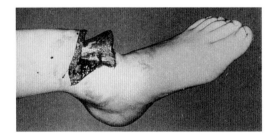

Figure 15.52. Open fracture of the distal end of the tibia. The protruding tibial fragment has penetrated the skin from within and the skin has been further torn by severe displacement at the moment of injury.

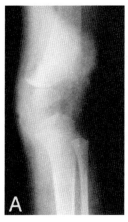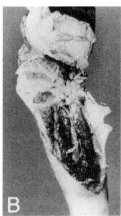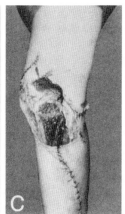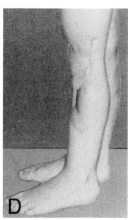

Figure 15.54.   **A.** An open fracture of the distal end of femur and proximal end of tibia in a child. A power saw has lacerated and avulsed skin and has cut out a portion of femur and tibia. **B.** Clinical appearance of the limb showing the extensive skin lacerations, avulsion of skin, extensive damage to underlying soft tissues and bones. **C.** After debridement and partial closure of the wound. The residual skin deficit was covered later by a split thickness skin graft. **D.** One year later, there is extensive scarring but good function. Nevertheless, further reconstructive surgery will be required because of an inevitable growth disturbance in the injured epiphyseal plates (physes).

ing classification system based on the severity of the soft tissue injury: type 1—a clean wound less than 1 cm in length (usually from within with little soft tissue injury); type 2—a laceration more than 1 cm in length but without extensive soft tissue damage, skin flaps, or avulsions and with a simple transverse or oblique fracture; type 3—extensive soft tissue damage such as skin flaps, avulsions, and muscle and nerve injuries. More recently, Gustilo has described three categories of type 3 open fractures: 3A—extensive soft tissue damage but adequate bone coverage, segmental fractures, and gunshot wounds; 3B—extensive soft tissue damage with extensive periosteal stripping and devascularized bone that requires skin flaps or free grafts. This type is usually associated with gross contamination; 3C—associated vascular injury requiring repair.

The authors recommended primary closure of the skin in types 1 and 2 open fractures (this is controversial) but delayed primary closure in type 3 open fractures. In many trauma centers, open fractures are left open initially, that is, for the first 4 to 7 days. Using antibiotics (usually one of the cephalosporins) before,

during, and after operation, the overall infection rate was 2.4% whereas the infection rate for type 3 injuries alone was 10%.

Open fractures represent a surgical emergency. They require expert treatment based on well-established guidelines to minimize the risk of infection. The following aspects of treatment for open fractures are particularly important.

Cleansing the Wound. Gross dirt, bits of clothing, and other foreign material should be literally washed away by extensive pulsating irrigation as well as by mechanical cleansing with copious amounts of sterile water or isotonic saline (rather than merely camouflaged by strong antiseptics that cause further tissue damage). Residual material should be carefully picked out of the wound. The wound may even have to be opened further to allow adequate assessment of the degree of contamination and to deal with it.

Excision of Devitalized Tissue (Debridement). Because tissues that have lost their blood supply prevent primary wound healing and enhance infection, the meticulous surgical excision of all devitalized tissue, such as skin, subcutaneous fat, fascia, muscle, and loose fragments of bone, is essential. Foreign material such as bits of clothing and dirt should also be removed. It also is wise to obtain a culture of the wound at the time of operation.

Treatment of the Fracture. When the open wound is small, such as a puncture wound from within, the fracture can usually be treated by closed means, after the wound has been cleansed, debrided, and left open. When the wound is extensive, the fracture may require either skeletal traction or open reduction with skeletal fixation. External skeletal fixation "at a distance" above and below the fracture by an external fixator is often of value. In general, internal fixation may be used unless it is thought that its mere insertion would tend to traumatize and devitalize more tissue and increase the risk of infection. Under certain circumstances, such as excessive instability of the fracture or an associated vascular injury, internal fixation is completely justified because the risks of its application are less serious than the risks of alternative methods.

Closure of the Wound. Even when the open fracture is treated within "the golden period" of the first 6 or 7 hours and contamination is not extensive, *immediate primary closure* of the wound is usually contraindicated, in keeping with the aphorism "leave open fractures open." After the first 4 to 7 days, provided no infection has developed, *delayed primary closure* of the wound is indicated. Loss of skin may necessitate the delayed application of split thickness skin grafts. Suction drainage should be used to prevent accumulation of blood and serum in the depths of the wound. Delayed primary closure is particularly applicable in grossly contaminated open fractures sustained on the battlefield or in major disasters.

Antibacterial Drugs. To be effective in the prevention of infection, antibacterial drugs must be administered in large doses before, during, and after treatment of the wound. Even so, antibacterial treatment is no guarantee against infection because many bacteria are resistant to various drugs. Furthermore, antibacterial drugs cannot reach any wound tissue that has lost its blood supply. The surgical care of the wound is of even greater importance than the antibacterial therapy.

Prevention of Tetanus. All patients with open fractures require preventive measures against the uncommon but serious complication of tetanus. If the patient has been previously immunized by tetanus toxoid, a booster dose of toxoid should be given. If there has been no previous immunization, or if inadequate information is available, immediate passive immunity can be achieved by the use of 250 units of tetanus immune globulin (human). Active immunity with tetanus toxoid is initiated at the same time.

Anesthesia for Patients with Fractures

During the first hour after a fracture has occurred, the patient's tissues are somewhat numb and under these circumstances only, it may be possible to reduce certain fractures without anesthesia. Even then, however, reduction without anesthesia should be performed only if the physician or surgeon is confident that it can be accomplished with one deft manipulation and the patient is not unduly tense and nervous. There is no justification for the use of "vocal" anesthesia: a combination of the physician's or surgeon's futile vocal reassurances and the patient's anguished vocal complaints!

Certain fractures, such as a Colles' fracture at the lower end of the radius in adults, are amenable to reduction after *infiltration* of a local anesthetic agent in and around the fracture site. Other fractures in the limbs can be reduced under regional anesthesia such as a brachial plexus block for the upper limb and a spinal anesthetic for the lower limb.

In general, the majority of fractures requiring reduction are best treated under general anesthesia, which provides complete comfort and the muscle relaxation necessary in reducing a fracture. The risk of aspiration of stomach contents during the induction of general anesthesia as well as during the recovery period merits special mention in relation to patients with fractures. After a significant injury, such as a fracture, gastric motility virtually ceases for many hours and consequently, if the patient has ingested food or drink shortly before or after the injury, the stomach retains a mixture of undigested food and gastric acid, either of which can cause death if aspirated into the trachea or lungs. Under these circumstances (unless there is a serious complication such as an open fracture or a vascular injury), general anesthesia should be delayed until at least 6 hours after the ingestion of food or drink; even after this period, special precautions (such as removal of gastric contents through a tube) are necessary to prevent the serious complication of aspiration. The welfare of the patient must always take precedence over the convenience of his or her physician or surgeon. Temporary splints should not be removed nor the fractured part be moved during the preliminary stages of anesthesia, or the painful stimulus could initiate either cardiac arrest or laryngeal spasm.

After-Care and Rehabilitation for Patients with Fractures

You will recall that four aims of all fracture treatment are: 1) to relieve pain; 2) to obtain and maintain satisfactory position of the fracture fragments; 3) to allow and if necessary to encourage bony union; 4) to restore optimum function. The most important is restoration of function, for what does it profit patients if they gain union of their fracture in a satisfactory position but fail to regain useful function of their injured part?

The more function that can be preserved during the treatment of the patient's fracture, the less function that will have to be restored. For intra-articular fractures that have been reduced by open operation and then completely stabilized by rigid internal fixation, the immediate application of CPM postoperatively and its continuation for 2 or 3 weeks maintains an excellent range of joint motion and stimulates the healing of the fractured articular cartilage, as discussed in an earlier section of this chapter (Fig. 15.24). Thus, rehabilitation of a patient begins with the immediate care of his or her injury, continues through the emergency treatment, the definitive treatment and beyond until the patient is restored to normal or as near normal as the injury permits.

Excessive and persistent edema in soft tissues produces glue-like adhesions with resultant joint stiffness. It should be prevented or minimized by appropriate elevation of the

fractured limb during the early phase of fracture healing, as well as by improvement of venous return through active exercises of all regional muscles. Muscles that are not used soon exhibit disuse atrophy, which can be prevented by active static (isometric) exercises of those muscles that control the immobilized joints, and active dynamic (isotonic) exercises of all other muscles of the limb or trunk. Supervised physiotherapy is particularly important in the after-care of adults with fractures; the patients must be helped to help themselves. All joints that are not immobilized by the fracture treatment should be put through a full range of motion daily—by the patient (Fig. 15.55).

In addition to preservation of function in the muscles and joints after a fracture, healthy function in the *patient's mind* must also be preserved, because the patient's attitude toward his or her injury determines to a considerable extent the rate at which recovery will progress. Indeed, *psychological considerations*

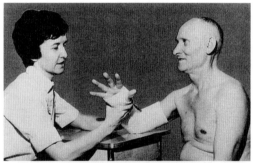

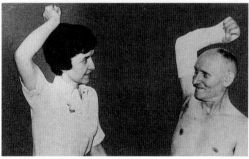

Figure 15.55. Supervised physiotherapy. The physiotherapist is teaching and encouraging the patient (who has a fracture of radius and ulna) to actively move all joints in the fractured limb that are not immobilized.

added to good care of the patient's fracture can usually prevent unnecessary despondency, depression, and undue concern about the future. Many patients regain function readily, some need help, and others who are more timid and self centered need constant encouragement in their efforts.

After the period of external immobilization of the fracture, active exercises should be continued even more vigorously until normal muscle power and joint motion have been regained. If necessary, the patient should be retrained in the activities of daily living and occupation, usually through supervised *occupational therapy* (Fig. 15.56). After a period away from work the patient's general condition has often deteriorated and he or she may need to embark on a program of general physical fitness before returning to work; this

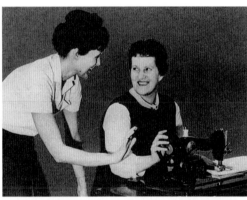
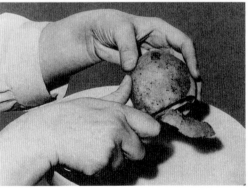

Figure 15.56. Supervised occupational therapy. The occupational therapist is retraining and encouraging this patient (who is recovering from a Colles' fracture of the distal end of her radius) in activities of daily living appropriate for her occupation as a homemaker.

is often best accomplished in a rehabilitation center.

Rehabilitation of the whole person, as discussed in Chapter 6, is always important, especially when the fracture has required a particularly long period of treatment or has been associated with serious complications.

Complications of Fracture Treatment

Complications of the original injury are classified in a previous section of this chapter. Complications that are iatrogenic in that they are caused by the treatment of the fracture are classified below. These complications are mostly preventable; they are related to three main factors: excessive local pressure, excessive traction, and infection.

Classification of Complications of Fracture Treatment

1. Skin Complications
   Tattoo effect from abrasions
   Pressure lesions (pressure sores)
      Bed sores (decubitus ulcers)
      Cast sores (cast ulcers)
2. Vascular Complications
   Traction and pressure lesions
   Volkmann's ischemia (compartment syndromes)
   Gangrene and gas gangrene
   Venous thrombosis and pulmonary embolism
3. Neurological Complications
   Traction and pressure lesions
4. Joint Complications
   Infection (septic arthritis) complicating open operative treatment of a closed injury
5. Bony Complications
   Infection (osteomyelitis) complicating open operative treatment of a closed injury

Recognition and Treatment of Complications, from Both the Initial Injury and Its Treatment

Some of the complications discussed below are caused by the initial injury that produced the fracture, whereas others are iatrogenic, having been caused by the treatment of the fracture. Both groups of complications have been classified previously.

The total care of the injured must include constant diligence and vigilance, so that the initial presence or subsequent development of a significant complication is not overlooked. The detection of complications requires that you attend to every complaint of the patient, examine the patient clinically at frequent intervals, assess any positive clinical findings, and when necessary, proceed with special investigations.

Initial and Early Complications
Local Complications

Skin Complications. The skin may have sustained an abrasion (friction burn), with particles of dirt having been ground into the dermis. Such abrasions must be thoroughly

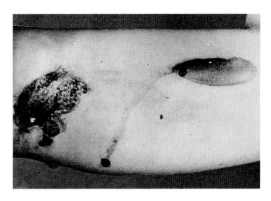

Figure 15.58. Blisters, or blebs, in the skin of the forearm in association with a fracture of the radius and ulna. One bleb has ruptured and the other is seeping serum.

cleansed under anesthesia to prevent the late unsightly tattoo effect of residual pigmentation from dirt under the re-epithelialized surface (Fig. 15.57).

The management of associated lacerations, puncture wounds, penetrating missile wounds, avulsion of skin, and skin loss have been discussed in relation to the treatment of open fractures.

Gross swelling within a fractured limb may stretch the overlying skin and compromise the circulation to its superficial layers with resultant *blister* or *bleb* formation (Fig. 15.58).

During fracture treatment, an area of skin may be constantly compressed between a firm surface on the outside and an underlying bony prominence. Thus, a patient who is not turned regularly or is insensitive to pain may develop a *bed sore* (decubitus ulcer), particularly over the sacrum and heels (Fig. 15.59). Excessive local pressure from an incorrectly applied plaster-of-Paris cast may produce a pressure sore (cast sore) (Fig. 15.60). These iatrogenic complications, which are preventable, may necessitate extensive skin grafting.

Vascular Complications

Arterial complications (injury to a major artery). Small blood vessels are torn at the time of all fractures, but injury to a major artery is uncommon. Nevertheless, such a complicating injury is serious because of the sequelae of persistent arterial occlusion. Major arteries are particularly vulnerable to injury in association

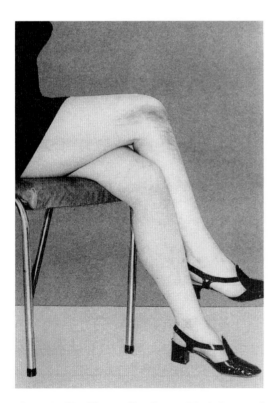

Figure 15.57. Tattoo effect from residual pigmented dirt that should have been removed from the abrasion during the initial treatment and is now covered by epithelium. This unsightly blemish is preventable.

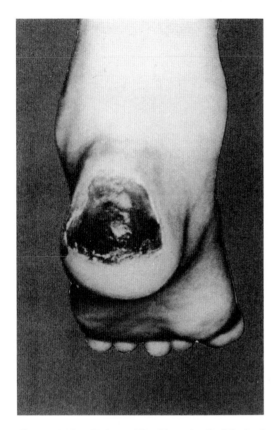

Figure 15.59. Bed sore (decubitus ulcer) of the heel in an elderly comatose patient. This lesion is preventable by frequent turning of the patient by the nursing staff.

with certain specific fractures and dislocations (Fig. 15.61).

Arterial division. A major artery may be completely or incompletely divided, either by the sudden displacement of a sharp fracture fragment from within or by an object or missile that has penetrated the deep tissues from without. A completely torn artery usually retracts and stops bleeding spontaneously, whereas one that is incompletely torn tends to continue bleeding. In either instance there is a residual hematoma locally and ischemia distally. In addition, incomplete division of an artery may lead to the development of a pulsating hematoma (false aneurysm).

Arterial spasm. When a major artery is subjected to sudden and severe traction, either at the time of fracture or during treatment of the fracture, it may react by *persistent spasm* of its

muscular coat with resultant occlusion. Although the artery has not been divided, there is usually a tear in the intima that leads to thrombosis. Secondary arterial spasm may spread both proximally and distally to include collateral arteries, in which case the resultant ischemia distally becomes even more extensive.

Arterial compression. Occasionally a major artery becomes trapped and compressed between two fracture fragments. Compression of an artery can also be iatrogenic due to the combination of an excessively tight encircling plaster-of-Paris cast or bandage externally, and progressive swelling within a closed space internally.

Arterial thrombosis. After any arterial injury that results in persistent occlusion, thrombosis is a potential sequela. As might be expected, the presence of pre-existing arterio-

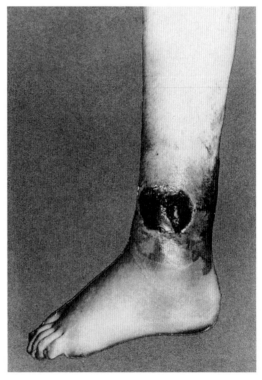

Figure 15.60. Pressure sore (cast sore) over the lateral aspect of the leg from excessive local pressure of an ineptly molded plaster cast. This iatrogenic complication, which is preventable by appropriate padding and molding, required a skin graft.

Doppler probe is very helpful in detecting a peripheral pulse that is too weak to be palpable. Arteriography is useful in localizing the precise site of arterial occlusion (Fig. 15.63).

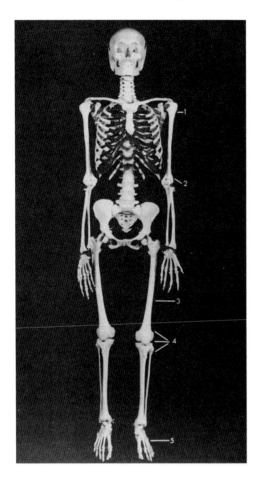

Figure 15.61.   Sites of vascular complications in relation to fractures. 1, axillary artery—fracture-dislocations and dislocations of the shoulder. 2, brachial artery—supracondylar fractures of the humerus. 3, femoral artery—fractures of the shaft of the femur. 4, popliteal artery—fractures of the distal end of femur and proximal end of tibia, dislocation of the knee. 5, dorsalis pedis artery—fractures in the forefoot.

sclerosis increases the risk of posttraumatic arterial thrombosis.

Recognition of arterial complications. External hemorrhage from a divided artery is obvious, whereas internal hemorrhage is evidenced only by a progressively enlarging local swelling. Complete arterial occlusion in a limb is associated with initial pallor of the skin distally, loss of arterial pulse, coolness of the skin and later, mottled, dark discoloration that heralds gangrene (Fig. 15.62). If the presence of a palpable peripheral pulse is questionable, it is probably absent. Nevertheless, a surface

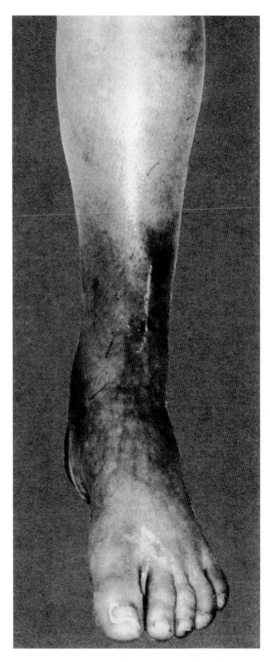

Figure 15.62.   Impending gangrene of the foot and distal part of the leg in a 15-year-old boy who had sustained a closed fracture of the proximal end of the tibia. No pulse could be detected below the knee and the skin was cool with mottled dark discoloration.

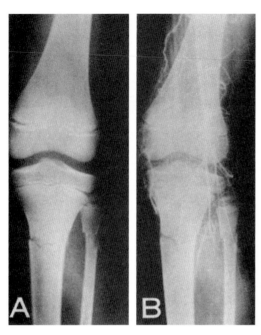

Figure 15.63. The value of arteriography in vascular occlusion. **A.** The knee region of a 15-year-old boy with a relatively undisplaced fracture of the proximal end of the tibia and fibula. The fracture, which was said to have been angulated, had been reduced 8 hours previously; the foot immediately became white and pulseless. The appearance of the boy's foot on admission is shown in Figure 15.62. **B.** An arteriogram immediately after admission reveals the exact site of vascular occlusion just distal to the bifurcation of the popliteal artery. Exploration of the arteries was performed forthwith. The arteries were decompressed after which blood flow was restored. The boy's foot did not become gangrenous but because of the 8-hour delay before arterial exploration, he did develop Volkmann's ischemia (compartment syndrome) of the leg muscles requiring fasciotomies.

Because this is usually at the site of the fracture, arteriography is not always essential. It should not be allowed to delay surgical exploration and repair of the arterial injury.

Compartment syndromes. When the increased pressure of progressive edema within a rigid osteofascial compartment of either the forearm or the leg (between the knee and the ankle) threatens the circulation to the enclosed (intracompartmental) muscles and nerves, the phenomenon is called a *compartment syndrome.* Any condition that either increases the content of a given compartment, decreases its volume, or both, causes an in-

creased intracompartmental pressure. Formerly known as *Volkmann's ischemia,* compartment syndromes most frequently involve the flexor compartment of the forearm and the anterior tibial compartment of the leg (although any osteofascial compartment may be affected). Because tissues outside the compartment are spared, the skin and the distal part of the limb, although transiently affected, survive and hence, the disorder is different from gangrene.

The progressive intracompartmental pressure from edema initially compromises capillary blood flow to muscle. This produces more edema and a vicious cycle is established. Peripheral nerves within the compartment can withstand only 2 to 4 hours of ischemia, but they do have some potential for regeneration. By contrast, muscle can survive up to 6 hours of ischemia but cannot regenerate. In due course, necrotic muscle is replaced by dense fibrous scar tissue that gradually shortens to produce a *"compartmental contracture"* or Volkmann's ischemic contracture (Fig. 15.64).

A compartment syndrome may be secondary to one of two different phenomena: 1) proximal (extracompartmental) occlusion of the main artery supplying the compartment; 2) intracompartmental injury to either bone, soft tissue, or both with resultant hemorrhage. In both types, the intracompartmental pressure rises rapidly to dangerous levels, and unless this pressure is relieved by a complete surgical fasciotomy, ischemic *necrosis* and consequent ischemic *contracture* are inevitable.

The injuries that are most frequently complicated by a compartment syndrome are: 1) displaced supracondylar fractures of the humerus with damage to the brachial artery in children; 2) excessive longitudinal traction in the treatment of fractures of the femoral shaft in children with resultant arterial spasm; 3) fractures (as well as surgical osteotomies) of the proximal third of the tibia; 4) drug-induced coma with resultant pressure on major arteries from lying on a hard surface in an awkward position for a prolonged period.

The *clinical picture* of a compartment syndrome with impending compartmental ischemia, or Volkmann's ischemia, is character-

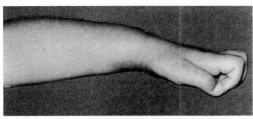

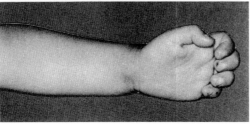

Figure 15.64. Volkmann's ischemic contracture (post compartment syndrome) of muscles of the forearm in a 6-year-old child. After reduction of a supracondylar fracture of the humerus the child had complained of severe pain in the forearm. Regrettably, his surgeon prescribed large doses of analgesics that relieved the pain somewhat. In the meantime the child developed severe Volkmann's ischemia (compartment syndrome) of nerves and muscles in the forearm. In these photographs taken 6 months later, it is apparent that he has severe deformities and serious disability as a result of progressive contracture of the necrotic muscles that have been replaced by fibrous tissue. This tragic outcome could have been prevented by early recognition of this serious complication, removal of all encircling bandages and cast, fasciotomies, and stabilization of the supracondylar fracture by percutaneous pinning.

ized by severe pain after a pain-free internal (from muscle ischemia), transient decrease in peripheral circulation with relative pallor and coolness of the skin as well as puffy swelling of the hand or foot, and ischemic disturbance of the involved peripheral nerve function as evidenced by paresthesia, hypoesthesia, and paralysis. Thus the clinical warnings of impending intracompartmental ischemia are pain, pallor, puffiness, and paresthesia. The involved compartment feels tense or tight, and tender. Muscle paralysis is a late manifestation. If the underlying cause is extracompartmental, the peripheral pulse is likely to be absent, but if the cause is intracompartmental, the peripheral pulse may be palpable. If the extracompartmental injury also involves serious damage to major peripheral nerves supplying sensation

to the compartment, pain may not be a feature; this can be dangerously misleading. When the peripheral nerves are intact, passive extension of the fingers and wrist (or toes and ankle) dramatically aggravates the pain.

The injudicious use of analgesics for severe and persistent pain after a fracture may well mask the compartmental ischemia and should be avoided.

In recent years, it has become possible to measure intracompartmental interstitial fluid pressure by means of the transcutaneous insertion of a catheter such as the slit catheter (Rorabeck). Commercial pressure monitors are also available. The normal resting intracompartmental pressure is from 0 to 8 mm Hg. Pressures above 30 to 40 mm Hg (or within 30 mm Hg of the patient's diastolic blood pressure) represent an absolute indication for immediate decompression of the compartment by complete surgical fasciotomy throughout the complete length of the compartment. The fascia must be left wide open; the skin also should be left open, for at least 7 days, after which time delayed primary closure can be performed. Surgical stabilization of any associated fracture is an important part of the treatment of a compartment syndrome.

Treatment of vascular complications. Occlusion of a major artery represents a surgical emergency inasmuch as within a few hours of onset, the results of the associated ischemia become irreversible. Treatment of the vascular complication takes precedence over treatment of the associated fracture itself. A series of therapeutic measures must be instituted immediately, in the following order: 1) any constricting cast or bandage must be *completely* removed (and not just cut); 2) any distortion of the fractured limb or extreme position of a nearby joint should be lessened; 3) if the fracture is being treated by continuous traction, the amount of traction should be decreased; 4) if these measures fail to restore adequate peripheral circulation, an emergency arteriogram is indicated; if there is no improvement within half an hour, the artery should be explored surgically. Sympathetic denervation by anesthetic block is of doubtful value.

At operation, if the artery has been divided, it should be repaired by direct suture; if this is not possible, continuity can be achieved either by means of an autogenous vein graft or a plastic arterial prosthesis. Associated division of a major vein should also be repaired. If the artery is merely compressed it can be released, and provided there is no associated arterial spasm, flow will be re-established. An arterial thrombus should be removed. If the artery is severely contused or if there has been an intimal tear, it may be necessary to resect the damaged portion of the vessel and restore its continuity by direct suture, vein graft, or prosthesis. Persistent arterial spasm may be more difficult to relieve; if the local application of warm papaverine does not relieve the spasm, the constricted portion of the artery can sometimes be permanently dilated by means of intra-arterial injection of saline, beginning proximally and dilating the vessel a segment at a time as described by Mustard. Severe arterial spasm can be overcome by meticulous microsurgical excision of the encircling adventitia (outer layer) of the spastic segment of the artery under the magnification of the operating microscope (Chapter 6, Fig. 6.31).

Even after re-establishment of the arterial blood flow there is likely to be a residual compartment syndrome; consequently the compartment(s) supplied by that artery may need to be decompressed by surgical fasciotomy as described above.

After operative treatment for a vascular complication, internal fixation of the fracture is indicated to prevent further movement at the site of the arterial injury and resultant disruption of the repair.

Sequelae of arterial complications

1. **Gangrene.** Persistent total ischemia distal to an arterial lesion results in necrosis of all tissues including skin (*gangrene*). The ischemic tissues become mummified and the skin eventually comes to resemble dark leather. This irreversible complication necessitates early amputation through viable tissues.

2. **Compartment syndrome (Volkmann's ischemic contracture).** Persistent occlusion of deep arteries for approximately 6 hours or longer produces ischemia of mus-

cles and nerves with resultant necrosis. Necrotic muscle is subsequently replaced by fibrous scar tissue, which causes the involved muscle to become permanently short (contracture) (Fig. 15.64). After the establishment of persistent Volkmann's ischemia of muscle, but before the development of muscle contracture, surgical resection of the infarcted area of muscle decompresses the nerves and may prevent contracture. Established Volkmann's contracture necessitates major reconstructive operations including muscle release, nerve grafts, and tendon transfers to minimize the severe disability. The most important aspect of Volkmann's ischemia is its prevention. Impending Volkmann's ischemia, if recognized and treated very early, can be reversed.

3. **Intermittent claudication.** When an arterial lesion has not been sufficiently severe or persistent to produce either gangrene or Volkmann's ischemic contracture, but has not been completely repaired, the sequelae of the persistent relative ischemia include pain, which is initiated by muscle activity and relieved by rest (intermittent claudication). There also may be persistent muscle weakness, numbness, and coldness in the limb.

4. **Gas gangrene.** The uncommon but serious and even life-threatening complication of fulminating infection by an anaerobic bacteria, *Clostridium welchii*, produces rapidly progressive edema and gas formation in the local tissues. The blood supply is soon occluded with the resultant development of gas gangrene.

   After an incubation period of 24 to 48 hours, the patient experiences severe and constant local pain and becomes acutely and seriously ill. There is a characteristic foul, fetid odor associated with gas gangrene. Physical examination may reveal local soft tissue crepitus indicating the presence of gas; the gas can also be detected radiographically as demonstrated in Chapter 5 (Fig. 5.16).

   The local wound should be reopened and debrided immediately. The patient should be given systemic antibacterial therapy, usually penicillin and one of the tetracyclines. Treatment in a hyperbaric oxygen chamber for several 2-hour periods usually results in dramatic improvement in the clinical picture, both locally and systemically. The late diagnosis of gas gangrene is associated with irreversible gangrene and a life-threatening infection that necessitates immediate amputation.

Venous complications: division of a major vein. A major vein may be completely or incompletely divided, either by the displacement of a fracture fragment from within or by an object or missile that has penetrated the deep tissues from without. Injuries to major veins should be repaired surgically to prevent the late sequelae of persistent venous congestion distally.

Venous thrombosis and pulmonary embolism. The combination of deep vein thrombosis (DVT) and pulmonary embolism (PE) is a common cause of morbidity and mortality in adult orthopaedic patients. The veins of the lower limbs and pelvis are more susceptible to thrombosis after a fracture than those of the upper limbs. Adults are more susceptible to thrombosis than children. The main factor that precipitates thrombosis is *venous stasis,* which can be caused by local pressure on a vein from prolonged bed rest or from a tight encircling plaster-of-Paris cast or bandage. Other factors include increased coagulability and vessel wall damage. Venous stasis is aggravated by inactivity of muscles that normally have a pumping action on venous return from the limb. After a fracture, the venous lesion is usually a phlebothrombosis, as opposed to an inflammatory thrombosis (thrombophlebitis). The thrombus is only loosely adherent to the wall of the vein. It may come loose and pass to the lungs to produce *pulmonary embolism.* Approximately one half of pulmonary emboli arise from a previously undetected thrombosis (i.e., silent thrombosis). There is an increased risk of DVT and PE in smokers and in women who are taking oral contraceptives.

Diagnosis. When the venous thrombosis is in the calf, the patient complains of local pain; there is tenderness in the midline posteriorly and distal swelling due to congestion. Passive dorsiflexion of the ankle aggravates the pain (Homan's sign). When the thrombosis is in the thigh, the entire lower limb becomes swollen. However, less than 50% of DVTs can be diagnosed clinically. A venogram is most helpful in localizing the site of thrombosis. Other useful methods of investigation include impedance plethysmography and Doppler ultrasound.

The complication of pulmonary embolism varies in severity. A small pulmonary embolus may go undetected or may cause only mild chest pain. An embolus of moderate size is manifest by the sudden onset of chest pain, dyspnea, and sometimes hemoptysis. A friction rub may be heard and radiographic examination reveals a triangular-shaped area of increased density in the lung, representing the infarcted segment (Fig. 15.65).

A massive pulmonary embolus, however, produces a dramatic onset of severe chest pain. The patient immediately blanches and literally drops dead.

Prevention of venous thrombosis. The venous stasis underlying venous thrombosis can

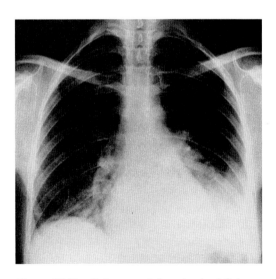

Figure 15.65. Pulmonary infarct in the left lower lobe of the lung due to pulmonary embolism in a 35-year-old woman. Five days after closed reduction of a fractured tibia, the patient experienced the sudden onset of severe pain in the left side of the chest as well as left shoulder-tip pain (referred from the left diaphragm). This radiograph reveals a triangular area of density representing the infarcted segment as well as evidence of a pleural effusion.

be prevented to a large extent by avoiding constant local pressure on veins and by encouraging the patient to actively contract all muscles in the injured limb and to move about as much as possible given the limits imposed by the treatment of the fracture. For adults confined to bed, the use of the elastic compressive stocking, CPM, and cyclic external pneumatic compression help in the prevention of DVT. Patients at high risk of developing a DVT should be given a prophylactic anticoagulant such as low-molecular-weight heparin.

Treatment of venous thrombosis. As soon as this complication is recognized, the patient should be treated with appropriate anticoagulant drugs such as heparin or warfarin. Recent thrombosis in the femoral vein is best treated by surgical thrombectomy to decrease the risk of PE and to prevent the late sequelae of persistent venous obstruction in the lower limb. Deep vein thromboses below the knee are much less likely to embolize to the lung than those above the knee.

Neurological Complications. Complicating injuries to brain, spinal cord, or peripheral nerves associated with a fracture may be caused either by the original injury or, less often, by inept treatment of the fracture itself. Neurological complications are relatively common in association with specific fractures and dislocations (Fig. 15.66). The etiology, diagnosis, and treatment of these injuries are discussed in Chapter 12.

Visceral Complications. Thoracoabdominal viscera may be injured at the time of an accident independent of any fractures; they may also be injured by penetration by a sharp fracture fragment from a nearby bone. Thus, displaced fractures of the ribs may damage the heart and produce a hemopericardium with resultant cardiac tamponade, or they may perforate the pleura to produce a hemothorax. They may even perforate the lung to produce a hemopneumothorax. Displaced fractures of the lower ribs may perforate the liver, spleen, or kidneys. Fractures of the thoracic and lumbar spine may result in paralytic ileus and gastric dilatation. Displaced fractures of the pelvis may rupture the bladder or urethra, and sometimes the colon or rectum.

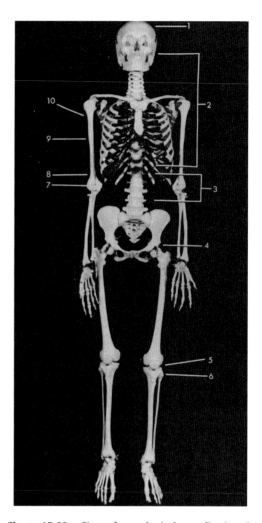

Figure 15.66. Sites of neurological complications in relation to fractures. 1, brain—skull fractures. 2, spinal cord—cervical and thoracic spine fractures and dislocations. 3, cauda equina—lumbar spine fractures and dislocations. 4, sciatic nerve—posterior dislocations and fracture-dislocations of the hip. 5, medial and lateral popliteal nerves—dislocations of the knee. 6, lateral popliteal nerve—vulnerable to external pressure from bandages and casts. 7, ulnar nerve—avulsion fracture-separation of the medial epicondyle. 8, median nerve—supracondylar fractures of the humerus. 9, radial nerve—fractures of the shaft of the humerus. 10, circumflex nerve—dislocations and fracture-dislocations of the shoulder.

Joint Complications

Infection of a joint (septic arthritis). After an open intra-articular fracture—less often after open operation on a closed intra-articular fracture—the serious complication of *septic*

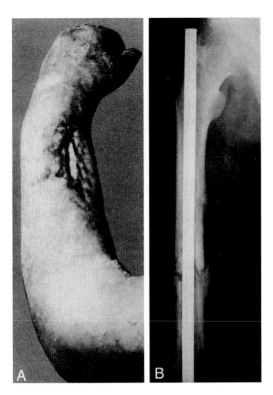

Figure 15.67. Osteomyelitis complicating open reduction of fractures. **A.** Severe osteomyelitis of the radius complicating open reduction of a closed fracture in a young man. The wound has broken open (dehisced) and necrotic infected bone is exposed in its depths. The patient's disability will be greatly increased and prolonged as a result of this serious complication. **B.** Severe osteomyelitis of the shaft of the femur complicating open reduction and intramedullary rod fixation of a closed fracture in a young woman. Subperiosteal new bone can be seen at each end of a necrotic, infected fragment (sequestrum). This infection will be exceedingly difficult to control. The sequestrum will have to be excised and the entire area irrigated continuously with a combination of antibiotic and a detergent such as alevaire. The intramedullary nail will have to be removed as soon as there is sufficient new bone formation to provide stability at the fracture site.

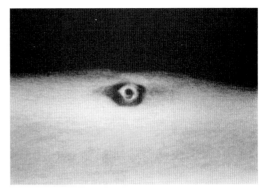

Figure 15.68. A typical ring sequestrum in the anterior cortex of the tibia due to the complication of a pin track infection at the site of a pin that had been used for continuous skeletal traction. The radiopaque ring-shaped sequestrum is surrounded by a radiolucent area of osteolytic resorption of bone. The infection subsided after removal of the sequestrum.

tion, which involves all layers of the soft tissues and bone at the fracture site. The treatment of open fractures is discussed in an earlier section of this chapter. Its aim is to minimize the risk of acute osteomyelitis and its sequelae—chronic osteomyelitis, delayed union, and even nonunion.

A closed fracture may become infected after open operation—a terrible tragedy (Fig. 15.67). Furthermore, bone may become infected locally along the track of a metal pin used either for continuous skeletal traction or external skeletal fixation (pin track osteomyelitis). Indeed, a ring of bone surrounding the pin track may become infected and necrotic, forming a *ring sequestrum* (Fig. 15.68).

Avascular necrosis of bone. Posttraumatic avascular necrosis of bone is usually caused by disruption of the nutrient vessels at the time of the original injury. It also may be iatrogenic as a result of excessive dissection during open reduction of fractures and dislocations. It is a serious complication because it leads to delayed union and to subsequent joint incongruity and degenerative arthritis (Fig. 15.69). The complication of avascular necrosis usually occurs after certain specific fractures and dislocations because of the precarious blood supply to bone at these sites (Fig. 15.70). Posttraumatic avascular necrosis of bone is also discussed in Chapter 13.

arthritis may ensue. Unless treated early and effectively, septic arthritis leads to destruction of articular cartilage, which results in degenerative joint disease. The diagnosis and treatment of septic arthritis are discussed in Chapter 10.

Bony Complications
Infection of bone (osteomyelitis). Open fractures are particularly susceptible to infec-

Remote Complications

Fat Embolism Syndrome. Fat globules can be found in the circulation of most adults after a major fracture of the long bone. Fortunately, only about 9% of such patients develop detectable systemic fat embolization and a significant respiratory distress syndrome with severe arterial hypoxia, the combination of which constitutes the *fat embolism syndrome*. It is probably relatively common in mild, clinically undetected (subclinical) forms. Small fat emboli are frequently an unsuspected finding at postmortem examination of adult accident victims who may have died *with* fat emboli but not necessarily *because of* fat emboli. Most susceptible to the serious complication of clinical fat embolism syndrome are previously healthy young adults who have sustained severe fractures, especially when associated with other injuries (multiple injuries, or polytrauma). Elderly individuals who sustain fractures of the upper end of the femur are also susceptible. This syndrome, although rare in previously normal children, may complicate fractures in those who have some type of preexisting systemic collagen disease with or without corticosteroid therapy.

Etiology and pathogenesis. Although fat embolization from bone marrow has been proven to occur, its precise pathogenesis is both conjectural and controversial. However, it would seem that stress-induced changes in lipid metabolism and in blood coagulation (as

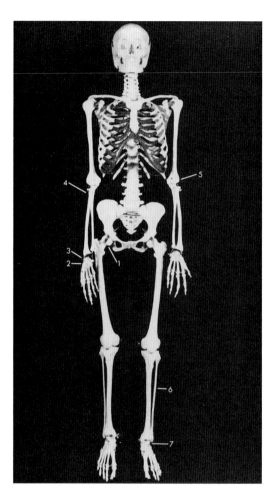

Figure 15.70. Sites of avascular necrosis of bone in relation to fractures. 1, femoral head—fractures of the femoral neck, dislocations of the hip. 2, lunate—dislocations of the lunate. 3, scaphoid—fractures of the scaphoid. 4, radial head—fractures of the neck of the radius. 5, lateral condyle (capitellum)—fractures of the lateral condyle (especially after excessive soft tissue dissection during open reduction). 6, middle segment of a comminuted fracture. 7, body of the talus—fractures of the neck of the talus.

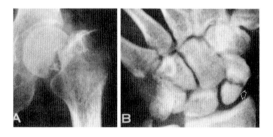

Figure 15.69. Posttraumatic avascular necrosis of bone. **A.** Avascular necrosis of the femoral head complicating a fracture of the femoral neck in a 40-year-old woman. Note also that there is nonunion of the fracture. **B.** Avascular necrosis of the proximal half of the scaphoid complicating a fracture in a 22-year-old man (*arrow*). The fracture has failed to unite 1 year after injury and will require bone grafting.

may result from severe trauma) may cause coalescence of chylomicrons to form macroglobules of fat that produce fat embolization and resultant arterial hypoxia with metabolic and respiratory acidosis. Fat emboli can deform and thereby pass through the lung, causing fat embolism through the systemic circulation to the brain (which accounts for the cerebral manifestations).

Clinical features. A detectable fat embolism usually develops after a latent period of 2 or 3 days, although in very severe cases it may appear within a few hours of injury. Because the symptoms and signs are manifestations of emboli in various organs, they might be anticipated. Pulmonary emboli cause respiratory distress with dyspnea, hemoptysis, tachypnea, and cyanosis. Cerebral emboli are manifest by headache, confusion, and irritability followed by delirium, stupor, and coma. Cardiac emboli cause tachycardia and a drop in blood pressure. Transient skin lesions become apparent as multiple petechial hemorrhages (possibly due to a transient thrombocytopenia rather than to emboli), particularly in the skin of the upper chest and axillae as well as in the conjunctivae (Fig. 15.71). The patient also becomes febrile. The prognosis in patients who exhibit pulmonary insufficiency and coma is grave in that the mortality rate is approximately 20%, a fatal outcome usually being related to a combination of pulmonary and cerebral lesions. Fat embolism syndrome has been estimated to be the major cause of death in 20% of fatalities associated with fractures.

Radiographic features. In well-established fat embolism, radiographic examination of the lungs reveals multiple areas of consolidation—a "snow storm" appearance.

Laboratory features. Because there is no pathognomonic laboratory test for fat embolism syndrome, the diagnosis is primarily clinical. In approximately half the patients with clinically recognizable fat embolism, the serum fatty acids are elevated because of hydrolyzation of neutral fat by an elevated serum lipase. There is free fat in the sputum and urine. The hemoglobin usually drops sharply very early in the process. The partial pressure of oxygen in the blood (PO_2) is reduced well below the normal level of 100 mm—sometimes as low as 60 mm. Thrombocytopenia is often present.

Prevention of fat embolism. Inasmuch as fat embolism is related at least in part to disturbed metabolism, efforts should be made to prevent metabolic and respiratory acidosis by good general care of the injured patient, including high carbohydrate intake plus constant maintenance of fluid and electrolyte balance. Such care of all adults who have sustained two or more fractures definitely decreases the incidence of fat embolism. The early operative fixation of associated fractures would also seem to decrease the incidence of this complication.

Treatment of established fat embolism. Once fat embolism is established, the use of heparin increases the rate of hydrolysis and removal of emboli. Large doses of corticosteroids may decrease the tissue injury in the lungs. Blood volume and electrolytes should be restored. Intravenous alcohol is of doubtful value and may even mask the cerebral symptoms. Low-molecular-weight dextran infusion may help to improve the microcirculation in the involved organs. In the presence of respiratory distress, endotracheal intubation or a tracheostomy followed by mechanically as-

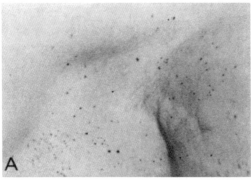
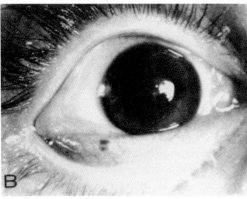

Figure 15.71. Petechial hemorrhages associated with fat embolism: **A,** over the lateral chest wall and axilla and **B,** in the conjunctiva of the lower lid (which has been everted). Two days previously the patient had sustained fractures of both femora in an automobile accident.

sisted intermittent positive pressure ventilation (IPPV) with oxygen improves the patient's clinical condition by decreasing cerebral anoxia. Constant monitoring of PO_2, partial pressure of carbon dioxide (PCO_2) and arterial pH provides the best appraisal of the patient's metabolic status and guides corrective therapy.

Pulmonary Embolism. This complication has been discussed in a previous section of this chapter dealing with venous thrombosis.

Pneumonia. When treatment of a patient's fracture involves complete and prolonged bed rest (which should be avoided whenever possible), the convalescent period may become complicated by *hypostatic pneumonia*. The elderly are particularly susceptible. Likewise, painful fractures of the ribs with associated limitation of respiratory excursion may lead to the development of pneumonia. Treatment includes antibiotic therapy, deep breathing exercises, frequent turning of the bedfast patient and, if necessary, bronchoscopic suction.

Tetanus. Tetanus, which is caused by *Clostridium tetani,* is a preventable complication of open wounds. Nevertheless, at least 300 individuals die each year in North America as a result of this tragic complication that, even with treatment, has a mortality rate of 50%.

Etiology and pathogenesis. Clostridium tetani, being an anaerobic organism, thrives in devitalized or dead tissue where it produces a powerful neurotoxin that is carried by the lymphatics and bloodstream to the central nervous system. Once there, it soon becomes fixed in anterior horn cells, after which it can no longer be neutralized by antitoxins. The site of entry may vary from an apparently insignificant puncture wound to a severe open fracture wound. Although the incubation period may vary considerably, it is usually from 10 to 14 days.

Clinical features. The effect of the powerful neurotoxin is to initiate tonic, and later clonic, contractions of skeletal muscles (*tetanic spasms*). Spasms of the neck and trunk muscles produce the characteristic arched back posture (*opisthotonus*), spasms of the jaw muscles produce trismus ("*lock jaw*"), whereas spasms in the fascial muscles account for the sardonic grin (*risus sardonicus*) (Fig.

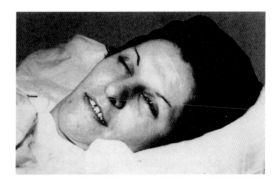

Figure 15.72.   Risus sardonicus of severe tetanus in a 35-year-old woman. The sardonic grin is caused by tetanic spasms of her facial muscles. She was acutely ill and at this stage was semicomatose.

15.72). Eventually involvement of intercostal muscles and diaphragm leads to fatal asphyxia.

Prevention. The prevention of tetanus has been described in the preceding section of this chapter in relation to the treatment of open fractures.

Treatment. Established tetanus requires the intravenous administration of large doses of tetanus immune globulin (human), heavy sedation and, in the presence of severe muscle spasms and respiratory involvement, endotracheal intubation and mechanically assisted respiration. Antibacterial therapy is of little value in the treatment of established tetanus but may be helpful in preventing or controlling associated infections.

Delirium Tremens. When a chronic alcoholic sustains a major injury and is admitted to hospital, the source of alcohol is abruptly withdrawn. During the ensuing few days, the patient may exhibit dramatic and even alarming withdrawal symptoms, characterized by disorientation, anxiety, agitation, and disturbing visual hallucinations. Understandably the development of delirium tremens (the "DTs") interferes with treatment of the patient's injuries and may also mimic such complications as head injury and fat embolism.

Late Complications
Local Complications
Late Joint Complications
Joint stiffness. Transient stiffness is an anticipated sequela in any joint that has been

immobilized during fracture healing. It can be minimized by active contraction of all muscle groups controlling the joint and can usually be successfully treated by active movement of the joint after the immobilization has been discontinued. This transient type of joint stiffness is not considered a complication.

Persistent joint stiffness, by contrast, is a significant complication because it retards restoration of normal function in the injured limb. It is most likely to complicate fractures that are close to a joint or those that actually involve a joint surface. Rare in childhood, the incidence of persistent joint stiffness rises with advancing years and is particularly common in joints that have had pre-existing degenerative changes.

The most common causes are periarticular adhesions, intra-articular adhesions, adhesions between the muscles and bone, and posttraumatic myositis ossificans (posttraumatic ossification in muscle).

Periarticular adhesions. After a fracture near a joint, adhesions may develop between the fibrous capsule and ligaments as well as between these structures and nearby muscles and tendons. Such adhesions impair the normal gliding between these structures. Forceful passive movement at this stage may actually cause more adhesions. After a period of extensive physiotherapy (involving active movements only), when no further improvement in joint motion is being obtained, a gentle manipulation of the joint under general anesthesia frequently yields a considerable increase in joint movement that then must be retained by further physiotherapy. Under these circumstances, CPM is also useful.

Intra-articular adhesions. Intra-articular fractures, dislocations, and fracture-dislocations are invariably associated with a hemarthrosis and subsequent fibrinous deposits on the synovium and articular cartilage. These deposits lead to firm adhesions within the joint between folds of synovium and between the synovium and cartilage. After a period of extensive physiotherapy, any persistent joint stiffness in large joints such as the knee and shoulder may respond to gentle manipulation under anesthesia. If it does not respond, then surgical excision of the adhesions (arthrolysis) is indicated.

As with periarticular adhesions, CPM is helpful in the prevention and treatment of intra-articular adhesions.

Adhesions between muscles and between muscles and bone. Severely displaced fractures are always associated with extensive tearing of surrounding muscles. Likewise, during open reduction of fractures, the surrounding muscles may be damaged. Subsequent formation of fibrous scar tissue binds muscles to each other as well as to the underlying bone. This phenomenon is particularly common after fractures of the lower end of the femur, where the adhesions involving the quadriceps muscle result in persistent limitation of knee flexion. Physiotherapy helps to restore joint motion, but manipulation is contraindicated because it may cause additional muscle tears and adhesions. Surgical release of the adhesions sometimes becomes necessary for this type of persistent joint stiffness. We have used CPM immediately after such operations with much benefit.

Posttraumatic degenerative joint disease or arthritis. Any residual incongruity of joint surfaces after an intra-articular fracture, dislocation, or fracture-dislocation, particularly in weightbearing joints, leads inevitably to the development of degenerative arthritis, as discussed in Chapter 11 (Fig. 15.73). This complication emphasizes the importance of perfect restoration of joint surfaces after injury. Another cause of posttraumatic degenerative arthritis in the weightbearing joints is malunion, especially malalignment, of fractures with residual excessive stresses being applied to one area of the joint (Fig. 15.74). The treatment of degenerative arthritis of various joints is discussed in Chapter 11.

Bony Complications

Abnormal healing of fractures. The healing of a fracture may be abnormal in one of three ways: 1) union may occur in the usual time but in an abnormal position (malunion); 2) union may be delayed beyond a reasonable time (delayed union); 3) union may fail to occur (nonunion). It has been estimated that 5% to 10% of the approximately 6 million frac-

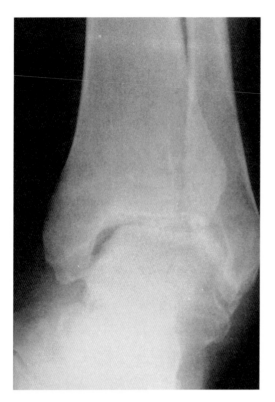

Figure 15.73. Posttraumatic degenerative joint disease in the ankle of a 57-year-old man who had sustained an intra-articular fracture of his ankle 25 years previously.

tures that occur in North America each year are either slow to heal or fail to heal.

Malunion. As the term *malunion* implies, union has occurred, but badly, in the sense that the fracture has united in an unsatisfactory position of significant deformity. Minor degrees of residual deformity (angulation, rotation, shortening, lengthening) are common and do not present significant problems in either appearance or function. Major degrees of residual deformity, particularly angulatory deformity, are significant in both appearance and function, as well as in the late complication of degenerative arthritis (Fig. 15.75). Malunion frequently requires a corrective osteotomy; however, it can be prevented by obtaining and maintaining an acceptable reduction of the fracture.

Delayed union. Under certain circumstances, healing of a fracture is much slower than the estimated rate of healing for that par-

ticular fracture. This slow type of fracture healing is referred to as *delayed union.* Successive clinical and radiographic examinations reveal evidence of slow but steady progression toward union with no radiographic sclerosis of the bone ends. Patience is required by both the patient and the surgeon (Fig. 15.76). Occasionally, the surgeon must encourage union by means of an autogenous bone graft.

Nonunion. Complete failure of a fracture to unite by bone after a much longer period than normal is referred to as *nonunion* of which there are two types. In one type, the fracture has healed by fibrous tissue only (*fibrous nonunion*). It may have some potential for bony union provided it has been rigidly immobilized internally for long enough and that any local deterrent to fracture healing, such as infection, has been eradicated (Fig. 15.77). Once radiographic examination reveals that the bone ends have become sclerosed, the surgeon should encourage union by autogenous bone graft.

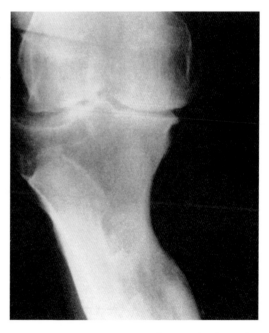

Figure 15.74. Posttraumatic degenerative joint disease in the knee of a 60-year-old man. The degenerative joint disease is secondary to excessive wear on the medial side of the knee joint, which in turn has resulted from the long-standing varus malalignment of a malunited tibia. The deformity had been present for 20 years.

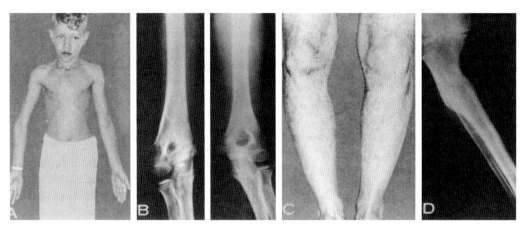

Figure 15.75. Malunion of fractures. **A.** Cubitus varus ("gunstock deformity") of the right elbow of a boy due to malunion of a supracondylar fracture of the humerus. Notice also the congenital cataract of his right eye. **B.** Cubitus varus of the right elbow. The loss of carrying angle of the right elbow is apparent when compared with the normal carrying angle of the left elbow. **C.** Genu varum ("bow leg") of the right leg in a 60-year-old man due to malunion of a fractured tibia 20 years previously. **D.** Marked varus deformity of a malunited tibia. Note the degenerative arthritis of the knee, especially in the medial compartment. (This is the same patient whose radiograph is depicted in Fig. 15.74.)

In the second type of nonunion, continued movement at the fracture site stimulates the formation of a false joint (*pseudarthrosis*) complete with a synovial-like capsule, synovial cavity, and synovial fluid (Fig. 15.78). An established nonunion cannot possibly unite, even with prolonged immobilization, and therefore requires bone grafting. Autogenous cancellous bone grafts are much more effective than large cortical grafts.

A variety of methods may be used to enhance fracture healing that is either delayed

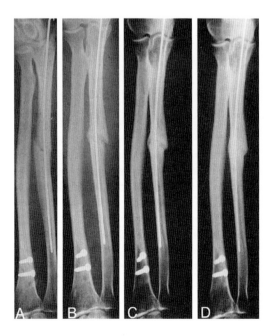

Figure 15.76. Delayed union of an oblique fracture of the shaft of the ulna in a 35-year-old woman. The fracture had been treated by open reduction and intramedullary nailing. A coexistent fracture of the distal end of the radius had been treated by open reduction and screw fixation. **A.** Two months after injury the fracture line in the ulna is clearly visible and there is little callus. **B.** Four months after injury, union in the ulna is delayed but still progressing. The fracture of the radius has united. **C.** Nine months after injury, the ulna is still not united but union is progressing slowly. **D.** One year after injury, union, though delayed, has finally occurred.

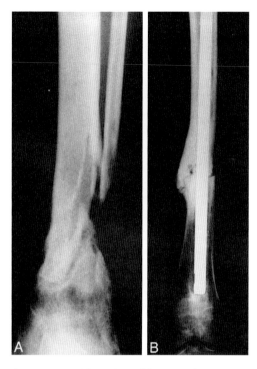

Figure 15.77. Nonunion of fractures. A. Nonunion of a comminuted fracture of the tibia in a 24-year-old woman despite 18 months of immobilization. Note the sclerosis of the bone ends. This is an atrophic fibrous nonunion that requires bone grafting. **B.** Infected nonunion of the closed femoral shaft fracture that had been treated 1 year previously by open reduction and intramedullary nailing in a 30-year-old man. The fracture line is still apparent, the bone ends are sclerosed, and there is rarefaction around both the medial and lateral sides of the distal end of the nail. This is referred to as the "windshield wiper phenomenon" and it is evidence of persistent movement around the nail in the distal fragment. This fracture will not unite until the infection has been eradicated.

or has failed. These include autogenous bone grafts, the use of allogeneic bone grafts, osteoconductive methods (such as calcium-based ceramic grafts), and osteoinductive methods (such as freeze-dried demineralized allogeneic bone combined with collagen, transforming growth factor-betas, bone morphogenetic proteins, fibroblast growth factors, and platelet-derived growth factor).

Electrical Stimulation of Fracture Healing. During the past 2 decades, one facet of biophysics that has become particularly relevant to fracture healing has been the electrical

stimulation of osteogenesis as an alternative to bone grafting in the treatment of delayed union and nonunion of fractures (as discussed in Chapter 6). When bone is stressed by bending forces, *stress-generated electrical potentials* develop—electronegative on the concave (compression) side and electropositive on the convex (tension) side. Furthermore, *bioelectrical potentials* that depend on cellular viability occur in living unstressed bone—electronegative in sites of bone growth and repair, and electropositive in other sites. It also has been shown that the application of relatively small amounts of electrical currents to bone stimulates osteogenesis around the negative electrode (cathode).

On the basis of these biophysical data, the following three systems of electrical stimulation have been developed for the treatment of delayed union and nonunion of fractures in humans: 1) constant direct current through percutaneous wire cathodes (semi-invasive) and more recently capacitative coupling (noninvasive) (Brighton); 2) constant direct current through implanted electrodes and an implanted power pack (invasive) (Dwyer and Paterson); 3) inductive coupling through electromagnetic coils (noninvasive) (Bassett and deHaas).

Although each of these systems has advantages and disadvantages, all three have been proven to be effective in that, for properly selected patients, they provide an overall success rate comparable to that of bone grafting operations. All three systems are effective in the treatment of delayed unions and fibrous nonunions, but they are ineffective when there is an established false joint (pseudarthrosis).

Another method of treatment of delayed unions and nonunions that is thought to be as effective as bone grafting operations is the local injection into the fracture site of autogenous bone marrow as reported by Connolly.

Success in the treatment of nonunions and defects in bones using human bone morphogenetic protein (1 BMP) combined with autolyzed, antigen-extracted, allogeneic (AAA) bone has been reported by Johnson, Urist, and Finerman.

The factors that favor delayed union and nonunion include the following: 1) severe dis-

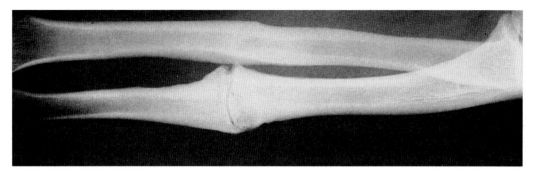

Figure 15.78.   A hypertrophic nonunion of the ulna with formation of a pseudarthrosis in a 60-year-old man whose fracture had occurred 20 years previously. The patient still complained of pain and local tenderness. This type of nonunion requires bone grafting and internal fixation.

ruption of the periosteal sleeve at the time of the original fracture, or subsequently at the time of open operation; 2) loss of blood supply to one or both fracture fragments; 3) inadequate immobilization of the fracture; shearing forces are particularly harmful; 4) an inadequate period of immobilization; 5) distraction of fracture fragments by excessive traction; 6) persistent interposition of soft tissues in the fracture site; 7) infection at the fracture site from an open fracture (or from an open operation); 8) a local and progressive disease of bone (certain types of pathological fractures).

Persistent Infection of Bone.   If osteomyelitis that has complicated an open fracture or open reduction of a closed fracture is not completely eradicated, it persists and becomes chronic osteomyelitis, which may be extremely resistant to treatment, as discussed in Chapter 10. Furthermore, local chronic osteomyelitis frequently leads to delayed union or even nonunion (infected nonunion) and the fracture cannot heal until the infection is completely controlled (Fig. 15.77B).

Posttraumatic Osteoporosis.   During the period of immobilization of a fractured limb, particularly if the patient has failed to maintain good tone in muscles controlling immobilized joints, the bones atrophy (disuse atrophy, disuse osteoporosis), because bone resorption exceeds bone deposition (Fig. 15.79). Minor degrees of disuse osteoporosis are common, but if the osteoporosis is severe and persistent

it retards restoration of normal function of the limb. Intensive physiotherapy and gradual increase in the stresses applied to the osteoporotic bones tend to reverse the process.

Sudeck's Posttraumatic Painful Osteoporosis (Reflex Sympathetic Dystrophy).   Certain individuals, particularly those who are somewhat fearful and inhibited, seem predisposed to develop the troublesome complication of Sudeck's posttraumatic painful osteoporosis, a sympathetically mediated pain syndrome. The initial injury, which is usually in the distal part of a limb, may or may not include a fracture and may even be trivial.

This complication is usually detected by the unexpected failure of the patient to regain normal function in the hand or foot a few months after the injury when most patients would have recovered fully. The patient complains of severe pain in the hand or foot and is disinclined to use it. The joints become stiff, the soft tissues are edematous, and the skin is moist, mottled, smooth, and shiny (Fig. 15.80A). Radiographic examination reveals an exaggerated degree of disuse osteoporosis (Fig. 15.80B).

Sudeck's posttraumatic painful osteoporosis is a prolonged complication that is difficult to treat. Local warmth and active exercises are helpful. Occasionally, repeated sympathetic blocks are required to relieve the symptoms. Recovery is slow and may take many months but is relatively sure.

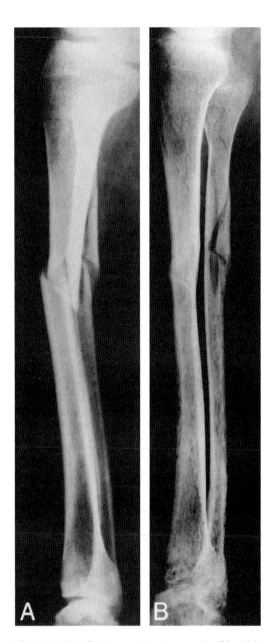

Figure 15.79. Posttraumatic osteoporosis of the tibia and fibula after a period of immobilization. **A.** Spiral fracture of the tibia and fibula in a young adult. **B.** Three months later, the fractures are uniting but note the marked osteoporosis, particularly in the distal fragments. This is an example of disuse osteoporosis caused by the combination of immobilization and non-weightbearing.

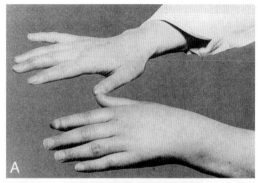

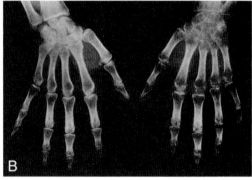

Figure 15.80.   Sudeck's painful posttraumatic osteoporosis (reflex sympathetic dystrophy) in the left hand of a 30-year-old woman 3 months after a fracture of the radius. **A.** Note that the left hand is swollen and the skin is smooth and shiny. **B.** An exaggerated degree of osteoporosis in the left hand, most striking in the areas of cancellous bone.

Refracture. The bone at the site of a completely healed fracture that has become remodeled and consolidated is just as strong as it was before the fracture. Nevertheless, during the relatively long period between clinical union and complete consolidation, the fracture is still relatively susceptible to *refracture*. This complication is uncommon in adults but occasionally occurs in children who, with few inhibitions and little fear, return to vigorous activity including sports at the earliest possible opportunity (Fig. 15.81).

A different type of refracture, seen in both children and adults, occurs not at the exact site of the original fracture but at the site of a screw, a site that is always weaker than normal bone (Fig. 15.82).

Metal Failure. A metallic device that is used to obtain internal fixation of a fracture serves

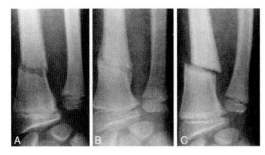

Figure 15.81. Refracture. **A.** Fracture of the distal end of the radius in a 13-year-old boy. **B.** Six weeks after injury, the fracture had become clinically united but not yet radiographically consolidated. **C.** Three months after the initial injury and before the fracture had become consolidated, the boy sustained a second injury and a refracture through the still relatively weak area of the original fracture.

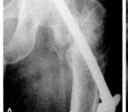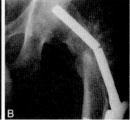

Figure 15.83. Metal failure. **A.** Nonunion of a fracture of the femoral neck in an elderly adult. The metal nail was unable to withstand the repeated stresses of continual movement at the fracture site and was beginning to bend. **B.** Two months later, the metal had fatigued, had failed completely, and had broken. (This type of internal fixation device is no longer used.)

only as a temporary internal splint to maintain reduction of the fracture fragments during the early weeks or months of healing. When fracture healing proceeds normally, the metal is subjected to diminishing stress until the fracture is completely united after which the metal

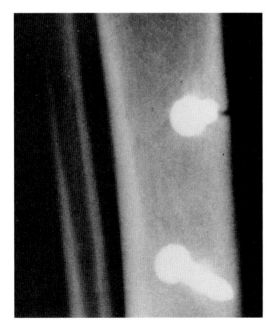

Figure 15.82. Refracture of the tibia that had occurred 5 years after the original injury, not through the site of the original fracture but through the weakened site of a screw.

is no longer stressed. By contrast with delayed union and non-union, there is persistent movement, causing repeated stress on the metal at the fracture site over a period of many months or even years. Under these circumstances, the metal may "fatigue" as a result of local rearrangement of its molecular structure. A crack develops and eventually the metallic device fails completely and breaks (Fig. 15.83).

Muscular Complications
Traumatic myositis ossificans (posttraumatic ossification). Occasionally after a fracture, a dislocation, or even an isolated muscle injury, particularly in the region of the elbow and thigh of children and young adults, a rapidly enlarging painful tender mass develops in the injured tissues. This mass, which is in part a hematoma, is initially radiolucent; soon radiographic examination reveals evidence of extensive ossification (Fig. 15.84). This new bone formation in an abnormal site is referred to as *heterotopic ossification* and develops between (rather than within) the torn muscle fibers. Patients with severe head injuries or paraplegia are particularly prone to develop this complication. Understandably, this painful lesion is accompanied by considerable limitation of motion in the related joint. The complication can be prevented to some extent by the drug, indocid, or by prophylactic radiation.

The treatment for posttraumatic myositis ossificans consists of local rest by splinting

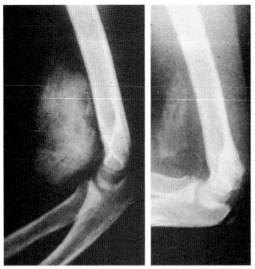

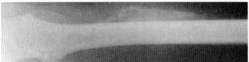

Figure 15.84. Posttraumatic myositis ossificans. **Left,** 3 weeks after a posterior dislocation of the elbow that had been reduced but not immobilized, radiographic examination of the child's elbow reveals evidence of extensive ossification in the soft tissues. At this stage there was marked limitation of elbow motion. **Right,** 6 months later, after no treatment other than active exercises, the area of myositis ossificans has been to a large extent resorbed. The range of elbow motion had returned to near normal. **Bottom,** posttraumatic myositis ossificans in the anterior aspect of the thigh of a 20-year-old football player 4 weeks after he had sustained a direct blow to this area. This type of posttraumatic ossification also tends to be resorbed spontaneously.

during the active stage. Passive stretching or manipulation of the related joint is contraindicated, because it tears more muscle fibers and aggravates the entire process. The same is true of attempts to excise the lesion in the early stages. The microscopic appearance of the lesion at this stage is dangerously similar to that of osteosarcoma for which it could be tragically mistaken. Left completely alone, the heterotopic new bone is to a large extent resorbed spontaneously over the ensuing months. The residual lesion is no longer painful and joint motion usually improves.

Late rupture of tendons. In the region of the wrist and ankle, tendons glide along

smooth bony grooves but after a metaphyseal fracture that heals with an irregularity in the cortex, these grooves are no longer smooth. Consequently, over a period of months a tendon may gradually become frayed from the friction and finally rupture. This complication of a fracture is uncommon, but it occasionally occurs in the extensor pollicis longus tendon after a Colles' fracture of the distal end of the radius.

Neurological Complications

Tardy nerve palsy. A residual valgus deformity of the elbow after either malunion or nonunion of a fracture of the lateral condyle results in excessive stretching of the ulnar nerve as well as friction between the nerve and the distal end of the humerus during flexion and extension of the elbow (Fig. 15.85). Gradually, over a period of 10 to 20 years, the nerve becomes thickened by intraneural fibrosis, at which time symptoms and signs of an ulnar nerve lesion become apparent. The only effective treatment for this late complication is surgical transposition (relocation) of the ulnar nerve to the anterior aspect of the elbow.

Remote Complications

Renal Calculi. Patients, particularly adults, who are confined to bed for many weeks or

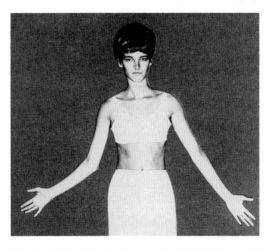

Figure 15.85. Tardy ulnar palsy. This 20-year-old girl had residual right cubitus valgus secondary to malunion of a fractured lateral condyle 15 years previously. She had recently developed symptoms and signs of an incomplete tardy ulnar nerve palsy.

months as a result of multiple complicated fractures, have a tendency to develop radiopaque renal calculi of the calcium type. The combined underlying factors responsible for this complication are inadequate drainage of urine from the dependent calyces and the hypercalcemia associated with generalized disuse osteoporosis. Renal calculi can be prevented by an increased fluid intake (at least 4000 ml per day) and frequent turning of the patient. As soon as it is feasible, the patient should be allowed out of bed, not only to facilitate renal drainage but also to minimize disuse osteoporosis.

Accident Neurosis. When a fracture or dislocation has resulted from an accident for which a patient is entitled to industrial compensation or accident or liability insurance, the patient may either wittingly or unwittingly develop patterns of neurotic behavior. Such a patient, although not necessarily a malingerer, consistently denies being able to return to his or her former occupation. Even extensive rehabilitation may fail to accelerate the patient's recovery and occasionally psychiatric assessment is required. In some instances, recovery becomes possible only after legal settlement of the patient's claim in his or her favor.

SPECIAL TYPES OF FRACTURES

Four types of fractures merit separate consideration. These fractures, which are "special" in that they are significantly different from ordinary fractures, include *stress fractures, pathological fractures, birth fractures,* and *fractures that involve the epiphyseal plate.* The latter two types of fractures are discussed in Chapter 16.

Stress Fractures (Fatigue Fractures)

Just as metal may fatigue as a result of repeated stresses and consequently may develop a small crack or fatigue fracture, so also may bone, particularly if it is subjected to unaccustomed stresses for which it has not had time to become conditioned by the normal process of work hypertrophy. Thus, when an individual who is out of condition begins to participate in activities such as long marches, track and field activities, or ballet dancing, one of the weightbearing bones may fatigue as a result

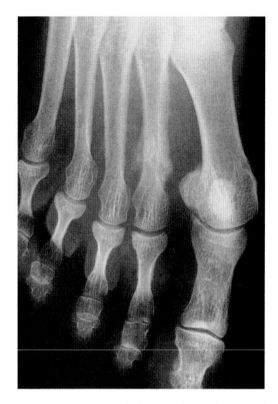

Figure 15.86.   Stress fracture, or fatigue fracture, of the neck of the second metatarsal in a 45-year-old woman who had recently undertaken an exercise program, including long walks. She had complained of pain for 3 weeks prior to this radiograph, which reveals abundant callus surrounding the stress fracture. In the metatarsals, such fractures are usually referred to as "march fractures."

of the repeated stresses and develop a small crack (*stress fracture* or *fatigue fracture*). Unlike metal, living bone can react to fatigue by healing and the crack does not proceed to a displaced fracture.

The more common clinical examples of stress or fatigue fractures are: the second, third, or fourth metatarsals in military recruits ("march fracture") (Fig. 15.86); the lower end of the fibula in runners; and the upper third of the tibia in jumpers and ballet dancers.

Clinically, when the fatigue fracture first develops, the patient experiences the insidious onset of local pain that is aggravated by activity and relieved by rest; local deep tenderness can be readily detected. The tiny crack may not become apparent radiographically until

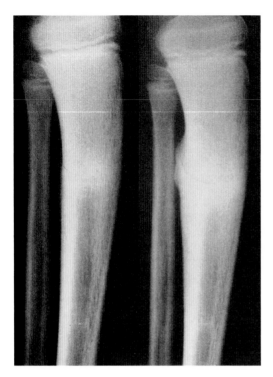

Figure 15.87.   Stress fracture of the upper end of the tibia in a 10-year-old boy who had recently become involved in strenuous track and field activities. **Left,** the initial radiograph, taken after the boy had been complaining of local pain for only 1 week, reveals only a tiny crack and slight sclerosis. **Right,** 5 weeks later radiographic examination reveals the stress fracture more clearly as well as the subperiosteal and endosteal new bone of the healing process.

subperiosteal and endosteal new bone appears during the healing process (Figs. 15.86 and 15.87).

Treatment consists of desisting from the responsible activity until the crack has healed. Subsequently, gradual resumption of activity results in sufficient work hypertrophy of the bone to increase its strength and gradually condition it for the stresses of the particular activity involved.

Pathological Fractures

Whereas an ordinary fracture occurs through ordinary or normal bone, a *pathological fracture* is one that occurs through abnormal bone—bone that is pathological, weaker, and more susceptible to fracture than normal bone. The pathological bone may be so weak

that it is fractured by a trivial injury, or even by normal use. Nevertheless, even if the pathological bone breaks as a result of a major injury, it is still a pathological fracture.

Pathological fractures can occur in a variety of disorders, some localized, some disseminated, and others generalized. The following is a classification of disorders in which pathological fractures are most likely to occur.

Classification of Disorders That Predispose Bone to Pathological Fracture

  I. Congenital abnormalities (Chapter 8)
        Localized
            Congenital defect of tibia (leading to pseudarthrosis)
        Disseminated
            Enchondromatosis
        Generalized
            Osteogenesis imperfecta (fragile bones)
            Osteopetrosis (chalk bones)
 II. Metabolic bone disease (Chapter 9)
        Rickets
        Osteomalacia
        Scurvy
        Osteoporosis
        Hyperparathyroidism
III. Disseminated bone disorders of unknown etiology (Chapter 9)
        Polyostotic fibrous dysplasia
        Skeletal reticuloses
        Langerhans' cell histiocytoses (Hand-Schüller-Christian disease, eosinophilic granuloma)
        Gaucher's disease
 IV. Inflammatory disorders (Chapter 10)
        Hematogenous osteomyelitis
        Osteomyelitis secondary to wounds
        Tuberculous osteomyelitis
        Rheumatoid arthritis
  V. Neuromuscular disorders (with disuse osteoporosis) (Chapter 12)
        Paralytic disorders
            Poliomyelitis, paraplegia (spina bifida and acquired paraplegia)
        Disorders of muscle
            Muscular dystrophy
 VI. Avascular necrosis of bone (Chapter 13)
        Posttraumatic avascular necrosis
        Postirradiation necrosis

VII. Neoplasms of bone (Chapter 14)
    Neoplasm-like lesions of bone
    A. Osteogenic
        The various neoplasm-like lesions of bone of osteogenic cell origin are not listed here because they do not weaken the bone and consequently do not render it susceptible to fracture.
    B. Chondrogenic
        1. Enchondroma
        2. Multiple enchondromata (Ollier's dyschondroplasia)
    C. Fibrogenic
        1. Subperiosteal cortical defect (metaphyseal fibrous defect)
        2. Nonosteogenic fibroma (nonossifying fibroma)
        3. Monostotic fibrous dysplasia
        4. Polyostotic fibrous dysplasia
        5. Osteofibrous dysplasia (Campanacci syndrome)
        6. "Brown tumor" (hyperparathyroidism; see Chapter 9)
    D. Angiogenic
        1. Angioma of bone (hemangioma and lymphangioma)
        2. Aneurysmal bone cyst (ABC)
    E. Uncertain origin
        1. Simple bone cyst (unicameral bone cyst [UBC])
    True Primary Neoplasms of Bone
    A. Osteogenic
        1. Osteosarcoma (osteogenic sarcoma)
        2. Surface osteosarcoma (parosteal sarcoma; periosteal sarcoma)
    B. Chondrogenic
        1. Benign chondroblastoma
        2. Chondromyxoid fibroma
        3. Chondrosarcoma
    C. Fibrogenic
        1. Fibrosarcoma of bone
        2. Malignant fibrous histiocytoma of bone
    D. Angiogenic
        1. Angiosarcoma of bone
    E. Myelogenic
        1. Myeloma of bone (multiple myeloma)
        2. Ewing's sarcoma (Ewing's tumor)
        3. Hodgkin's lymphoma of bone
        4. Non-Hodgkin's lymphoma (reticulum cell sarcoma)
        5. Skeletal Reticuloses (Langerhans' cell histiocytoses) (see Chapter 9)
        6. Leukemia
    F. Uncertain Origin
        1. Giant cell tumor of bone (osteoclastoma)
    Metastatic Neoplasms In Bone
        Metastatic carcinoma
        Metastatic neuroblastoma

Clinical Features and Diagnosis

Occasionally a pathological fracture is the first manifestation of an abnormality of bone, in which case further investigation is required to establish the precise nature of the underlying disorder. The clinical features are those of the underlying condition and have been described in preceding chapters indicated in the classification.

Prognosis of Pathological Fractures

Most pathological fractures will unite, because the rate of bone deposition in fracture healing is usually more rapid than the rate of bone resorption of the underlying pathological process (Fig. 15.88). A pathological fracture through an area of osteomyelitis, however, will not usually unite until the infection has been controlled. In certain highly malignant primary neoplasms such as osteosarcoma, the rate of bone destruction and resorption may be almost as great as that of bone deposition. Under these circumstances, union will be markedly delayed and amputation is indicated (Fig. 15.89). Pathological fractures through metastatic neoplasms in the limbs usually merit internal fixation with or without methyl-methacrylate combined with irradiation and, if indicated, hormone therapy. The pathological fracture treated in this way will usually unite and the patient, whose prognosis is hopeless, will be spared much misery, pain, and disability during the remaining months of life (Fig. 15.90).

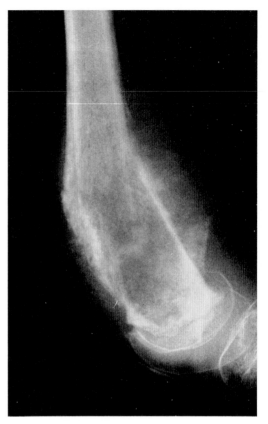

Figure 15.89.   Pathological fracture through an osteosarcoma in the lower end of the femur in a 9-year-old girl. Because of the rapidly growing malignant neoplasm, union will be delayed and refracture is likely. Consequently, amputation is indicated.

DISLOCATIONS AND ASSOCIATED INJURIES

Much of the discussion about fractures in the preceding section of this chapter is equally applicable to dislocations and associated injuries. Certain special features of joint injuries, however, merit special consideration.

Normal Joint Stability

Synovial joints are designed to permit smooth movement through a normal range that is specific for each joint. Three structural factors are responsible for preventing an abnormal range of motion and thereby, for providing *joint stability:* 1) the reciprocal contours of the opposing joint surfaces; 2) the integrity of the fibrous capsule and ligaments; 3) the protective

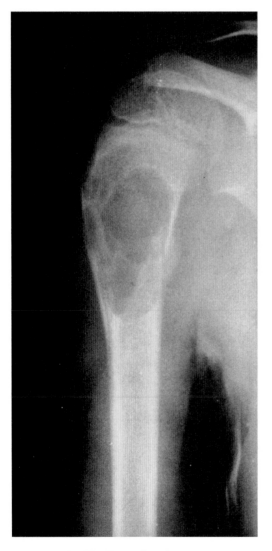

Figure 15.88.   Simple or solitary bone cyst in the metaphyseal region of the upper end of the humerus in a 10-year-old boy. Note the healing pathological fracture through the weakened cortex on the medial side. The boy had sustained a minor injury 3 weeks previously.

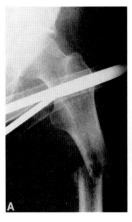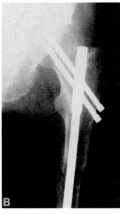

Figure 15.90. Pathological fracture through a metastatic neoplasm. **A.** Pathological subtrochanteric fracture of the femur through a metastasis from carcinoma of the breast in a 55-year-old woman. **B.** The same pathological fracture after reduction and internal fixation with a reconstruction intramedullary nail. The patient was thereby relieved of her pain.

power of muscles that move the joint. Thus, a defect in any one or combination of these structures may result in loss of joint stability.

The relative importance of these stabilizing factors varies with each type of joint. For example, in a ball-and-socket joint, such as the hip, the joint contours are the most important factor. In a hinge joint such as the knee, ligaments are the most important factor; in a freely mobile joint such as the shoulder, however, joint stability depends mostly on the integrity of the fibrous capsule and the protective power of surrounding muscles.

Physical Factors in the Production of Joint Injuries

Whereas a fracture of a bone is a break in its continuity, dislocation of a joint is a *structural loss of its stability*. The physical factors that suddenly force a joint beyond its normal range of motion cause a tension failure, either in the bony components of the joint, in the fibrous capsule and ligaments, or in both the bone and the soft tissues. These structures are particularly vulnerable to tension failure when the muscles controlling the joint are either weak or caught off guard at the moment of injury. The causative force of tension failure is usually an indirect injury in which the initial force is

transmitted through the bones to the involved joint.

Descriptive Terms Pertaining to Joint Injuries

A direct blow to a joint usually produces a *contusion* but, if sufficiently severe, may produce an *intra-articular fracture*. An indirect injury produces sudden tension on a ligament that may cause severe stretching of the ligament, resulting in minor tears and some hemorrhage (*ligamentous sprain*) without loss of joint stability. A more severe injury produces a major *ligamentous tear* that may be either partial or complete with resultant loss of joint stability. If the ligament itself does not tear, it may avulse a fragment of its bony attachment at either end (*ligamentous avulsion*). A ligamentous strain, by contrast, refers to the gradual elongation of a ligament that results

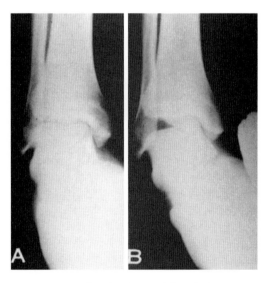

Figure 15.91. Occult joint instability. **A.** Anteroposterior radiograph of the ankle of a football player who, after an inversion injury of his ankle had pain, swelling, and local tenderness over the lateral aspect of the joint. The radiograph is normal but this does not exclude occult joint instability. **B.** Anteroposterior radiograph of the same ankle while it is being stressed (stress radiograph) with the patient under general anesthesia. Note the marked opening up of the ankle joint (talar tilt) on the lateral side, indicating joint instability associated with a complete tear of the lateral ligament of the ankle. The stress simulates the original injury.

from repeated mild stretching over a prolonged period.

There are three degrees of joint instability: 1) *occult joint instability* (apparent only when the joint is stressed) (Fig. 15.91); 2) *subluxation* (less than a luxation), in which the joint surfaces have lost their normal relationship but still retain considerable contact (Fig. 15.92); 3) *dislocation* (luxation), in which the joint surfaces have completely lost contact with each other (Fig. 15.93).

Either a dislocation or a subluxation may have occurred only momentarily at the time of injury and may have reduced spontaneously, leaving no radiographic evidence of the seriousness of the injury unless the joint is stressed (Fig. 15.91). When the dislocation is accompanied by either an intra-articular or extra-articular fracture, it is referred to as a *fracture-dislocation* (Fig. 15.94). As with fractures, a

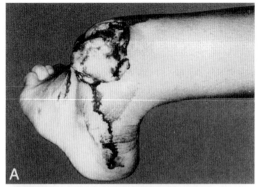
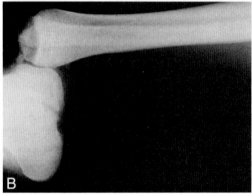

Figure 15.93.   Open traumatic dislocation (luxation) of the ankle joint. **A.** The distal ends of the fibula and tibia have burst through the skin from within at the time of the dislocation. **B.** The radiograph (taken in the same projection as the photograph) reveals that the joint surfaces of the ankle joint have completely lost contact.

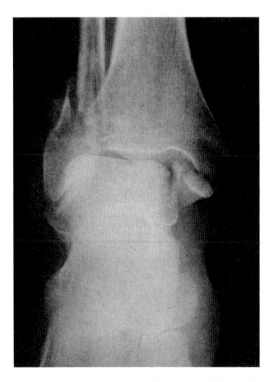

Figure 15.92.   Traumatic subluxation of the ankle joint associated with a fracture of the medial malleolus and the distal end of the fibula—a fracture-subluxation. The talus has become displaced laterally in the ankle mortice so that the joint surfaces have lost their normal relationship but still retain considerable contact.

joint injury may be closed (simple) or open (compound), either from within or from without (Fig. 15.93).

Most susceptible to traumatic dislocation are the shoulder, elbow, interphalangeal, hip, and ankle joints. Internal derangements of the knee joint due to a torn meniscus are discussed in Chapter 17.

Associated Injury to the Fibrous Capsule

The fibrous capsule and contiguous periosteum may be stripped up from the bony margin of the joint and stretched by the causative injury resulting in an *intracapsular dislocation*. More often, the fibrous capsule is torn and one bone end perforates the rent in the capsule to produce an *extracapsular disloca-*

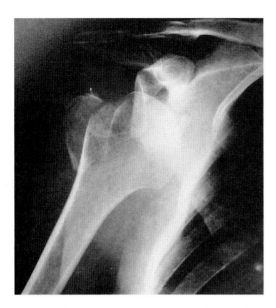

Figure 15.94. Fracture-dislocation of the right shoulder in an adult. Note the fracture of the greater tuberosity of the humerus and the dislocation of the humeral head in relation to the glenoid cavity.

tion. Occasionally, the large bone end becomes trapped in the dislocated position by the small rent in the capsule, and this phenomenon is referred to as a *buttonhole dislocation,* which may be impossible to reduce by closed methods. Occasionally, at the time of closed reduction of a dislocation, a flap of torn capsule becomes trapped between the joint surfaces, preventing perfect reduction and resulting in residual subluxation of the joint. Such a subluxation, which is most often seen after closed reduction of a posterior dislocation of the hip, is an absolute indication for open reduction.

Diagnosis of Joint Injuries

Many of the clinical features of traumatic dislocation and subluxation are comparable to those already discussed in a previous section of this chapter in relation to the clinical features of fractures. Because of normal proprioceptive sensation in joints, the patient is usually aware that a given joint has "gone out of place." The associated joint instability and stretching of the injured structures cause pain and muscle spasm. Also, there is decreased function of the involved part.

Physical examination in the presence of a complete dislocation usually reveals *swelling* (unless the dislocated joint is deep, as in the hip), *deformity* (angulation, rotation, loss of normal contour, shortening), and *abnormal movement* (occurring through the unstable joint) (Fig. 15.95). There is local tenderness over a sprained or torn ligament. Dislocations and subluxations may go unrecognized because of inadequate physical examination and consequent failure to obtain the appropriate radiographic examination. Physical examination must also include a diligent search for any associated injuries to spinal cord, peripheral nerves, or major vessels.

Radiographic examination reveals the typical features of a subluxation (Fig. 15.92) or dislocation (Fig 15.93). At least two projections at right angles to each other (anterioposterior and lateral) are essential for accurate diagnosis (Fig. 15.96). In the absence of radiographic evidence of a dislocation or subluxation, despite clinical evidence of significant ligamentous injury, additional radiographs taken while the joint is being stressed (under local or general anesthesia) are helpful in the diagnosis of occult joint instability (Fig. 15.91).

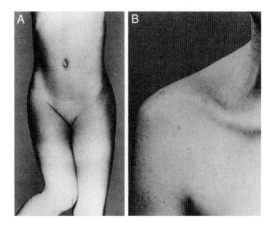

Figure 15.95. Clinical deformity associated with traumatic dislocations. **A.** The typical clinical deformity of traumatic posterior dislocation of the right hip—flexion, adduction, internal rotation, and apparent shortening. **B.** The typical clinical deformity of traumatic inferomedial dislocation of the right shoulder. The normal round contour of the shoulder has been lost and the shoulder looks square.

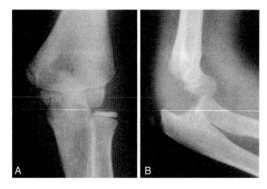

Figure 15.96.   The importance of at least two radiographic projections at right angles to each other (anteroposterior and lateral). **A.** The anteroposterior projection reveals some evidence of disturbance in this child's elbow (the radial head is not in correct relationship with the capitellum) but it is not striking. **B.** The lateral projection clearly reveals a posterior dislocation of the elbow.

Normal Healing of Ligaments

Unlike bone, which heals without a scar, torn ligaments heal by fibrous scar tissue that is not as strong as the normal ligament. Partial tears in a ligament heal reasonably well provided the ligament is protected during the healing process. With complete tears of ligaments, there is usually a considerable gap between the shredded ends of the ligament—a gap that can heal only with fibrous scar tissue. Under these circumstances, even if the torn ligament heals, it is both elongated and relatively weak.

The time required for normal healing of a torn ligament varies according to its size and the forces to which it is normally subjected. Thus, the ligaments of the finger joints may be healed in 3 weeks, whereas the major ligaments of the knee may require 3 months. The healing time for torn ligaments is somewhat shorter in children than in adults, but the influence of age is much less significant in ligamentous healing than in fracture healing.

Complications of Dislocations and Associated Injuries

The complications of the original injury that produced the dislocation or subluxation are much the same as those of fractures that have been classified and discussed in an earlier section of this chapter. The immediate local complications include associated injury to skin, blood vessels, peripheral nerves, and spinal cord as well as multiple injuries. The early local complications include infection (septic arthritis), after either an open joint injury or an open reduction of a joint injury, and avascular necrosis of one of the articulating bone ends (especially the head of the femur). Late complications of dislocations, subluxations, and occult joint instability include persistent joint stiffness, persistent joint instability and recurrent dislocation, posttraumatic arthritis (degenerative joint disease), posttraumatic osteoporosis, reflex sympathetic dystrophy and posttraumatic myositis ossificans.

General Principles of Treatment for Joint Injuries

The six general principles of fracture treatment discussed in an earlier section of this chapter are equally applicable to the treatment of dislocations and associated injuries. Dislocations and subluxations must be reduced perfectly to restore normal congruity of the joint surfaces and prevent posttraumatic arthritis. The drug treatment of soft tissue injuries includes the short-term use of nonsteroidal antiinflammatory drugs (NSAIDS) that reduce the severity and duration of the associated inflammation and pain. The systemic use of corticosteroids is not indicated. Furthermore, steroids should not be injected directly and repeatedly into tendons, ligaments, or joints because of their deleterious effects.

Specific Types of Joint Injuries
Contusion
When a joint receives a direct blow, the synovial membrane reacts to the injury by producing an effusion; synovial vessels may even rupture with a resultant hemarthrosis. Radiographic examination is necessary to exclude the possibility of an associated intra-articular fracture.

Ligamentous Sprain
An acute sprain is caused by a sudden stretching of the ligament with a minor, incomplete tear and local hemorrhage but no loss of continuity. The sprain is manifest by local swelling, tenderness, and pain that is aggravated by

movements of the joint that stretch the sprained ligament. Because the ligament has not been unduly elongated, there is no joint instability.

Radiographic examination is required to exclude a dislocation, subluxation, or fracture. Additional radiographs taken while the joint is being stressed are essential to exclude occult joint instability (Fig. 15.91).

Treatment of a simple ligamentous sprain is aimed at protecting the injured ligament from further stretching during the healing process. Complete immobilization is seldom necessary except for severe pain, but appropriately applied adhesive strapping can serve as a temporary ligament that relieves pain by restricting undesired motion while permitting other movements of the joint (Fig. 15.97). Active exercises are important to maintain joint motion and to increase the protective power of the muscles that control the involved joint.

Dislocations and Subluxations

To restore normal congruity to the joint surfaces, perfect reduction of dislocations and subluxations must be achieved, either by closed manipulation or, when necessary, by open reduction. After reduction of the dislocation or subluxation, consideration must be given to the torn ligaments to prevent the complication of residual joint instability and resultant recurrent dislocation of the joint.

Torn Ligaments

A complete tear of certain major ligaments, such as the collateral ligaments of the knee, should be repaired surgically as soon as possible after the injury, because the results of delayed or late repair are less satisfactory than those of immediate repair. For many other ligaments, such as the lateral ligament of the ankle or the collateral ligaments of the fingers, the reduced joint needs to be immobilized to protect the injured ligaments and capsule from further stretching during the healing process. Immobilization of a joint after reduction of a dislocation is necessary to obtain stability. In the elbow and hip, immobilization is also helpful in preventing the complication of posttraumatic myositis ossificans.

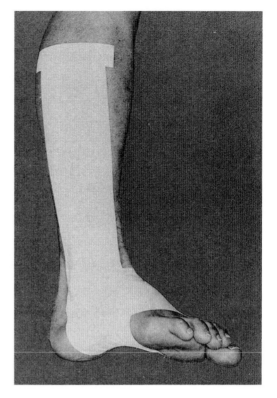

Figure 15.97.   Adhesive strapping on an ankle in the treatment of a lateral ligamentous sprain. Each strip of adhesive begins on the lateral aspect of the ankle, encircles the foot, and extends up the lateral aspect of the leg while the foot is held in eversion (to relieve tension on the sprained ligament). The adhesive strapping, which serves as a temporary external ligament, restricts inversion at the subtalar joint but permits dorsiflexion and plantar flexion at the ankle joint, as well as full weightbearing.

MUSCLE INJURIES

When severe tension is suddenly applied to an already contracted muscle, some of the muscle bundles may rupture and produce the painful local lesion well known to athletes and trainers as a "charley horse." Occasionally, a more extensive rupture occurs at the musculotendinous junction of a major muscle such as the quadriceps femoris or the gastrocnemius (Fig. 15.98).

A strain refers to a chronic overstretching of a muscle or its tendon due to overuse. It usually resolves after modification of the offending physical activity. The most common site of a strain is the musculotendinous junction.

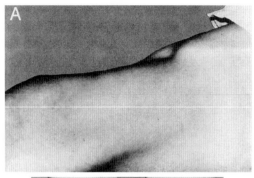

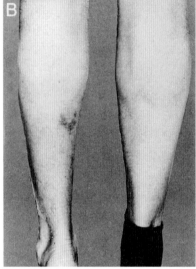

Figure 15.98. Rupture of muscles. **A.** Rupture of the musculotendinous junction of the left quadriceps muscle in the suprapatellar region of a hockey player (as seen from the lateral aspect). Note the retracted muscle belly proximally and the gap distally. This injury required surgical repair. **B.** Rupture of the musculotendinous junction of the medial head of the left gastrocnemius of a tennis player. Note the ecchymosis and loss of normal contour of the calf. Because only part of one head of the gastrocnemius muscle has ruptured, it retracts relatively little. Elevation of the heel of the shoe reduces the tension on the calf muscles and relieves pain on walking during the healing process. A more serious injury is a complete rupture of the entire Achilles tendon.

TENDON INJURIES
Closed Tendon Injuries

A normal tendon seldom ruptures even with strenuous activity. However, if it has become frayed by friction or has degenerated, it may rupture with even normal activity. In either case, reconstructive operations are required to repair or replace the abnormal part of the ruptured tendon. Sudden tension on a normal tendon may avulse a fragment of its bony insertion. The most common example of this injury is the mallet finger (baseball finger, cricket finger) (Fig. 15.99).

Open Tendon Injuries

Clean, open division of tendons in most sites should be treated by immediate surgical repair. The complex and intricate arrangement of flexor tendons in the hand, however, presents special problems because adhesions between injured tendons interfere significantly with hand function. Such injuries are best treated by an experienced hand surgeon. When both the profundus and sublimis tendons are divided at the wrist or in the proximal part of the palm, both tendons should be repaired. Even when both tendons are divided in the critical area ("no man's land") between the distal palmar crease and the proximal interphalangeal joint (Fig. 15.100), both should be repaired, especially in children. Distal to this area, the lacerated profundus tendon should be repaired if possible. If not, the proximal end should be advanced and secured to

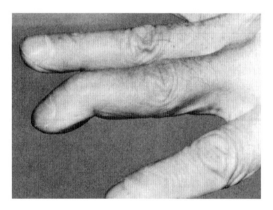

Figure 15.99. Mallet finger (baseball finger, cricket finger). The distal interphalangeal joint of this man's right middle finger was suddenly forced into acute flexion as he miscaught a ball. A small fragment of the insertion of the long extensor tendon into the base of the distal phalanx was avulsed so that he lost active extension of the joint. Alternatively, the thin extensor tendon may rupture proximal to its insertion. The resultant deformity bears some resemblance to a mallet. Treatment is discussed in Chapter 17.

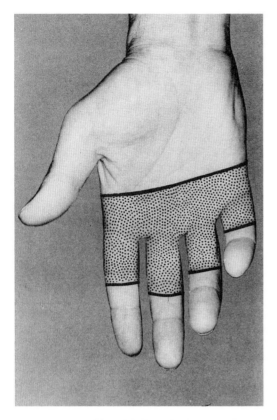

Figure 15.100.   The critical area for flexor tendon injuries in the hand ("no man's land"). In this area, both the profundus and sublimus tendons for each finger pass through an unyielding fibrous tunnel. Consequently, adhesions between repaired tendons and the fibrous tunnel are a potential complication.

the distal phalanx with a "pull-out" wire. In the postoperative management of open tendon injuries in the hand, the use of early controlled and supervised finger motion is valuable in the prevention of adhesions.

SUGGESTED ADDITIONAL READING

Aaron AD. Bone grafting and healing. In: Kasser JR, ed. Orthopaedic knowledge update 5. Rosemont, IL: American Academy of Orthopaedic Surgeons, 1996:21–28.

Alexander RH, Proctor HS, eds. ATLS: advanced trauma life support—program for physicians. 5th ed. Committee on trauma. Chicago: American College of Surgeons, 1993.

Allgower M, Spiegel PG. Internal fixation of fractures. Evolution of concepts. Clin Orthop 1979; 138:26–29.

Apley AG. Fixation is fun (editorial). J Bone Joint Surg 1992;74B:485.

Apley AG, Solomon L. Fracture pathology and diagnosis. In: Concise system of orthopaedics and fractures. 2nd ed. London: Butterworth's, 1994: 211–230.

Apley AG, Solomon L. Principles of fracture treatment. In: Apley's system of orthopaedics and fractures. 7th ed. Oxford: Butterworth Heinemann, 1993:515–565.

Bassett CAL, Valdes MG, Hernandez E. Modification of fracture repair with pulsing electromagnetic fields. J Bone Joint Surg 1982;64A: 888–895.

Becker RO. The significance of electrically stimulated osteogenesis. Clin Orthop 1979;141: 266–274.

Behrens F, Shepard N, Mitchell N. Alteration of articular cartilage by intra-articular injections of glucocorticoids. J Bone Joint Surg 1975;57-A: 70–76.

Bone LB. Emergency treatment of the injured patient. In: Browner BD, Jupiter JB, Trafton PG, eds. Skeletal trauma. Fractures dislocations. Ligamentous injuries. Vol 1. Philadelphia: WB Saunders, 1992:127–156.

Bone LB, Babikian G, Border JR, et al. Multiple trauma: pathophysiology and management. In: Frymoyer JW, ed. Orthopaedic knowledge update 4. Rosemont, IL: American Academy of Orthopaedic Surgeons, 1993:141–153.

Bone LB, McNamara K, Shine B, et al. Mortality in multiple trauma patients and fractures. J Trauma 1994;37:262–264.

Brighton CT. The biology of fracture repair. In: Murray JA, ed. Principles of fracture healing. Vol. 33. AAOS instructional course lectures. St. Louis: CV Mosby, 1984:60.

Brighton CT. The treatment of non-unions with electricity. Current concepts review. J Bone Joint Surg 1981;63A:847–851.

Brighton CT, Hunt RM. Early histological and ultrastructural changes in medullary fracture callus. J Bone Joint Surg 1991;73A:832–847.

Brighton CT, Pollack SR. Treatment of recalcitrant non-union with a capacitively coupled electrical field—a preliminary report. J Bone Joint Surg 1985;67A:577–585.

Browner BD, Jupiter JB, Levine AM, et al. Skeletal trauma. Vols. 1 and 2. Philadelphia: WB Saunders, 1992.

Buckwalter JA. Pharmacologic treatment of soft-tissue injuries (current concepts review) J Bone Joint Surg 1995;77A:1902–1914.

Bullough PG. Bullough and Vigorita's orthopaedic pathology. 3rd ed. London: Mosby-Wolfe, 1997.

Carter DR, Blenman PR, Beaupre GS. Correlation between mechanical stress history and tissue differentiation in initial fracture healing. J Orthop Res 1988;6:736.

Charnley J. The closed treatment of common fractures. 3rd ed. New York: Churchill Livingstone, 1961.

Clark CR, Bonfiglio M, eds. Orthopaedics: essentials of diagnosis and treatment. New York: Churchill Livingstone, 1994.

Connolly JF, Guse R, Lippiello L, et al. Development of an osteogenic bone-marrow preparation. J Bone Joint Surg 1989;7A:684–691.

Connolly JF, Guse R, Tiedeman J, et al. Autologous marrow injection for delayed unions of the tibia: a preliminary report. J Orthop Trauma 1989;3:276–282.

Connolly JF, Mendes M, Browner BD. Principles of closed management of common fractures. In: Browner BD, Jupiter JB, Levine AM, et al, eds. Skeletal trauma: fractures dislocations. Ligamentous injuries 1992;1:211–230.

Court-Brown CM, McQueen MM, Quaba AA, eds. Management of open fractures. London: Martin Dunitz, 1996.

deHaas WG, Watson J, Morrison DM. Noninvasive treatment of ununited fractures of the tibia using electical stimulation. J Bone Joint Surg 1980; 62B:465–470.

Dehne E, Metz CW, Deffer PA, et al. Nonoperative treatment of the fractured tibia by immediate weightbearing. J Trauma 1961;1:514–533.

Dwyer AF, Wickham GG. Direct current stimulation in spine fusion. Med J Aust 1974;1:73–75.

Einhorn TA. Enhancement of fracture-healing. (Current concepts review). J Bone Joint Surg 1995;77A:940–956.

Frank CB, Jackson DW. The science of reconstruction of the anterior cruciate ligament. J Bone Joint Surg 1997;79A:1556–1576.

Garrett WE Jr. Muscle strain injuries: clinical and basic aspects. Med Sci Sports Exerc 1990;22:436–443.

Goodship AE, Lawes TJ, Harrison L. The biology of fracture repair. In: Hughes SPF, McCarthy ID, eds. Sciences basic to orthopaedics. London: Mosby-Wolfe, 1997;128–143.

Goodship AE, Kenwright J. The influence of induced micromovement upon the healing of experimental tibial fractures. J Bone Joint Surg 1985;65B:650.

Gossling HR, Polsburg SL, eds. Complications of fracture management. Philadelphia: JB Lippincott, 1984.

Green NE, Swiontkowski MF. Skeletal trauma in children. Vol. 3. Philadelphia: WB Saunders, 1994.

Gustilo RB, Anderson JT. Prevention of infection in the treatment of one thousand and twenty-five open fractures of long bones. J Bone Joint Surg 1976;58A:453–458.

Gustilo RB, Merkow RL, Templeman D. The management of open fractures. (Current concepts review). J Bone Joint Surg 1990;72A:299–304.

Hansen ST Jr, Swiontkowski MF, eds. Orthopaedic trauma protocols. New York: Raven Press, 1993.

Heckman JD, ed. Emergency care and transportation of the sick and injured. 5th ed. Chapter 7 Park Ridge, IL: American Academy of Orthopaedic Surgeons, 1992.

Johnson EE, Urist MR, Finerman AM. Resistant non-unions and partial or complete segmental defects of long bones. Treatment with implants of a composite of human bone morphogenetic protein (1 BMP) and autolyzed, antigen-extracted, allogeneic (AAA) bone. Clin Orthop 1992;277:229–237.

Johnson KD. Hard-tissue trauma. In: Poss R, ed. Orthopaedic knowledge update 3. Park Ridge, IL: American Academy of Orthopaedic Surgeons, 1990:75–80.

Lane JM, ed. Fracture healing. New York: Churchill Livingstone, 1987.

McRae R. Practical fracture treatment. 2nd ed. London: Churchill Livingstone, 1989.

Muëller ME. The role of internal and/or extraskeletal fixation: probable future refinements of techniques and their applications. In: Straub LR, Wilson PD Jr, eds. Clinical trends in orthopaedics. New York: Thieme-Stratton, 1982.

Muëller ME, Allgower M, Schneider R et al; Schatzker J, trans. Manual of internal fixation—techniques recommended by the AO Group. 2nd ed. Berlin: Springer-Verlag, 1979.

Mustard WT, Bull C. A reliable method for relief of traumatic vascular spasm. Ann Surg 1962;155:339–344.

Pan WT, Einhorn TA. The biochemistry of fracture healing. Curr Orthop 1992;6:207–213.

Paterson DC, Lewis GN, Cass CA. Treatment of delayed union and nonunion with an implanted direct current stimulator. Clin Orthop 1980;148:117–128.

Peltier LF. Fat embolism: I: an appraisal of the problem. Clin Orthop 1984;187:3–17.

Perren SM. Physical and biological aspects of fracture healing with special reference to internal fixation. Clin Orthop 1979;138:175–196.

Ranney D. Chronic musculoskeletal injuries in the workplace. Toronto: WB Saunders, 1996.

Richards RR. Fat embolism syndrome. Can J Surg 1997;40:334–339.

Rockwood CA, Green DP, Bucholz RW, et al., eds. Rockwood and Green's fractures in adults. Vols. 1 and 2. 4th ed. Philedelphia: Lippincott Raven, 1996.

Rodgrigo JJ. Orthopaedic surgery, basic science and clinical science. Boston: Little Brown, 1986.

Rorabeck CH. Compartment syndromes. In: Browner BD, Jupiter JB, Levine AM, et al., eds. Skeletal trauma: fractures dislocations. Ligamentous injuries. Philadelphia: WB Saunders, 1992; 1;285–309.

Salter RB, Hamilton HW, Wedge JH, et al. Clinical application of basic research on continuous passive motion for disorders and injuries of synovial joints: a preliminary report of a feasibility study. J Orthop Res 1984;1:325–342.

Salter RB. Continuous passive motion (CPM). A biological concept for the healing and regeneration of articular cartilage, ligaments and tendons: from origination to research to clinical application. Baltimore: Williams & Wilkins, 1993.

Salter RB, Gross A, Hall JH. Hydrocortisone arthropathy—an experimental investigation. Can Med Assoc 1967:97:374–377.

Salter RB, Harris DJ. The healing of intra-articular fractures with continuous passive motion. In: American Academy of Orthopaedic Surgeons Instructional Course Lecture Series. St. Louis: CV Mosby, 1979;28:102–117.

Sarmiento A, Latta LL. Closed functional treatment of fractures. Berlin: Springer-Verlag, 1981.

Sarmiento A, Mullis DL, Latta LL, et al. A quantitative comparative analysis of fracture healing under the influence of compression plating vs. close weight bearing treatment. Clin Orthop 1980;149:232–239.

Sarmiento A, Latta LL. Functional fracture bracing: tibia, humerus, and ulna. Berlin: Springer-Verlag, 1995.

Schatzker J, Tile M. The rationale of operative fracture care. 2nd ed. Berlin: Springer-Verlag, 1996.

Schenk RK. Biology of fracture repair. In: Browner BD, Jupiter JB, Levine AM, et al., eds. Skeletal trauma: fractures, distortions. Ligamentous injuries. Vol 1. Philadelphia: WB Saunders, 1992: 31–75.

Schultz RJ. The language of fractures. 2nd ed. Baltimore: Williams & Wilkins, 1990.

Schutzer SF, Gossling HR. The treatment of reflex sympathetic dystrophy syndrome. (Current Concepts Review). J Bone Joint Surg 1994;66A: 625–629.

Scott G, King JB. A prospective double-blind trial of electrical capacitative coupling in the treatment of non-union of long bones. J Bone Joint Surg 1994;76A:820–826.

Shuler TE. Trauma, Section 1, Adult Trauma. In: Miller MD, ed. Review of orthopaedics. 2nd ed. Philadelphia: WB Saunders, 1996:350–392.

Tibbles PM, Edelsberg JS. Hyperbaric-oxygen therapy (medical progress). N Engl J Med 1996; 334:1642–1648.

Urist MR. Bone formation by osteoinduction. Science 1965;150:893–899.

Urist MR. Bone morphogenetic protein with special reference to bone transplants, implants and the bone-bone marrow consortium. In: Peck IVA, ed. Bone and mineral research. Vol. 6. New York: Elsevier Science Publishers, 1989.

Urist MR, Silvermann BF, Büring K, et al. The bone induction principle. Clin Orthop 1967;53: 243–283.

16 Specific Fractures and Joint Injuries in Children

Before beginning this chapter, you may wish—if you have not already done so—to review Chapter 15, *General Features of Fractures and Joint Injuries.*

Indeed, your knowledge of the general features, combined with your good sense, will enable you to deduce, and therefore anticipate, the appropriate methods of treatment for specific injuries in children.

Before considering specific injuries in children, however, you should consider some of the special features of fractures and dislocations during the growing years. Just as in all other clinical fields of medicine and surgery, so also in the field of fractures, children cannot be considered simply as "little adults." As you will see, fractures in children, and the reactions of children's tissues to these fractures, differ greatly from those in adults. Blount deserves special credit for emphasizing the fact that "fractures in children are different."

SPECIAL FEATURES OF FRACTURES AND DISLOCATIONS IN CHILDREN

The special features of fractures and dislocations in children are listed and then discussed individually. The differences are most striking in the infant and young child; they become progressively less striking as the child approaches adulthood. Terms such as "more" and "less" refer to a comparison between fractures and dislocations in children and adults.

1. Fractures more common
2. Stronger and more active periosteum
3. More rapid fracture healing
4. Special problems of diagnosis
5. Spontaneous correction of certain residual deformities
6. Differences in complications
7. Different emphasis on methods of treatment

8. Torn ligaments and dislocations less common
9. Less tolerance of major blood loss

1. Fractures More Common

The higher incidence of fractures in children is explained by the combination of their relatively slender bones and their carefree capers. Some of these injuries, such as crack or hairline fractures, buckle fractures, and greenstick fractures, are not serious. Others, such as intra-articular fractures and epiphyseal plate fractures, are very serious indeed. In children not yet walking who have a fracture or joint injury, you must consider the possible but tragic diagnosis of child abuse.

2. Stronger and More Active Periosteum

The stronger periosteum in children is less readily torn across at the time of a fracture; consequently there is more often an intact periosteal hinge that can be used during closed reduction of the fracture as described in Chapter 15 (Figs. 15.11 and 15.36). Furthermore, the periosteum is much more osteogenic in children than it is in adults (Fig. 16.1).

3. More Rapid Fracture Healing

As mentioned in Chapter 15, the rate of healing in bone varies much more with age, particularly during childhood than it does in any other tissue in the body. This is closely related to the osteogenic activity of the periosteum and endosteum, a process that is remarkably active at birth, becomes progressively less active with each year of childhood, and remains relatively constant from early adult life to old age.

Fractures of the shaft of the femur serve as an example of this phenomenon. A femoral

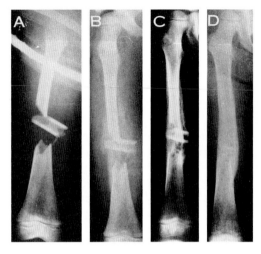

Figure 16.1. The importance of the strong and actively osteogenic periosteum in the healing process of children's fractures is demonstrated in this series of radiographs of a fractured femoral shaft in a 4-year-old child. **A.** The day of injury; a double fracture with the middle segment lying almost transversely. The strong periosteal sleeve would not be completely torn across. Note the metal ring of the Thomas splint. **B.** Three weeks after injury, abundant callus is forming from the actively osteogenic periosteum. At this stage traction was replaced by a hip spica cast. **C.** Ten weeks after injury, the middle segment is well incorporated in the callus and is being resorbed. The fracture was clinically united at this stage and the child was allowed to walk. **D.** Six months after injury, the contour of the femur is returning to normal through the process of remodeling.

various secondary centers of ossification appear at relatively constant ages, these are not easy to remember. Likewise, the radiographic appearance of the various epiphyseal plates may be puzzling to the inexperienced and may be mistaken for fracture lines. These radiographic problems of diagnosis can be readily resolved in limb injuries if you are uncertain about the presence or absence of a fracture or an epiphyseal plate injury. Just as you would naturally compare an injured limb with its normal uninjured mate during the clinical examination, so also can you compare areas of the two limbs in similar positions during the radiographic examination (Fig. 16.2).

5. Spontaneous Correction of Certain Residual Deformities

In adults, the deformity of a malunited fracture is permanent, but in children certain residual deformities tend to correct spontaneously either by extensive remodeling or epiphyseal plate growth, and sometimes by a combination of both. Just how much spontaneous correction of the healed fracture deformity can be anticipated depends on the age of the child (hence the number of years of skeletal growth remaining) and the type of deformity (angulation, incomplete apposition,

shaft fracture occurring at birth will be united in 3 weeks; a comparable fracture at the age of 8 years will be united in 8 weeks; at the age of 12 years, it will be united at 12 weeks; and from the age of 20 years to old age it will be united in approximately 20 weeks.

Nonunion of children's fractures is rare, unless an open operation has damaged the blood supply to the fracture fragments or has introduced the complication of infection. An exception is a widely displaced fracture of the lateral condyle of the humerus.

4. Special Problems of Diagnosis

The varying radiographic appearance of a given epiphysis, both before and after the development of a secondary center of ossification, can be quite confusing, and although the

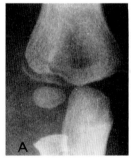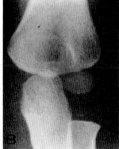

Figure 16.2. The value of a comparable radiographic examination of the opposite uninjured limb. **A.** Does the radiolucent line just proximal to the capitellum of this child's right humerus represent a fracture or just part of the epiphyseal plate? **B.** Comparison with the radiograph of the opposite elbow clarifies the situation. The child has a slightly displaced fracture of the lateral condyle of the right humerus, a potentially serious fracture as will be seen in a subsequent section of this chapter.

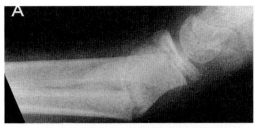

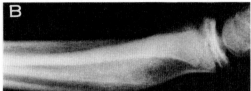

Figure 16.3.   Spontaneous improvement in a residual fracture deformity with subsequent growth. **A.** Lateral projection of the distal end of the radius of a 10-year-old boy 6 weeks after injury. Unfortunately the metaphyseal fracture had been allowed to unite with 35 degrees of anterior angulation. **B.** Six months later, there is only 15 degrees of anterior angulation and the corners of the angulation deformity have remodeled. Note that the epiphysis has grown away from the fracture site during these 6 months.

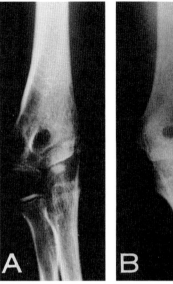
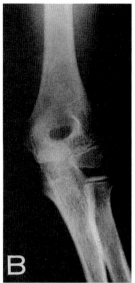

Figure 16.4.   Failure of spontaneous correction of a residual fracture deformity. **A.** A supracondylar fracture of the humerus in a 9-year-old girl had been allowed to unite with 20 degrees of lateral angulation 2 years previously. **B.** The opposite elbow has a normal carrying angle of 15 degrees. On the injured side, the normal carrying angle has been lost and reversed so that there are 5 degrees of varus and a total of 20 degrees of residual lateral angulation deformity. This deformity of malunion is permanent.

shortening, rotation). This phenomenon is best considered in relation to specific deformities.

Angulation

Residual angulation near an epiphyseal plate will tend to correct spontaneously with subsequent growth, provided that the plane of the deformity is the same as the plane of motion in the nearest joint. For example, residual anterior angulation at the site of a healed fracture in the distal end of the radius is in the same plane as the flexion and extension motion in the wrist joint. Thus, in a young child it can be expected to correct to a large extent (Fig. 16.3). By contrast, residual angulation at right angles to the plane of motion of the nearest joint, such as a lateral angulation or varus deformity in the supracondylar region of the humerus which is at right angles to the flexion and extension motion of the elbow, cannot be expected to correct (Fig. 16.4). In angulation in the middle third of a long bone, being well away from an epiphyseal plate, complete correction cannot be expected to occur spontaneously (Fig. 16.5A).

Another type of injury, and one that can

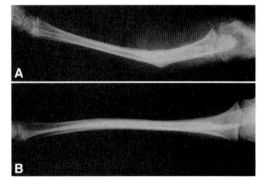

Figure 16.5.   **A.** Failure of spontaneous correction of a residual fracture deformity. The fractures of the middle third of the radius and ulna of an 8-year-old girl had been allowed to unite in the unsatisfactory position of 35° of posterior angulation one year previously. This deformity of malunion is, at least to some extent, permanent. **B.** Plastic deformation of the shafts of the radius and ulna in a child. Note that there are no radiographically detectable fractures.

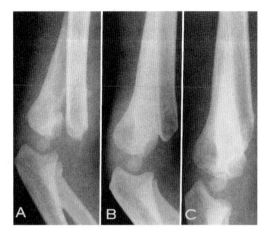

Figure 16.6. Spontaneous correction of incomplete apposition through remodeling. **A.** An unreduced supracondylar fracture of the humerus in a 4-year-old child 3 weeks after injury. Note the new bone formation in the periosteal tube through which the proximal fragment is protruding. **B.** Five months after injury the periosteal tube has formed a new shaft and the original shaft is becoming resorbed. **C.** One year after injury the contour of the fracture site has been greatly improved by the process of remodeling. Note that the epiphysis has grown away from the fracture site.

cause a gentle bend in the middle of a growing bone without an obvious fracture, is known as "plastic deformation" of bone, a phenomenon that is probably associated with occult microfractures (Fig. 16.5B). This type of deformity does not often correct completely, but it is usually too mild to require treatment.

Incomplete Apposition

With incomplete apposition of the fracture fragments, or even side-to-side (bayonet) apposition in children, the contour of the healed fracture improves greatly through the active process of remodeling—an example of Wolff's law (Fig. 16.6).

Shortening

After a displaced fracture of a long bone in a growing child, the associated disruption in the nutrient artery results in a compensatory increase in the blood flow at the epiphyseal ends of the bone. This phenomenon produces a temporary acceleration of longitudinal growth in the bone for as long as 1 year after the fracture (Fig. 16.7). This is most striking after dis-

placed femoral shaft fracture; therefore, overriding is a desirable aim in the treatment of such fractures, because the shortening will be corrected spontaneously by temporary overgrowth and the two femora will become almost the same length (Fig. 16.8).

Rotation

Residual rotational deformity at the site of a healed fracture in a long bone does not usually correct spontaneously regardless of the child's age or the site of the deformity.

6. Differences in Complications

Most of the complications discussed in Chapter 15 can occur in both children and adults,

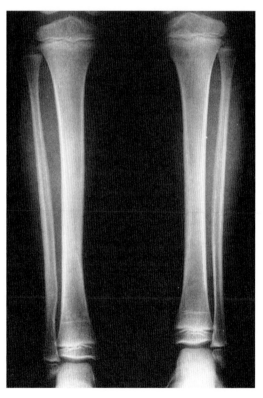

Figure 16.7. Overgrowth of a long bone after a displaced fracture. One year previously, the right tibia of this 8-year-old boy had been fractured and during the ensuing year it had overgrown 1 cm. The transverse radiopaque lines in the distal tibial metaphyses represent the site of the epiphyseal plate at the time of injury. Note that there has been more growth from the epiphyseal plate of the right tibia than from the left. The resultant leg-length discrepancy will be permanent.

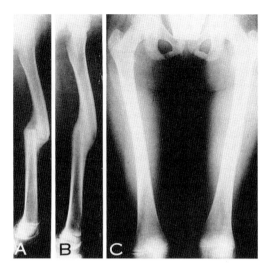

Figure 16.8. Overgrowth of the left femur after a displaced fracture of the shaft in a 9-year-old girl. **A.** Lateral projection 8 weeks after injury. The fracture had been allowed to unite with 1 cm of overriding intentionally. **B.** Six months after injury the united fracture is becoming remodeled. **C.** Eighteen months after injury the femora are virtually equal in length as a result of overgrowth of the left femur. If the fracture had been allowed to unite end to end, the femur would have been 1 cm too long 18 months later and the leg-length discrepancy would have been permanent.

but certain differences merit consideration. Of course, growth disturbances after epiphyseal plate injuries occur only in children. Osteomyelitis secondary to either an open fracture or open reduction of a closed fracture tends to be more extensive in a child and the infection may even destroy an epiphyseal plate with resultant growth disturbance. Volkmann's ischemia (compartment syndrome) of nerves and muscles is much more common in children, as are posttraumatic myositis ossificans and refracture.

By contrast, persistent joint stiffness after fracture is relatively uncommon in children, unless the period of immobilization of a joint has been unduly prolonged or the fracture has involved the joint surface. Consequently, physiotherapy and occupational therapy are seldom required in the after-care of children with fractures. Likewise, fat embolism, pulmonary embolism, and accident neurosis are rare in childhood.

7. Different Emphasis on Methods of Treatment

Although the principles of fracture treatment described in Chapter 15 apply equally to children and adults, the methods of treatment in the two age groups differ. Virtually all fractures of the long bones in young children can and should be treated by means of closed reduction, either by manipulation or by continuous traction. Of course, the emotional exuberance and physical vigor of children recovering from fractures demand that their plaster-of-Paris casts be particularly strong.

Certain fractures in children do necessitate open reduction and internal skeletal fixation; for example, displaced intra-articular fractures, femoral neck fractures, and certain types of epiphyseal plate injuries, which are described in a subsequent section. In recent years (mostly because of health cost constraints necessitating shorter hospital stays), there has been a growing tendency, at least in older children, to treat some diaphyseal fractures, especially in the radius, ulna, and femur by operative means. There is no indication for excision of a fracture fragment and replacement by an endoprosthesis in children. The results of treatment of children's fractures must be optimal because they have to last a long lifetime.

8. Torn Ligaments and Dislocations Less Common

Children's ligaments are strong and resilient. Furthermore, because they are stronger than the associated epiphyseal plates, sudden powerful traction on a ligament at the time of injury results in a separation of the epiphyseal plate rather than a tear in the ligament (Fig. 16.9). This is also true, although to a lesser extent, of fibrous joint capsules; for example, the type of injury that would produce a traumatic dislocation of the shoulder in an adult will produce a fracture-separation of the proximal humeral epiphysis in a child.

9. Less Tolerance of Major Blood Loss

The importance of percentage blood loss in relation to shock is well known. Obviously,

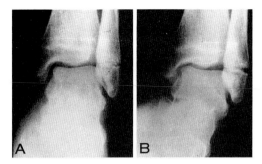

Figure 16.9. Traumatic separation of the distal fibular epiphysis in a 14-year-old boy. **A.** This radiograph appears normal because after the injury, the fibular epiphysis had been returned to its normal position by the elastic recoil of the soft tissues. **B.** In this stress radiograph (taken while a varus stress is being applied to the ankle joint with the child under anesthetic), there is a tilt of the talus and the separation of the fibular epiphysis is apparent.

the total blood volume is proportionately smaller in a child than in an adult. A formula for estimating the approximate blood volume in a child is 75 ml/kg/body weight. Thus, the approximate blood volume of a child who weighs 20 kg (44 lb) is 1500 ml. Consequently, external hemorrhage of 500 ml in such a child represents 33% of the total blood volume, whereas a similar hemorrhage in an average adult would represent only 10% of the total blood volume of 5000 ml. Trauma accounts for 50% of deaths in children, making it the most common cause of death in this age group.

SPECIAL TYPES OF FRACTURES IN CHILDREN

In addition to *stress fractures* and *pathological fractures,* which occur in both children and adults as discussed in Chapter 15, there are two special types of fractures that are limited to childhood, namely, *fractures that involve the epiphyseal plate* and *birth fractures.*

Fractures That Involve the Epiphyseal Plate (Physis)

Epiphyseal plate fractures, or physeal fractures, present special problems in relation to both diagnosis and treatment. They also carry the risk of becoming complicated by a serious

disturbance of local growth and the consequent development of progressive bony deformity during the remaining years of skeletal growth.

Although the term "physis" is a relatively recent and acceptable synonym for the epiphyseal plate, the latter term is still more widely used in many countries and hence is used throughout this textbook.

Anatomy, Histology, and Physiology

The anatomy and histology of pressure and traction types of epiphyses and their epiphyseal plates have been discussed in Chapter 2, but a few pertinent points merit emphasis. The types of epiphyses are shown in Figure 16.10.

The weakest area of the epiphyseal plate is the zone of calcifying cartilage (also known as the zone of provisional calcification). When the epiphysis is separated by injury, the line of separation is through this zone (Fig. 16.11). Thus, the epiphyseal plate, which is radiolucent and not radiographically visible, always remains attached to the epiphysis.

The blood supply of the epiphyseal plate enters from its epiphyseal surface and, there-

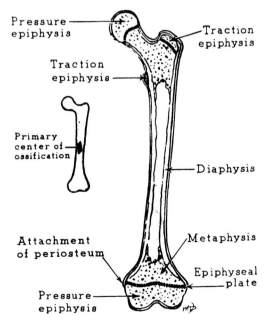

Figure 16.10. Types of epiphyses (secondary centers of ossification) in the femur. Note the attachment of the periosteum to the epiphysis.

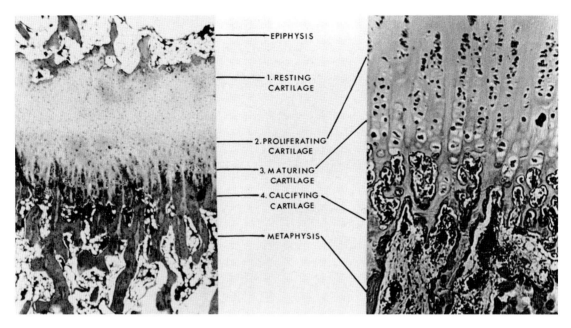

EPIPHYSIS

1. RESTING
   CARTILAGE

2. PROLIFERATING
   CARTILAGE

3. MATURING
   CARTILAGE

4. CALCIFYING
   CARTILAGE

METAPHYSIS

Figure 16.11.   Left. Low power magnification photomicrograph of an epiphyseal plate from the proximal end of the tibia of a child. **Right.** Higher power magnification photomicrograph.

fore, if the epiphysis loses its blood supply and becomes necrotic, the plate also becomes necrotic and growth ceases. In most sites, the blood supply to the epiphysis is not damaged at the time of injury, but in the proximal femoral epiphysis and the proximal radial epiphysis, the blood vessels course along the neck of the bone and cross the epiphyseal plate peripherally. Consequently in these sites, epiphyseal separation frequently damages the blood supply and leads to avascular necrosis of the epiphysis and the epiphyseal plate with cessation of growth.

The cartilaginous epiphyseal plate is weaker than bone and yet epiphyseal injuries account for only 15% of all fractures in childhood. The explanation for this apparent paradox is that the epiphysis is firmly attached to its metaphysis peripherally by the union of perichondrium and periosteum (Fig. 16.10). Nevertheless, as mentioned previously, epiphyseal plates are also weaker than their associated ligaments and joint capsule. For this reason, injuries that would result in a torn ligament or a dislocation in an adult usually produce a traumatic separation of the epiphysis in a child (Fig. 16.9).

In the lower limb, more longitudinal growth takes place at the epiphyseal plates in the region of the knee than of the hip or ankle. In the upper limb by contrast, more growth takes place in the region of the shoulder and the wrist than of the elbow.

Diagnosis of Epiphyseal Plate Injuries
You should suspect an epiphyseal plate fracture clinically in any injured child who exhibits signs (such as local swelling and tenderness) suggestive of a fracture near the end of a long bone, a traumatic dislocation, or a ligamentous injury (including a sprain). Precise diagnosis, however, depends on radiographic examination; at least two projections at right angles to each other are essential. Furthermore, if you are uncertain whether a radiolucent line represents a fracture or an epiphyseal plate, you should also obtain comparable projections of the same region of the opposite uninjured limb (Fig. 16.2).

Salter-Harris Classification of Epiphyseal Plate Injuries
The following classification, which the author developed with W. Robert Harris, is based on

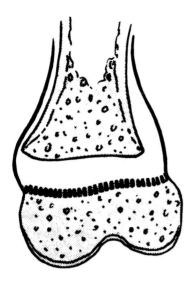

Figure 16.12.   Type I epiphyseal plate injury. Separation of the entire epiphysis.

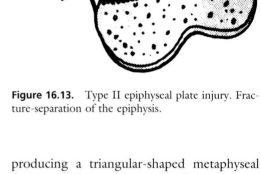

Figure 16.13.   Type II epiphyseal plate injury. Fracture-separation of the epiphysis.

the mechanism of injury as well as the relationship of the fracture line to the growing cells of the epiphyseal plate. It is correlated as well with the method of treatment and the prognosis of the injury concerning growth disturbance.

Type I (Fig. 16.12)

There is complete separation of the entire epiphysis without any fracture through bone. The growing cells of the epiphyseal plate remain with the epiphysis. This type of injury, the result of a shearing force, is more common in newborns (from birth injury) and in young children in whom the epiphyseal plate is relatively thick.

Closed reduction is not difficult because the periosteal attachment is intact around most of its circumference. The prognosis for future growth is excellent provided the blood supply to the epiphysis is intact, which it usually is in sites other than the proximal femoral epiphysis and the proximal radial epiphysis.

Type II (Fig. 16.13)

In this, the most common type, the line of fracture-separation extends along the epiphyseal plate to a variable distance, then out through a portion of the metaphysis thereby

producing a triangular-shaped metaphyseal fragment. The growing cells of the plate remain with the epiphysis. This type of injury, the result of shearing and bending forces, usually occurs in the older child in whom the epiphyseal plate is relatively thin. The periosteum is torn on the convex side of the angulation but is intact on the concave side; thus the intact periosteal hinge is always on the side of the metaphyseal fragment.

Closed reduction is relatively easy both to obtain and maintain. The intact periosteal hinge and the metaphyseal fragment both prevent overreduction. The prognosis for growth is excellent, provided the blood supply to the epiphysis is intact, which it nearly always is in sites where type II injuries occur.

Type III (Fig. 16.14)

The fracture is intra-articular, extends from the joint surface to the deep zone of the epiphyseal plate, then along the plate to its periphery. This uncommon type of injury is caused by an intra-articular shearing force and is usually limited to the distal tibial epiphysis in a teenager in whom one part of the epiphyseal plate has already closed and the other part is still open.

A variant of this epiphyseal plate injury and

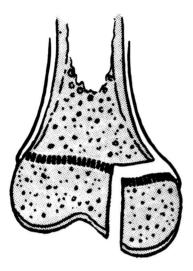

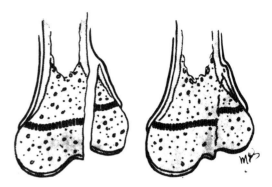

Figure 16.15.   Type IV epiphyseal plate injury. **Left.** Fracture of the epiphysis and also of the epiphyseal plate. **Right.** Unless the fracture is perfectly reduced, bony union will cause premature closure of the plate.

Figure 16.14.   Type III epiphyseal plate injury. Fracture of part of the epiphysis.

one that also occurs in teenagers is what is known as a *triplane fracture*. In the antero-posterior projection, it resembles a type III injury, but in the lateral projection, it resembles a type II injury. The precise anatomy of a triplane fracture is best assessed by a CT scan.

For type III injuries as well as for intra-articular triplane fractures, open reduction and internal fixation are usually necessary to restore a perfectly normal joint surface. The prognosis for growth is good provided the blood supply to the separated portion of the epiphysis has not been disrupted.

Type IV (Fig. 16.15)

The fracture, which is intra-articular, extends from the joint surface through the epiphysis, across the entire thickness of the epiphyseal plate, and through a portion of the metaphysis. The most common type IV injury is the fracture of the lateral condyle of the humerus.

Open reduction and internal skeletal fixation are absolutely necessary to restore a normal joint surface and to obtain perfect apposition of the epiphyseal plate. Unless the fractured surfaces of the epiphyseal plate are kept perfectly reduced, fracture healing occurs across the plate and renders further longitudinal growth impossible. The prognosis for growth after a type IV injury is bad unless per-

fect reduction is both obtained and maintained.

Type V (Fig. 16.16)

This uncommon injury results from a severe crushing force being applied through the epiphysis to one area of the epiphyseal plate. It is most likely to occur in the region of the knee and ankle.

Because the epiphysis is not usually displaced, the diagnosis of a type V injury is difficult. Weightbearing must be avoided for at least 3 weeks in the hope of preventing further compression of the epiphyseal plate. The prognosis of type V injuries is decidedly poor

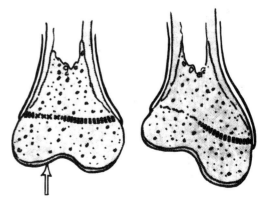

Figure 16.16.   Type V epiphyseal plate injury. **Left.** Crushing of one side of the epiphyseal plate. **Right.** Premature closure of the plate on one side with a resultant angulatory deformity.

because premature cessation of growth is almost inevitable.

To these five basic types of epiphyseal plate injuries, Rang has added a sixth type, namely the rare injury to the peripheral perichondrial ring, or zone of Ranvier, that encircles the plate. Although this type of injury can be caused by a direct blow, it is more often due to an open slicing mechanism by a sharp object such as the blade or blades of a power lawn mower. This type VI injury carries a bad prognosis for subsequent growth because a local bony bridge tends to form across the epiphyseal plate.

Recently, Ogden published an encyclopedic classification of epiphyseal injuries that comprises 9 types and 18 subtypes.

Healing of Epiphyseal Plate Injuries

After reduction of a separated epiphysis, as in types I, II, and III injuries, endochondral ossification on the metaphyseal side of the epiphyseal plate is only temporarily disturbed. Within 2 or 3 weeks of replacement of the epiphysis, endochondral ossification has resumed and has united the epiphyseal plate to the metaphysis. This special type of fracture healing accounts for the clinical observation that these three types of epiphyseal separations heal in only half the time required for union of a fracture through the metaphysis of the same bone in a child of the same age. Type IV injuries by contrast must heal in the same manner as any other fracture through cancellous bone, and type V injuries usually heal by a bony bridge across the epiphyseal plate.

Prognosis Concerning Growth Disturbance

The following factors will help you to estimate the prognosis of an epiphyseal plate injury in a child.

1. Type of Injury

The prognosis for each of the five classified types of epiphyseal plate injury has been discussed above.

2. Age of the Child

This is really an indication of the amount of growth normally expected in the particular epiphyseal plate Obviously, the younger the child at the time of injury, the more serious any growth disturbance will be.

3. Blood Supply to the Epiphysis

Disruption of the blood supply to the epiphysis is associated with a poor prognosis for reasons already discussed.

4. Method of Reduction

Unduly forceful closed manipulation or unskilled open reduction of a displaced epiphysis may crush the epiphyseal plate and increase the likelihood of growth disturbance.

5. Open or Closed Injury

Open injuries of the epiphyseal plate carry a risk of infection that may destroy the plate and result in premature cessation of growth.

6. Velocity and Force of the Injury

Regardless of the type of the epiphyseal plate injury, the prognosis concerning possible growth arrest is worse if the injury has been incurred by a high velocity and/or high force mechanism (such as an automobile accident or a fall from a great height).

Possible Effects of Growth Disturbance

Fortunately, 85% of epiphyseal plate injuries are uncomplicated by growth disturbance. In the remaining 15%, the clinical problem associated with the dread complication of premature cessation of growth depends on several factors, including the bone involved, the extent of the disturbance in the epiphyseal plate, and the amount of growth normally expected from that particular epiphyseal plate.

If the entire epiphyseal plate ceases to grow in a single bone, the result is a progressive limb-length discrepancy (Fig. 16.17). If the involved bone is one of a parallel pair (such as tibia and fibula, or radius and ulna), progressive length discrepancy between the two bones will produce a progressive angulatory deformity in the neighboring joint (Fig. 16.18). If growth ceases in only one part of the plate (for example on the medial side) but continues in the remainder, the result will be a progressive angulatory deformity (Fig. 16.19).

Premature cessation of growth does not necessarily occur immediately after an injury

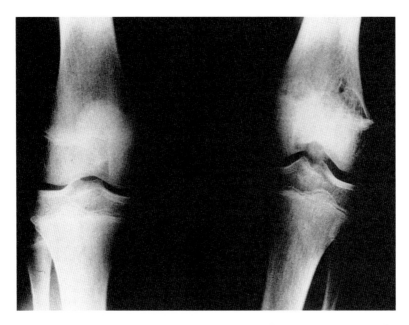

Figure 16.17. Progressive leg-length discrepancy secondary to premature cessation of growth in the entire left distal femoral epiphyseal plate. A type IV epiphyseal plate injury had occurred 2 years previously in this 11-year-old boy. The discrepancy will continue to increase during the remaining years of growth.

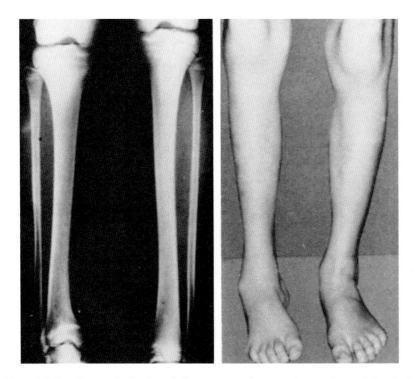

Figure 16.18. Progressive leg-length discrepancy and progressive angulatory deformity in a 9-year-old girl 18 months after a type IV epiphyseal plate injury of the right medial malleolus. Growth has ceased in the medial part of the tibial epiphyseal plate and has continued in the lateral part, as well as in the epiphyseal plate of the fibula. The result is a progressive varus deformity of the ankle. Note also that the right tibia is shorter than the left.

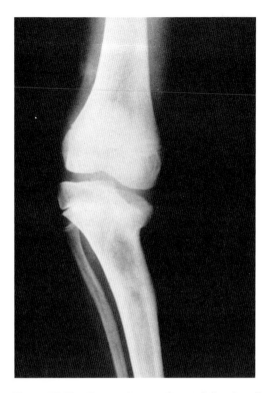

Figure 16.19.   Progressive angulatory deformity of the knee in a 15-year-old boy 3 years after a type V injury involving the medial part of the upper tibial epiphyseal plate. Growth has ceased on the medial side but has continued on the lateral side, with a resultant progressive varus deformity of the knee.

to the epiphyseal plate. In fact, growth may be retarded only for a period of 6 months, or even longer, before it ceases completely.

Resection of Bony Bridges

On the basis of experimental investigations in animals, Langenskiold has devised the surgical procedure of resection of an established bony bridge that is tethering the epiphyseal plate and causing a growth disturbance, either peripherally or centrally. The resultant defect is then filled with an autogenous fat graft to prevent recurrence of the bridge. Provided that the bony bridge has not already extended to cover more than one half of the surface of the epiphyseal plate (as demonstrated by CT scans in the anteroposterior and lateral projections), this procedure usually enables resumption of symmetrical growth and sometimes even achieves some correction of the existing angu-

latory deformity. The smaller the bony bridge, the better the result from its resection. More recently, Peterson and others have recommended filling the defect with a variety of materials including cranioplast (which is methylmethacrylate without the barium), with results that are comparable to those of autogenous fat grafts.

On the orthopaedic horizon is the technical possibility, through microvascular surgery, of transplantation of an expendable autogenous epiphyseal plate (such as that of the proximal end of the fibula) to the site of a prematurely closed plate.

Special Considerations in the Treatment of Epiphyseal Plate Injuries

From the foregoing discussion, you will appreciate that injuries involving the epiphyseal plate must be treated gently and as soon after injury as possible. Types I and II injuries can nearly always be treated by closed reduction. Displaced type III injuries and displaced type IV injuries always require open reduction and internal fixation. The period of immobilization required for types I, II, and III injuries is only half that required for a metaphyseal fracture of the same bone in a child of the same age.

The parents of a child who has sustained an epiphyseal plate injury should always be given some indication of the prognosis concerning future growth without causing them undue anxiety. The parents should also be comforted with the assurance that if a growth disturbance does develop, it can be treated. Furthermore, the child should be carefully examined both clinically and radiographically at six-month intervals for at least 1 year, and often longer, to detect any growth disturbance. As with the follow-up management of all children's fractures, it is important to have a well-established "call-back system" to contact those families that fail to keep an appointment.

Specific epiphyseal plate injuries are discussed on a regional basis, along with specific fractures and dislocations in a subsequent section of this chapter.

Avulsion of Traction Epiphyses

A sudden traction force applied through either a ligament or a tendon to a traction epiphysis (apophysis) may result in an avulsion of the epiphysis through its epiphyseal plate. Examples of such injuries are avulsion of the medial epicondyle of the humerus and the lesser trochanter of the femur. Because the epiphyseal plates of these traction epiphyses do not contribute to the longitudinal growth of the bone, such injuries are not complicated by a growth disturbance.

Birth Fractures

During the difficult delivery of a large baby, especially a breech presentation, when the threat of fetal anoxia may necessitate rapid extraction of the baby, one limb may be difficult to disengage from the birth canal and a bone may be inadvertently fractured or an epiphysis separated. Only rarely is a previously normal joint dislocated by a birth injury. This usually unavoidable mishap is uncommon but when it does occur it is often the proximal bones of the limbs that are injured.

Multiple birth fractures are nearly always pathological and the cause seen most often is osteogenesis imperfecta (Chapter 8). Birth fracture of the tibia is rare and when it does occur it is nearly always a pathological fracture that fails to unite—congenital pseudarthrosis of the tibia (Chapter 8).

When either the humerus or the femur is fractured during delivery, the obstetrician feels and usually hears the bone break. When an epiphysis is separated, it tends to slide off the metaphysis and the obstetrician may neither feel nor hear it. Thus the diagnosis of epiphyseal separations requires careful and repeated physical examination of the newborn.

Parents are understandably distressed when their new baby has sustained a birth fracture—and so is the obstetrician. The physician or surgeon who treats the newborn infant's injury should gently inform the parents that such an injury is unavoidable under the circumstances and that it is much less serious than fetal anoxia, which the obstetrician had undoubtedly prevented by rapid delivery of their baby.

Specific birth injuries are discussed below in order of decreasing incidence.

Specific Birth Fractures
Clavicle

The slender newborn clavicle is the bone most susceptible to fracture during delivery, particularly in a broad-shouldered baby. The infant tends not to move the affected limb during the first week. This "pseudo paralysis" can be differentiated from the true paralysis of a brachial plexus injury by clinical examination (although, of course, the two may coexist). Radiographic examination confirms the presence of a fractured clavicle.

The fracture unites with remarkable rapidity, a strikingly large callus becoming apparent both clinically and radiographically within 10 days. Simple protection with a sling for comfort is the only treatment required.

Humerus

The humeral shaft is particularly susceptible to a birth fracture during a difficult breech delivery. The complete fracture is in the shaft and is frequently associated with a radial nerve injury. The latter, being only a neuropraxia, recovers completely. The newborn infant's fractured arm is obviously floppy and the diagnosis is readily confirmed radiographically (Fig. 16.20).

The infant's arm should be bandaged to the

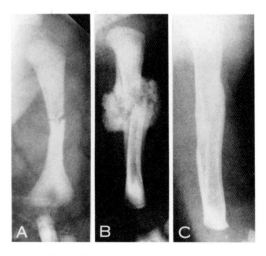

Figure 16.20. Birth fracture of the humerus. **A.** The day of birth. **B.** Ten days later, there is profuse callus formation. The fracture at this stage was clinically united. **C.** Ten weeks later a remarkable amount of remodeling has occurred.

chest for a period of 2 weeks, by which time the fracture is always clinically united. Mild residual angulatory deformities improve with subsequent growth, but rotational deformities are permanent. Rarely, the proximal humeral epiphysis is separated by a birth injury.

Femur

Birth fractures of the femur are most likely to occur during the delivery of a baby who has presented as a frank breech. The clinical deformity and floppiness of the lower limb are apparent and radiographic examination confirms the diagnosis of a fracture, which is usually in the midshaft. Overhead (Bryant's) skin traction on both lower limbs provides adequate alignment of the fracture, which is clinically united within 3 weeks (see Fig. 16.76). An alternative form of treatment is an immediate hip spica cast for a full-term baby or a Pavlik harness for a tiny premature baby.

Traumatic separation of the distal femoral epiphysis is more difficult to recognize clinically and may escape detection until the knee becomes enlarged by extensive new bone formation (Fig. 16.21). Overhead (Bryant's) skin traction is required for 10 days. Being a type

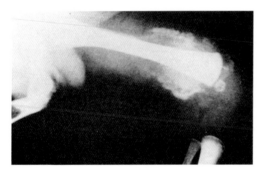

Figure 16.21. Birth injury of the distal femoral epiphysis. In this radiograph taken 10 days after birth, the center of ossification of the distal femoral epiphysis is seen to be displaced posteriorly (normally it is in line with the central axis of the femoral shaft). The significant new bone formation from the elevated periosteum would have taken approximately 10 days to develop; therefore, by deduction, this type I epiphyseal plate injury probably occurred at birth. The injury had been unsuspected at the time of the difficult breech delivery but the radiograph was taken 10 days later because of the gross clinical swelling of the infant's knee.

I epiphyseal plate injury in an epiphysis that has a good blood supply, the prognosis for subsequent growth is excellent. A long leg cast is a reasonable alternative.

Traumatic separation of the proximal femoral epiphysis is difficult to differentiate clinically from dislocation of the hip, but the latter is rare as a birth injury. Radiographically, the differentiation also may be difficult inasmuch as at birth, the head, neck, and greater trochanter are completely unossified. The radiographic differentiation from a congenitally dislocated hip at birth may require either an arthrogram or MRI. Within 3 weeks, a radiographic examination reveals evidence of new bone formation in the metaphyseal region indicating a traumatic epiphyseal separation (Fig. 16.22). Treatment consists of immobilization of the hip in abduction and flexion in a spica cast for 2 weeks. The prognosis for subsequent growth is good because at birth, the proximal femoral epiphysis consists of the head, neck, and greater trochanter, and at this stage, separation of the entire epiphysis does not jeopardize its blood supply.

Spine

Fortunately, birth injuries of the spine are rare but they are extremely serious because they may be complicated by complete paraplegia.

SPECIFIC FRACTURES AND DISLOCATIONS

The Hand

Apart from crush injuries of the distal phalanges, fractures of the hand are much less common in children than in adults.

In children, a hyperflexion injury of the distal interphalangeal joint may produce a fracture-separation through the epiphyseal plate, a childhood type of mallet finger that can be differentiated from avulsion of the extensor tendon by a lateral radiograph. This becomes an open injury if the nailbed has been disrupted. The finger should be immobilized with the distal joint in extension for 3 weeks.

Phalangeal fractures must be accurately reduced to avoid a persistent angulatory deformity (Fig. 16.23). Rotational deformity in a finger, which is most likely to occur through

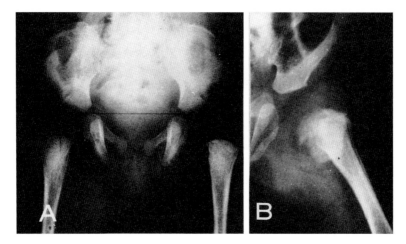

Figure 16.22. Birth injury of the proximal femoral epiphysis. **A.** Six days after birth there is obvious lateral displacement of the metaphysis of the left femur in relation to the acetabulum (the normal hip serves as a helpful comparison). Clinically, the infant was thought to have congenital dislocation of the left hip. The center of ossification does not appear until approximately 6 months of age. Note the slight new bone formation around the metaphysis. This differentiates an epiphyseal plate injury from a dislocation of the hip. **B.** Eight weeks later there is further new bone formation and early remodeling.

a separation of the proximal phalangeal epiphyseal plate, should also be corrected because it seriously impairs function of the hand (Fig. 16.24). Either angulatory or rotational malunion of a proximal phalanx will cause that finger to cross over its neighbor when the fingers are completely flexed.

Displaced *intra-articular fractures of finger joints* merit open reduction and internal fixation with fine Kirschner wires to restore a perfect joint surface.

Metacarpophalangeal dislocation of the thumb is common in children as a result of a hyperextension injury (Fig. 16.25). The first metacarpal head escapes through a small tear in the joint capsule that then tends to grip the narrow neck of the metacarpal and act as a "buttonhole." For this reason, the dislocation may be frustratingly difficult to reduce by closed manipulation and frequently requires open reduction, followed by immobilization of the joint in the stable position of moderate flexion for 3 weeks.

Older boys who fight with more force than finesse may sustain a *fracture of the neck of the mobile fifth metacarpal,* which is usually referred to as a "boxer's fracture" but is more appropriately called a "street-fighter's fracture." (A boxer strikes the opponent with the heads of the stronger second and third metacarpals). This fracture responds well to closed reduction. The depressed metacarpal head can be elevated by pressure along the axis of the proximal phalanx with the metacarpophalangeal joint flexed to a right angle. The fracture should be immobilized for 4 weeks with the finger in moderate flexion.

Fractures of the carpal bones are rare in childhood, possibly because of their relatively large cartilaginous component during the growing years. Nevertheless, *fractures of the carpal scaphoid* sometimes occur in adolescents and may require the same prolonged immobilization as they do in adults.

Severe injuries of the hand, particularly tendon injuries and open fractures, should be treated by a surgeon who has a special interest and skill in surgery of the hand.

The Wrist and Forearm

Fractures in the region of the wrist and forearm are extremely common in childhood because of frequent falls in which the forces are transmitted from the hand to the radius and ulna.

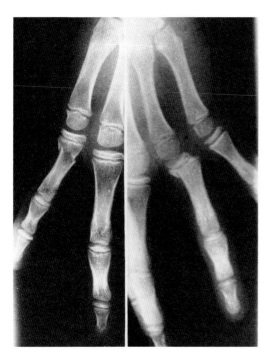

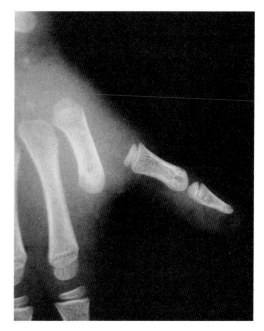

Figure 16.23.   Left. Fracture through the metaphysis of the proximal phalanx of the little finger with angulation. If this angulatory fracture deformity is not reduced, there will be a permanent deformity of the finger.

Figure 16.25.   Traumatic dislocation of the metacarpophalangeal joint of the thumb of a child. In this particular child, the dislocation could not be reduced by closed manipulation and open reduction was required.

Figure 16.24.   Right. Type II fracture-separation of the epiphysis of the proximal phalanx of the ring finger. Only slight displacement is apparent in this radiograph, which was taken 3 weeks after injury. Clinical examination at this time, however, revealed a 45-degree rotational deformity of the finger. As a result, this finger crossed over its neighbor during flexion. Because the epiphyseal plate injury had unfortunately been allowed to heal with this deformity, a corrective osteotomy of the phalanx was required to restore normal function in the child's hand.

Distal Radial Epiphysis

A type II fracture-separation of the distal radial epiphysis is by far the most common epiphyseal plate injury in the body, accounting for approximately half the total. This injury occurs frequently in older children and may be accompanied by a greenstick fracture of the ulna. It is a type II injury, as indicated by the separation of the entire epiphysis with a small triangular-shaped metaphyseal fragment (Fig. 16.26). Because this fracture-separation results from a forced hyperextension and supination injury, it can be reduced by a combination of flexion and pronation. The reduced fracture-separation should be immobilized in an above-elbow cast with the forearm in pronation for a period of 3 weeks (epiphyseal separations heal twice as rapidly as fractures through the cancellous area of the same bone in the same child). Being a type II injury, the prognosis for subsequent growth is excellent.

Distal Third of Radius and Ulna
Incomplete Fractures
In young children the most frequent fracture in this region is the *buckle type* (Fig. 16.27), which requires protection alone for three weeks.

Greenstick fractures of the distal metaphyseal region of the radius and ulna require closed reduction by manipulation if the angulation is significant. The angulation is gradually corrected to the point where the remaining intact part of the cortex is heard and felt to crack through, but not become displaced (Fig. 16.28). Indeed, if this is not done, the angulatory deformity will not be corrected com-

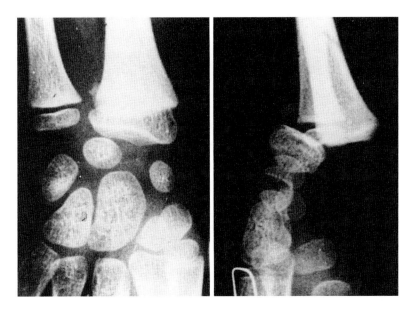

Figure 16.26.   Type II fracture-separation of the distal radial epiphysis. In the anteroposterior projection, the epiphyseal plate of the radius is not apparent because the epiphysis is displaced and angulated. In the lateral projection, the backward displacement and angulation of the epiphysis are apparent. Note the small triangular-shaped metaphyseal fragment that is attached to the epiphysis and its epiphyseal plate.

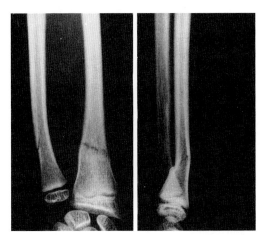

Figure 16.27.   Buckle fracture of the distal metaphysis of the radius and a crack fracture of the ulna in a child. The angulation deformity with buckling or crumpling of the thin dorsal cortex is apparent in the lateral projection. This is sometimes referred to as a "torus" fracture because of the ridge on the cortex (from the Latin, torus: a ridge or protuberance, as seen at the base of a column of a building).

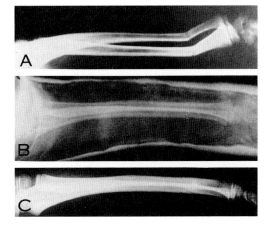

Figure 16.28.   **A.** Greenstick fractures of the distal third of the radius and ulna in a 7-year-old boy with anterior angulation. **B.** Reduced position of the fractures in a plaster cast. The remaining intact portion of the cortex of each bone was deliberately cracked through at the time of reduction. **C.** Six weeks later, both fractures have united in a satisfactory position.

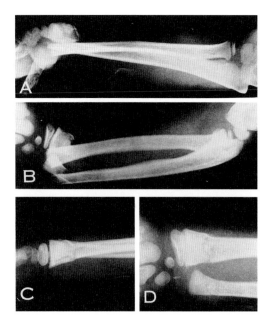

Figure 16.29. Displaced fractures of the distal metaphysis of the radius and ulna with marked overriding. **A and B.** Before reduction. **C and D.** Immediately after closed reduction using the intact periosteal hinge (as depicted in Figs. 15.11 and 15.36).

Middle Third of Radius and Ulna

Greenstick fractures of the middle third of the radius and ulna can be completely reduced by closed manipulation, provided the aforementioned practice of cracking through the remaining intact part of the cortex is used (Fig. 16.30). Indeed, unless the angulatory deformity is well corrected, the normal rotation of the radius around the ulna during supination and pronation will be permanently restricted.

Displaced fractures of the middle third of the radius and ulna are unstable and may be difficult to reduce as well as to keep reduced. Just how much of the fracture deformity is due to angulation and how much to rotation often is better assessed by looking at the child's forearms than by looking at the radiographs.

Both angulation and rotation at the fracture site must be corrected, but side-to-side (bayonet) apposition of both fractures is acceptable. Nevertheless, it is usually possible to obtain end-to-end apposition, first of one

pletely and may even recur during the period of immobilization.

Complete Fractures

Displaced fractures of the distal metaphyseal region of the radius and ulna are particularly common in childhood (Fig. 16.29). They may be difficult to reduce unless the significance of the intact periosteal hinge, as discussed in Chapter 15, is appreciated (Figs. 15.11 and 15.36). When the radius alone is fractured, the injury has been one of supination; consequently the reduction is most stable in pronation. When both the radius and ulna are fractured, the reduction may be more stable with the forearm in the neutral position. In either case a well-molded, above-elbow plaster cast is required for 6 weeks.

Moderate residual angulation, either anterior or posterior, although not desirable, is acceptable since it tends to correct spontaneously to a remarkable degree with subsequent growth, as already mentioned (Fig. 16.3).

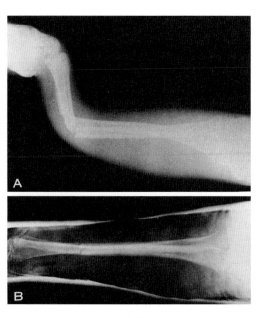

Figure 16.30. Greenstick fractures of the middle third of the radius and ulna of a 14-year-old boy. **A.** Note the gross angulation. **B.** Reduced position of the fractures in a plaster cast. The remaining intact portion of the cortex of each bone was deliberately cracked through at the time of reduction.

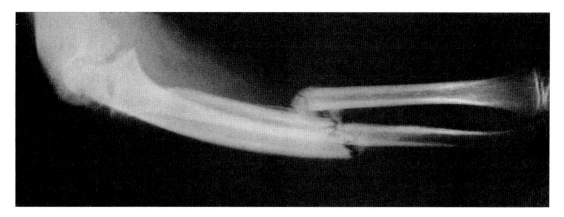

Figure 16.31.   Displaced fractures of the middle third of the radius and ulna of a 15-year-old child. Six weeks after injury, the position of the fragments is obviously unsatisfactory. The ulna is out to length but there is significant overriding of the radial fracture and a rotational deformity at both fractures. At this time (after 6 weeks of healing), the fractures could not be reduced by closed manipulation and consequently open reduction and internal fixation were required. Closed reduction would have been possible at an earlier stage had the loss of position of the fragments been detected by repeated radiographic examinations during the first few weeks.

fracture and then of the other, after which the most stable position of the reductions can be assessed. It is usually, but not invariably, the midposition between supination and pronation. Immobilization in a well-molded, above-elbow cast with the forearm in the most stable position should be maintained for 8 weeks (healing through cortical bone is slower than through cancellous bone).

Unstable fractures of both bones of the forearm should be examined radiographically each week for at least 4 weeks to detect any deterioration in the position of the fragments (Fig. 16.31). If angulation recurs during the period of immobilization, remanipulation is best performed about 2 weeks after the injury, at which time the fracture sites have become "sticky" and the reduction is likely to be more stable. Loss of apposition with resultant overriding should be corrected by remanipulation as soon as it is recognized.

Fractures of both bones of the forearm in children may be difficult to treat and are often not treated well. There is virtually no indication for open reduction of these fractures in young children. Some of the avoidable pitfalls of treatment are depicted as examples (Figs. 16.32 and 16.33).

In older children with unstable fractures of both bones of the forearm, intramedullary flexible nails or Kirschner wires after closed reduction, or if necessary open reduction, are an acceptable alternative to closed reduction.

Proximal Third of Radius and Ulna
Fracture of the shaft of the ulna combined with dislocation of the radiohumeral joint (Monteggia fracture-dislocation) is a serious injury because it is a fracture-dislocation and because the dislocation component of the injury is so frequently unrecognized and consequently remains untreated (Fig. 16.34). Because of the firm attachment of the radius to the ulna through the fibrous interosseous membrane, a fracture of the middle or proximal third of the ulna cannot become angulated unless its attached mate, the radius, either fractures also or dislocates at its proximal end. Thus, as was pointed out in Chapter 15, whenever you see a child with an angulated fracture of the ulna, you should be certain that the radiographic examination includes the full length of the forearm (see Fig. 15.15).

In children, closed reduction of a Monteggia fracture-dislocation can usually be obtained by correcting the angulation of the ulnar fracture, thereby replacing the radial

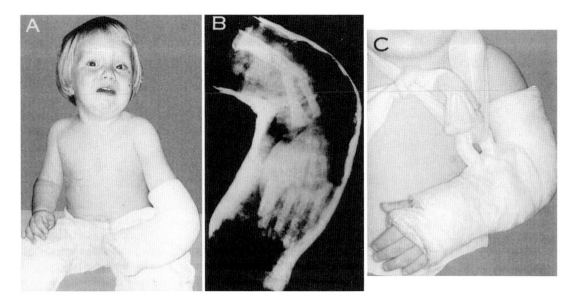

Figure 16.32.   Avoidable pitfall in the treatment of fractures of both bones of the forearm in a child. **A.** This 2-year-old child has reason to cry. The incorrectly applied above-elbow cast for her fractured forearm had been gradually slipping off during the preceding 3 days. Note that the fingers have disappeared into the cast and the elbow of the cast is no longer at the level of the child's elbow. It is on the way to becoming a "shopping bag cast," one which the mother brings back in her shopping bag. **B.** The child's fractures have become angulated because they are now at the level of the elbow of the cast. A second reduction was required. **C.** After the second reduction, a well-molded cast was applied and suspended from the child's neck. These precautions prevent the cast from slipping off.

head in proper relationship with the capitellum (Fig. 16.35). Immobilization of the limb in a cast with the elbow in flexion is necessary for 6 weeks to ensure union of the fracture of the ulna as well as to maintain the reduction of the radial head. Active exercises may be required to help regain elbow motion after removal of the cast.

Neglected residual dislocation of the radiohumeral joint is difficult to treat even a few months after the injury and necessitates an ex-

tensive reconstructive operation (Fig. 16.34). If more than 1 year has elapsed from the time of injury, the dislocation is better left unreduced because elbow stiffness after surgical correction may be more troublesome than the joint instability associated with the residual dislocation.

The Elbow and Arm

Fractures and dislocations of the elbow in children are common injuries. They are also seri-

Figure 16.33.   Avoidable pitfalls in the treatment of unstable fractures of both bones of the forearm in an 8-year-old girl. **A.** Initial radiographs. **B and C.** The position obtained by closed reduction was unsatisfactory. The treating surgeon did not appreciate the rotational deformity at the fracture sites. **D.** The surgeon then performed an open reduction of both fractures but failed to secure the reduction of both fractures by means of internal fixation. **E.** Six weeks after injury the fractures have united with an unacceptable amount of angulation (malunion). The surgeon apparently felt this would correct spontaneously with subsequent growth. **F.** One year later the angulation remains unchanged. In addition to an ugly clinical deformity, there was gross restriction of pronation and supination of the forearm.

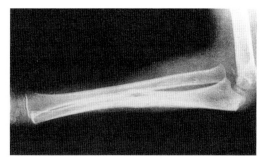

Figure 16.34.   Healed fracture of the shaft of the ulna combined with dislocation of the radial head (Monteggia fracture-dislocation). The radial head should always be opposite the capitellum. The child had been treated for the fractured ulna 3 months previously but the dislocated radial head had not been recognized. Unfortunately, at this stage, reconstructive surgery on the ulna and radiohumeral joint was required.

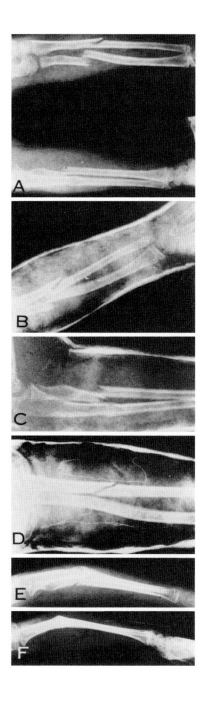

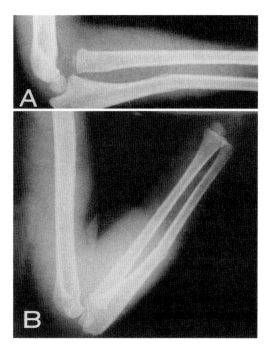

Figure 16.35.   Fresh fracture of the shaft of the ulna combined with dislocation of the radial head. **A.** Before reduction. **B.** After closed reduction of the angulated ulna and the dislocated radial head.

ous because of inherent difficulties in obtaining adequate reduction and the high incidence of complications. In very young children in whom many of the structures of the elbow are still cartilaginous, arthroscopy or MRI may be required to determine the precise diagnosis.

One very common but minor injury, "pulled elbow," also merits discussion in this section.

Pulled Elbow

Children of preschool age are particularly vulnerable to a sudden longitudinal pull or jerk on their arms and frequently sustain the common minor injury well known to family physicians and pediatricians as a "*pulled elbow.*"

Clinical Features

The history is characteristic: a parent, nursemaid, nanny, or older sibling, while lifting the small child up a step by the hand or pulling him or her away from potential danger, exerts a strong pull on the extended elbow. The resulting injury of pulled elbow is sometimes referred to as "nursemaid's elbow"; although the nursemaid may cause the injury, it is the child who suffers it (Fig. 16.36).

The child begins to cry and refuses to use the arm, which he or she protects by holding it with the elbow flexed and the forearm pronated.

Understandably, the parent fears that "something must be broken" and seeks medical attention.

Diagnosis

Physical examination reveals a crying or fretting child but the only significant local finding is painful limitation of forearm supination. Radiographic examination is consistently negative.

Pathological Anatomy

Pulled elbow is essentially a *transient subluxation of the radial head*. For years it was assumed that in children under the age of 5 years, the diameter of the cartilaginous radial head was no larger than that of the radial neck and that in this age group, the radial head could easily be pulled through the annular ligament. This assumption is incorrect. Anatom-

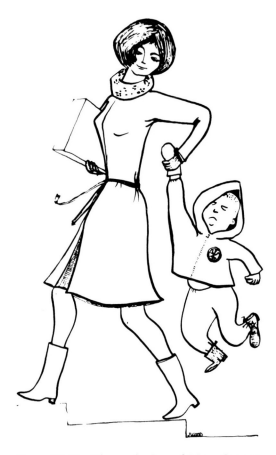

Figure 16.36. The mechanism of injury that produces a pulled elbow in a young child.

ical studies in our postmortem room reveal that in children of all ages, the diameter of the radial head is always larger than that of the neck. In young children, however, the distal attachment of the annular ligament to the radial neck is thin and weak.

In postmortem studies that we have conducted with the elbow joint exposed, we demonstrated that in young children, a sudden pull on the extended elbow while the forearm is pronated produces a tear in the distal attachment of the annular ligament to the radial neck. The radial head penetrates only part way through this tear as it is distracted from the capitellum but then the proximal part of the annular ligament slips into the radiohumeral joint, where it becomes trapped between the joint surfaces when the pull is released (Fig. 16.37). The subluxation, therefore, is tran-

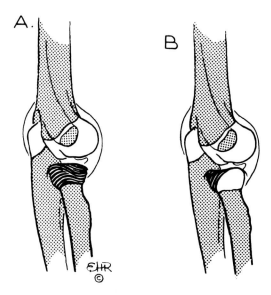

Figure 16.37.   Schematic representation of the pathological anatomy of a pulled elbow. **A.** Normal arrangement of the annular ligament. **B.** In the pulled elbow, there is a tear in the distal attachment of the annular ligament through which the radial head has protruded slightly. The proximal portion of the annular ligament has slipped into the radiohumeral joint where it has become trapped.

sient and this explains the normal radiographic appearance of the elbow. The source of pain is the pinched annular ligament. Postmortem studies also revealed that with the elbow flexed, sudden supination of the forearm frees the incarcerated part of the annular ligament, which then resumes its normal position.

Treatment
On the basis of the foregoing explanation of the pathological anatomy of pulled elbow, its rational treatment simply consists of a deft supination of the child's forearm while the elbow is flexed. A slight "click" can usually be felt over the anterolateral aspect of the radial head as the annular ligament is freed from the joint. Within moments, the child's pain is relieved and normal use of the arm is restored.

If the child has been sent to the radiology department prior to treatment, the radiographic technician frequently, and unwittingly, "treats" the pulled elbow while the forearm is being passively supinated to obtain the anteroposterior projection.

After-treatment consists of a sling for 2 weeks to allow the tear in the distal attachment of the annular ligament to heal. In addition, the parents are advised about the harmful effects of pulling or lifting their small child by the hand.

Proximal Radial Epiphysis
Fracture-separation of the proximal radial epiphysis is produced by a fall that exerts a compression and abduction force on the elbow joint. It is a type II epiphyseal plate injury with a characteristic metaphyseal fragment and the radial head becomes tilted on the neck (Fig. 16.38).

Treatment
Satisfactory closed reduction can usually be obtained by pressing upward and medially on the tilted radial head while an assistant holds the arm with the elbow extended and adducted. If this proves to be impossible, a Kirschner wire can be inserted percutaneously into the displaced radial head and then used as a "joystick" to reduce the fracture-separation. Because of subsequent remodeling, residual angulation of less than 40 degrees is compatible with acceptable function. Occasionally, open reduction is necessary to restore congruity between the joint surface of the radial head and that of the capitellum. Internal fixation is usually not necessary. Even if the radial head has lost all its soft tissue attachments, it should *never* be excised during childhood. Removal of the radial epiphysis also includes its epiphyseal plate from the proximal end of the radius. As you might anticipate, this produces a progressive discrepancy in length between the radius and ulna due to loss of the radial head and to relatively less growth in the radius. Consequently, the hand becomes progressively deviated toward the radial side. After either closed or open reduction, the child's elbow should be immobilized for 3 weeks at a right angle with the forearm supinated, as this is the most stable position.

Complications
Because the blood supply to the intra-articular radial head is precarious, displaced fracture-separations through the epiphyseal plate may

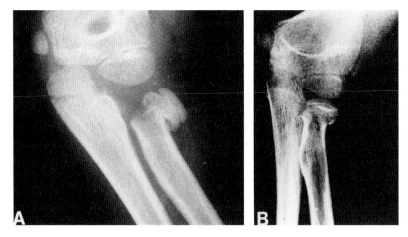

Figure 16.38.   Type II fracture-separation of the proximal radial epiphysis in a child. **A.** Note the valgus deformity of the elbow, the angulation at the fracture site, and the loss of contact of the radiohumeral joint surfaces. **B.** The position of the fragments after closed reduction is satisfactory.

be complicated by avascular necrosis of the epiphysis. The small volume of the radial epiphysis permits fairly rapid revascularization and regeneration. Little deformity of the replaced radial head ensues, but necrosis of the epiphyseal plate results in the aforementioned premature cessation of growth at this site and a length discrepancy between the radius and ulna. Nevertheless, this result is far superior to the results of removing the radial head in children.

Dislocation of the Elbow

Posterior dislocation of the elbow joint occurs relatively frequently in young children as a result of a fall on the hand with the elbow flexed. The distal end of the humerus is driven through the anterior capsule as the radius and ulna dislocate posteriorly (Fig. 16.39).

Treatment

Closed reduction is readily accomplished by reversing the mechanism of injury. Traction is applied to the flexed elbow through the forearm, which is then brought forward. The reduced elbow should be maintained in the stable position of flexion above a right angle in a plaster cast for 2 weeks after which gentle active exercises are begun.

Fracture-dislocations of the elbow are dis-

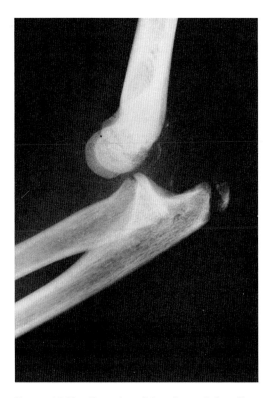

Figure 16.39.   Posterior dislocation of the elbow joint in a child. The apparently separated fragment of bone at the proximal end of the ulna is a traction epiphysis (apophysis) of the olecranon rather than a fracture fragment.

cussed in relation to the specific fractures of the medial epicondyle and lateral condyle of the humerus.

Complications
The complication of *posttraumatic myositis ossificans,* which may develop after dislocation of the elbow, is discussed in Chapter 15 (see Fig. 15.84).

Medial Epicondyle
Avulsion of the medial epicondyle (a traction epiphysis) results from a sudden traction force through the attached medial ligament in association with two types of injuries. In one type, the medial epicondyle is avulsed at the time of a posterior dislocation of the elbow and is carried posteriorly; as the dislocation is reduced, so also is the separation of the medial epicondyle.

More frequently, the injury that avulses the medial epicondyle is severe abduction of the extended elbow with or without a transient lateral dislocation of the joint; the medial epicondyle is carried distally. There is significant local swelling and tenderness. In the absence of a permanent lateral dislocation of the elbow, radiographic examination reveals only moderate separation of the medial epicondyle from the distal end of the humerus (Fig. 16.40). If there is doubt about the diagnosis, comparable radiographic projections of the opposite elbow are helpful.

Treatment
Stability of the elbow joint is the most important aspect of this second type of avulsion injury and should always be assessed under either regional or general anesthesia to determine the optimum form of treatment. If the elbow is stable when subjected to an abduction force, the relatively slight separation of the medial epicondyle requires only immobilization with the elbow in flexion for 3 weeks. Under these circumstances, even if the epicondyle heals by fibrous union, there is no growth disturbance and the long-term result will be satisfactory. If, however, the elbow is grossly unstable when subjected to an abduction force, open reduction and internal fixa-

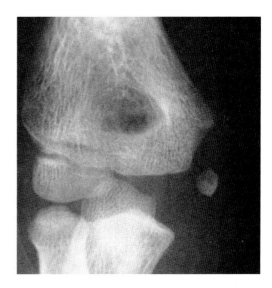

Figure 16.40. Avulsion of the medial epicondyle (a traction epiphysis) from the distal end of the humerus in a 6-year-old child. The medial epicondyle has shifted distally approximately 1 cm to reach the level of the joint line of the elbow.

tion are indicated to restore stability of the joint (Fig. 16.41).

Complications
A traction injury of the ulnar nerve is a frequent complication of the abduction type of avulsion of the medial epicondyle. The prognosis for recovery of the nerve lesion is excellent and the presence of such a lesion in itself is not an indication for open reduction.

Occasionally, at the moment of spontaneous reduction of a lateral dislocation (due to the elastic recoil of the soft tissues), the avulsed medial epicondyle is trapped in the elbow joint. Under these circumstances, the medial epicondyle can sometimes be freed from the joint by closed manipulation, but because open reduction and internal fixation are indicated to restore stability to the elbow, the trapped medial epicondyle is best freed at the time of operation.

Lateral Condyle
Fractures of the lateral condyle of the humerus in children are relatively common, frequently complicated, and regrettably, often inadequately treated. The fracture line begins at the

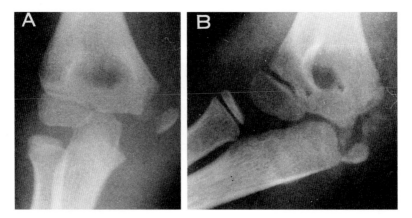

Figure 16.41.   Instability of the right elbow joint of a 7-year-old boy in association with avulsion of the medial epicondyle. **A.** Anteroposterior projection of the elbow showing moderate separation of the medial epicondyle. **B.** This stress radiograph taken with the boy under anesthetic and with an abduction force being applied to the elbow reveals gross instability of the joint. The medial epicondyle has been pulled further distally.

joint surface, passes through the cartilaginous portion of the epiphysis medial to the capitellum, crosses the epiphyseal plate, and extends into the metaphysis. Thus, a fracture of the lateral condyle represents a type IV epiphyseal plate injury, the serious significance of which is discussed in an earlier section of this chapter (Fig. 16.15).

These fractures are inherently unstable because they are predominantly intra-articular. The only periosteal covering is on the metaphyseal fragment and this is frequently completely disrupted. Consequently, even when the fracture appears undisplaced initially, it has a tendency to become displaced subsequently with serious sequelae.

In a less serious variation of a fractured lateral condyle described by Rang, at least part of the articular cartilage remains intact, and this prevents significant lateral displacement of the condyle.

Radiographically, an undisplaced fracture of the lateral condyle may escape detection unless comparable projections of the opposite elbow are obtained (Fig. 16.2). The lateral condyle, which includes the capitellum and the lateral portion of the metaphysis, may be undisplaced, slightly displaced, moderately displaced and angulated, or even completely distracted and rotated (Fig. 16.42). With severe injuries, there even may be an associated

dislocation of the elbow and, hence, a fracture-dislocation.

Treatment
Even undisplaced fractures of the lateral condyle are potentially serious because of their instability. They may be treated initially by immobilization of the arm in a plaster cast with the elbow at a right angle. During the first 2 weeks, repeated radiographic examinations are essential because even during immobilization, the fracture may become displaced in which case immediate open reduction and internal fixation are indicated. A more effective method of treatment is percutaneous pinning of the undisplaced lateral condyle in situ, which prevents subsequent displacement.

Displaced fractures of the lateral condyle represent one of the relatively few absolute indications for open reduction and internal fixation in children. Because these fractures are type IV epiphyseal plate injuries, even a slight displacement must be perfectly reduced and the reduction must be constantly maintained by internal fixation with pins to avoid an otherwise inevitable growth disturbance (Fig. 16.42D). After operation, the arm should be immobilized in a plaster cast with the elbow at a right angle for 3 weeks. The metallic internal fixation (usually Kirschner wires) should then

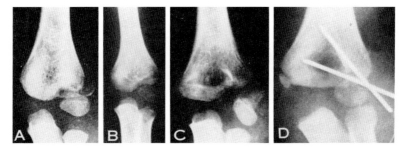

Figure 16.42.   Fractures of the lateral condyle of the humerus in children: a type IV epiphyseal plate injury. **A.** Slightly displaced. **B.** Moderately displaced and angulated. **C.** Completely distracted and rotated. **D.** After open reduction and internal fixation of the fracture with Kirschner wires.

be removed and gentle active exercises should be started.

Complications

If union is delayed because of inadequate fixation, the associated hyperemia may cause an overgrowth on the lateral side of the elbow with resultant cubitus varus (loss of carrying angle) (Fig. 16.43A). Failure to obtain and maintain perfect reduction of a fractured lateral condyle of the humerus leads to a growth disturbance in the central part of the epiphyseal plate (Fig. 16.43B). If the fracture is complicated by avascular necrosis of the capitellum, there is not only a growth disturbance and deformity but also a significant secondary enlargement of the radial head (Fig. 16.44). Inadequate treatment of a fractured lateral condyle may even result in a complete nonunion, one of the few examples of this complication of fractures in childhood (Fig. 16.45). The resultant cubitus valgus (increased carry-

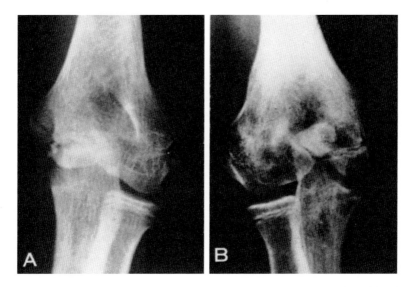

Figure 16.43.   Growth disturbances complicating fractures of the lateral condyle of the humerus. **A.** Cubitus varus 1 year after a fracture of the lateral condyle due to overgrowth of the lateral part of the epiphyseal plate. **B.** Notch in the distal end of the humerus 2 years after a fracture of the lateral condyle (due to premature cessation of local epiphyseal plate growth).

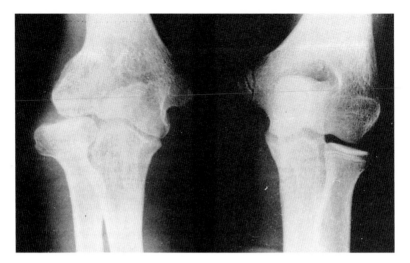

Figure 16.44. The late effects of avascular necrosis of the right capitellum that occurred 5 years previously as a complication of a fracture of the lateral condyle of the humerus. Note the growth disturbance of the distal end of the humerus, the deformity of the capitellum, and the secondary enlargement of the radial head.

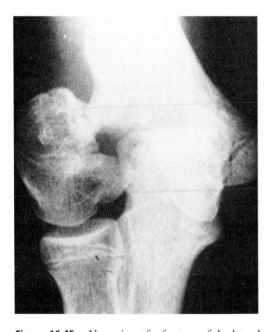

Figure 16.45. Nonunion of a fracture of the lateral condyle in a 12-year-old boy 6 years after an injury that had been thought to be a "sprained elbow." The boy's elbow was deformed and unstable but had a reasonable range of motion. Reconstructive surgery at this stage would be unlikely to improve the unfortunate situation.

ing angle) is complicated further by the gradual development of a tardy ulnar palsy as discussed in Chapter 15 (Fig. 15.85).

Supracondylar Fracture of the Humerus

Of the significant injuries about the elbow, displaced supracondylar fractures of the humerus are the most common and certainly the most serious. They are associated with a high incidence of malunion with residual deformity and, more importantly, with the serious risk of Volkmann's ischemia (compartment syndromes) of nerves and muscles of the forearm with resultant contracture.

The following discussion refers to the extension type of supracondylar fracture, which comprises 99% of the total.

Pathological Anatomy

The flared but flat distal metaphysis of the humerus is indented posteriorly (the olecranon fossa) and also anteriorly (the coronoid fossa), making it a relatively weak site in the upper limb. As a result of either a hyperextension injury or a fall on the hand with the elbow flexed, the forces of injury are transmitted through the elbow joint, which grips the distal end of the humerus like a right-angled mon-

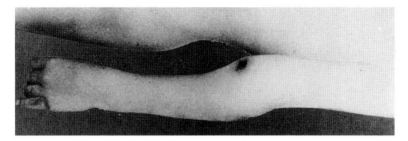

Figure 16.46.   Clinical appearance of a child's arm with an open supracondylar fracture of the humerus. Note the wound in the antecubital fossa (the fracture was open from within), the gross swelling, and the striking anterior angulation deformity just proximal to the elbow joint.

key wrench. Thus, the resultant fracture is consistently immediately proximal to the elbow joint. When the injury is severe, there is considerable "follow-through" of the fragments at the moment of fracture. The jagged end of the proximal fragment is driven through the anterior periosteum and the overlying brachialis muscle into the plane of the brachial artery and median nerve and comes to rest in the subcutaneous fat of the antecubital fossa. It may even penetrate the skin from within, thereby creating an open fracture (Fig. 16.46).

Diagnosis

Clinically there is an obvious deformity in the elbow region that soon becomes grossly swollen and tense as a result of extensive internal hemorrhage (Fig. 16.46). The state of the peripheral circulation and the function of the peripheral nerves should be assessed immediately. Impairment of the circulation demands urgent reduction of the fracture. Radiographic examination provides striking evidence of the displacement of the fragments but little evidence of the severe soft tissue damage (Fig. 16.47). The distal fragment lies posteriorly, and there is an intact posterior hinge of periosteum. In addition, the distal fragment is displaced either medially or laterally, more often the former. When it is displaced medially, there is an intact medial hinge of periosteum, whereas when it is displaced laterally there is an intact lateral hinge. These facts are important in relation to treatment, as you will see.

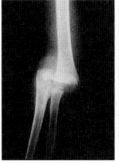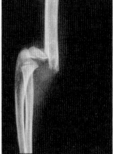

Figure 16.47.   Displaced supracondylar fracture of the left humerus in a 7-year-old boy. **Left.** In the anteroposterior projection, the distal fragment of the humerus is displaced medially and proximally. **Right.** In the lateral projection the distal fragment is displaced posteriorly and proximally. The jagged end of the proximal fragment is lying in the soft tissues of the antecubital fossa.

Treatment

Undisplaced supracondylar fractures require only immobilization of the arm with the elbow flexed for 3 weeks. Most displaced supracondylar fractures of the humerus can be treated by closed reduction, which is made possible by using the intact periosteal hinge. Gentle traction on the forearm (with the elbow slightly flexed to avoid traction on the brachial artery) brings the fragments into general alignment, after which any rotational deformity and any medial or lateral displacement are corrected. At this stage—and not before—the elbow is flexed beyond a right angle. This maneuver tightens the posterior hinge of periosteum and helps to maintain the

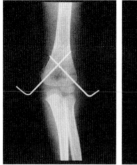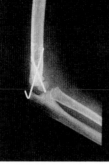

Figure 16.48. After closed reduction of the supracondylar fracture shown in Figure 16.47, the position of the fragments is satisfactory. The reduction is being maintained by percutaneous pinning of the fracture using two crossed Kirschner wires, the bent distal ends of which are left protruding outside the skin.

reduction. If the distal fragment was originally displaced medially, the forearm is then pronated because this tightens the medial hinge and closes the fracture line on the lateral side, preventing any varus deformity at the fracture site. If the distal fragment had been displaced laterally, the forearm is supinated because this tightens the lateral hinge and closes the fracture on the medial side, which prevents any valgus deformity at the fracture site.

After reduction of the fracture, anteroposterior and lateral radiographs (or images provided by an image intensifier) are obtained by rotating the tube of the x-ray machine (rather than by rotating the child's arm) so that the reduction is not lost. At this stage, the reduction is maintained by percutaneous pinning under an image intensifier (Fig. 16.48). This method also avoids the risks to the circulation associated with immobilization of the swollen elbow in acute flexion. The child's upper limb is then immobilized in less than 90 degrees of flexion in a posterior plaster splint (nonencircling) that is held in place by a soft bandage (Fig. 16.49).

Children who require closed reduction of a supracondylar fracture of the humerus should be admitted to the hospital for at least a few days for observation of peripheral circulation in the limb. A well-reduced and pinned fracture is stable and comfortable. Persistent pain may be a warning signal of Volkmann's

ischemia (compartment syndromes) and should not be masked by sedation.

Healing of supracondylar fractures is rapid and the cast should always be removed after only 3 weeks. Immobilization for a longer period is nearly always followed by prolonged elbow joint stiffness even in children because of the extensive soft tissue damage.

After removal in 3 weeks of the posterior plaster splint and the pins, the child's elbow always lacks extension. Active exercises are the only safe way of regaining joint motion and may have to be carried out for several months or even longer before full range of motion is regained. Passive stretching of the joint is decidedly deleterious and should always be avoided.

Supracondylar fractures in which the reduction is grossly unstable as well as those with excessive soft tissue swelling may be

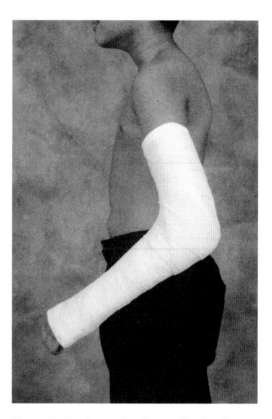

Figure 16.49. A posterior plaster splint that does not encircle the upper limb. This splint, which maintains the patient's elbow at only 70 degrees of flexion, is held in place loosely by a soft encircling bandage.

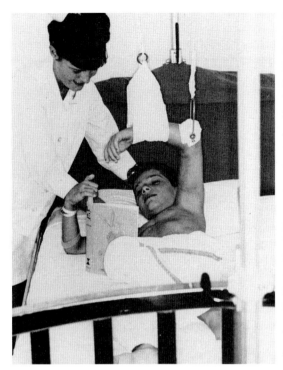

Figure 16.50. Continuous skeletal traction through a pin in the olecranon for a grossly unstable supracondylar fracture of the humerus. The position of the fragments must be monitored every few days by radiographic examination during the first 2 weeks so that the line and amount of traction may be adjusted as necessary to prevent malunion.

treated by continuous skeletal traction through either a transverse pin or a vertical screw in the olecranon (Fig. 16.50). Except in the circumstance of extreme instability of the reduction, this method has been supplanted by percutaneous pinning.

The rare flexion type of supracondylar fracture in which the distal fragment is displaced anteriorly is not serious. It requires only closed reduction and immobilization of the elbow in extension.

Complications

Volkmann's Ischemia (Forearm Compartment Syndrome). The most serious complication of displaced supracondylar fractures of the humerus in children is Volkmann's ischemia of nerves and muscles of the forearm. This is a form of compartment syndrome due to vascular occlusion, either extracompartmental or intracompartmental. The brachial artery may be caught and kinked in the fracture site, a complication that can be relieved only by reduction of the fracture. Moreover, the brachial artery, often contused at the moment of fracture, and with or without an intimal tear, is prone to develop severe arterial spasm, particularly if the subsequent manipulation of the fracture has been forceful, or if there is rapidly progressive swelling within the unyielding fascial compartment of the arm. Excessive flexion of the elbow aggravates the tightness of the deep fascia in the antecubital fossa and may also compress the brachial artery. A tight encircling cast may have the same effect. Consequently, both of these methods of postreduction management should be avoided.

The dread vascular complications including Volkmann's ischemia (compartment syndrome), its recognition and urgent treatment, as well as subsequent Volkmann's contracture, are fully discussed in Chapter 15 under the headings of Vascular Complications (Arterial Division, Spasm, Compression, Thrombosis, Recognition, Compartment Syndrome, Treatment, and Sequelae of Vascular Complications). This should be reviewed in Chapter 15 at this time because it is particularly pertinent to supracondylar fractures of the humerus in children (see Fig. 15.64).

Peripheral Nerve Injury. Although the median nerve and less commonly the radial and ulnar nerve may be injured at the moment of fracture, they are not divided and consequently the prognosis for recovery is excellent (unless one of these nerves is caught in the fracture site).

Malunion. A common complication of displaced supracondylar fractures of the humerus is malunion, particularly residual cubitus varus (Fig. 16.51). Once thought to be the result of an epiphyseal growth disturbance, this unsightly deformity is now known to be the result of fracture healing in an unsatisfactory position (malunion). It can and should be prevented by accurate reduction of the fracture.

Malunion, if sufficiently severe, necessitates a supracondylar osteotomy of the humerus

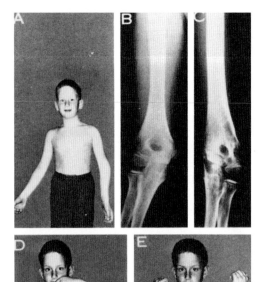

Figure 16.51. Cubitus varus (reversal of the carrying angle) of the left elbow of a 9-year-old boy due to malunion of a supracondylar fracture of the humerus 1 year previously. **A.** Note the unsightly deformity (sometimes referred to as a "gun stock" deformity). **B and C.** Radiographs of this boy's upper limbs. Unfortunately the supracondylar fracture of the left humerus had been allowed to unite in a position of varus. **D.** Because of the altered plane of the elbow joint the boy cannot put the left hand to his mouth without abducting his shoulder. **E.** For the same reason his hand and forearm are deviated laterally when he keeps his elbow to his side (which could create problems for a dinner partner seated on his left side during the soup course). The appearance and function of this boy's arm can be improved by a supracondylar osteotomy of the humerus.

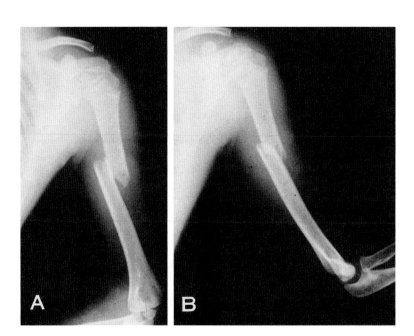

Figure 16.52. Unstable fracture of the midshaft of the left humerus in a 7-year-old boy. Before the radiographic examination, this boy's arm should have been splinted so that it could not be moved through the fracture site. **A.** An anteroposterior projection of both the proximal and the distal fragments. **B.** This is a lateral projection of the distal fragment but an anteroposterior projection of the proximal fragment. Obviously, between the two exposures the child's arm was rotated approximately 90 degrees through the unstable fracture site by the technician. The child would have experienced much pain at that time and might even have sustained further injury to the related soft tissues.

after the child has regained a full range of elbow motion. Because this deformity is not caused by a growth disturbance, its correction does not need to await the end of skeletal growth.

Shaft of the Humerus

Fractures of the humeral shaft are not common in childhood and when they do occur, they are the result of a fairly severe injury. The fracture is usually in the midshaft—less commonly in the proximal metaphysis—and tends to be unstable (Fig. 16.52).

Relatively undisplaced stable fractures of the humeral shaft or proximal metaphysis can be adequately treated by a sling and a thoracobrachial bandage that binds the arm to the chest. Most displaced fractures can be managed by closed reduction followed by a shoulder spica cast for 6 weeks (Fig. 16.53). Significantly unstable fractures, particularly those in older children, may require continuous skeletal traction (as shown in Fig. 16.50) for a few weeks to maintain alignment and correct rotation, after which the fracture is sufficiently sticky that the traction can be replaced by a sugar-tong plaster cast from the axilla, including the flexed elbow in combination with a sling. An above-elbow cast suspended by a loop around the neck (a so-called "hanging cast") is an inefficient method of providing traction during the first few weeks, especially during sleep, and is uncomfortable for a child.

The most common complication of a fracture of the midshaft of the humerus is an associated injury of the radial nerve that winds around the humerus at this level. The prognosis for spontaneous recovery is good.

The Shoulder

Proximal Humeral Epiphysis

The type of injury that in an adult would produce a dislocation of the shoulder produces a type II *fracture-separation of the proximal humeral epiphysis* with a large metaphyseal fragment in a child, because the joint capsule is stronger than the epiphyseal plate (Fig. 16.54).

If the displacement is only slight, reduction is not necessary. Furthermore, only a sling and a

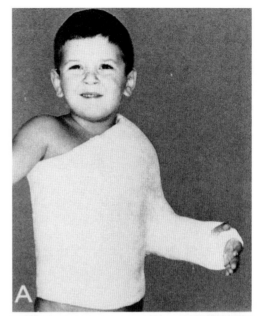

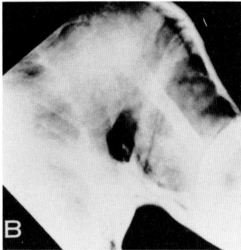

Figure 16.53. **A.** Shoulder spica cast for immobilization of an unstable fracture of the midshaft of the humerus in a 5-year-old boy. **B.** Anteroposterior projection through the cast showing the satisfactory position of the fragments. For older children, a shoulder spica cast has been replaced by a "sugar-tong" plaster splint.

thoracobrachial bandage are used to immobilize the shoulder for 3 weeks.

If the displacement is considerable, closed reduction can be difficult unless the intact periosteal hinge is used. Because there is anterolateral angulation at the fracture site, this necessitates applying traction to the arm while

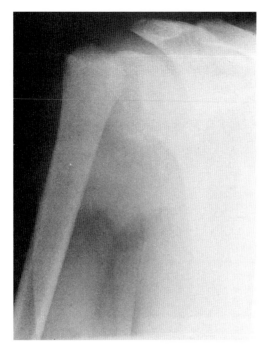

Figure 16.54. Type II fracture-separation of the right humeral epiphysis in a 14-year-old boy. Note the large metaphyseal fragment and the significant displacement of the fracture. The humeral head has retained its normal relationship with the glenoid cavity of the scapula.

it is held directly over the child's head in line with the trunk, a maneuver that pulls the distal fragment into line with the epiphysis. The reduction is frequently most stable in this position, which is known as the Statue of Liberty or "forward (football) pass" position. Rather than immobilize the reduced fracture in this awkward position, the reduction should be maintained by means of percutaneous pinning (Fig. 16.55).

Even with imperfect reduction of the separated epiphysis, union occurs through the intact portion of the periosteal tube. Spontaneous correction of a significant deformity (up to 60 degrees) through remodeling of the proximal end of the humerus usually produces a satisfactory result. There is virtually no indication for open reduction of these type II epiphyseal injuries unless a soft tissue structure such as the long head of the biceps is trapped in the fracture site.

The axillary (circumflex) nerve may be injured with this fracture and because it has not been divided, the prognosis for recovery is excellent.

Clavicle

Fractures of the clavicle are the most common but the least serious of all childhood fractures.

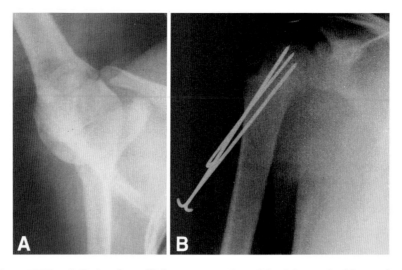

Figure 16.55.   A. Reduced type II fracture-separation of the right proximal humeral epiphysis in the boy whose initial radiograph is shown in Figure 16.54. Note that the arm is in the overhead position and looks "upside down." **B.** The reduction has been maintained by percutaneous pinning.

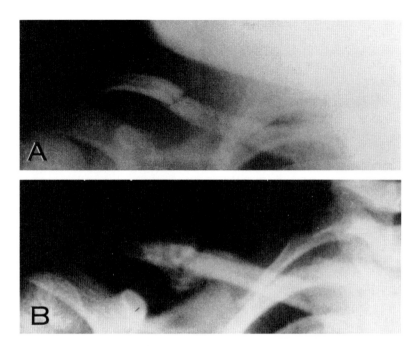

Figure 16.56.   A. Undisplaced fracture of the right clavicle in a 2-year-old boy. **B.** Three weeks after injury, there is abundant callus formation. The fracture callus was both visible and palpable as a lump.

Preschool children tumble almost daily and when they land on their hands, elbows, or shoulders, their slender clavicles are subjected to indirect forces that may produce a fracture. The reason that these fractures are not serious in children is that they virtually all unite rapidly and there are almost no permanent sequelae (Fig. 16.56).

Greenstick fractures of the clavicle require only a sling to provide protection from further injury for 3 weeks. Displaced fractures of the clavicle in young children (under the age of 10 years) usually do not require reduction. They are best treated by means of a snug figure-eight bandage, not so much to hold the fragments in perfect position as to hold them relatively still to make the child more comfortable (Fig. 16.57). The parents are instructed to tighten the bandage each day as it becomes loose from stretching. Within 2 weeks, fracture callus is abundant in young children. The callus is even apparent clinically as a lump, but remodeling of the healed clavicle is remarkably complete within 3 months. The parents and the child need to be reassured about this.

In children older than 10 years of age, fractures of the clavicle are more often displaced. In this age group, an attempt should be made to align the fracture fragments by pulling the shoulders up and back before applying the figure-eight bandage (Fig. 16.58). For older boys, particularly those who are very active, the addition of plaster-of-Paris over the figure-eight bandage provides additional stability of the fracture. Even in older children, the clinical results are consistently good and any residual deformity corrects spontaneously by growth and remodeling during the ensuing year.

There is absolutely no justification for open reduction and internal fixation in closed, uncomplicated fractures of the clavicle in children.

The Spine

The spinal column is much more flexible in children than it is in adults and, therefore, is less susceptible to fractures or dislocations. Indeed, because of this flexibility and the resultant elastic recoil of the soft tissues of the spine,

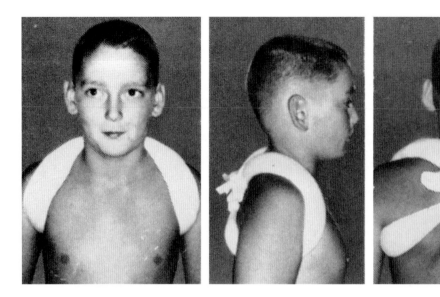

Figure 16.57.   Figure-eight bandage for treatment of a fractured clavicle in a child. The bandage, which consists of stockinette filled with cotton wool, is adjustable so that the parent can tighten it each day.

children may sustain a serious "spinal cord injury without radiographic abnormality," which is referred to by the acronym SCIWORA. With the exception of automobile accidents and falls from considerable heights, injuries to the spine during childhood tend to be less violent than those during adult life.

When a spinal injury is suspected clinically by local tenderness, muscle spasm, and deformity, radiographic examination must be thor-

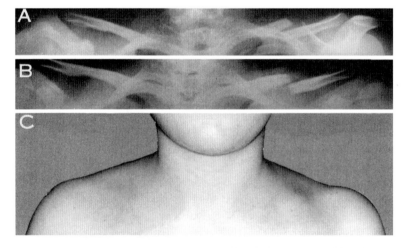

Figure 16.58.   **A.** Displaced fracture of the left clavicle in a 15-year-old girl. Note the overriding of the fracture fragments. **B.** Three weeks after closed reduction and application of a snug figure-eight bandage, the clavicle is almost out to normal length. The side-to-side (bayonet) apposition of the fragments is satisfactory, callus formation is apparent, and at this stage the fracture was clinically united. **C.** The same girl 3 weeks after injury showing a lump over the left clavicle. This became inconspicuous over the ensuing 6 months.

ough: at least four projections are required (anteroposterior, lateral, right and left oblique) and sometimes special projections, CT scans, MRI, or even cineradiography are indicated.

Cervical Spine
Rotatory Subluxation of the Atlantoaxial Joint

Movement at the atlantoaxial joint (C1-2) is principally rotation that allows the head to turn from side to side. If this joint is forced beyond its normal range of rotation by a sudden twisting type of injury, it may become "locked" in a position of *rotatory subluxation,* a phenomenon that is relatively common in childhood. Rotatory subluxation of the atlantoaxial joint is particularly prone to develop in a child who has had a recent throat infection because secondary inflammation in the deep cervical glands may soften the ligaments of the upper cervical spine, rendering the atlantoaxial joint less stable than normal. Under these circumstances, a rotatory subluxation may occur even without injury.

Diagnosis

The child develops an acute and painful wry-neck deformity that persists because of muscle spasm. The uncomfortable child may prefer to support his or her head with the hands or to lie down. The radiographic examination may be difficult to interpret, but a projection taken through the open mouth usually reveals persistent asymmetry at the atlantoaxial joint (Fig. 16.59).

Treatment

Although it is possible to reduce the rotatory subluxation by manipulation of the neck, there is a slight risk of producing further displacement and even spinal cord injury, particularly when the ligaments have been previously softened by inflammation. The safest form of treatment is mild continuous traction through a head halter. Spasm soon subsides as the subluxation is reduced and in a few days, the child's neck can be supported by a cervical "ruff" for a few weeks (Fig. 16.60).

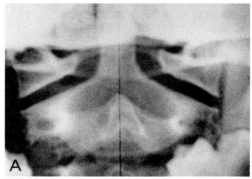
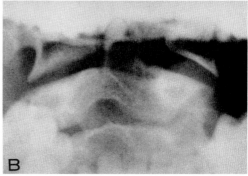

Figure 16.59.   Anteroposterior projections of the atlantoaxial joint taken through the open mouth. **A.** Normal atlantoaxial joint. Note the symmetrical relationship of the lateral masses of the atlas (C1) to the odontoid process as well as to the lateral masses of the axis (C2). **B.** Rotatory subluxation of the atlantoaxial joint. Note the asymmetrical relationship of the lateral masses of the atlas to the odontoid process as well as to the lateral masses of the axis.

Anterior Subluxation of the Atlantoaxial Joint

A severe fall on the top of the head may cause a forward subluxation of the atlas (C-1) on the axis (C-2). Such injuries may be incurred from diving into shallow water, from falls on the head from a considerable height, and from body contact sports.

Because the spinal cord is jeopardized by the injury, reduction of the subluxation and maintenance of the reduction are essential. Reduction is more effectively obtained by continuous traction through a "halo" (as depicted in Chapter 15, Fig. 15.39C) than through a head halter. After reduction, the C1-2 joint should be stabilized by arthrodesis (fusion) to prevent recurrence of the subluxa-

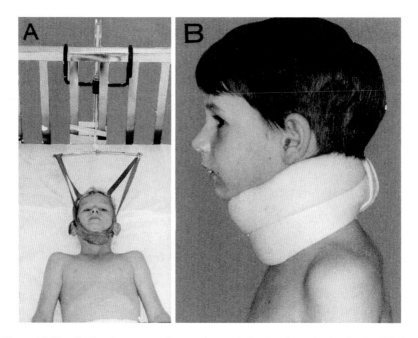

Figure 16.60.   **A.** Continuous traction on the cervical spine through a leather head halter. **B.** A cervical "ruff" made of stockinette filled with cotton wool to provide temporary support for the cervical spine.

tion, or even a dislocation, from a subsequent injury.

Subluxations at Other Levels of the Cervical Spine

After any neck injury in children, cervical radiographs must be interpreted with caution. The increased mobility of the child's cervical spine may produce an appearance of subluxation, particularly between C2 and C3. Nevertheless, true subluxations, or even dislocations, may occur as the result of a severe injury (Fig. 16.61).

Such injuries are best reduced by "halo" traction. The reduction is maintained by means of a "halo vest" or a "halocast" for 8 weeks. If the injured segment is still unstable at the end of this time, local posterior spinal arthrodesis is indicated (Fig. 16.62).

Thoracic Spine

Because fractures of the normal thoracic spine are relatively uncommon in childhood, the presence of such a fracture should always raise the possibility that the fracture is of the pathological type.

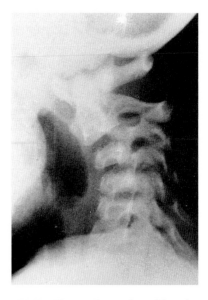

Figure 16.61.   Traumatic anterior subluxation of C2 on C3 in a 5-year-old boy who had fallen on his head during a fight. He had marked muscle spasm in his neck and a tingling sensation (paresthesia) in one arm.

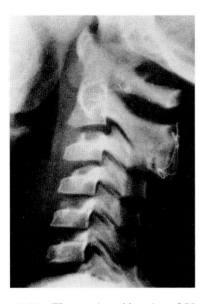

Figure 16.62. The anterior subluxation of C2 on C3 shown in Figure 16.61 had been reduced by halo traction but was still unstable despite 8 weeks immobilization in a halo vest brace. Consequently, a local posterior C2-3 spinal arthrodesis (fusion) was performed to provide permanent stability of the joint.

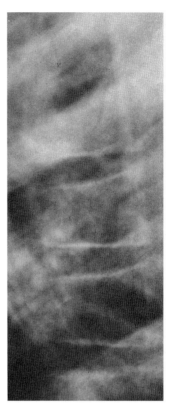

Figure 16.63. Compression fractures of two thoracic vertebrae in a 14-year-old boy who had sustained a severe fall while skiing. Note that the two vertebral bodies have been crushed anteriorly and are somewhat wedge shaped.

A compression fracture of a thoracic vertebral body may result from a severe fall (Fig. 16.63). The posterior longitudinal ligaments of the spine remain intact and there is no injury to the spinal cord. The prognosis is excellent and no attempt at reduction of the slight deformity is necessary. Whereas such an injury in a responsible adult can be treated by protection alone, it is wiser in active, uninhibited children to immobilize the spine in a body cast for 8 weeks (as depicted in Chapter 15, Fig. 15.34A).

Lumbar Spine

In children, the lumbar segments of the spine are particularly mobile. Thus, violent trauma is required to produce either a fracture or a dislocation in this region. Such violent trauma tends to produce a fracture-dislocation of the lumbar spine with resultant injury to the cauda equina (Fig. 16.64).

When a child who is wearing a lap seat belt is involved in a head-on automobile accident, the resultant acute flexion of the lumbar spine can produce a flexion-distraction fracture that shears off a vertebral body end-plate and frac-

tures the pedicles. This is known as a "Chance" fracture. Burst fractures of the lumbar spine occur more often in adults and are described in Chapter 17.

After closed reduction of the displacement of any type of displaced thoracolumbar fracture in a child, immobilization in a body cast for 8 weeks may be sufficient to stabilize the spine, particularly if there has been an associated fracture. If there is any residual instability of the spine at the end of this time, spinal instrumentation and arthrodesis are indicated. An alternative, especially for older children, is spinal instrumentation and arthrodesis within a few days of the injury.

The Foot
Fractures of the Metatarsals
An isolated fracture of a single metatarsal is not common in childhood. More common are

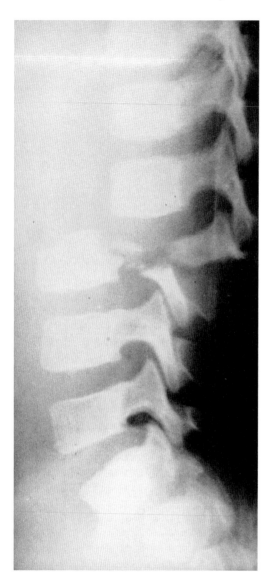

Figure 16.64. Severe fracture-dislocation of the lumbar spine in a child who had been struck by an automobile. The injury was complicated by damage to the cauda equina.

fractures of several metatarsals, usually the result of a crushing injury such as a heavy object dropped on the child's foot. The local arteries and veins are usually injured also. Realignment of the metatarsals by manipulation is important, but even more important is elevation of the foot to minimize soft tissue swelling, which tends to be excessive. Tight encircling bandages (especially those that are elasticized) and casts are contraindicated because of the

associated vascular injury with the risk of ischemia and a resultant compartment syndrome. Furthermore, the child should not be weightbearing for at least 3 weeks, after which a walking cast should be applied and retained for an additional 3 weeks.

Avulsion Fracture of the Base of the Fifth Metatarsal

Occasionally in an older child, a sudden inversion injury of the foot causes an avulsion of the bony insertion of the peroneus brevis tendon into the base of the fifth metatarsal, an insertion that may be into a separate center of ossification. Local tenderness and comparable radiographic projections of the opposite foot are helpful in assessing the injury. A walking cast applied with the foot in a position of eversion provides comfort for the child during the 4 weeks required for healing.

Fracture of the Os Calcis

In children, the cancellous bone of the os calcis is relatively resistant to fracture. Nevertheless, a crush or compression type of fracture may occur when a child falls from a considerable height and lands on his or her heels. Under these circumstances, the child's spine should also be examined both clinically and radiographically because of the likelihood of a coexistent compression fracture of a vertebral body. The precise fracture pattern of the os calcis is best determined by a CT scan.

After a few days of bed rest with the foot elevated, the child may be allowed up on crutches without bearing weight on the injured foot for several weeks. Active exercises during this period help to regain a normal range of motion in the subtalar joint. In older children, as in adults, an intra-articular fracture of the os calcis may require open reduction and internal fixation.

The Ankle and Leg

During childhood, all significant fractures around the ankle involve an epiphyseal plate and should be considered in relation to the particular type of epiphyseal plate injury, as classified and described earlier in this chapter.

Type I Injury of the Distal Fibular Epiphysis

Avulsion of the distal fibular epiphysis may be caused by a sudden inversion injury of the ankle. If the epiphysis returns immediately to its normal position, the child may seem to have merely sprained his or her ankle inasmuch as radiographic examination will be negative. Significant local tenderness at the site of the epiphyseal plate is an indication to obtain stress radiographs, which may reveal evidence of occult joint instability due to separation of the epiphysis as previously described (Fig. 16.9).

Treatment consists of a below-knee walking cast for 3 weeks. The prognosis for subsequent growth is excellent.

Type II Injury of the Distal Tibial Epiphysis

Even severely displaced type II epiphyseal plate injuries around the ankle can be readily reduced by closed means. Furthermore, the reduction can be well maintained, provided there is appropriate molding of the plaster cast (Fig. 16.65). Healing is usually complete within 3 weeks and the prognosis for subsequent growth is excellent.

Type III Injury of the Distal Tibial Epiphysis

In older children who are almost fully grown, a severe ankle injury may fracture the antero-lateral corner of the distal tibial epiphysis—the last part of the epiphysis to become fused to the metaphysis.

This injury is more readily detected in the lateral radiographic projection than in the anteroposterior projection (Fig. 16.66). Because the fracture is intra-articular, open reduction and internal fixation are indicated to obtain perfect restoration of the joint surfaces.

The *triplane fracture* is a variant of a type III epiphyseal plate injury combined with a type II injury. This epiphyseal plate injury, which occurs primarily in the distal tibial epiphysis, is described in an earlier section of this chapter.

Type IV Injury of the Distal Tibial Epiphysis

A severe inversion injury of the ankle may produce a type IV intra-articular fracture through the medial portion of the distal tibial epiphyseal plate. The fracture line, which begins at the ankle joint surface, crosses the epiphyseal plate and extends into the metaphysis. As with

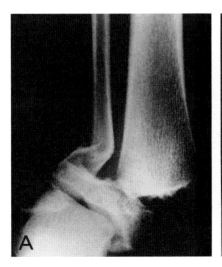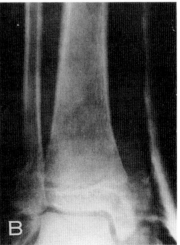

Figure 16.65. **A.** Severely displaced type II fracture-separation of the distal tibial epiphysis combined with a green-stick fracture of the distal third of the fibula in a 13-year-old boy. The intact periosteal hinge is on the lateral aspect of the tibia. **B.** After closed reduction the fragments. are in satisfactory position and the reduction is maintained by a well-molded plaster cast.

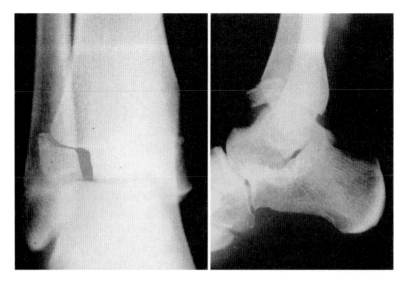

Figure 16.66. Type III injury of the distal tibial epiphysis in a 14-year-old boy. Note that the displacement of the anterolateral corner of the epiphysis is more obvious in the lateral projection than in the anteroposterior projection.

type IV injuries elsewhere, the fracture is unstable.

This treacherous injury requires open reduction and internal fixation to obtain and maintain perfect apposition of the fracture fragments. Even a slight residual disparity at the level of the fractured surfaces of the epiphyseal plate leads inevitably to a serious growth disturbance (Fig. 16.67).

Type V Injury of the Distal Tibial Epiphysis

When a child gets one foot caught, between the pickets of a fence for example, and then falls, the severe angulation of the ankle produces a tremendous compression force on the distal tibial epiphysis and epiphyseal plate. The result may be a type V epiphyseal plate injury.

Despite the paucity of clinical and radiographic evidence of the injury, the prognosis concerning subsequent growth is very poor indeed (Fig. 16.68). When a type V injury is suspected, the child should be kept from bearing weight on the ankle for at least 3 weeks in an attempt to prevent further compression of the epiphyseal plate. Regardless of treatment, subsequent growth disturbance is almost inevitable. As soon as this complication becomes apparent, it should be treated by ex-

cision of the bony bar that crosses the epiphyseal plate (as described in an earlier section of this chapter).

Fracture of the Tibia

The majority of tibial shaft fractures in children are relatively undisplaced and this may be explained in part by the strong periosteal sleeve that is not readily torn across. Consequently, such fractures are relatively stable and can be adequately treated by closed reduction (Fig. 16.69A, B). Widely displaced open fractures of the tibia and fibula can result from major trauma such as an automobile accident (Fig. 16.69C).

Closed reduction of a fractured tibial shaft must correct both angulatory and rotational deformities. The reduction is best maintained by the application of a long-leg cast with the knee flexed to a right angle not only to control rotation but also to prevent the child from bearing weight. After 4 weeks in such a cast, the fracture is usually sufficiently healed that a long-leg walking cast can be applied and retained for an additional 4 weeks. There is virtually no indication for open reduction of an uncomplicated fracture of the tibial shaft in children.

Correction of alignment by closed reduc-

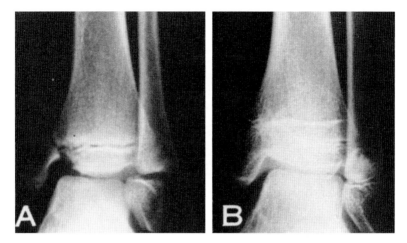

Figure 16.67.   Type IV injury of the distal tibial epiphysis. **A.** Note that the fracture line begins at the joint surface, crosses the epiphyseal plate, and extends into the metaphysis. The entire medial malleolus is shifted medially and proximally. This fracture should have been treated by open reduction and internal fixation. Notice also the type I injury of the distal fibular epiphysis. **B.** One year after injury, a growth disturbance is apparent. The medial part of the distal tibial epiphysis has ceased growing whereas the lateral part has continued to grow. The varus deformity of the ankle will be progressive.

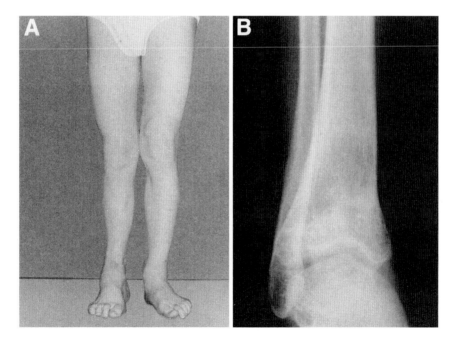

Figure 16.68.   Type V injury of the distal tibial epiphysis. **A.** Clinical varus deformity of the ankle in a 9-year-old boy 5 years after a fall from a considerable height. He landed on his right foot and was thought to have sustained "only a sprained ankle." One year later. he began to develop a progressive deformity of his ankle. Note also the shortening of the right leg. **B.** A radiograph of the ankle reveals a growth disturbance of the distal tibial epiphysis. Growth had ceased in the medial part of the epiphyseal plate due to a type V crushing injury but had continued in the lateral part and also in the fibular epiphysis with a resultant varus deformity and shortening.

tion is particularly important when the fracture is in the proximal metaphysis of the tibia, because neither valgus nor varus deformities can be expected to correct spontaneously with subsequent growth (Fig. 16.70). In this particular site, a flap of interposed pes anserinus and periosteum in the fracture site may prevent accurate reduction, in which case the flap should be surgically released to prevent the combination of malunion and progressive growth disturbance. The child should not be allowed to bear weight on the tibia until the fracture is united. Displaced fractures of the proximal third of the tibia and fibula are potentially serious because of the risk of injury to the anterior and posterior tibial arteries at the upper border of the interosseous membrane and resultant compartment syndromes as previously described in Chapter 15 (Fig. 15.63).

The Knee and Thigh

The most significant injuries about the knee in children involve the epiphyseal plate or the

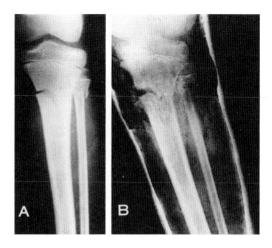

Figure 16.70.   A. Slightly angulated fracture in the metaphyseal region of the upper end of the left tibia of a 9-year-old boy. Even this slight angulation should be corrected by manipulation and no weightbearing should be allowed in the early stages of healing. Regrettably, the boy was treated with a long-leg walking cast. **B.** With weightbearing, the angulation increased over the ensuing 6 weeks. This angulatory deformity cannot be expected to correct spontaneously.

epiphysis of either the proximal tibia or the distal femur.

Avulsion Fracture of the Anterior Tibial Spine

Because the anterior cruciate ligament (ACL) is inserted into the anterior tibial spine, and because in children the ligaments are stronger than the epiphyses, the mechanism of injury that tears the ACL in an adult produces an avulsion fracture of the anterior tibial spine in a child. Being an intra-articular fracture, it is associated with a hemarthrosis. The fracture extends both medially and laterally into the articular cartilage; consequently, the reduction must be complete.

If the avulsed anterior tibial spine is only slightly elevated or if it is elevated anteriorly and hinged posteriorly, it can usually be pushed back into place by extending the knee joint, which should then be immobilized in a cylinder cast in complete extension for 4 weeks. If, however, the anterior tibial spine cannot be reduced by this means, often because of an entrapped meniscus, then either

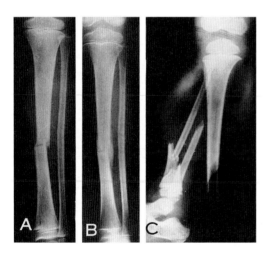

Figure 16.69.   Fractures of the tibial shaft. **A.** A relatively undisplaced and stable fracture of the tibial shaft in a 6-year-old girl. No reduction was required. **B.** Six weeks later, the fracture is clinically united. **C.** Widely displaced open fracture of the tibia and fibula of a 5-year-old boy who was run over by a truck. The skin was split open from the ankle to the knee and there was extensive soft tissue damage. Note the significant overriding and external rotation at the fracture site. After thorough debridement, the fractures were reduced and the soft tissues were repaired. Both bones and soft tissues healed without infection.

open or arthroscopic reduction and internal fixation are indicated.

Type II Injury of the Proximal Tibial Epiphysis

The attachment of the proximal tibial epiphysis to the metaphysis is particularly strong because of its irregular contour. Consequently, a severe injury is required to separate it. A severe hyperextension injury of the knee may produce a type II fracture-separation of the proximal tibial epiphysis that, although not common, is serious because of the risk of injury to the popliteal artery (Fig. 16.71).

Type II Injury of the Distal Femoral Epiphysis

The distal femoral epiphysis is more often separated from its metaphysis than is the proximal tibial epiphysis. A hyperextension injury may produce a type II fracture-separation of the epiphysis: the metaphysis of the femur tears the posterior periosteum and is driven posteriorly into the soft tissues of the popliteal

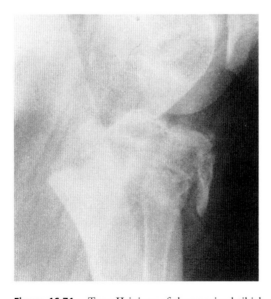

Figure 16.71.   Type II injury of the proximal tibial epiphysis in a 14-year-old boy who was hit on the anterior aspect of the tibia by an automobile. This injury was complicated by severe damage to the popliteal artery, which necessitated local resection of the damaged portion of the artery and replacement by a vein graft.

fossa, where it may injure the popliteal artery and the medial or lateral popliteal nerves.

Clinical examination reveals a grossly swollen knee because of the associated hemarthrosis. Radiographic examination reveals a striking displacement of the epiphysis (Fig. 16.72).

This fracture-separation may be difficult to reduce unless the child is lying face-down. Reduction then becomes comparable to that for a supracondylar fracture of the humerus. Traction is applied to the leg with the knee slightly flexed after which the epiphysis can be pushed into its normal position. The reduction is maintained by the method of percutaneous pinning combined with a long-leg cast with the knee slightly flexed for only 3 weeks, after which active exercises are begun. Because this is a type II injury, the prognosis concerning subsequent growth is excellent, provided it has not been incurred by a high velocity or high force mechanism (such as an automobile accident or a fall from a great height).

Type IV Injury of the Distal Femoral Epiphysis

Fortunately, this serious type of epiphyseal plate injury is uncommon at the knee. Being a type IV fracture that traverses the joint surface as well as the epiphyseal plate, the prognosis concerning subsequent growth is very poor unless the reduction is perfect (Fig. 16.73).

This type of injury is extremely important to recognize because with accurate open reduction and secure internal fixation, the otherwise inevitable growth disturbance can be prevented.

Traumatic Dislocation of the Patella

Older children and adolescents, particularly girls who have some degree of genu valgum and generalized ligamentous laxity, may sustain a lateral dislocation of the patella due to an abduction, external rotation injury to the knee. The patient experiences sharp pain, her knee gives way completely, and she falls.

Diagnosis

Physical examination reveals a grossly swollen knee due to a gross hemarthrosis. The patella can be felt lying on the lateral aspect of the

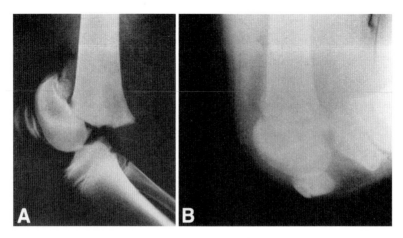

Figure 16.72.   A. Type II injury of the distal femoral epiphysis in a 13-year-old boy as the result of a hyperextension injury of the knee. Note the large triangular-shaped fragment anteriorly, the side of the intact periosteal hinge. **B.** After reduction, the epiphysis is in good position and the reduction is maintained by the flexed position of the knee.

knee. Sometimes the patella has slid back into its normal position spontaneously before the patient is seen. Radiographic examination must include a tangential superoinferior (skyline) projection to detect the presence of an

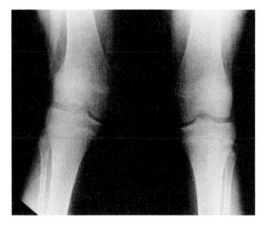

Figure 16.73.   Type IV injury of the right distal femoral epiphysis of a 12-year-old boy 1 year after injury. The fracture began at the joint surface of the lateral femoral condyle, crossed the epiphyseal plate, and extended into the metaphysis. The lateral condyle was displaced proximally and should have been treated by open reduction and internal fixation but unfortunately it was not. One year after injury, growth has ceased in the lateral part of the epiphyseal plate but has continued in the medial part with a resultant progressive valgus deformity.

associated osteochondral fracture of either the medial edge of the patella or the lateral lip of the patellar groove, the site of impact as the patella dislocates laterally.

Treatment
If there is no osteochondral fracture, the dislocated patella should be reduced by closed manipulation with the knee in the extended position. The knee is then immobilized in a cylinder cast (ankle to groin) in extension for a period of 6 weeks. The presence of an osteochondral fracture is an indication for open operation with removal of the fragment and repair of the torn soft tissues. During and after the period of immobilization, quadriceps exercises are important in attempting to prevent recurrence of the dislocation.

Complications
Recurring dislocation of the patella is a troublesome complication of this injury (Fig. 16.74). Moreover, with each dislocation, the articular cartilage of the patella is reinjured and this leads to the development of chondromalacia of the patella and eventually to degenerative joint disease (degenerative arthritis) of the knee. Recurring dislocation of the patella is an indication for a reconstructive operation that involves the release of tight structures on the lateral side of the joint, repair of the fi-

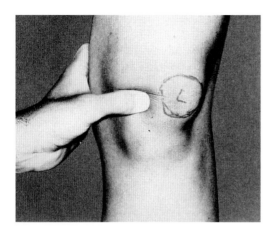

Figure 16.74.   Recurring dislocation of the left patella in a 14-year-old girl who exhibited generalized ligamentous laxity. The patella could almost be dislocated by simply pushing it laterally with the thumb.

mains intact, a point of considerable importance to treatment as well as to healing of the fracture.

Diagnosis
The diagnosis is obvious from clinical examination alone because of the typical deformity (Fig. 16.75). Because these fractures are extremely unstable, it is essential to apply a temporary splint (such as a Thomas splint) before radiographic examination is undertaken to spare the child unnecessary pain and to prevent further injury to the femoral artery.

Treatment
During the past decade, the treatment of fractures of the femoral shaft in children has

brous joint capsule on the medial side, and redirection of the line of pull of the patellar tendon by means of a tenodesis (using the semitendinosus tendon). In a growing child, this type of operation is safer than that in which the tibial tubercle is transplanted because interference with the tibial tubercle (which includes part of the proximal tibial epiphyseal plate) may cause a serious growth disturbance.

Internal Derangements of the Knee
The semilunar cartilages (menisci) of the knee in children are resilient and relatively resistant to disruption. For this reason, torn menisci are uncommon in young children. Nevertheless, they may occur in older children and adolescents as a result of injuries incurred in such sports as skiing, football, and hockey. Meniscal injuries and their treatment are discussed in Chapter 17.

Fractures of the Femoral Shaft
Displaced fractures of the femoral shaft are common in childhood and merit special consideration. Usually involving the middle third of the femur, the fracture may be transverse, oblique, spiral, or even comminuted depending on the mechanism of injury. Even with significant displacement of the fragments, at least part of the strong periosteal sleeve re-

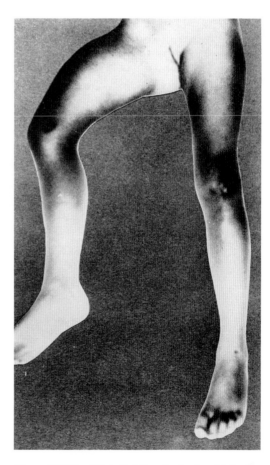

Figure 16.75.   Clinical deformity in the thigh of a child with a displaced fracture of the right femoral shaft. Note the angulation, external rotation, and shortening.

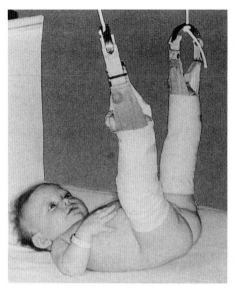
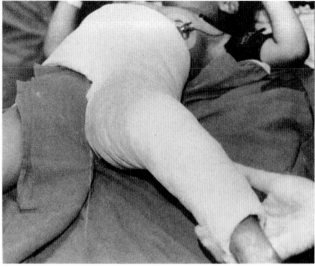

Figure 16.76.   Left. Continuous overhead (Bryant's) skin traction in the treatment of a fracture of the shaft of the left femur in a 6-month-old infant girl. Note that both lower limbs are included in the traction and that the infant's buttocks are just clear of the bed. **Right.** Hip spica cast that has been applied immediately after closed reduction of a fracture of the femoral shaft (under general anesthesia) for a 2-year-old child.

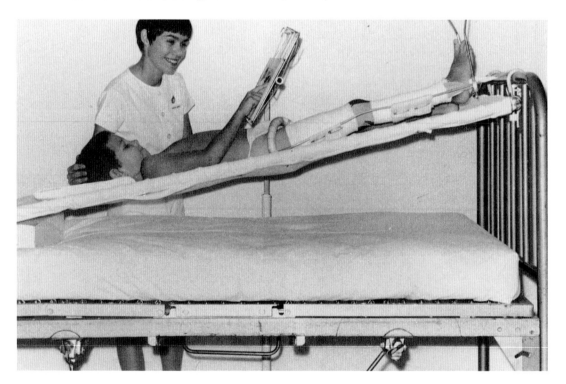

Figure 16.77. Continuous skin traction combined with a Thomas splint slightly bent at the knee for the treatment of an unstable fracture of the midshaft of the right femur in an 8-year-old boy. This type of traction is used only for a few days pending definitive treatment.

changed dramatically, the main reason being the reduction in the number of hospital beds and the need to use methods of treatment that enable the child to be discharged within a few days rather than a few weeks. The former method of traction for several weeks followed by a hip spica cast was both safe and sound, but it had to be replaced for the aforementioned reasons.

Although the details of treatment vary from one center to another, the general consensus, which is based on the age of the child, is as follows:

1. From Birth to 5 Years. Initial skin traction for a few days followed by the application of a carefully molded hip spica cast with the hip and the knee in slight flexion. (Fig. 16.76-Right) For children up to the age of 2 years, temporary overhead (Bryant's) traction is appropriate (Fig. 16.76-Left). For children from 2 to 5 years, the brief period of traction is with the involved limb in a Thomas splint and the child on an inclined frame (Fig. 16.77). The child is then allowed to go home in the hip spica cast. Important contraindications to this early hip spica treatment include initial shortening of more than 3 cm at the fracture site, multiple injuries, and an associated head injury. After the early discharge from hospital, the child should be seen regularly for outpatient radiographic assessment (through the cast) to make certain that the alignment of the fracture fragments is being maintained.

2. From 5 to 10 Years. After a few days in skin traction, the fracture is treated by closed reduction followed either by hip spica treatment or the blind insertion of flexible intramedullary nails (Fig. 16.78). An alternative is external skeletal fixation (Fig. 16.79).

3. Older Than 10 Years. After a brief period in traction, the femoral shaft fracture is treated by the blind insertion of a rigid, locked intramedullary nail. These nails are locked both proximal and distal to the fracture by screws that traverse the bone and pass through transverse holes in the rod, thereby controlling rotation at the fracture site (Fig. 16.80). The advantage of this method, which is also used in adults, is that the patient can begin to bear full weight on the involved limb the next day.

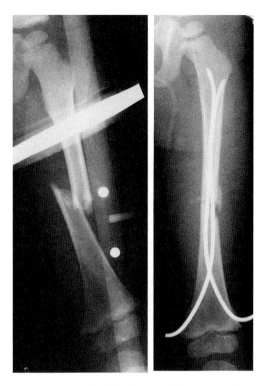

Figure 16.78. Flexible intramedullary nails of the Nancy type as an alternative form of treatment after closed reduction of a fracture of the shaft of the femur in a child from 5–10 years. These nails are inserted blindly from below under image intensification. They prevent redisplacement of the fracture while allowing some motion at the fracture site. This controlled type of motion will stimulate osteogenesis from the periosteum with resultant abundant callus formation.

An alternative method of treatment in this age group is open reduction and internal fixation with a plate and screws.

Temporary Overgrowth of the Fractured Femur

For reasons discussed at the beginning of this chapter, temporary overgrowth always occurs after displaced fractures of the femoral shaft. The average amount of overgrowth is 1 cm and any residual discrepancy in length 1 year after the fracture is permanent (Fig. 16.81). It will be obvious to you, therefore, that the ideal position in which to allow the fragments to unite with nonoperative treatment is side-to-side (bayonet) apposition with approximately 1 cm of overriding. This intentional

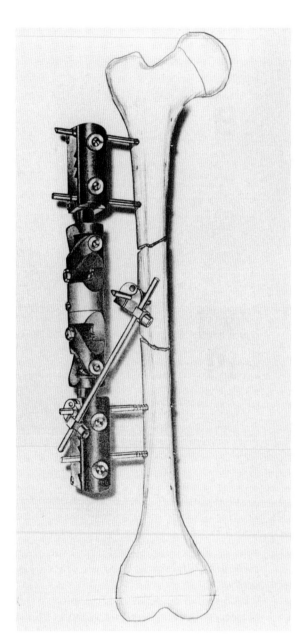

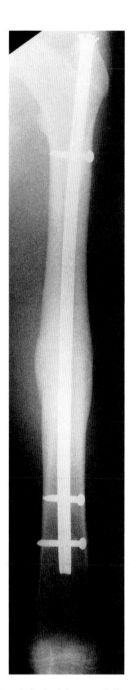

Figure 16.79. External skeletal fixation as an alternative form of treatment after closed reduction of a fracture of the shaft of the femur in a child from 5 to 10 years.

Figure 16.80. A locked intramedullary nail for the treatment after closed reduction of a fracture of the shaft of the femur in a 14-year-old boy. Note that the fracture has healed well with excellent external callus.

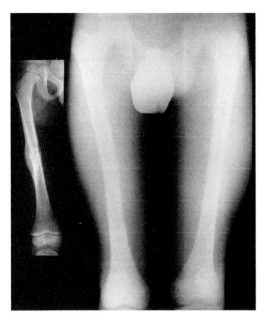

Figure 16.81. Overgrowth of the right femur after a perfectly reduced fracture of the midshaft at age 5 years (*inset*). Eight years later, the right femur is 1.2 cm longer than the left.

shortening is compensated within 1 year by the overgrowth, as discussed in an earlier section of this chapter (Fig. 16.8).

Complications

The most serious complication of femoral shaft fractures in children is Volkmann's ischemia (compartment syndrome) of nerves and muscles due either to femoral arterial spasm or to hemorrhage and edema within a soft tissue compartment. The spasm, which in turn may be secondary to a tear of the intima, is further aggravated by excessive traction on the fractured limb. The clinical manifestations of impending Volkmann's ischemia in the lower limb are the same as those in the upper limb—pain, pallor, puffiness, pulselessness, paresthesia, and paralysis. Children being treated for a fracture of the femoral shaft should not be given analgesics. A well-controlled fracture should not be a source of pain, and if the child has severe and constant pain, especially pain in the calf, the most likely cause is impending ischemia (compartment syndrome). Analgesics may mask this important warning signal and are contraindicated.

The moment impending Volkmann's ischemia is suspected, all encircling bandages should be removed. The skin traction should be replaced by skeletal traction through the distal metaphysis of the femur with the hip and knee flexed. If the peripheral circulation has not been re-established within half an hour, exploration of the artery is indicated, as described in Chapter 15 in relation to Volkmann's ischemia. Associated compartment syndromes must be treated urgently by fasciotomies. The permanent effects of Volkmann's ischemia (compartment syndrome) and subsequent Volkmann's ischemic contracture are tragic (Fig. 16.82).

Fractures of the Subtrochanteric Region of the Femur

When the femoral fracture is just distal to the trochanters, that is, subtrochanteric, the muscles inserted into the proximal fragment, particularly the iliopsoas and the glutei, pull it into a position of acute flexion, external rotation, and abduction (Fig. 16.83). Therefore, to obtain correct alignment of the fracture fragments, the temporary continuous traction must be so arranged as to bring the distal fragment up to and in line with the proximal fragment. This is best accomplished by continuous skeletal traction through the distal metaphysis of the femur with the thigh flexed, externally rotated, and abducted (Figs. 16.84 and 16.85). Most subtrochanteric fractures of the femur, however, occur in children older than age 10. In these older children, the preferred treatment is either blind, locked intramedullary rod or an open reduction with internal fixation with a nail plate (Fig. 16.86).

The Hip and Pelvis

Fractures of the Femoral Neck

The femoral neck in the child, unlike that in the elderly adult, is extremely strong and, consequently, a severe injury is required to fracture it. Fractures of the femoral neck are not common but they are serious. The combination of the severe injury and the precarious blood supply to the femoral head leads, as you might expect, to a high incidence of posttraumatic avascular necrosis. Femoral neck fractures are as highly unstable in children as they

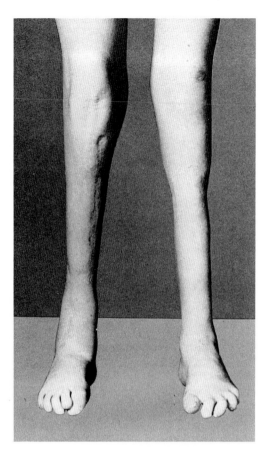

Figure 16.82. Residual Volkmann's ischemic contracture of both lower limbs in a 7-year-old boy who had been treated in overhead (Bryant's) traction for bilateral fractured femora at age 5 years, much beyond the age when overhead traction is safe. During the first 2 days of traction, the boy had complained of severe pain in both legs. The ill-advised use of analgesics relieved the pain somewhat and this masked the relentless development of severe Volkmann's ischemia (compartment syndromes in both lower limbs) until the nerve and muscle damage was irreversible. This is a preventable tragedy!

are in adults and cannot be adequately treated either by closed reduction and external immobilization or by continuous traction.

Treatment

Displaced femoral neck fractures in children represent an absolute indication for closed reduction combined with internal skeletal fixation using percutaneous pinning with threaded pins (Fig. 16.87). Because a child cannot be expected to refrain from

weightbearing during the healing phase of the fracture, it is necessary to supplement the internal fixation with a hip spica until the fracture is clinically united, which usually requires 3 months.

Complications

If internal skeletal fixation has not been used or if it has been inadequate, fractures of the femoral neck in children are likely to be complicated by nonunion and a progressive coxa vara deformity (Fig. 16.88).

When the femoral head has lost its blood supply by disruption of its vessels at the time of a fracture, the result is *posttraumatic avascular necrosis,* a complication that occurs in approximately 30% of children with this in-

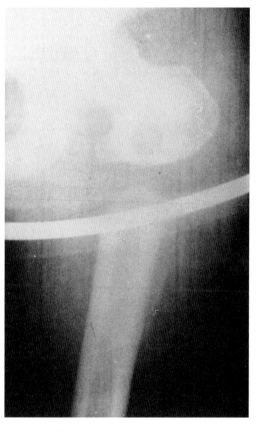

Figure 16.83. Subtrochanteric fracture of the left femur of a 14-year-old girl. Note the ring of the Thomas splint. In this anteroposterior projection, the proximal fragment is flexed to 90 degrees. You are looking into its medullary cavity, which is represented by the round radiolucent area.

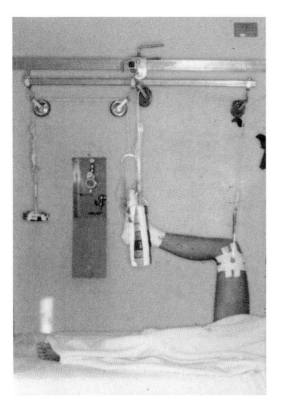

Figure 16.84. Continuous skeletal traction through a pin in the distal metaphysis for treatment of a subtrochanteric fracture of the femur. The distal fragment is brought into line with the flexed proximal fragment.

Type I Injury of the Proximal Femoral Epiphysis

This uncommon but serious injury carries the same risk of avascular necrosis of the femoral head and resultant premature closure of the underlying epiphyseal plate as do fractures of the femoral neck, and for the same reasons (Fig. 16.89). Like the femoral neck fracture, a type I injury of the proximal femoral epiphysis should be treated by internal skeletal fixation, usually with two or more threaded wires.

Traumatic Dislocation of the Hip

The normal hip joint is most vulnerable to dislocation when it is in a position of flexion and

jury. There is little radiographic evidence of this complication until several months have elapsed. The ossific nucleus stops growing for at least 6 months after the injury and at first appears *relatively* radiopaque (relative to the posttraumatic osteoporosis of the living bone in the acetabulum and femoral shaft). Later, when the ossific nucleus is being revascularized and reossified, it appears *absolutely* radiopaque as new bone is laid down on dead trabeculae. Subsequently, the femoral head may become deformed, as described in the section on Legg-Perthes' disease in Chapter 13. The treatment of the complication of posttraumatic avascular necrosis of the femoral head in children is the same as that previously described for Legg-Perthes' disease in Chapter 13.

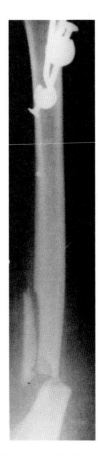

Figure 16.85. Lateral projection of the same fractured femur as shown in Figure 16.83 (*inverted*). Note the metal pin and stirrup in the region of the distal end of the femur. The distal fragment has been brought into line with the flexed proximal fragment. The comminution was not apparent in the anteroposterior projection.

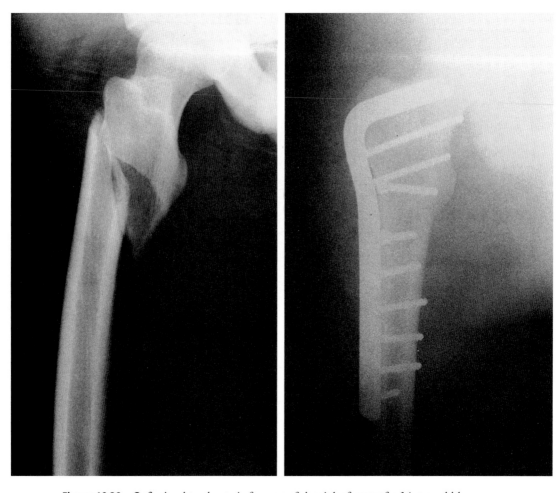

Figure 16.86. **Left.** A subtrochanteric fracture of the right femur of a 14-year-old boy. **Right.** The fracture has been treated by open reduction and internal fixation with a nail plate and screws.

adduction. In this position, a force transmitted along the shaft of the femur (as may occur from a dashboard injury or a fall on the flexed knee) may drive the femoral head posteriorly over the labrum, or lip, of the acetabulum to produce a posterior dislocation. Less force is required to dislocate the hip in a child than in an adult. Because the femoral head escapes through a rent in the capsule, it is an extracapsular type of dislocation (as opposed to congenital dislocation, which is intracapsular).

Diagnosis

The clinical deformity of a posterior dislocation of the hip—flexion, adduction, and inter-

nal rotation—is characteristic (Fig. 16.90). Traumatic anterior dislocation of the hip is rare in childhood but when it does occur, the hip is held in the opposite position—extension, abduction, and external rotation. Posterior dislocation is obvious radiographically (Fig. 16.91).

Treatment

As long as the hip is dislocated, the torn capsule and surrounding structures constrict the femoral neck vessels and jeopardize the blood supply to the femoral head. For this reason, traumatic dislocation of the hip represents an emergency. The dislocation should be re-

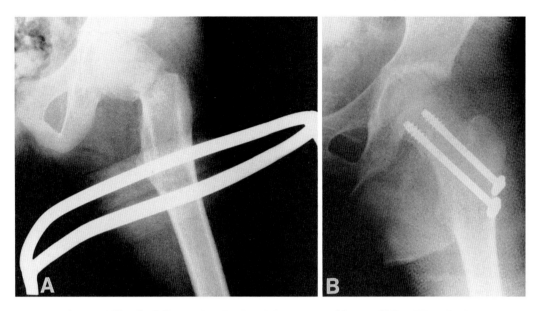

Figure 16.87.   A. A fractured neck of the left femur in a 10-year-old boy. Note the ring of the Thomas splint. **B.** The fracture has been treated by closed reduction and internal fixation with two cannulated threaded screws that have been inserted percutaneously under an image intensifier.

duced as soon as possible to prevent the serious complication of avascular necrosis of the femoral head. Indeed, in children whose hips are reduced within 8 hours from the time of injury, the incidence of avascular necrosis is low, whereas in those whose hips have remained unreduced for longer than 8 hours, the incidence of this complication is high (approximately 40%).

Closed reduction is accomplished by applying upward traction on the flexed thigh and forward pressure on the dislocated femoral head from behind. After reduction, which must be perfect both clinically and radiographically, a hip spica cast is applied with the hip in its most stable position—extension, abduction, and external rotation. Immobilization of the reduced hip is maintained for 6 weeks to allow strong healing of the torn capsule.

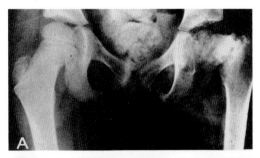

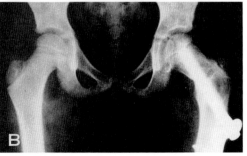

Figure 16.88.   A. Nonunion of a fracture of the left femoral neck in a 9-year-old boy. Note the sclerosis at the fracture site and the coxa vara deformity with resultant shortening of the limb. This fracture should have been treated by internal skeletal fixation. **B.** Correction of the deformity and union of the fracture were obtained by means of an operation that included bone grafting and the use of a nail and plate. The device shown is no longer used. It has been replaced by a dynamic hip screw.

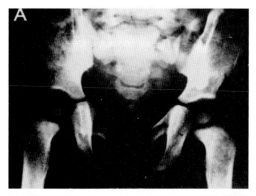

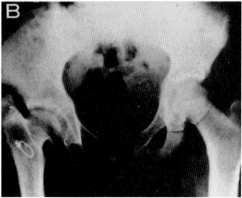

Figure 16.89.   Type I injury of the proximal femoral epiphysis in a 1-year-old child who had been struck by a truck. **A.** Note the obvious fractures of the pelvis. Less obvious is the increased distance between the proximal femoral epiphysis and metaphysis on the right side, indicating a type I epiphyseal separation. **B.** Ten years later there is deformity of the femoral head (coxa plana), noticeable shortening of the femoral neck, and coxa vara, which are the sequelae of avascular necrosis as a complication of the type 1 injury. (The wire loop is at the site of a previous osteotomy of the femur.)

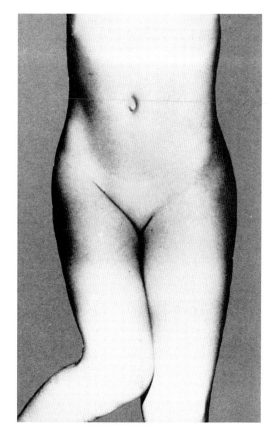

Figure 16.90.   The typical clinical deformity of a child with traumatic posterior dislocation of the right hip—flexion, adduction, internal rotation, and apparent shortening.

Complications

The acetabular margin, being largely cartilaginous in children, is seldom fractured, and the sciatic nerve is seldom injured. The complication of posttraumatic avascular necrosis of the femoral head has been described above in relation to fractures of the femoral neck.

The longer the hip remains dislocated, especially after 8 hours, the higher the incidence of this complication.

Soft tissue interposition of capsule or labrum in the joint prevents perfect reduction. The residual subluxation leads to degenerative

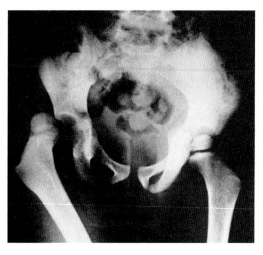

Figure 16.91.   Traumatic posterior dislocation of the right hip suffered by the same patient shown in Figure 16.90.

arthritis; such soft tissue interposition, often best detected by CT, should be removed surgically.

Pelvis

The pelvis of a child is more flexible and more yielding than an adult's because of the cartilaginous components at the sacroiliac joints, triradiate cartilages, and symphysis pubis. Consequently, serious fractures of the pelvis are not common in childhood, but they do occur as the result of a severe injury such as occurs in an automobile accident.

The most important aspects of fractures of the pelvis in children are not the fractures themselves but rather the associated complications—extensive internal hemorrhage from torn vessels and extravasation of urine from rupture of the bladder or urethra.

Diagnosis

Physical examination reveals local swelling and tenderness, and in unstable fractures there may also be deformity of the hips as well as instability of the pelvic ring. Special radiographic projections are required to assess the precise nature of a pelvic fracture because the anteroposterior projection provides only a two-dimensional concept of the injury. The lateral projection, which would normally provide the third dimension, is unsatisfactory because of overlap of the two innominate bones. Thus, to obtain a three-dimensional concept of the disturbed anatomy of the injury, it is necessary to obtain: 1) an anteroposterior projection; 2) a tangential projection in the plane of the pelvic ring (with the tube directed upward 50 degrees); 3) an inlet projection looking down into the pelvic ring with the tube directed downwards 60 degrees. Computed tomography is useful in obtaining a three-dimensional appreciation of the precise sites of the fractures and the position of the fragments in the pelvis, including the acetabulum.

Treatment

The emergency care of a child with a fractured pelvis centers on the two major complications.

The pelvis is a particularly vascular area, and displaced fractures of the pelvis may tear vessels (such as the large superior gluteal artery

in the sciatic notch) with resultant major hemorrhage. A child may lose as much as 60% of circulating blood volume into the peripelvic and retroperitoneal tissues, resulting in severe hemorrhagic shock. The recognition and treatment of shock have been discussed in Chapter 15.

While the child's shock is being treated, a catheter should be inserted into the bladder to investigate the possibility of associated injury to the bladder or urethra. If there is blood in the urethra and a catheter cannot be passed, the urethra is almost certainly torn. Hence a suprapubic cystotomy must be performed pending surgical repair of the urethra. If the catheter can be passed into the bladder and the urine contains blood, a cystogram should be carried out immediately to determine if the bladder has been ruptured, in which case it should be repaired as soon as possible.

Because the bone of the pelvis is principally of the cancellous type, and because its blood supply is abundant, fractures of the pelvis unite rapidly. Treatment of the various types of fractures is aimed at correcting significant fracture deformities to prevent malunion and resultant disturbance of function.

Stable Fractures of the Pelvis

Fractures that do not transgress the pelvic ring do not interfere with stability of the pelvis in relation to weightbearing and do not require reduction.

In children, particularly in athletic boys, a sudden violent pull on the hamstring muscles may avulse their origin, the ischial apophysis. This injury usually heals well but may result in a fibrous union.

Isolated fractures of the ilium are of little significance and require only protection from weightbearing until pain subsides within a few weeks.

A "straddle" injury of the pelvis (which may occur as a child loses his or her footing while walking along the top of a fence) may cause one or more fractures of the inferior pubic rami but, more importantly, is likely to produce a tear of the urethra.

Unstable Fractures of the Pelvis

Complete separation of the symphysis pubis and opening out of the pelvic ring is best re-

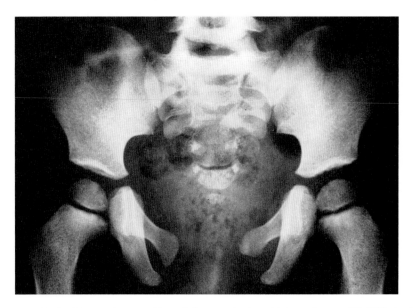

Figure 16.92.   Traumatic separation of the symphysis pubis in a 2-year-old child. Both sacroiliac joints have been spread open also. The separation was reduced by internal rotation of both hips and the reduction was maintained in a hip spica cast.

duced by internally rotating both hips. The reduction is maintained in a well-molded hip spica cast (Fig. 16.92).

Lateral compression of the pelvis may produce a "bucket-handle" fracture in which the fractured half of the pelvis rolls forward and inward (Fig. 16.93). In children, this type of fracture can usually be managed by externally rotating the lower limb, and the reduction can be maintained by the application of a well-molded hip spica cast.

Unstable fractures in which one half of the pelvis is driven proximally by an upward thrust require continuous skeletal traction through the femur to obtain and maintain reduction.

Alternative methods of treatment for complex and markedly unstable fractures of the pelvis as well as those that involve the acetabulum include external skeletal fixation and open reduction and internal fixation with plates.

CHILD ABUSE

Distasteful and difficult to understand as it may be, the tragic truth remains that some infants and small children are, in fact, physically abused within their own homes by a disturbed parent, an older brother or sister, or even a baby sitter. Such child abuse tends to be repeated and often results in multiple musculoskeletal injuries, frequently referred to by the sickening synonym "battered baby syndrome," a repulsive yet realistic term. A more euphemistic synonym is "nonaccidental injury."

Fractures in children under younger than 3 years are not very common, but it has been estimated that at least 25% of fractures in this age group are caused by child abuse.

Diagnosis

The victim of such pathological behavior may not be brought for medical attention immediately. When the child is brought, the history of injury given by the parents is often vague and may even be deliberately misleading. There is usually something mysterious about the mishap in that the severity of the injury or injuries is incompatible with a history of a simple fall and this should arouse your suspicion.

Physical examination may reveal multiple bruises, often in varying stages of resolution, which suggests multiple assaults over time. The child usually has a sad countenance—and for good reason (Fig. 16.94).

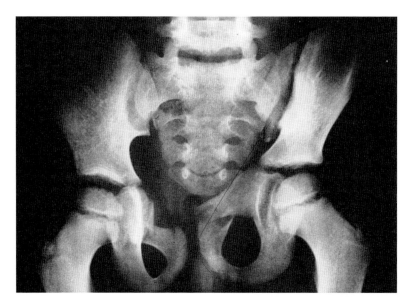

Figure 16.93.   A bucket-handle type of unstable fracture of the pelvis of a 9-year-old boy who was run over by a truck. Note the vertical fracture just lateral to the left sacroiliac joint and the fractures of the superior pubic rami. The left half of this child's pelvis has been displaced forward and inward. The displacement was reduced by external rotation of the left hip and the reduction was maintained in a hip spica cast.

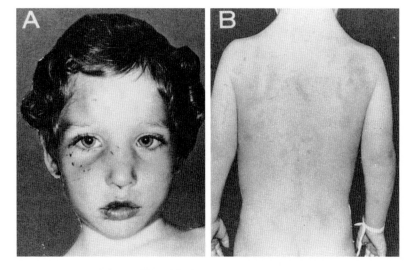

Figure 16.94.   Child abuse. This sad-looking 5-year-old girl was brought to hospital with a history of having "fallen in the garden." Note the bruising and abrasions over the right side of her face. Further examination revealed multiple bruises in various stages of resolution over the girl's trunk and limbs. These physical findings suggest repeated assaults.

Radiographic and scintigraphic (bone scan) examinations under such circumstances need to be extensive and should include the skull, chest, and all four limbs. Skull fractures, multiple rib fractures, "corner" metaphyseal fractures (close to the epiphyseal plate), epiphyseal separations (rarely), and periosteal new bone formation in the limbs are the most characteristic skeletal injuries. These multiple fractures may also be in varying stages of healing, an observation that usually indicates repeated assaults (Fig. 16.95). These musculoskeletal injuries from child abuse are often forerunners of more serious injuries. Magnetic resonance

imaging is useful in the assessment of any associated soft tissue injuries.

Treatment

Infants and children suspected of having been physically abused should be admitted to hospital for complete investigation (as well as photographic documentation). The physician or surgeon who suspects child abuse has a moral, and legal, obligation to report the *suspicion* of such abuse to the local authorities, including a Suspected Child Abuse and Neglect (SCAN) Program and the police, who then proceed with the necessary investigation and action. Records of previous attendance at the hospital should be studied. Indeed, if a central registry of physically abused children is kept in the community, this should also be consulted because the parents may not consistently bring their child to the same hospital, particularly in a large community.

Sadly, if these protective and preventive steps are not taken, a significant percentage of these helpless and hapless little children will eventually succumb to multiple injuries of increasing severity—particularly potentially fatal cerebral injuries—that are wittingly and willfully being inflicted upon them.

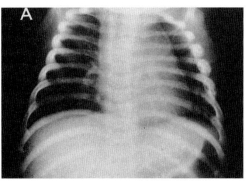

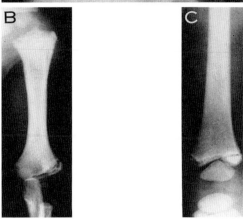

Figure 16.95.   Child abuse. A 1-year-old child suspected of being the victim of child abuse. **A.** Note the multiple rib fractures on the left side of the chest, some of which are fresh and others partially healed. **B.** Note the callus formation in the region of the proximal metaphysis of the humerus as well as the partially healed fracture of the lateral condyle. **C.** A healing metaphyseal fracture close to the epiphyseal plate is apparent in the distal end of the child's femur. These multiple radiographic findings are typical of child abuse.

SUGGESTED ADDITIONAL READING

Akbarnia BA. The role of the orthopaedic surgeon in child abuse. In: Morrissy RT, Weinstein, SL, eds. Lovell and Winter's pediatric orthopaedics. 4th ed. Philadelphia: Lippincott-Raven, 1996.

Aronson DD, Prager BI. Supracondylar fractures of the humerus in children. A modified technique for blind pinning. Clin Orthop 1987;219: 174.

Aronson J, Tursky EA. External fixation of femur fractures in children. J Pediatr Orthop 1992;12: 157–163.

Bailey DA, Wedge JH, McCulloch RG, et al. Epidemiology of fractures of the distal end of the radius in children associated with growth. J Bone Joint Surg 1989;71A:1225–1231.

Baxter MP, Wiley JJ. Fractures of the proximal humeral epiphysis: their influence on humeral growth. J Bone Joint Surg 1986;68B:570.

Beaty JH. Fractures of the proximal humerus and shaft in children In: Eilert RE, ed. Instructional course lectures, vol. 41, American Academy of Orthopaedic Surgeons, pp. 369–372, 1992.

Beaty JH, Austin SM, Warner WC, et al. Interlocking intramedullary nailing of femoral shaft fractures in adolescents. Preliminary results and complications. J Pediatr Orthop 1994;14: 178–183.

Beaty JH, Kasser JR. Fractures about the elbow. In: Instructional course lectures, vol. 44, American Academy of Orthopaedic Surgeons, 1995.

Benson MKD, Fixen JA, MacNicol MF. Children's orthopaedics and fractures. Edinburgh: Churchill Livingstone, 1994.

Bernstein SM, McKeever P, Berstein L. Percutaneous reduction of displaced radial neck fractures in children. J Pediatr Orthop 1993;13:85–88.

Best TN. Management of old unreduced Monteggia fracture dislocations of the elbow in children. J Pediatr Orthop 1994;4:193–199.

Blount W. Fractures in children. Baltimore: Williams & Wilkins, 1955.

Broughton NS, ed. A textbook of pediatric orthopaedics. Philadelphia: WB Saunders, 1997.

Buchler KC, Thompson JD, Sponseller PD, et al. A prospective study of early spica casting outcomes in the treatment of femoral shaft fractures in children. J Pediatr Orthop 1995;15:30–35.

Canale ST, Tolo VT. Fractures of the femur in children. J Bone Joint Surg 1995;77A:294–315.

Carty HML. Fractures caused by child abuse. J Bone Joint Surg 1993;75B:849–857.

Chip Routt ML, Jr. Fractures of the femoral shaft. In: Green NE, Swiontkowski MF, eds. Skeletal trauma in children. Philadelphia: WB Saunders, 1994;3:345–365.

Christodoulou AG, Colton CL. Scaphoid fractures in children. J Pediatr Orthop 1986;6:37–39.

Clement DA. Assessment of a treatment plan for managing acute vascular complications associated with supracondylar fractures of the humerus in children. J Pediatr Orthop 1990;10:97–100.

Cooperman DR, Spiegel PG, Laros GS. Tibial fractures involving the ankle, the so-called triplane epiphyseal fracture. J Bone Joint Surg 1978; 60A:1040.

Cramer KE. The pediatric polytrauma patient. Clin Orthop 1995;318:125–135.

Crawford AH. Operative treatment of spine fractures in children. Orthop Clin North Am 1990; 21:325–339.

Czitrom AA, Salter RB, Willis RB. Fractures involving the distal femoral epiphyseal plate. International Orthop 1981;4:269.

Davison BL, Weinstein SL. Hip fractures in children: a long-term follow-up study. J Pediatr Orthop 1992;12:355–358.

Devito DP. Management of fractures and their complications. In: Morrissy RT, Weinstein SL, eds. Lovell and Winter's pediatric orthopaedics. 4th ed. Philadelphia: Lippincott-Raven, 1996;2: 1229–1334.

Dickman CA, Zambranski JM, Hadley MN, et al. Pediatric spinal cord injury without radiographic abnormalities (SCIWORA): report of 26 cases and review of the literature. J Spinal Disord 1991;4:296–305.

Dormans JP, Azzoni M, Davidson RS, et al. Major lower extremity lawn mower injuries in children. J Pediatr Orthop 1995;15:78–82.

Ertl JP, Barrack RL, Alexander AH, et al. Triplane fracture of the distal tibial epiphysis. Long-term follow-up. J Bone Joint Surg 1988;70A: 967–976.

Feldman DS, Otsuka NY, Hedden DM. Extra-articular triplane fracture of the distal tibial epiphysis. J Pediatr Orthop 1995;15:479–481.

Fowles JV, Kassab MT. Observations concerning radial neck fractures in children. J Pediatr Orthop 1986;6:51–57.

Garbuz DS, Lietch K, Wright JG. The treatment of supracondylar fractures in children with an absent radial pulse. J Pediatric Orthop 1996;16: 594–596.

Garvin KL, McCarthy RE, Barnes CL, et al. Pediatric pelvic fractures. J Pediatr Orthop 1990;10: 577–582.

Glasgow JFT, Graham HK. Management of injuries in children. London: BMJ Publishing Group, 1997.

Green NE. Child abuse. In: Green NE, Swiontkowski, MF, eds. Skeletal trauma in children. Volume 3. Philadelphia: WB Saunders, 1994.

Green NE, Swiontkowski MF. Skeletal trauma in children. 2nd ed. Volume 3. Philadelphia: WB Saunders, 1998.

Gustilo RB, Merkow RL, Templeman D. Current concepts review: the management of open fractures. J Bone Joint Surg 1990;72A:299.

Hansen ST Jr. Internal fixation of children's fractures of the lower extremity. Orthop Clin North Am 1990;21:353.

Hope PG, Cole WG. Open fractures of the tibia in children. J Bone Joint Surg 1992;74B: 546–553.

Hughes LO, Beaty JH. Fractures of the head and neck of the femur in children. J Bone Joint Surg 1994;76A:283–291.

Hynes D, O'Brien T. Growth disturbance lines after injury of the distal tibial physis: their significance in prognosis. J Bone Joint Surg 1988; 70B:23.

Jakob R, Foules JV, Rang M, et al. Observation concerning fractures of the lateral humeral condyle in children. J Bone Joint Surg 1975;57B: 430–436.

Kallio PE, Foster BK, Paterson DC. Difficult supracondylar fractures in children: analysis of percutaneous pinning technique. J Pediatr Orthop 1992;12:11–15.

Kasser JR. Forearm fractures. In: Eilert RE, ed. Instructional course lectures, vol. 41, American Academy of Orthopaedic Surgeons, pp. 391–396, 1992.

Kreder HJ, Armstrong P. A review of open tibia fractures in children. J Pediatr Orthop 1995; 15:482–488.

Langenskiold A, Videman T, Nevalainen T. The

fate of fat transplants in operations for partial closure of the growth plate: clinical examples and an experimental study. J Bone Joint Surg 1986;68B:234.

Letts M, ed. Management of pediatric fractures. Edinburgh: Churchill Livingstone, 1994.

Letts M, Locht R, Weins J. Monteggia fracture—dislocations of the elbow in children. J Pediatr Orthop 1994;14:193–199.

Leventhal JM, Thomas SA, Rosenfield NS, et al. Fractures in young children. Distinguishing child abuse from unintentional injuries. American Journal of Diseases of Children 1993;147:87–92.

Loder RT, Bookout C. Fracture patterns in battered children. J Orthop Trauma 19981;5:428–433.

MacEwen GD, Kasser JR, Heinrich SD. Pediatric fractures. A practical approach to assessment and treatment. Baltimore: Williams & Wilkins, 1993.

Mehserle WL, Meehan PL. Treatment of the displaced supracondylar fracture of the humerus with closed reduction and percutaneous pinning. J Pediatr Orthop 1992;12:11–15.

Mubarak SJ, Owens CA, Hargens AR. Acute compartment syndromes. Diagnosis and treatment with the aid of the Wick catheter. J Bone Joint Surg 1978;60A:1091.

Ogden JA. Skeletal injury in the child. 2nd ed. Philadelphia: WB Saunders, 1990.

Peterson HA. Partial growth plate arrest. In: Morrissy RT, ed. Lovell and Winter's pediatric orthopaedics. 3rd ed. Philadelphia: JB Lippincott, 1990.

Pirone AM, Graham HK, Krajbich JI. Management of displaced extension type supracondylar fractures of the humerus in children. J Bone Joint Surg 1988;70A:641–650.

Rang M. Children's fractures. 2nd ed. Philadelphia: JB Lippincott, 1983.

Rockwood CA, Wilkins K, Beaty JH, eds. The textbook: fractures in children, 4th ed. Philadelphia: Lippincott-Raven, 1996.

Rooker G, Salter RB. Prevention of valgus deformity following fracture of the proximal metaphysis of the tibia in children. J Bone Joint Surg 1980;62B:527.

Rorabeck CH. A practical approach to compartment syndromes. Part III, Treatment, Instructional course lectures, vol. 32, Chicago: American Academy of Orthopaedic Surgeons, p 102, 1983.

Rumball K, Jarvis J. Seat-belt injuries of the spine in young children. J Bone Joint Surg 1992;74B:571–574.

Salter RB. Epiphyseal plate injuries. In: Letts M, ed. Management of pediatric fractures. New York: Churchill Livingstone, 1994:11–26.

Salter RB, Best TN. The pathogenesis and prevention of valgus deformity following fractures of the proximal metaphyseal region of the tibia in children. In: Uhthoff HK, Wiley JJ, eds. Behaviour of the growth plate. New York: Raven Press, 1988:289–293.

Salter RB, Harris WR. Injuries involving the epiphyseal plate. J Bone Joint Surg 1963;45A:587–622.

Salter RB, Zaltz C. Anatomic investigations of the mechanism of injury and pathological anatomy of "pulled elbow" in young children. Clin Orthop 1971;77:134–143.

Shapiro F. Fractures of the femoral shaft in children. The overgrowth phenomenon. Acta Orthop Scand 1981;52:649–655.

Shaw BA, Kasser JR, Emans JB, et al. Management of vascular injuries in displaced supracondylar humerus fractures without arteriography. J Orthop Trauma 1990;4:25–29.

Shuler TE. Trauma—section 2. Pediatric trauma. In: Miller MD, ed. Review of orthopaedics. 2nd ed. Philadelphia: WB Saunders, 1996:394–420.

Sponseller PD, ed. Section IV, Trauma. Orthopaedic knowledge update. Pediatrics. In: Richards BS, ed. Pediatric orthopaedic society of North America. Rosemont: American Academy of Orthopaedic Surgeons, 1996.

Staheli LT. Fundamentals of pediatric orthopaedics. New York: Raven Press, 1992.

Tolo VT. External skeletal fixation in children's fractures. J Pediatr Orthop 1983;3:435.

Walker JL, Rang M. Forearm fractures in children: cast treatment with the elbow extended. J Bone Joint Surg 1991;73B:299–301.

Wilber JH, Thompson GH. The multiply injured child. In: Green NE, Swiontkowski MF, eds. Skeletal trauma in children, vol. 3. Philadelphia: WB Saunders, 1994.

Wiley JJ, Baxter MP. Tibial spine fractures in children. Clin Orthop 1990;255:54–60.

Woods GM, Tullos HG. Elbow instability and medial epicondyle fracture. Am J Sports Med 1977;5:23–30.

17 Specific Fractures and Joint Injuries in Adults

Your knowledge and understanding of the *general features* of fractures, dislocations, and soft tissue injuries gained from Chapter 15—combined with your own good sense—will enable you to deduce and anticipate the appropriate methods of treatment for *specific injuries* in adults. You may wish to review Chapter 15 before learning about specific fractures and joint injuries in adults in the present chapter.

From Chapter 16, you will have learned about the special features of fractures and dislocations in children as compared to adults. The differences between fractures in children and adults are sufficiently important to your understanding of fracture treatment to merit further emphasis.

SPECIAL FEATURES OF FRACTURES AND DISLOCATIONS IN ADULTS

The special features of fractures and dislocations in adults are first listed and then discussed individually. These features are relatively constant in both young and middle-aged adults. Special problems associated with fractures in the elderly are discussed in a separate section at the end of this chapter.

In the present section, terms such as "more" and "less" refer to a comparison between fractures and dislocations in adults and in children. The following features pertain to adults.

1. Fractures less common but more serious.
2. Weaker and less active periosteum.
3. Less rapid fracture healing.
4. Fewer problems of diagnosis.
5. No spontaneous correction of residual fracture deformities.
6. Differences in complications.
7. Different emphasis on methods of treatment.

8. Torn ligaments and dislocations more common.
9. Better tolerance of major blood loss.

1. Fractures Less Common But More Serious

Buckle fractures and greenstick fractures—so common in children—do not occur in adults, and crack or hairline fractures are relatively uncommon. More force is required to break a bone in the adult. Consequently, when a fracture does occur, it tends to be significantly displaced and to be associated with extensive soft tissue injury. It is also more likely to be complicated. Added to these features are the slower rate of fracture healing and the greater socioeconomic loss due to time away from work and other responsibilities of adulthood.

2. Weaker and Less Active Periosteum

In adults the periosteum is relatively thin and weak. Consequently, it is readily torn across at the time of fracture, often with no intact periosteal hinge left that can be used during closed reduction of the fracture. This is particularly true in sites where the bone lies subcutaneously (such as the shafts of the ulna and tibia) or where a portion of the bone (such as the neck of the femur) lies within a synovial joint. The periosteum is much less osteogenic in adults than in children, an important biological factor that accounts largely for the less rapid fracture healing in adults.

3. Less Rapid Fracture Healing

Throughout adult life, the rate of normal fracture healing in a given bone is relatively constant, but always considerably slower than during childhood. Fractures of the shaft of the femur serve as an example. A femoral shaft fracture occurring at birth will be united in 3 weeks. A comparable fracture at the age of 8 years will be united in 8 weeks. At the age of 12 years it will be united in 12 weeks. From the age of 20 years to old age, it will be united in approximately 20 weeks.

Related to the slower rate of union of fractures in adults is the higher incidence of delayed union and nonunion. Thus, fracture healing is not only slower in adults than in children; it is also less certain.

4. Fewer Problems of Diagnosis

Because in adults there are no separate centers of ossification and all epiphyseal plates have closed, there are fewer problems of radiographic diagnosis of fractures than in children. Nevertheless, at least two radiographic projections at right angles to each other are just as important in the diagnosis of fractures in adults as in children.

5. No Spontaneous Correction of Residual Fracture Deformities

In adults, unlike in children, the deformity of a malunited fracture is permanent because residual angulation, shortening, or rotation at the site of a healed fracture cannot correct spontaneously. The process of remodeling in the shaft of a long bone can still occur in the adult, albeit more slowly and less completely than in the child. The sharp corners of an incompletely reduced shaft fracture gradually become smooth through the process of remodeling, an example of Wolff's law. Nevertheless, residual angulation, shortening, and rotation persist. In adults, these deformities must be adequately corrected during the initial treatment of the fracture.

6. Differences in Complications

Most of the complications discussed in Chapter 15 can develop in both children and adults but certain differences merit consideration. Open fractures are more common in adults, as are major arterial injuries, gangrene, venous thrombosis, pulmonary embolism, fat embolism, pneumonia, and renal calculi. Delirium tremens and accident neurosis are virtually confined to adult life. Persistent joint stiffness after fracture is a more common complication in adults than in children, and its prevention requires vigorous measures throughout the period of fracture treatment and aftercare. [We are currently conducting prospective investigations concerning the clinical application of the biological concept of continuous passive motion (CPM) to the care of patients immediately after open reduction and internal fixation of intra-articular fractures and ligament reconstruction.] As mentioned above, delayed union and nonunion are also more common in adults than in children. The complication of growth disturbance, of course, does not occur during adult life.

7. Different Emphasis on Methods of Treatment

Although the *principles* of fracture treatment described in Chapter 15 are equally applicable to children and adults, there is a different emphasis on the *methods* of treatment in the two age groups. Adults tend to be more cooperative during treatment, and consequently, their undisplaced and impacted fractures can be more reasonably treated by protection alone. Such is not the case in children. On the other hand, displaced and unstable fractures (particularly of the forearm bones and femur) in adults frequently require open reduction and internal fixation, whereas such long bone fractures in young children can be treated by closed means. In an elderly person who has sustained a severely displaced fracture of the neck of the femur with disruption of blood supply to the femoral head, the most reasonable initial method of treatment may be excision of the femoral head and neck fragment and replacement by an endoprosthesis. This method, of course, would not be indicated for any type of fracture in a child.

In recent decades, there has been growing use of three specific methods of fracture treatment in adults: functional fracture-bracing, external skeletal fixation, and the AO/ASIF, or AO, system of rigid internal fixation. Before proceeding further in this chapter, you may wish to review the discussions of these three methods in Chapter 15.

8. Torn Ligaments and Dislocations More Common

Ligaments and fibrous joint capsules are less resilient in adults than in children. Consequently, they are more often either completely torn across or avulsed with a small fragment of attached bone. Moreover, the type of injury that produces a separation of an epiphysis through its epiphyseal plate in a child is likely to produce a dislocation, or even a fracture-dislocation, in an adult. These observations account for the increased incidence of major ligamentous tears and dislocations in adults.

9. Better Tolerance of Major Blood Loss

Hemorrhage, either external or internal, of 500 ml in a child who weighs 20 kg (44 lb) represents 33% of the total blood volume, whereas a similar hemorrhage in an average adult would represent only 10% of the total blood volume. It must be remembered, though, that the elderly do not tolerate major blood loss as well as young and middle-aged adults.

SPECIFIC FRACTURES AND DISLOCATIONS

The Hand

General Features

Fractures and dislocations in the adult hand are both common and potentially serious. Such injuries are often considered to be minor and consequently are treated with indifference. These important injuries should always be treated with deference rather than with indifference to prevent permanent disability.

Hand function is closely related to anatomical form, especially in the fingers and thumb. Because of the close relationship of gliding tendons to bones, fractures involving the phalanges in particular must be accurately reduced. There is only a small margin of tolerable imperfection in the treatment of hand injuries.

The injured hand is prone to become grossly swollen and, because the damaging effects of persistent edema are particularly disabling in the fingers and thumb, the injured hand must always be kept elevated to prevent

this complication. Fractured digits should be immobilized for as short a time as possible, almost never more than 3 weeks, lest adhesions produce a permanent loss of joint motion. In general, fingers should be immobilized in the flexed position of function and *never* in an extended position, as on a straight splint. After the period of immobilization, the patient should actively exercise the fingers, if necessary under supervision of a physical therapist or an occupational therapist. Fingers should *never* be forcibly manipulated, because manipulation of such small joints usually produces an excessive reaction and leads to permanent stiffness of the injured finger.

Phalanges
Distal Phalanx

Crush injuries of the distal phalanx are common, particularly in industry. They are also frequently caused by the fingertip being caught in a closing door. Because the fingertips have such highly developed sensation, crush injuries are particularly painful. The fracture of the distal phalanx is usually comminuted, and the soft tissues are infiltrated by an enlarging hematoma in a relatively closed space. A tense subungual hematoma may require decompression through a small drill hole in the fingernail for relief of pain. Treatment of the fracture is of secondary importance to treatment of the injured soft tissues. A simple aluminum splint serves to protect the crushed fingertip from further injury during the healing phase.

Mallet Finger
(Baseball Finger, Cricket Finger)

Sudden, unexpected passive flexion of the distal interphalangeal joint with the extensor tendon under tension may avulse a fragment of bone from the base of the distal phalanx into which the tendon is inserted. Alternatively, the extensor tendon may rupture just proximal to its insertion. In either case, the distal interphalangeal joint remains flexed and can no longer be actively extended—the typical mallet finger deformity (Fig. 17.1). Treatment of the acute injury consists of splinting the finger in a molded plaster cast with the distal interphalangeal joint extended and the proximal interphalangeal joint flexed (the position in which there is least tension on the extensor tendon). Immobilization is continued for 3 weeks. Because healed bone is stronger than healed tendon, the results are more satisfactory when a fragment of bone has been avulsed than when the tendon ruptures. If the bony fragment is sufficiently large that it includes a significant part of the joint surface, open reduction and fine Kirschner wire fixation of the avulsion fracture are indicated.

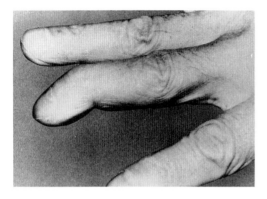

Figure 17.1. Mallet finger ("baseball finger," "cricket finger"). The distal interphalangeal joint of this man's right middle finger was suddenly forced into acute flexion as he miscaught a ball. A small fragment of the insertion of the long extensor tendon into the base of the distal phalanx was avulsed so that he lost active extension of the joint. The resultant deformity bears some resemblance to a mallet.

Middle and Proximal Phalanges

Most fractures of the middle and proximal phalanges are the result of either crushing or hyperextension injuries. Because of the close relationship of the fracture to the flexor tendons, accurate skeletal alignment is essential.

Undisplaced phalangeal fractures are usually stable because of the relatively intact periosteal tube. They are best treated by strapping the injured finger to an adjacent finger—the "buddy system"—which protects the fractured phalanx, yet allows movement of the finger joints (Fig. 17.2).

Displaced phalangeal fractures tend to be unstable (Fig. 17.3). There is frequently anterior angulation at the fracture site. After closed manipulation (using the principle of the intact

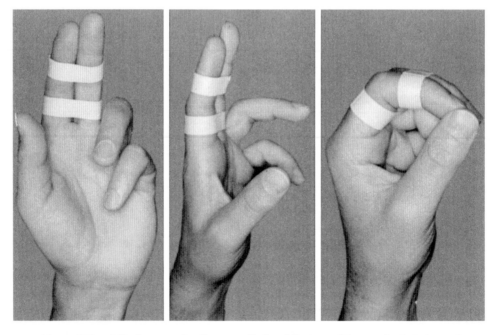

Figure 17.2.   Adhesive strapping for an undisplaced fracture of the proximal phalanx of the index finger. The adjacent uninjured finger serves as a splint and the two fingers are free to move together as a unit: the "buddy system."

periosteal hinge), the reduction can usually be maintained by means of a padded malleable aluminum splint that extends above the wrist (Fig. 17.4). Unstable oblique fractures that tend to slip with simple immobilization require either continuous traction through the fingertip (with the finger held in flexion by a cast) or, preferably, open reduction of the fracture and internal fixation with fine Kirschner wires.

Intra-articular phalangeal fractures involve the joint surface and, if displaced, should be treated by open reduction and internal fixation with either fine Kirschner wires or tiny AO screws.

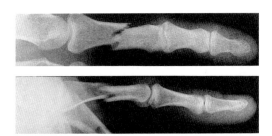

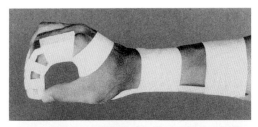

Figure 17.3. Displaced and unstable fracture of the proximal phalanx of the index finger of a working man. The alignment is satisfactory.

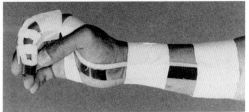

Figure 17.4. Padded malleable aluminum splint taped to the injured finger and the forearm. The splint immobilizes the wrist as well as the finger in the position of function and reduces tension on the long flexor and extensor tendons.

Sprains and Dislocations of the Interphalangeal Joints

A sudden abduction or adduction injury to a finger may either partially or completely tear a collateral ligament. If the ligamentous tear is incomplete, the finger is painful and swollen but the injured joint is stable. The sprained finger should be immobilized in flexion by means of a malleable aluminum splint for 3 weeks.

Lateral or medial dislocation of the interphalangeal joint indicates a complete tear of the collateral ligament. The dislocation is readily reduced by traction, often performed either by the patient or another person immediately after the injury. It is likely that some so-called sprains of interphalangeal joints have been associated with a momentary subluxation or dislocation, in which case a complete tear of a collateral ligament has occurred. After reduction of a dislocated interphalangeal joint, the finger should be immobilized in the flexed position for 3 weeks.

Recovery of a full range of painless motion is notoriously slow after dislocation of an interphalangeal joint and may take as long as 6 months or even 1 year. With persistent active exercises, full function is eventually regained. In the meantime, the patient requires reassurance and encouragement.

Dislocation of the Metacarpophalangeal Joints

A metacarpophalangeal joint is usually dislocated by a severe hyperextension injury. The metacarpal head is driven through a rent in the anterior capsule of the joint and comes to lie immediately under the skin of the palmar surface (Fig. 17.5). Closed reduction may be possible by a combination of hyperextension of the joint followed by traction. Sometimes, closed reduction is impossible because of the "buttonhole" effect of a relatively small tear in the capsule, the edges of which grip the metacarpal neck tightly and do not permit it to be reduced. Under these circumstances, open reduction becomes necessary. After reduction, the metacarpophalangeal joint is immobilized in a position of flexion for 3 weeks.

Metacarpals

The metacarpal bones (with the exception of the first metacarpal of the thumb) are closely bound to one another and isolated fractures of the metacarpals tend to be stable. Furthermore, because the metacarpals are covered to a large extent by muscle, they have a good blood supply and, therefore, metacarpal fractures usually heal rapidly. Undisplaced fractures of a metacarpal require protection from

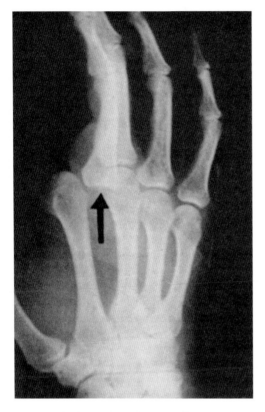

Figure 17.5.   Posterior dislocation of the metacarpophalangeal joint of the right index finger (*arrow*). The head of the metacarpal was easily palpable immediately under the skin of the palmar surface. Closed reduction was possible in this particular patient.

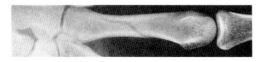

Figure 17.6.   Undisplaced fracture of a metacarpal. No immobilization was required.

further injury for a period of 3 weeks (Fig. 17.6).

Fracture of the Neck of the Fifth Metacarpal

Sometimes referred to as a "boxer's fracture," this injury is more appropriately considered a "street fighter's fracture" inasmuch as it results from an unskillful blow with the clenched fist (a boxer punches with the second and third metacarpals rather than with the more mobile fifth metacarpal). There is characteristic depression of the metacarpal head and posterior angulation at the fracture site (Fig. 17.7). Reduction can be accomplished by flexing the metacarpophalangeal joint and the proximal interphalangeal joint to a right angle and then pushing the metacarpal head back into position by means of pressure along the long axis of the proximal phalanx. The reduced fracture should be immobilized with the finger in this position in a padded plaster cast, but never for longer than 2 weeks for fear of a flexion contracture of the finger. If the

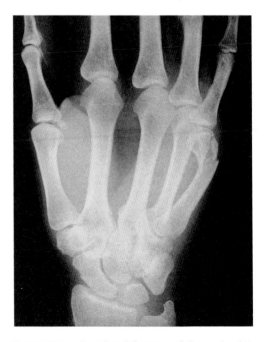

Figure 17.7.   Angulated fracture of the neck of the right fifth metacarpal ("street fighter's fracture") in a man who had become engaged in a brawl with more vigor than skill.

fracture is unstable, the distal fragment can be transfixed by a transverse percutaneous Kirschner wire to the fourth and third metacarpals, the protruding portion of the wire being incorporated in a below-elbow cast.

Fracture of Multiple Metacarpals

Severe crushing injuries of the hand may produce multiple metacarpal fractures with resultant instability. Such fractures are best stabilized by means of longitudinal intramedullary Kirschner wires.

Fracture-Dislocation of the First Carpometacarpal Joint (Bennett's Fracture)

In adults, a longitudinal force along the axis of the first metacarpal with the thumb flexed may produce a serious intra-articular fracture-dislocation of the carpometacarpal joint. A small triangular-shaped fragment of the base of the metacarpal remains in proper relationship with the trapezium. The remainder of the metacarpal, which carries with it the major portion of the joint surface, is dislocated and assumes a position of flexion (Fig. 17.8). Clinically, there is significant local swelling, tenderness, and reluctance to use the thumb.

Closed reduction, although not easy, is usually possible, provided the first metacarpal is extended and the below-elbow cast is carefully molded to press the base of the metacarpal inward and the head of the metacarpal outward. If the reduction cannot be maintained in a cast, continuous tape traction on the thumb may have to be added, the traction being attached to an outrigger loop that is incorporated into the cast (Fig. 17.9). Occasionally, the fracture-dislocation is so unstable that open reduction and internal fixation with either a Kirschner wire or a small AO screw are indicated (Fig. 17.10). Residual incongruity of the first carpometacarpal joint may lead to posttraumatic degenerative joint disease, but this complication is seldom disabling.

Fractures of the Scaphoid

Fractures of the carpal scaphoid are relatively common in young adults, particularly in males. The responsible injury is usually a fall on the open hand with the wrist dorsiflexed and radially deviated. The scaphoid, which

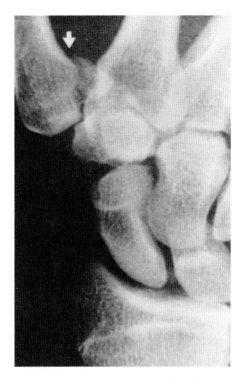

Figure 17.8. Fracture-dislocation of the first carpometacarpal joint (Bennett's fracture) in the hand of a young man who fell on his hand with the thumb flexed. Note the oblique intra-articular fracture line (*arrow*), the small triangular fragment that has remained in its normal relationship with the joint, and the dislocation of the main portion of the first metacarpal, which is in a position of flexion.

spans the joint line between the proximal and distal rows of carpal bones, bears the brunt of injury at this level.

No other fracture in adults is more frequently overlooked at the time of injury than a fracture of the scaphoid. Sometimes the patient dismisses the injury as a "sprain," an uncommon injury at the wrist, and does not seek medical attention. Occasionally the physician or surgeon makes the same error, but more often radiographs are obtained and the error lies in the interpretation of the radiographs. Fractures of the scaphoid are potentially serious in that they have a high incidence of complications, and hence, accurate diagnosis is most important.

Clinical Features

The patient experiences pain on the radial side of the wrist, particularly on dorsiflexion and

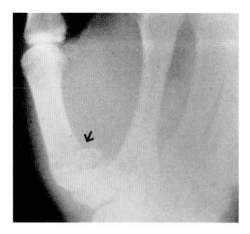
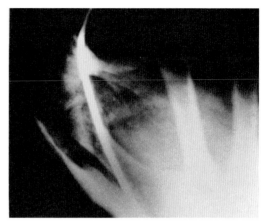

Figure 17.9. Fracture-dislocation of the first carpometacarpal joint (Bennett's fracture). **Left.** Initial radiograph. **Right.** Postreduction radiograph. The first metacarpal has been extended at the carpometacarpal joint. The wire seen in this radiograph is part of an outrigger to which traction was applied. Careful molding of the cast is more important than traction.

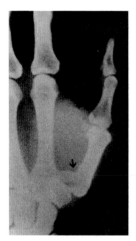
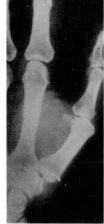

Figure 17.10. Fracture-dislocation of the first carpometacarpal joint (Bennett's fracture). **Left.** Initial radiograph showing considerable displacement of the first metacarpal. The small triangular-shaped fragment has remained in proper relationship with the joint. **Right.** This Bennett's fracture required open reduction and internal fixation with a wire loop. A more secure method of internal fixation would have been either a Kirschner wire or a small AO screw.

radial deviation. There is usually only slight swelling but significant local tenderness in the region of the anatomical "snuff box."

Radiographic Features

The scaphoid is not clearly outlined in anteroposterior projections of the wrist and requires special oblique projections. An undisplaced fracture of the scaphoid may not be apparent in the initial radiographs but becomes apparent after a week or more (Fig. 17.11).

Treatment

Because isolated fractures of the scaphoid are relatively undisplaced, no reduction is required, but the fragments should be immobilized in a below-elbow cast that incorporates all joints of the thumb (Fig. 17.12). Such treatment should be initiated on the basis of a clinical diagnosis even in the absence of initial radiographic confirmation of a fracture. The scaphoid has no muscle attachments and is covered to a large extent by articular cartilage. Consequently, its blood supply is precarious and fracture union may be seriously impaired. Furthermore, the relative absence of periosteum places the burden of fracture healing on endosteal callus formation alone. For these reasons, healing of a fractured scaphoid is characteristically slow, requiring at least 3 months and often much longer.

Complications

For reasons already mentioned, fractures of the scaphoid are prone to become complicated by *avascular necrosis, delayed union, nonunion,* and *posttraumatic degenerative joint disease.*

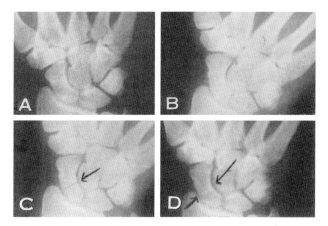

Figure 17.11.   Undisplaced fracture of the scaphoid in a young man who thought he had "sprained" his wrist. **A.** Two days after injury, there is no radiographic evidence of fracture. **B.** Eight days after injury, there is still no evidence of fracture. **C.** Twelve days after injury, a small crack fracture is visible through the waist of the scaphoid (*arrow*). **D.** Ten weeks after injury, the fracture has healed as indicated by the thin line of increased radiographic density (*arrows*). This series of radiographs emphasizes the importance of obtaining radiographs 1 week and if necessary, 2 weeks after a wrist injury if there is clinical suspicion of a fractured scaphoid. The hairline fracture becomes more apparent after 1 week or so, partly because of slight resorption of bone at the fracture site and partly because of slight separation of the fragments.

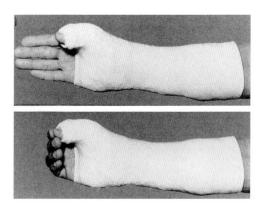

Figure 17.12.   Plaster cast for treatment of a fractured scaphoid. The cast immobilizes all joints of the thumb but in a functional position so that it can be opposed by the index and middle fingers for functions such as writing. The cast should be close fitting and well molded.

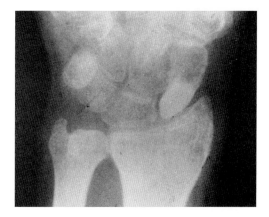

Figure 17.13.   Avascular necrosis of the proximal pole of the scaphoid 3 months after a fracture. The proximal pole is radiographically dense relative to the surrounding bone because, being avascular, it has not shared the immobilization-induced disuse osteoporosis of the remainder of the scaphoid and the neighboring bones.

Avascular necrosis of the proximal pole of the scaphoid complicates approximately one third of transverse fractures. The avascular fragment exhibits a relative radiographic density between 2 and 3 months after injury, inasmuch as it does not share in the disuse osteo- porosis of the surrounding vascular bones (Fig. 17.13). This complication may also lead to nonunion. Because revascularization of the proximal pole is exceedingly slow in adults and

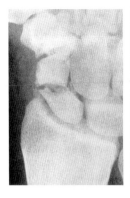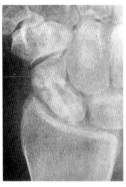

Figure 17.14.   Nonunion of a fractured scaphoid. **Left.** Nine months after the initial injury. Note the sclerosis at the fracture line and also the cyst formation in the proximal fragment. **Right.** The same man's scaphoid 3 months after bone grafting. The fracture has united and the bone graft is well incorporated. An even more effective method is the combination of a bone graft and a headless Herbert screw.

almost invariably results in degenerative joint disease of the wrist, painful established avascular necrosis may be treated by excision of the necrotic fragment, or, if necessary, by arthrodesis of the wrist.

Delayed union can be assumed if the fracture has not united within 4 months. It is an indication for an inlay bone graft.

Nonunion is a relatively common complication. Indeed, some patients seek medical attention after a recent injury (but many months after a previously undiagnosed injury) and are found to have an established nonunion that was merely aggravated by the recent injury. Thus, the symptoms of a nonunion of the scaphoid may be minimal. Radiographically, the unhealed fracture line is obvious and there may be cyst formation at the fracture site and sclerosis of the fracture surfaces (Fig. 17.14). If the nonunion is causing symptoms and is of 1 year's duration or less, inlay bone grafting is indicated with or without internal fixation with a headless Herbert screw (Fig. 17.14).

Degenerative joint disease usually supervenes 1 year or more after either avascular necrosis of the proximal pole or nonunion of the fracture. The arthritic changes involve the radiocarpal joint and the intercarpal joints and, if the associated pain is disabling, arthrodesis of the wrist is justified.

Dislocation of the Lunate

Anterior dislocation of the lunate is an uncommon but serious injury that may escape detection. Occurring as the result of a fall on the completely dorsiflexed wrist, the lunate is squeezed out of place toward the palmar surface where it comes to lie, rotated through 90 degrees, in the floor of the carpal tunnel.

Clinically, the wrist is swollen and the patient experiences pain when attempting to extend the fingers. There may be evidence of a median nerve lesion from compression within the carpal tunnel. Radiographic examination of the wrist requires two projections and the diagnosis is much more obvious in the lateral projection (Fig. 17.15).

Treatment of a recent anterior dislocation consists of strong traction on the hand and direct pressure over the lunate. Occasionally, open reduction is required to replace the lunate to its normal position in the carpus. For late, unrecognized dislocations, excision of the lunate may be required.

Complications include *median nerve compression* (which usually recovers completely after reduction of the lunate) and *avascular necrosis* of the lunate (similar to Kienböck's disease, which is discussed in Chapter 13). Degenerative joint disease of the wrist is a common sequela to avascular necrosis of the lunate and may even necessitate arthrodesis of the wrist.

Other less common injuries of the wrist include *perilunar dislocation of the carpus,* in which the lunate remains in its normal relationship with the distal end of the radius but the rest of the carpus is dislocated posteriorly in relation to the lunate. A variant of this injury, *transcaphoid perilunar dislocation,* is associated with a transverse fracture of the scaphoid.

The Wrist and Forearm

Distal End of the Radius
(Colles' Fracture)

A fracture through the flared-out distal metaphysis of the radius—the Colles' fracture—is the most common fracture in adults older than age 50 years; it occurs more frequently in women than in men. Thus, this fracture has the same age and sex incidence as

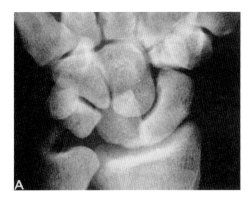

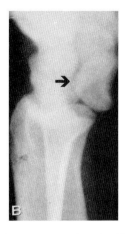
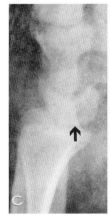

Figure 17.15. Anterior dislocation of the lunate. **A.** The anteroposterior radiograph reveals that the joint surfaces of the lunate are not congruous with those of the adjacent carpal bones, which always indicates a dislocation. The displacement, however, is not striking. **B.** In the lateral radiograph, dislocation of the lunate is obvious. The lunate has been rotated forward through 90 degrees. **C.** Post-reduction radiograph revealing that the lunate has been restored to its normal relationship to the distal end of the radius as well as to the carpal bones.

fractures of the neck of the femur and for the same reason. Both fractures occur through bone that has become significantly weakened by a combination of senile and postmenopausal osteoporosis.

The incidence of Colles' fracture is particularly high when walking conditions are slippery, because the typical mechanism of injury is as follows: the patient either slips or trips, and in an attempt to break her fall, lands on her open hand with the forearm pronated, breaking her wrist. The forces that fracture the

distal end of the radius involve dorsiflexion and radial deviation as well as supination, all of which account for the typical fracture deformity.

The fracture pattern is relatively constant, the main fracture line being transverse within the distal 2 cm of the radius. There may be only two major fragments, but comminution of the thin cortex is common, especially in the osteoporotic bone of the elderly. The ulnar styloid is frequently avulsed. The distal end of an intact radius extends beyond the distal end of the ulna and the joint surface is angulated 15 degrees toward the anterior (palmar) aspect of the wrist. After a Colles' fracture, these relationships are completely reversed and there is always some degree of subluxation of the distal radioulnar joint.

Clinical Features
The clinical deformity, frequently referred to as a "dinner fork deformity," is typical. In addition to swelling, there is an obvious jog just proximal to the wrist due to the posterior displacement and posterior tilt of the distal radial fragment (Fig. 17.16). The hand tends to be radially deviated and although often less obvious clinically, the wrist appears supinated in relation to the forearm.

Radiographic Features
Two main types of Colles' fracture can be differentiated radiographically. In the *stable type,* there is one main transverse fracture line with little cortical comminution (Fig. 17.17). In the *unstable type,* there is gross comminution, particularly of the dorsal cortex, and also significant crushing of the cancellous bone (Fig. 17.18). The intact periosteal hinge is on the dorsal aspect of the fracture in both types.

Treatment
Undisplaced Colles' fractures (which are uncommon) require only immobilization in a below-elbow cast for 4 weeks. *Displaced* fractures can usually be well reduced by closed manipulation, but the major problem is maintenance of reduction, particularly in the unstable type of Colles' fracture. In this type, with comminution of the dorsal cortex and crushing of the cancellous bone, the reduced

fracture tends to slip back toward the prere-duction position of deformity. The blood sup-ply to bone at the distal end of the radius is excellent and thus, bony union is assured. The main problem is not union but *malunion*.

Satisfactory analgesia for reduction of a Colles' fracture can be obtained by infiltration of the fracture hematoma with a local anes-thetic agent because muscle relaxation is not required. General anesthesia is preferred by some surgeons but carries a somewhat higher risk, especially for the elderly patient.

Closed reduction is obtained by using the principle of the intact periosteal hinge de-scribed in Chapter 15 (Fig. 15.36). The frac-ture deformity is first increased to disimpact the fragments and to slacken the intact perios-teal hinge on the dorsal surface, after which the distal fragment is moved distally to engage the proximal fragment. At this point, and not before, the dorsal displacement is corrected by pushing the distal fragment forward, the angulation is straightened, the radial deviation is corrected by placing the hand in ulnar devia-tion, and the supination deformity is corrected by placing the forearm in full pronation. These maneuvers bring the distal radius out to length, tighten the intact periosteal hinge and thereby help to maintain the reduction.

The plaster cast that is then applied must hold the reduced position of the fracture, just as the surgeon's hands do at the end of the reduction (Figs. 17.19 and 17.20). Thus, the cast, whether it be of the fully encircling type or the three quarters slab type held by band-ages, must be carefully molded (rather than tight and constricting) to maintain the reduc-tion. The thumb and fingers must be left free to move. Usually the cast extends only to the elbow, but if the fracture is very unstable, the elbow should be included in the cast, at least for the first 3 weeks, to maintain the forearm in complete pronation. Repeat radiographs are obtained 1 and 2 weeks after reduction because it is during this period that the frac-ture may slip into an unsatisfactory position. Also, up to the end of 2 weeks, the fracture is sufficiently mobile that the position can still be improved, if necessary, by remanipulation. Immobilization is continued for a total of 6 weeks.

Sarmiento recommends immobilizing the reduced Colles' fracture in supination for 2 weeks and the subsequent use of functional fracture-bracing.

For extremely comminuted and extremely unstable Colles' fractures, particularly in pa-tients younger than 60 years of age, the method of external skeletal fixation is of value in maintaining the reduction (Fig. 17.21).

Aftercare

Elevating the forearm to minimize swelling is extremely important after reduction of a Col-les' fracture. The thumb, fingers, elbow, and shoulder should be actively exercised hourly each day from the time of reduction. Indeed, for most patients, but especially for the frail and elderly, it is not only kinder but also more effective to admit them to hospital, at least for a few days, so that these important aspects of aftercare may be supervised. Physiotherapy and occupational therapy, as discussed in

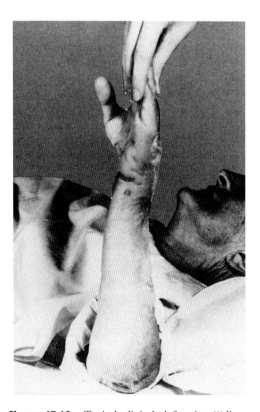

Figure 17.16. Typical clinical deformity ("dinner fork deformity") of a displaced fracture of the distal end of the radius (Colles' fracture) in an elderly woman. Note the jog just proximal to the wrist.

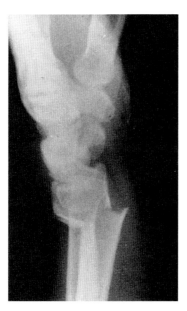 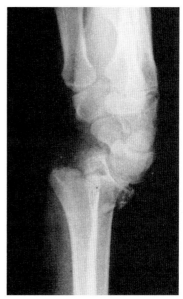

Figure 17.17.   Left. Lateral radiograph of a stable type of Colles' fracture. There is little comminution.

Figure 17.18.   Right. Lateral radiograph of an unstable type of Colles' fracture. There is gross comminution, particularly of the dorsal cortex, and also significant crushing of the cancellous bone.

Chapter 15, constitute an essential part of the total treatment.

Complications

Most Colles' fractures are well united in an acceptable position within 6 weeks. The complications, which are often preventable, include *finger stiffness, shoulder stiffness, malunion* with deformity and *residual subluxation of the distal radioulnar joint.*

Finger stiffness can be prevented by reducing swelling in the hand through elevation and by vigorous finger exercises.

Malunion can result either from imperfect reduction of the fracture or subsequent loss of a satisfactory reduction from inadequate immobilization of the reduced fracture. Associated with the ugly clinical deformity of malunion is a residual and painful *subluxation of the distal radioulnar joint* and limitation of wrist motion. If the symptoms are sufficiently disabling, the condition of the wrist can be improved by a corrective osteotomy of the radius with or without excision of the distal end of the

ulna. For an elderly patient, simple excision of the distal end of the ulna is more appropriate.

Less common complications of a Colles' fracture include *Sudeck's reflex sympathetic dystrophy* (discussed in Chapter 15) and *late rupture of the tendon of the extensor pollicis longus,* which has become frayed by friction at the level of the healed fracture. The latter complication, which usually develops from 1 to 2 months after the fracture, suddenly becomes apparent by the patient's inability to extend the thumb. Surgical repair of the ruptured tendon is ineffective and a tendon transfer is indicated.

Smith's Fracture of the Distal End of the Radius

Much less common than the Colles' fracture is the Smith's fracture, which is sometimes inaccurately referred to as a "reverse Colles' fracture." Occurring predominantly in young men, this fracture is a pronation injury, caused by a fall or blow on the back of the flexed wrist. The fracture line is transverse but may

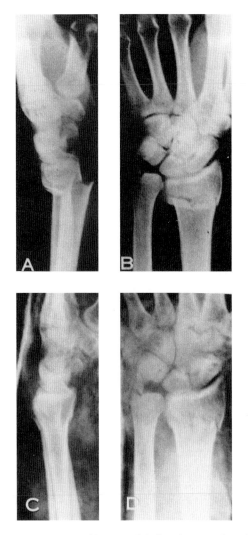

Figure 17.19. Stable type of Colles' fracture. **A and B.** Initial radiographs. There is little comminution. **C and D.** Postreduction radiographs. Note that the radius is out to length and that the tilt of the distal fragment has been corrected. Did you also notice the fracture through the styloid process of the ulna?

enter the wrist joint. Reduction requires strong supination of the wrist but open reduction and internal fixation are frequently necessary. An above-elbow cast is usually required during the 6-week period of immobilization to maintain the position of supination.

Fractures of the Shafts of the Radius and Ulna

Fractures of the shafts of the forearm bones present special problems in adults. One or

other may be fractured alone but more often both are fractured. Moreover, because these two bones are firmly bound to one another by the interosseous membrane, a fracture of only one bone is likely to be accompanied by a dislocation of the nearest joint. Thus, a fracture of the distal third of the radius is frequently associated with a dislocation of the distal radioulnar joint (a Galeazzi fracture-dislocation), whereas a fracture of the proximal half of the ulna is usually associated with a dislocation of the proximal radioulnar joint (a Monteggia fracture-dislocation).

The shafts of the radius and ulna have a relatively small cross-section, are composed of dense cortical bone, and are covered by rather thin periosteum (especially the ulna). For this reason, fractures of the forearm bones are much more likely to be displaced in adults than in children. Consequently they tend to be more unstable and heal much more slowly in adults than in children.

Fracture of the Shaft of the Radius and Dislocation of the Distal Radioulnar Joint (Galeazzi Fracture-Dislocation)

Displaced fractures of the distal third of the radial shaft are not common but when they do occur, they are associated with complete disruption and dislocation of the distal radioulnar joint. In this injury, which is usually sustained by young adults, the distal fragment of the radius is tilted posteriorly (anterior angulation at the fracture site). The carpus and hand are displaced with the radius and the resultant clinical deformity is striking (Fig. 17.22). Radiographically, the nature of the fracture-dislocation is most apparent in the lateral projection (Fig. 17.23).

The optimum form of treatment for the Galeazzi fracture-dislocation is open reduction and internal fixation of the radius, with either a plate and screws or an intramedullary nail. When the radius is perfectly reduced, so also is the dislocation of the distal radioulnar joint reduced (Fig. 17.24).

Isolated Fractures of the Proximal Two Thirds of the Radial Shaft

When the radial shaft is fractured in its upper two thirds, the fragments tend to override and

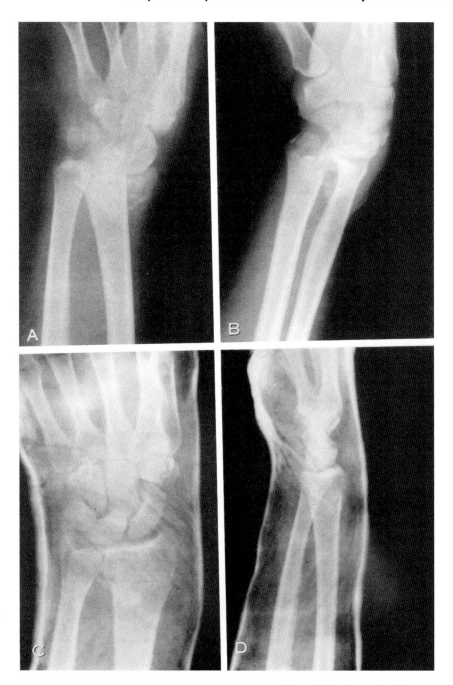

Figure 17.20.   Unstable type of Colles' fracture. **A and B.** Initial radiographs. Note the significant comminution and the shortening of the radius. **C and D.** Postreduction radiographs. Note that the wrist is ulnar-deviated but only slightly flexed. The radius has been restored to its correct length, and the angulation at the fracture site has also been corrected.

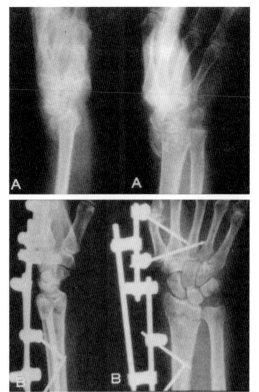

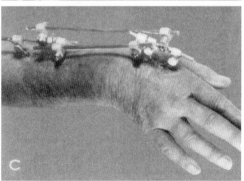

Figure 17.21. Extremely unstable comminuted Colles' fracture treated by closed reduction and external skeletal fixation. **A.** Initial radiographs. Note the marked tilting of the distal fragment, the severe comminution, and the shortening of the radius. **B.** Postreduction radiographs reveal that the fracture has been completely reduced. The reduction is being maintained by an external skeletal fixation device, the two pins of the proximal unit being in the radius and the two pins of the distal unit being in the metacarpals. **C.** Clinical appearance of this 50-year-old woman's wrist with the external skeletal fixation device still in place 6 weeks after closed reduction (the dressings around the pins had been removed temporarily for the purpose of taking the photograph).

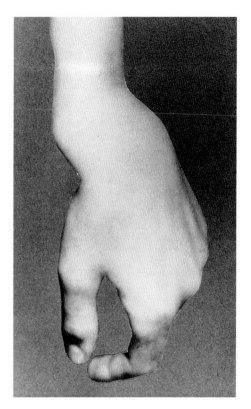

Figure 17.22. Typical clinical deformity of a severe fracture of the shaft of the radius and dislocation of the distal radioulnar joint (Galeazzi fracture-dislocation) in a 35-year-old man. The deformity is more proximal with this injury than it is with a Colles' fracture.

rotate. As a result of the shortening of the radius there is, of course, some degree of subluxation at the distal radioulnar joint. Isolated fractures of the radial shaft are difficult to reduce by closed means and reduction, if obtained, is difficult to maintain.

The most suitable form of treatment is open reduction of the radius and internal fixation with either an AO compression plate and screws or an intramedullary nail (Fig. 17.25).

Complications include *delayed union* and even *nonunion. Malunion* is a significant complication and usually involves a rotational deformity at the fracture site. If, for example, there is a 40-degree external rotational deformity (supination deformity) at the fracture site at the time of healing, the patient will have at least a 40-degree loss of pronation of the forearm (Fig. 17.26).

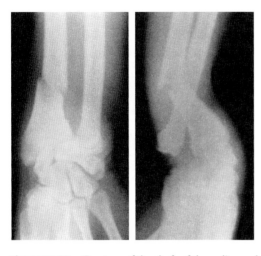

Figure 17.23.   Fracture of the shaft of the radius and dislocation of the distal radioulnar joint (Galeazzi fracture-dislocation) in the patient whose clinical deformity is shown in Figure 17.22. Note that the nature of the injury is much more obvious in the lateral projection than in the anteroposterior projection.

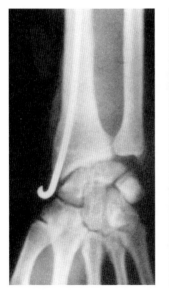
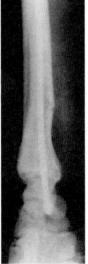

Figure 17.24.   Postreduction radiographs of the same patient illustrated in Figures 17.22 and 17.23. The radial fracture has been completely reduced and has been immobilized with a Rush intramedullary nail. A compression-type plate and screws are just as satisfactory in the treatment of this fracture and are sometimes easier to apply from a technical point of view. Note that the dislocation of the inferior radioulnar joint has also been reduced.

Fractures of the Radius and Ulna

For reasons already mentioned, fractures of both bones of the forearm in adults are more difficult to treat than comparable fractures in children. Usually the result of a severe injury, these fractures are most commonly sustained by young and middle-aged adults. A direct injury usually produces transverse fractures at the same level (most frequently in the middle third) whereas an indirect injury, which almost always involves rotation, tends to produce oblique or spiral fractures at different levels. Because of the relationship between the paired radius and ulna during supination and pronation, both fractures must be perfectly reduced in relation to alignment and rotation.

Closed reduction of both fractures *may* be possible using traction and varying degrees of pronation or supination depending on the deformity. In general, fractures of the distal third are most stable in pronation, those in the middle third are most stable in the midposition, and those in the proximal third are most stable in supination. The explanation for this generalization lies in the level of the fracture of the radius in relation to the insertion of the various muscles that normally pronate or supinate it. Even if accurate closed reduction can be obtained, fractures of both bones of the forearm are unstable and tend to redisplace despite a carefully molded above-elbow cast.

Nevertheless, Sarmiento recommends treating fractures of both bones of the forearm by functional fracture-bracing (after 3 to 5 weeks in an above-elbow cast) and has found that the position of supination is satisfactory regardless of the level of the fractures.

Open reduction is usually required for fractures of both bones of the forearm in adults, either as primary or secondary treatment after failure of closed reduction. The radius and ulna should be approached through separate incisions to minimize the risk of *cross-union* between the two bones. The most effective form of internal fixation for these fractures is an AO compression plate and screws (Fig. 17.27). The radius usually heals more rapidly than the ulna.

Complications include delayed union and even nonunion (especially in the ulna). In either case, autogenous cancellous bone graft-

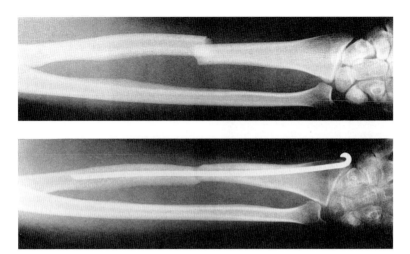

Figure 17.25.   Isolated fracture of the shaft of the radius in a 25-year-old man. **Top.** Initial radiograph revealing a transverse fracture with overriding of the fragments and consequent shortening of the radius. **Bottom.** The same patient's forearm 4 months after open reduction and intramedullary nailing with a Rush nail. The fracture has united satisfactorily.

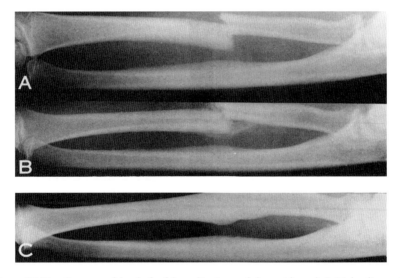

Figure 17.26.   Fracture of the shaft of the radius in an adolescent boy. **A.** Initial radiographs reveal that the distal fragment at the fracture site is broader than the proximal fragment, which indicates a rotational deformity. There is also loss of the normal bowing of the radial shaft. This fracture was left unreduced and was immobilized in an above-elbow plaster. **B.** Six weeks later, the radiograph reveals adequate callus formation. It was reported at the time of this radiograph that the fracture was clinically united. **C.** Six months later, the radiograph reveals consolidation of the fracture. Nevertheless, the rotational deformity persisted and at this stage, the patient was unable to pronate his forearm beyond the midposition. Supination was only slightly limited. This patient would have been better treated by open reduction and internal fixation of the fracture to prevent this malunion.

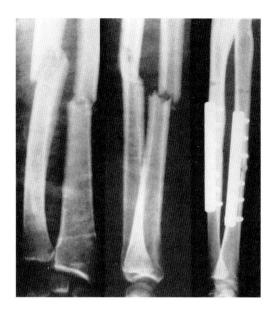

Figure 17.27.   Fracture of both bones of the forearm in a 20-year-old man. **Left and center.** Initial radiographs revealing displacement. **Right.** Postoperative radiograph. Both fractures were treated by open reduction and the application of AO compression plates and screws. Rigid fixation of the fractures was obtained at the time of operation and union progressed satisfactorily.

ing is indicated. Any residual deformity of angulation or rotation should be corrected at the same time and under these circumstances, a cortical onlay bone graft and screws may also be required. If cross-union develops between the radius and ulna (due to communication between the two fracture hematomata), there is a complete bony block to supination and pronation. Surgical treatment of this complication seldom yields satisfactory results.

Fracture of the Shaft of the Ulna and Dislocation of the Proximal Radioulnar Joint (Monteggia Fracture-Dislocation)

For reasons already mentioned, an angulated fracture of the proximal half of the ulna is invariably accompanied by a dislocation of the proximal radioulnar joint. Thus, radiographic examination for fractures in the forearm should always include both the wrist and elbow joints to avoid overlooking a fracture-dislocation, as described in Chapter 15 (Fig. 15.15).

In the common (extension) type of Monteggia fracture-dislocation, a hyperextension and pronation injury produces a fracture of the proximal half of the ulna with anterior angulation and anterior dislocation of the proximal radioulnar joint (Fig. 17.28). This injury can also be produced by a direct blow over the ulnar border of the forearm.

Monteggia fracture-dislocations in adults are best treated by open reduction of the ulna so that its length and alignment may be perfectly restored. Internal fixation of the fracture should be obtained by means of either a compression plate and screws or an intramedullary nail. Correction of the ulnar deformity usually results in a closed reduction of the radial head, in which case it is unnecessary to perform an open reduction of the dislocated proximal radioulnar joint or to repair the ruptured annular ligament. The limb should be immobilized in an above-elbow cast with the forearm in supination for approximately 3 months.

A rare variation of Monteggia fracture-dislocation is the flexion type, which is caused by a flexion injury and characterized by posterior angulation of the fractured ulna and posterior dislocation of the proximal radioulnar joint. This type of injury is treated using the same principles as the extension type of Monteggia fracture-dislocation.

The Elbow and Arm

Fracture of the Olecranon

The most common type of olecranon fracture occurs as the result of a fall with sudden passive flexion of the elbow combined with a sudden powerful contraction of the triceps muscle. The olecranon is literally pulled apart over the fulcrum of the trochlea. It is an *avulsion* type of fracture and in many ways is comparable to an avulsion fracture of the patella.

The fracture fragments are usually pulled far apart and the patient is no longer able to actively extend the elbow against gravity. Even when there is considerable swelling, a gap can be palpated at the fracture site. Radiographic examination reveals the widely separated fracture fragments (Fig. 17.29).

Closed treatment of avulsion fractures of the olecranon is only occasionally possible.

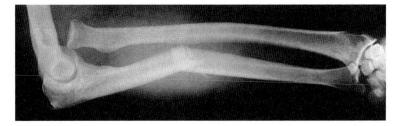

Figure 17.28. Fracture of the shaft of the ulna and dislocation of the proximal radioulnar joint (Monteggia fracture-dislocation). Note the overriding and anterior angulation at the fracture site in the ulna and the associated anterior and upward dislocation of the radial head. Unless the radiographic examination includes the elbow region, the dislocation of the radial head may escape detection.

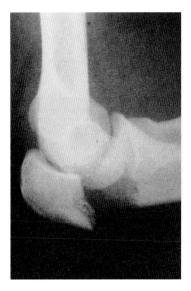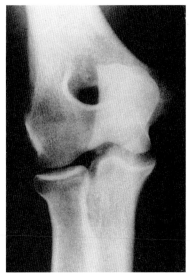

Figure 17.29. Avulsion fracture of the olecranon in a 21-year-old woman. The true nature of the injury is much more apparent in the lateral projection than in the anteroposterior projection, and this emphasizes the importance of always obtaining at least two projections at right angles to one another. Note also that in the anteroposterior projection, which was taken with the elbow extended, the fracture of the olecranon is only slightly displaced, whereas in the lateral projection, which was taken with the elbow flexed, the gap at the fracture site has widened. This patient's arm should have been immobilized in a temporary splint before the radiographic examination was carried out.

When the elbow is passively extended, the olecranon may fall back into normal position. Under these rare circumstances, the elbow should be immobilized in complete extension in a plaster cast for 6 weeks—an awkward position and one not well tolerated, particularly by the elderly.

The usual form of treatment is open reduction of the fracture and internal fixation using the AO principle of compression (Fig. 17.30). Unless the fixation is completely rigid, the elbow should be immobilized at a right angle for at least 3 weeks, after which active exercises are begun. This form of treatment is suitable

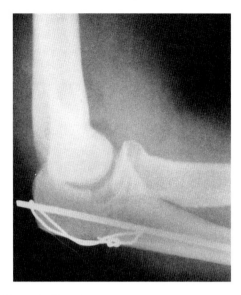
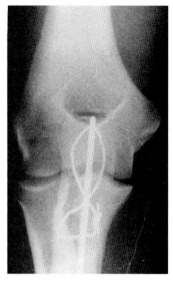

Figure 17.30.   Postoperative radiograph of the same elbow shown in Figure 17.29. The combination of an intramedullary pin and a figure-eight wire loop (tension band) maintained the reduction and compressed the fragments in accordance with the AO principle.

even in the elderly and is more satisfactory than excision of the olecranon and suture of the triceps to the ulna.

Complications of avulsion fractures of the olecranon include *nonunion* with resultant pain and weakness of extension and occasionally *degenerative joint disease* of the elbow secondary to the joint incongruity. Late operation to obtain union by bone grafting seldom provides a smooth joint surface and this emphasizes the importance of perfect reduction and rigid internal fixation in the primary treatment.

Fractures of the Radial Head

This relatively common injury in young adults is caused by a severe valgus (abduction) force applied to the extended elbow, usually at the time of a fall. The concave surface of the radial head is crushed against the convex surface of the capitellum and tends to split. The cartilage of both joint surfaces is damaged, but it is always the radial head that fractures. The medial ligament of the elbow is stretched and, if the valgus force is sufficient, the ligament may even be torn with a resultant momentary lateral dislocation of the elbow.

The patient experiences progressive pain in the elbow as a hemarthrosis develops. Supination and pronation are limited by pain and there is local tenderness over the radial head.

Radiographic examination usually reveals the fracture but, if the fracture is completely undisplaced, several radiographs taken with the radius in varying degrees of supination and pronation may be required for its detection.

Treatment depends on the severity of the damage to the radial head. It is important to remember that the actual damage to the joint surface, as well as to the underlying bone, is always more extensive than one would imagine from the appearance of the radiographs.

Undisplaced fractures without loss of joint congruity only require protection in a sling for 2 weeks, during which time active exercises (pronation and supination) are encouraged (Fig. 17.31). Single displaced fractures of the radial head can be treated by open reduction and internal fixation with a mini-AO screw.

Markedly depressed and comminuted fractures of the radial head are best treated by excision of the entire head (and not just the depressed portion) (Figs. 17.32 and 17.33). At the time of operation, the elbow joint should be carefully explored to remove any small fragments of bone or cartilage. Postoperatively, the elbow should be treated by CPM for 3 weeks. If the medial ligament of the elbow has been completely torn, the elbow will lack lateral stability after excision of the head of the radius. Under these circumstances it may be reasonable to replace the radial head with an endoprosthesis to provide stability, but this is seldom necessary.

Complications

The most significant complication of fractures of the radial head is *posttraumatic degenera-*

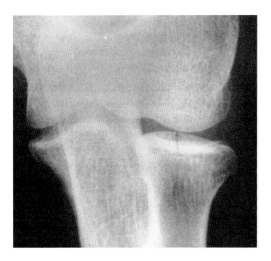

Figure 17.31. Undisplaced crack fracture of the radial head in a young woman who had a painful hemarthrosis and limitation of supination and pronation after a fall on the hand.

tive joint disease of the elbow—a complication of leaving a displaced fracture in situ. Once degenerative joint disease has developed, the pain and limitation of motion can be improved by excision of the head of the radius, followed by CPM. The results are not as satisfactory after late excision as after immediate excision.

Posterior Dislocation of the Elbow

There are two possible mechanisms of this fairly common injury in adults: a fall on the hand with the elbow slightly flexed or a severe hyperextension injury of the elbow.

The distal end of the humerus is driven forward through the anterior capsule as the radius and ulna dislocate posteriorly. Thus, there is always extensive soft tissue injury to the capsule and brachialis muscle (which may be torn from its insertion into the coronoid process). The brachial artery and median nerve may also be struck by the distal end of the humerus as it is driven forward. Occasionally associated with posterior dislocation of the elbow is a minor fracture of the coronoid process, capitellum, or radial head.

Clinically, the grossly swollen elbow is held in a position of semiflexion; the olecranon is readily palpable posteriorly. Radiographic examination is essential to confirm the clinical diagnosis and to detect any associated fractures (Fig. 17.34A).

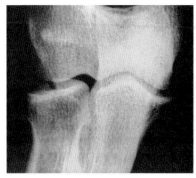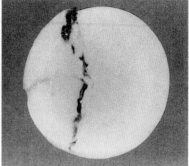

Figure 17.32. Depressed and comminuted fracture of the radial head in a young man. **Left.** Initial radiograph. Note the gap in the joint surface of the radial head. The depression is not obvious in this radiograph. **Right.** The excised radial head of the same patient reveals that the fracture is more comminuted and more extensive than one might think from the appearance of the radiographs. Nevertheless, this particular fracture of the radial head could have been treated by open reduction and internal fixation with a mini AO screw.

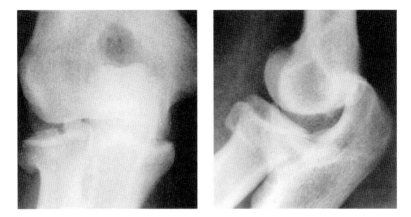

Figure 17.33.   Markedly depressed and comminuted fracture of the radial head in a 40-year-old man. This type of fracture is an indication for excision of the entire head of the radius.

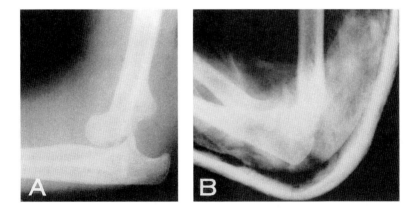

Figure 17.34.   Posterior dislocation of the elbow joint in a young man. **A.** Initial radiograph revealing the posterior displacement of the radius and ulna in relation to the distal end of the humerus. **B.** The postreduction radiograph revealing that the normal relationship between the distal end of the humerus and olecranon has been restored. The patient's elbow is immobilized in flexion in a plaster cast.

Reduction of the dislocation is readily accomplished by applying traction to the flexed elbow through the forearm, which is then brought forward. The reduced elbow is then flexed above a right angle to reduce tension on the torn anterior soft tissues and immobilized in a cast in this position, but only for 7 to 10 days (Fig. 17.34B).

Complications

After dislocation of the elbow in adults, *elbow stiffness* may persist for many months. The stiffness must be treated by active exercises only, because intermittent passive stretching of the soft tissues may aggravate the soft tissue injury and actually perpetuate the stiffness. *Median nerve injury* in association with dislocation of the elbow invariably recovers. The complication of *myositis ossificans* may occur after posterior dislocation of the elbow in adults—particularly if reduction is delayed or if the elbow has been repeatedly manipulated—but it is less common in adults than in children. This complication has been discussed in Chapter 15. Major *injury to the brachial artery* is not uncommon.

Fracture-Dislocations of the Elbow

An extremely severe fracture-dislocation of the elbow occurs when a driver or passenger has his or her elbow out the open window of a car at the moment the car is struck from the side by another vehicle. The elbow is dislocated and there are multiple comminuted fractures of the humerus, radius, and ulna—the "sideswipe injury" of the elbow (Fig. 17.35).

Treatment of this serious injury is understandably difficult. Open reduction of the dislocation and open reduction and internal fixation of the multiple fractures are best performed immediately to minimize late elbow stiffness.

Intercondylar Fractures of the Humerus

The intercondylar type of fracture of the distal end of the humerus in adults results from a severe fall on the point of the flexed elbow. In cross-section, the articular surface of the olecranon appears wedge shaped and hence, it is not surprising that with such a fall the olecranon is driven like a wedge between the

two condyles of the humerus and splits one or both from the shaft. Thus, the vertical component of the fracture is always intra-articular. Proximally there may be a transverse component in which case the comminuted fracture lines are T-shaped.

Clinically, the elbow region is grossly swollen and there is usually evidence of abrasions or bruises on the posterior aspect of the elbow indicating the mechanism of injury. Radiographic examination may require several projections to reveal the true extent of the injury. The comminution may be extreme.

Treatment

The form of treatment depends primarily on the degree of comminution of the fracture. Of course the most important fracture to be completely reduced is the vertical fracture that extends into the elbow joint (in keeping with the principle of obtaining and maintaining perfect reduction of intra-articular fractures). *Single fractures* that have split off only one condyle are best treated by open reduction and internal fixation with screws to restore the joint line (Fig. 17.36). *Double fractures* with a T-shaped component should also be treated by open reduction and internal fixation but with plates and screws. Provided the internal fixation is rigid, the elbow should be treated postoperatively by CPM for 3 weeks.

Severely comminuted fractures in the intercondylar region that are described as a "bag of bones" defy internal fixation and are best treated by immediate prosthetic elbow replacement. The complication of prolonged joint stiffness is particularly common when intercondylar fractures of the humerus have been immobilized in a plaster cast for longer than 3 weeks.

Fractures of the Shaft of the Humerus

Adults sustain fractures of the shaft of the humerus more readily than children. The common mechanism of injury is a direct blow, in which case the fracture tends to be transverse and somewhat comminuted. Indirect injury, as is sustained from a fall on the hand, is more likely to produce a spiral fracture. It must be remembered that the humeral shaft is a com-

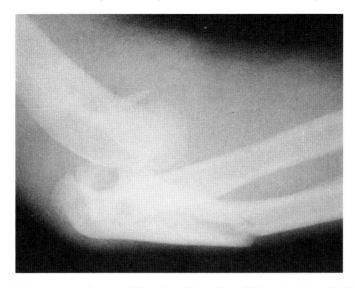

Figure 17.35.   A severe fracture-dislocation of the elbow ("sideswipe injury"). Note that there are fractures of the ulna, radial head, and distal end of the humerus. Note also the posterior dislocation of the elbow joint.

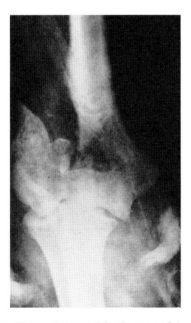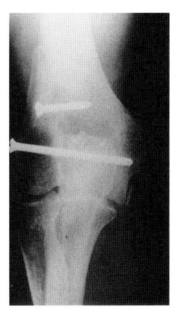

Figure 17.36.   Intercondylar fracture of the humerus in a 45-year-old man. **Left.** Initial radiographs (the elbow is immobilized in a temporary plaster splint). The lateral condyle has been split off from the distal end of the humerus and is displaced laterally and tilted. (The radiopaque areas seen medially and laterally distal to the elbow are in the plaster splint and not in the patient). **Right.** Postreduction radiograph showing the lateral condyle reduced and held in position with two screws. Note that the joint line has been completely restored.

mon site for metastases in the adult—particularly in the elderly.

The humerus, like the femur, being surrounded by muscle, has a fairly thick periosteum, and consequently fractures of the humerus usually unite well and rapidly, unless the fracture has been overdistracted (as it may be in a heavy "hanging cast"). The proximity of the radial nerve as it winds around the midshaft of the humerus accounts for the high incidence of radial nerve injury associated with fractures at this level.

Clinical examination reveals a flail arm that the patient tries to support with the opposite hand. A radial nerve lesion should always be sought and its presence or absence recorded at the time of the initial examination. The arm should be splinted before radiographic examination is carried out and the anteroposterior and lateral projections should be obtained by moving the radiographic tube rather than by moving the patient's fractured arm.

Treatment

Fractures of the shaft of the humerus respond well to closed treatment, the aim of which is to obtain and maintain reasonable alignment without rotational deformity. The reduction does not need to be perfect, and even side-to-side (bayonet) apposition with slight shortening is acceptable. Thus, nearly all fractures of the shaft of the humerus in adults can be adequately treated by closed means. Two indications for open reduction and internal fixation of the fracture are a coexistent injury to the brachial artery that requires arterial repair and a progressive loss of radial nerve function.

Transverse fractures of the humeral shaft should be reduced under anesthesia to get the fracture ends in contact and provide some stability. When the alignment and rotation have been corrected, a U-shaped plaster slab (sometimes referred to as a "sugar-tong splint") is applied and bandaged to the arm. A collar and wrist cuff sling are applied and for added comfort—particularly if the fracture is unstable—the upper limb can be bandaged to the chest (Fig. 17.37). Clinical union is usually achieved within 6 weeks, after which guarded movement of the elbow may be initiated. This form of treatment is preferable to a heavy "hanging cast," which hangs only when the patient is upright and may distract the fracture fragments, leading to delayed union. Because the hanging cast does not immobilize the fracture fragments, the patient experiences much discomfort during the early weeks of treatment.

Spiral and comminuted fractures of the humeral shaft do not require reduction or anesthesia. With the patient sitting upright, gravity alone is adequate to provide alignment of the fracture fragments, after which the above-mentioned U-shaped plaster sugar-tong splint with collar and cuff may be applied. Even slight residual angulation does not produce a clinically significant deformity at this level (Fig. 17.38).

Fractures of the shaft of the humerus can also be effectively treated by functional fracture-bracing (as described in Chapter 15) after an initial 2-week period of immobilization in a plaster cast.

Complications

For reasons already mentioned, *radial nerve injury* is frequent at the time of fracture. The nerve, however, is seldom divided (neurotmesis) and because the lesion is one in continuity (either neuropraxia or axonotmesis), recovery may be anticipated; therefore a radial nerve injury does not constitute an indication for open reduction unless the radial nerve deficit is increasing. If there has been no recovery of muscles innervated by the radial nerve within approximately 3 months (the estimated time required for regenerating nerve fibers to reach the first muscle after an axonotmesis), the nerve should be explored. Should the nerve be found to be irreparably damaged, function in the hand can be greatly improved by appropriate tendon transfers. *Delayed union* or *nonunion* may complicate a fracture of the humeral shaft, especially if the fracture has been operated on or has been overdistracted by a hanging cast. Although fresh fractures of the humerus usually unite rapidly and well, nonunion can be exceedingly difficult to treat and may need intramedullary nailing and autogenous cancellous bone grafting.

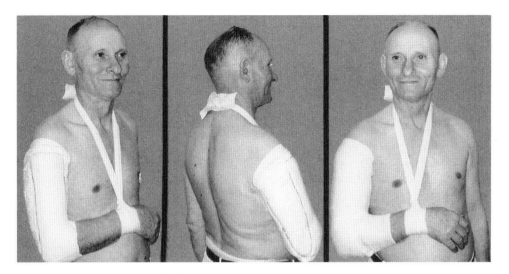

Figure 17.37. U-shaped plaster slab ("sugar tong splint") with a collar and wrist cuff sling for a fracture of the shaft of the humerus. One bandage separates the plaster from the skin and a second holds the plaster slab firmly in place. If the fracture is particularly unstable, the arm can then be bandaged to the trunk as well.

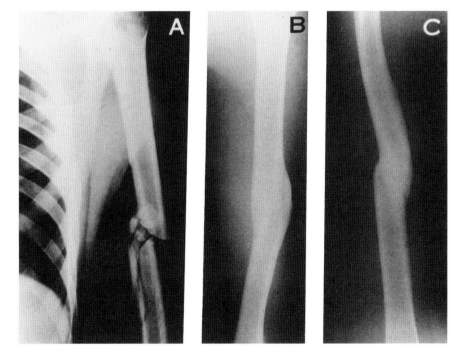

Figure 17.38. Spiral and comminuted fracture of the humeral shaft in a 44-year-old man. **A.** Initial radiograph taken with the patient sitting upright. The alignment is satisfactory. The fracture was treated with a U-shaped plaster ("sugar tong splint") with a collar and cuff sling. **B and C.** Anteroposterior and lateral radiographs one year later; the fracture is consolidated. The slight varus deformity was not apparent clinically.

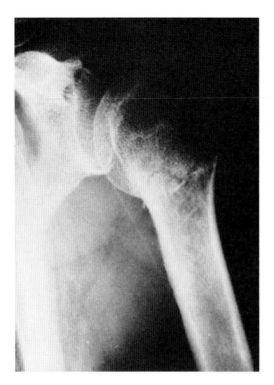

Figure 17.39. Impacted fracture of the neck of the humerus in an elderly woman. The impaction is easily seen on the medial side.

Fractures of the Neck of the Humerus

In elderly persons—especially women with a combination of senile and postmenopausal osteoporosis—impacted fractures of the neck of the humerus are relatively common. Resulting usually from a minor fall on the hand with forces being transmitted up the extended arm, the fracture line is transverse and the distal fragment is driven into, or *impacted*, in the proximal fragment.

Clinical examination may reveal relatively little evidence of the fracture, as it is sufficiently stable that the patient is able to move the arm reasonably well. There is local tenderness in the axilla but the arm can usually be moved passively with little pain. Radiographic examination reveals the extent of impaction of the fracture (Fig. 17.39).

Treatment

Because *impacted* fractures of the neck of the humerus are stable, the fracture need not be immobilized and requires only protection from further injury by means of a sling during the 6 weeks required for union. After 1 week, however, the patient should remove the sling daily for a period of pendulum exercises to prevent shoulder stiffness; while bending forward, the patient gently swings the dependent limb back and forth, and in a circle, like a pendulum. As soon as the patient no longer feels pain at the fracture site, he or she should be encouraged to abduct the arm against gravity (Fig. 17.40).

Fractures that are *not impacted* require more active treatment. Occurring more often in younger adults, these fractures may be markedly displaced. The short proximal fragment is usually abducted by the muscles inserted into the rotator cuff.

In young patients, the ideal treatment for unstable fractures of the neck of the humerus is open reduction and internal fixation. For the frail and the elderly, a more appropriate treatment is immediate prosthetic shoulder replacement of the hemiarthroplasty type.

Complications

In the elderly the most common complication of impacted fractures of the neck of the humerus that have not been treated by prosthetic replacement is *persistent shoulder stiffness,* a complication that is more easily prevented than treated. Prolonged physiotherapy is nec-

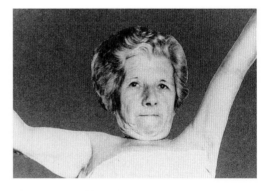

Figure 17.40. This elderly woman is abducting her shoulders 4 weeks after sustaining an impacted fracture of the neck of her right humerus. She will regain a useful, but not necessarily normal, range of shoulder motion.

essary to overcome such shoulder stiffness and occasionally, after several months of therapy, a gentle manipulation under anesthesia is required to regain shoulder motion. In younger adults with displaced fractures, there may be coexistent *injury to the circumflex (axillary) nerve,* manifest by deltoid muscle paralysis and a small area of diminished skin sensation over the outer aspect of the shoulder region. The prognosis for recovery of nerve function is good.

Fractures of the Greater Tuberosity of the Humerus

In middle-aged and elderly adults, a relatively common injury is an undisplaced fracture of the greater tuberosity of the humerus resulting from a fall directly on the point of the shoulder (Fig. 17.41). Treatment is identical to that described above for impacted fractures of the neck of the humerus.

In younger adults, the greater tuberosity is more often *avulsed* by an indirect injury such as a fall on the hand with the arm adducted. Under these circumstances, the greater tuberosity is usually retracted and abducted; reduction therefore necessitates abduction of the humerus and immobilization of the upper

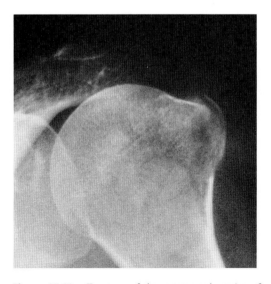

Figure 17.41.   Fracture of the greater tuberosity of the humerus of a 50-year-old woman who fell directly on the outer aspect of her shoulder.

limb and trunk in a shoulder spica cast or abduction splint for 6 weeks.

The Shoulder

Dislocations of the Shoulder

The shoulder joint is dependent for its stability on the joint capsule and surrounding muscles. The glenoid cavity, being small in relation to the head of the humerus, provides little bony stability. For this reason the shoulder joint is more often dislocated than any other joint in adults. The dislocation may be produced by either direct or indirect injury. Dislocation of a shoulder also may occur during the violent uncoordinated muscle contractions of a grand mal epileptic convulsion.

At the time of the initial shoulder dislocation, the joint capsule is usually avulsed from the margin of the glenoid cavity and, because there is little bony stability of the joint, a common sequela to the initial injury is recurrent dislocation. The dislocation usually is anterior and medial (subcoracoid) or, less often, posterior. Rarely, the injury is the inferior type of dislocation, in which the head of the humerus becomes caught under the glenoid cavity and the patient cannot bring his or her arm down to the side from the erect position (luxatio erecta).

Anterior Dislocation of the Shoulder

An injury predominantly of young adults (particularly athletes), anterior dislocation of the shoulder is usually caused by forced external rotation and extension of the shoulder. The humeral head is driven forward and frequently avulses the cartilaginous glenoid labrum and capsule from the anterior margin of the glenoid cavity (the Bankart lesion). Less commonly, anterior dislocation is caused by a fall on the hand or directly on the posterolateral aspect of the shoulder.

The patient is immediately aware that something has "given way" or "gone out of place" and is unable to use the arm, which he or she tends to support with the opposite hand. On physical examination, the shoulder appears strikingly square due to the anterior and medial displacement of the humeral head

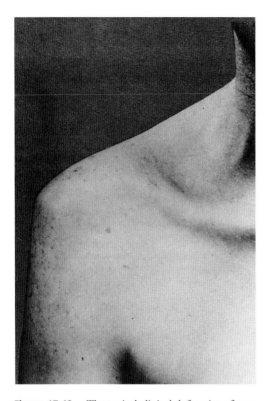

Figure 17.42.   The typical clinical deformity of anterior (inferomedial) dislocation of the right shoulder in a young athlete. The normal round contour of the shoulder has been lost and the shoulder looks square. The humeral head was palpable in the subcoracoid region.

into a subcoracoid location (Fig. 17.42). Circumflex (axillary) nerve function should always be assessed during the initial examination because this nerve may have been injured.

Radiographic examination confirms the diagnosis: the humeral head has lost contact with the glenoid cavity and is lying in the subcoracoid position (Fig. 17.43).

Treatment. The dislocation should be reduced as soon as possible, and this can usually be accomplished by one of two available methods. The simpler of these requires no anesthesia and is worth a trial unless the patient is unduly nervous; the patient merely lies face down on an operating room table with the injured arm (to which a weight is attached) hanging over the padded table edge. As the shoulder muscles relax over a period of several minutes, the humeral head usually slips back

to its normal position. If this method has not resulted in a reduction of the dislocation within 10 minutes, a general anesthetic may be required so that the following method may be performed. While an assistant applies constant traction to the upper limb with the shoulder in abduction, the surgeon can apply lateral and backward pressure on the dislocated humeral head with his or her hands, thereby reducing it. Complete reduction should be confirmed radiographically.

After reduction of the dislocation has been obtained by either of these methods, the patient's upper limb should be supported in a sling and bandaged to the chest to keep the shoulder adducted and internally rotated for 3 weeks. The avulsed capsule is thereby given a chance to heal and the risk of recurrent anterior dislocation is probably lessened, particularly in the young adult. For the elderly, 3 weeks' immobilization of the reduced shoul-

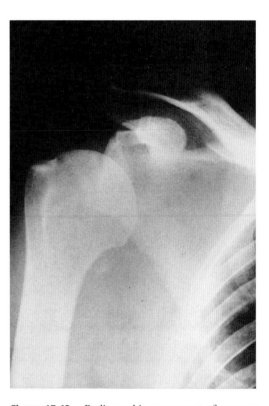

Figure 17.43.   Radiographic appearance of an acute anterior dislocation of the right shoulder. Note that the humeral head is no longer articulating with the glenoid cavity and is lying in the subcoracoid position.

der is neither necessary nor desirable. A simple sling is adequate.

Complications. In addition to *recurrent anterior dislocation* (which is discussed in the next section of this chapter), a relatively common complication of the initial dislocation is a *traction injury of the circumflex (axillary) nerve.* The patient is unable to abduct the shoulder because of deltoid paralysis, and there is a small patch of diminished skin sensation over the outer aspect of the shoulder. The prognosis for recovery is good. Occasionally a coexistent *tear of the musculotendinous cuff* of the shoulder complicates a dislocation, in which case the reduced shoulder should be immobilized for 3 weeks in an abducted position. Rarely, *interposition of the tendon of the long head of biceps* necessitates open reduction of the dislocation.

Recurrent Anterior Dislocation of the Shoulder

Because the stability of the shoulder depends to a large extent on the integrity of the joint capsule and because the capsule and anterior labrum are nearly always avulsed or stripped off the glenoid and neck of the scapula at the time of the initial dislocation of the shoulder, it is not surprising that, in some individuals, especially athletes, the dislocation may recur

more and more frequently with less and less violence. In addition to the unhealed soft tissue rent, which leaves an anterior pocket into which the humeral head may slip, there is often a "dent" in the posterior aspect of the head as the result of a compression fracture sustained during the initial dislocation. Such a dent (the Hill-Sachs lesion) allows the externally rotated humeral head to slip over the anterior margin of the glenoid cavity quite readily. Understandably, this dent cannot be detected radiographically in an anteroposterior projection but is easily seen in a special projection with the humerus internally rotated 60 degrees (Fig. 17.44).

Treatment. In young persons, recurrent anterior dislocation can be both irritating and disabling. The patient is constantly aware that if the arm is abducted and externally rotated the shoulder is likely to redislocate. Under these circumstances, surgical repair of the soft tissues is indicated. Of the large number and variety of operations designed to render such a shoulder stable, the two most often performed are the Bankart operation, in which the labrum and capsule are reattached to the anterior margin of the glenoid cavity; and the Putti-Platt operation, in which the capsule as well as the subscapularis muscle are divided and then reefed (overlapped), thereby limiting

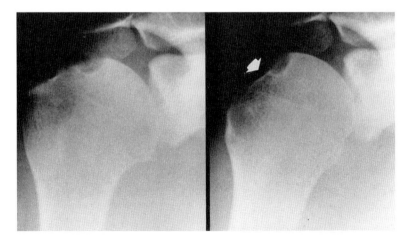

Figure 17.44.   Residual dent (Hill-Sachs lesion) in the posterior aspect of the humeral head after an acute anterior dislocation of the shoulder. **Left.** In this anteroposterior projection, the dent is not apparent. **Right.** In this projection (with the humerus internally rotated 60 degrees) the dent is obvious (arrow). It is rather like a dent in a ping-pong ball.

external rotation. After operation, the patient's arm should be supported in a sling and bandaged to the trunk with the shoulder internally rotated for 6 weeks. A successful repair enables the patient to return to full activities, including athletics.

Fracture-Dislocation of the Shoulder

The greater tuberosity of the humerus is sometimes avulsed at the time of an anterior dislocation of the shoulder (Fig. 17.45). Such a fracture-dislocation can usually be treated by closed reduction of the dislocation (as described above), which brings the humeral head back into reasonable relationship with the greater tuberosity. As with an associated tear of the musculotendinous cuff, fracture-dislocations of this type require immobilization of the reduced shoulder in a position of abduction.

An uncommon but serious type of fracture-dislocation is one in which a completely displaced fracture through the neck of the humerus is associated with complete dislocation of the humeral head. For this complex injury, open reduction of the dislocation and the fracture is necessary. The associated fracture can

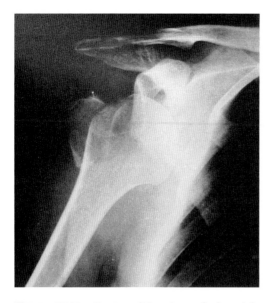

Figure 17.45. Fracture-dislocation of the right shoulder. Note the displaced fracture of the greater tuberosity of the humerus and the dislocation of the humeral head in relation to the glenoid cavity.

then be stabilized by internal fixation. In the elderly, a more appropriate treatment is immediate prosthetic shoulder replacement of the hemiarthroplasty type.

Posterior Dislocation of the Shoulder

Although much less common than anterior dislocation, posterior dislocation can occur from a fall on the front of the shoulder or on the hand with the shoulder adducted and internally rotated. It may also occur during an epileptic convulsion (including electric shock treatment for psychiatric disorders) and alcoholic intoxication; hence, the three "Es," *E*pilepsy, *E*lectric, and *E*thanol.

Clinically, the patient's arm seems locked in a position of adduction and internal rotation. Radiographically, the posterior dislocation is not readily detected in an anteroposterior projection because the humeral head slides only posteriorly and not medially. A special superoinferior (axillary) projection with the shoulder abducted is necessary to confirm that the humeral head is in fact lying posteriorly.

Treatment. Under anesthesia, the posterior dislocation can be reduced by externally rotating the shoulder and applying forward pressure on the dislocated humeral head. Reduction should be confirmed in both the anteroposterior and superoinferior (axillary) projections. The shoulder is then supported in a sling for 3 weeks.

Recurrent and Habitual Posterior Dislocation of the Shoulder

When a shoulder that previously dislocated posteriorly redislocates as a result of another injury, the second and subsequent dislocations are referred to as *recurrent* dislocations. Surgical repair of the posterior soft tissue is indicated. When, however, the patient is able to dislocate the shoulder posteriorly at will—and likewise reduce it—the condition is one of *habitual* dislocation, and is usually associated with generalized congenital laxity of ligaments. It also may be associated with an attention-seeking adolescent or adult. Such a patient should be discouraged from dislocating and reducing the dislocation as a "parlor trick." Should the shoulder dislocate involuntarily every time the patient's shoulder is flexed and adducted, surgical repair is justifiable.

Rupture of the Musculotendinous Cuff of the Shoulder

This relatively common injury, which is frequently preceded by degenerative changes in the musculotendinous rotator cuff, is described in Chapter 11.

Subluxation and Dislocation of the Acromioclavicular Joint

The term "shoulder separation" refers to either a subluxation or a dislocation of the acromioclavicular joint—injuries that are caused by a severe fall on the top of the shoulder and are therefore frequently encountered in young athletes engaged in body contact sports such as football, rugger, and hockey.

The acromion is driven downward while the clavicle is pulled upward by the action of the trapezius and sternomastoid muscles. The capsule of the acromioclavicular joint is torn. The coracoclavicular ligaments (trapezoid and conoid) normally bind the clavicle to the coracoid process of the scapula, and if these are not torn by the injury, the acromioclavicular joint is merely *subluxated*. If, however, these ligaments are completely torn, the result is a complete *dislocation* of the acromioclavicular joint.

The patient complains of severe pain over the shoulder and there is significant local tenderness over the acromioclavicular joint. Instability of the joint may be detected clinically, especially with a complete dislocation.

Radiographic examination, which should include both shoulders, is best conducted with the patient standing and holding a weight in each hand. In a subluxation, there is merely a slight depression of the acromion whereas in a dislocation, the joint surfaces have lost contact completely (Fig. 17.46).

Treatment

Nonoperative methods of strapping and plaster casts to depress the clavicle and elevate the acromion are frequently used and may relieve the acute symptoms but are of doubtful value in restoring and maintaining the normal rela-

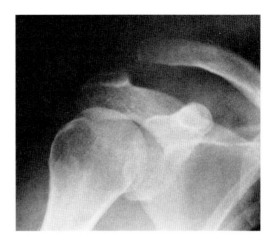

Figure 17.46. Complete dislocation of the right acromioclavicular joint in a football player. Note the marked depression of the acromion in relation to the outer end of the clavicle. The coracoclavicular ligaments (trapezoid and conoid) must be completely torn to permit this degree of displacement.

tionship of the clavicle to the acromion. For a subluxation, support of the arm in a sling for a few weeks—with or without strapping—is adequate in the realization that some degree of residual subluxation of the acromioclavicular joint is almost inevitable but nevertheless acceptable.

For a complete dislocation with severe displacement, most nonoperative methods are ineffectual. The most satisfactory form of treatment is open reduction, capsular repair, and the insertion of a *threaded* wire through the acromion, across the acromioclavicular joint and well into the clavicle. The distal (lateral) cut end of the threaded wire is left protruding through the skin and is bent through a right angle to prevent migration. The wire is removed after 6 weeks. (Smooth Kirschner wires should never be used because they may migrate medially and penetrate important structures). Another method involves screw fixation of the clavicle to the coracoid process.

Untreated or inadequately treated dislocation of the acromioclavicular joint leaves a permanent deformity as well as permanent weakness of the shoulder (Fig. 17.47).

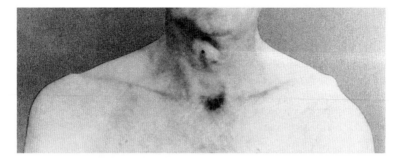

Figure 17.47.   Residual deformity of an untreated dislocation of the left acromioclavicular joint. This 52-year-old working man had weakness of shoulder abduction and experienced aching in the shoulder at the end of a day's work.

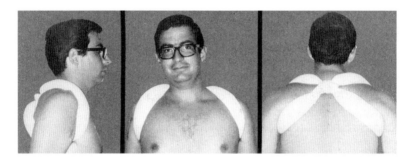

Figure 17.48.   Well-padded figure-eight bandage for the treatment of a fractured clavicle in an athletic adult. The bandage, which consists of stockinette filled with cotton wool, is adjustable so that it can be tightened as necessary each day. For additional support, this bandage can be reinforced by plaster-of-Paris bandages.

Dislocation of the Sternoclavicular Joint

A severe blow or fall on the front of the shoulder, which drives the outer end of the clavicle backward and the inner end forward, may produce an anterior dislocation of the sternoclavicular joint. This uncommon injury is more readily diagnosed clinically—by local tenderness and a prominence of the medial end of the clavicle—than radiographically. The dislocation can be reduced by local pressure over the dislocated medial end of the clavicle. The reduction can usually be maintained by the combination of a local pressure pad, strapping to hold the shoulder forward, and a sling for 3 weeks.

Recurrent anterior dislocation of the sternoclavicular joint is rare but if it causes pain or disability, it necessitates a reconstructive operation in which a "living suture" of fascia lata is used to retain the medial end of the clavicle in normal relationship with the sternum.

Posterior (retrosternal) dislocation of the sternoclavicular joint, a rare but very painful injury, may cause dangerous compression of the trachea or great vessels and necessitates urgent open reduction and internal fixation with a *threaded* pin, as described above, for acromioclavicular dislocations.

Fractures of the Clavicle

The relatively strong clavicles of adults are less frequently fractured than the slender clavicles of young children. The mechanism of injury in both groups is the same, namely a fall on the hand with forces being transmitted through the forearm and arm to the shoulder. The common site is the middle third of the clavicle and the lateral fragment is usually pulled inferiorly and medially by the weight

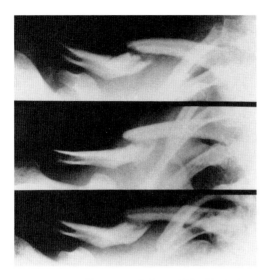

Figure 17.49.   Fracture of the middle third of the right clavicle in a young woman who had sustained multiple injuries in an automobile accident. Note that the segmental fracture is comminuted with an angulated middle segment and that the lateral fragment is displaced inferiorly and medially. **Top.** Three weeks after injury. The patient stated that her shoulder had not been immobilized in any way during the preceding 3 weeks. The alignment of this fracture could have been improved initially and maintained by treatment. **Center.** Three months after injury. New bone formation is apparent and although the fracture was clinically united at this time, bony union has been delayed. **Bottom.** Six months after injury. The fracture is now radiographically uniting and, although there has been some remodeling at the fracture site, there is still an obvious deformity of malunion.

of the shoulder and upper limb (Fig. 17.49). Less commonly the fracture occurs just medial to the acromioclavicular joint.

Treatment

Because fractures of the clavicle heal well, even in adults, and perfect reduction is not essential, closed manipulation under either local or general anesthesia is usually satisfactory. Both shoulders are pulled back as far as possible and are held in this position for 3 weeks by means of a stout figure-of-eight padded bandage with, or without, a sling (Fig. 17.48). Although the fracture is usually clinically united in 3 weeks, it is not radiographically united until much later.

Complications

Malunion of a fractured clavicle is common but is seldom a cause for cosmetic concern except for young and even not-so-young women (Figs. 17.49 and 17.50). For this group of patients the combination of careful alignment of the fracture fragments, the application of a well-molded double shoulder spica cast and a few weeks' rest in bed can prevent malunion and provide a more acceptable cosmetic result than the obvious surgical scar of an open reduction.

Delayed union may complicate a fractured clavicle that has been inadequately treated during the first few weeks (Fig. 17.49). *Nonunion* is relatively rare, unless the fracture has been complicated by infection after an open reduction.

The Spine

General Features

Fractures, dislocations, and fracture-dislocations of the spine have become increasingly more common in the present age of high-speed travel, the majority being caused by automobile accidents. Although 80% of spinal injuries are not accompanied by serious complications such as spinal cord injury, all spinal injuries must be considered initially to be potentially serious because 20% prove to be so. Thus, the preliminary (first-aid) care and transportation of individuals who have sustained such injuries, as discussed in Chapter 15, are extremely important.

In general, major injuries of the spinal column should be assessed in terms of their *sta-*

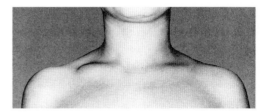

Figure 17.50.   Clinical deformity caused by malunion of the right clavicle of the young woman whose radiographs are shown in Figure 17.49. This permanent deformity, seen 6 months after injury, was a source of embarrassment to the patient.

bility. Stable injuries, such as wedge compression fractures and even compression burst fractures of vertebral bodies, are protected from significant displacement both initially and subsequently by intact posterior spinal ligaments. *Unstable injuries,* such as dislocations and fracture-dislocations, have been significantly displaced initially and may become further displaced because the posterior spinal ligaments have been torn. Assessment of stability sometimes requires that the radiographic examination be carried out with the injured part of the spine in varying degrees of flexion and extension—an example of very gentle stress radiography to detect occult joint instability—but always with the patient conscious and a physician or surgeon in control of the examination.

Initial and repeated neurological examination must be thoroughly conducted and recorded in all patients with spinal injury to determine the extent as well as the progress of complicating injuries to the spinal cord or nerve roots. *Traumatic paraplegia* has been discussed in Chapter 12.

Radiographic examination should always include a minimum of four projections (anteroposterior, lateral, right and left oblique). Sometimes, special projections or even special techniques, such as tomography (laminography), myelography, CT, and MRI are required to elucidate the nature and full extent of the injury.

Injuries of the Cervical Spine

The cervical segments, being the most mobile of the spinal column, are the most vulnerable to unstable injuries such as dislocations and fracture-dislocations; furthermore, the spinal cord in the cervical region is particularly vulnerable to either compression or transection. The most severe injuries of the upper part of the spinal cord are immediately fatal and the victim does not even reach a hospital.

Because many cervical spine injuries are associated with a severe blow on the head, all patients who have sustained a head injury should have a thorough clinical and diagnostic imaging examination of the cervical spine.

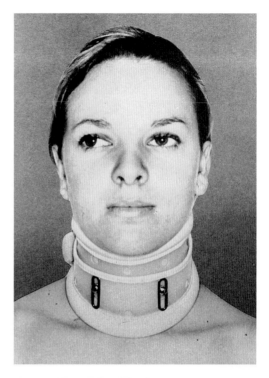

Figure 17.51. Adjustable plastic collar for the support of stable injuries of the cervical spine.

Fracture of the Atlas (C1)

When an individual falls from a height and lands on the top of the head with the cervical spine straight, the occipital condyles of the base of the skull may split or burst the ring of the atlas. Provided there is no angulatory or rotatory injury, the displacement is not severe and the spinal cord is not injured. Radiographic examination should include an anteroposterior view through the open mouth.

Treatment. Because a burst type fracture of the atlas is a stable injury, the only treatment required, in the absence of spinal cord injury, is immobilization of the cervical spine in a plaster collar or carefully fitted orthotic cervical collar for approximately 3 months (Fig. 17.51).

Displacements of the Atlantoaxial Joint (C1-C2)

The normal relationship between the atlas and axis is maintained to a large extent by the transverse ligament of the atlas that crosses behind the odontoid process (dens) of the axis.

Dislocation of the atlantoaxial joint as a result of trauma is seldom seen clinically because such a dislocation is likely to produce a fatal injury to the spinal cord. Gradual displacement of this joint, however, may complicate inflammatory disorders such as rheumatoid arthritis as a result of softening and subsequent stretching of the transverse ligament. Local spinal fusion of the completely reduced atlantoaxial joint is indicated to protect the spinal cord.

Fracture-dislocation of the atlantoaxial joint includes a fracture of the base of the odontoid process and either anterior or posterior dislocation of the atlas, usually the former. Because the transverse ligament is intact, the odontoid process moves with the atlas and the spinal cord may not be compressed. The patient quite understandably feels that his or her head is "about to fall off" and anxiously supports it with the hands.

The *treatment of undisplaced fractures of the base of the odontoid* requires only immobilization of the cervical spine in a plaster collar or well-molded plastic orthotic cervical collar (Fig. 17.51). Reduction of *displaced fracture-dislocations of the atlantoaxial joint* is best accomplished by continuous skull traction through a "halo" that is attached to the skull by screws (Fig. 17.52). After 1 month of skull traction, the fracture is usually sufficiently stable that a plaster cast or a plastic collar can be applied to immobilize the cervical spine for an additional 2 months. Even a fibrous union of the fracture may provide adequate stability; if it does not, however, local spinal fusion is indicated. In some patients, halo traction does not achieve adequate reduction of the fracture dislocation, in which case open reduction and internal fixation are required.

Compression Fracture of a Cervical Vertebral Body

A flexion injury of the cervical spine without disruption of the posterior spinal ligaments may cause a compression or crush-type fracture of the cancellous bone of a vertebral body. The compression is most significant anteriorly, so that the vertebral body becomes wedge-shaped. The spinal cord is not injured and the fracture is stable.

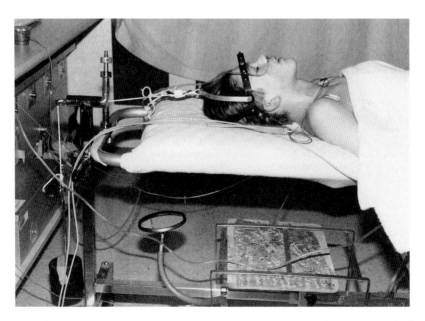

Figure 17.52.   Continuous skeletal traction through a "halo" attached to screws in the outer table of the skull for unstable fractures, dislocations, and fracture-dislocations of the cervical spine.

Treatment. Reduction of a wedge compression fracture of the cervical spine is neither necessary nor advisable. Support of the cervical spine in a plastic collar provides comfort for the patient during the 3 weeks required for bony healing (Fig. 17.51).

Flexion Subluxation of the Cervical Spine

When an individual's head moves forward suddenly and violently, as it does with the instant *deceleration* of a head-on collision or from a blow on the back of the head, one vertebral body in the lower half of the cervical spine may slide forward in relation to the subjacent vertebra. The posterior longitudinal ligaments are disrupted but, provided the posterior facet joints do not override, the injury is classified as a *subluxation*. The subluxation may reduce spontaneously, however, and initial radiographs may not reveal the true extent of the injury—hence the value of stress radiography to detect occult joint instability (Fig. 17.53A and B).

The spinal cord may be contused at the moment of injury but usually escapes serious injury unless the spinal canal has been narrowed by pre-existent osteophytes associated with degenerative joint disease of the cervical spine (cervical spondylosis).

Treatment. Passive extension of the cervical spine reduces the flexion type of subluxation and the reduction should be maintained by immobilization of the extended neck in a plastic collar for at least 2 months. If ligamentous healing is inadequate, the resultant residual instability of the injured segment may cause symptoms of sufficient severity that local spine fusion becomes necessary (Fig. 17.53C).

Flexion Dislocation and Fracture-Dislocation of the Cervical Spine

In these injuries, which are more severe and much more serious than a flexion subluxation but which arise from the same mechanisms of injury, the posterior longitudinal ligaments

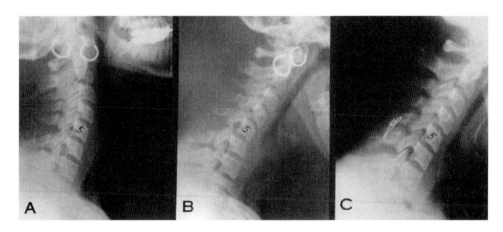

Figure 17.53. Flexion subluxation of the cervical spine at the C5-6 level in a young woman who had been injured in a head-on automobile collision. **A.** The initial lateral radiograph does not reveal any frank evidence of a fracture or a dislocation, but note the widening of the space between the spinous processes of C5 and C6 and the soft tissue swelling between the trachea and the cervical spine at the C5-C6 level. Both are clues that the cervical spine has been injured at this level. **B.** A lateral radiograph taken with the patient's neck in flexion (under the control of the surgeon and with the patient conscious) reveals a true flexion subluxation between C5 and C6. Note the gap between these two spinous processes indicating disruption of the posterior longitudinal ligaments. Note also that the posterior facet joints, although subluxated, have not overriden. These two radiographs serve as a good example of occult joint instability in the spine and emphasize the value of stress radiography. **C.** A lateral radiograph of the same woman's cervical spine after local posterior spinal fusion of C5 to C6. Fusion was necessitated by persistent segmental instability and pain. Stronger internal fixation devices for spinal fusion have replaced the wire loop seen in this radiograph.

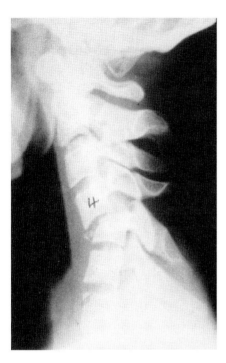 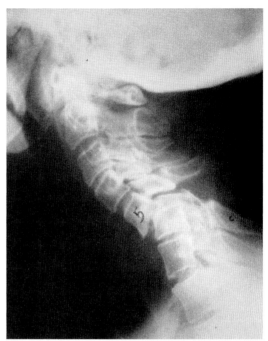

Figure 17.54.   Left. Flexion fracture-dislocation of the cervical spine at the C4-C5 level in a young man who had dived into shallow water and struck the back of his head on the bottom. He had an incomplete paraplegia. Note the forward displacement of C4 on C5, the fracture of the body of C5, the locked posterior facet joints, and the wide gap between the spinous processes of C4 and C5, indicating disruption of the posterior longitudinal ligaments.

Figure 17.55.   Right. Flexion dislocation of the cervical spine at the C5-C6 level in a young woman who at the time of a head-on automobile accident was thrown from her car and landed on the back of her head. She was not wearing a seat belt! The initial radiographs were said to have been normal, but 3 days after injury the patient became partially paraplegic; these radiographs reveal a complete dislocation. Note the forward displacement of C5 on C6, the complete loss of contact between the posterior facet joints, and the wide gap between the spinous processes, indicating complete disruption of the posterior longitudinal ligaments at this level. After gradual reduction of this extremely unstable dislocation by skull traction, a local posterior spinal fusion was performed and the patient's neurological lesion recovered.

are torn and the posterior facet on one or both sides has lost contact with its mate. The facet joints may be overriding and locked or they may be widely separated. There is usually a coexistent fracture of the anterior margin of the subjacent vertebra (Figs. 17.54 and 17.55).

This exceedingly unstable injury is frequently complicated by either complete transection or severe contusion of the spinal cord with resultant paraplegia.

If the dislocation or fracture-dislocation is at the C7-T1 level, it is difficult to visualize in a lateral radiograph because the patient's shoulders block the view. This problem can be overcome by taking the lateral radiograph with one shoulder elevated and the other depressed (the "swimmer's projection").

Treatment. Reduction of a flexion dislocation or fracture-dislocation of the cervical spine may be difficult, particularly if the facet joints are locked in an overriding position. Powerful continuous skull traction through a halo device (Fig. 17.52) under radiographic control is required—if necessary up to 40 lb. of traction—to distract the facet joints after which reduction is achieved by gradual extension of the neck and decreasing the amount of traction. The reduced dislocation or fracture-dislocation should then be immobilized in extension in a halo cast brace for at least 2 months.

Failure to obtain a complete reduction by continuous traction is an indication for open reduction. Residual instability after the period of immobilization is an indication for local spinal fusion. There is some justification for the opinion that local spinal fusion is indicated within a few days of the reduction of every major dislocation or fracture-dislocation of the cervical spine to prevent both residual symptoms and recurrent displacement from a subsequent injury.

Extension Sprains of the Cervical Spine

Whereas flexion injuries may produce a flexion subluxation, dislocation, or fracture-dislocation as described above, *extension* injuries tend to produce extension *sprains,* some of which may represent *momentary subluxations.*

Mechanism of Injury. By far the most common cause of significant extension injuries of the cervical spine in the present era is the rear-end collision. The mechanism of injury is as follows: an individual is sitting facing forward in a stopped automobile (for example at a traffic light), his or her back supported by the back of the seat but the head completely unsupported. At this moment, the automobile is suddenly struck from the rear by a moving automobile. It is shot forward with considerable force and is instantly *accelerated.* The body of the individual in the struck automobile is instantly accelerated also, but the unsupported head is momentarily left behind with the result that the cervical spine is suddenly forced into extreme extension. Thus, the soft tissues on the anterior aspect of the neck are stretched and sprained. The severity of the sprain depends on the rate of acceleration of the individual's body, which in turn depends on the force of impact and the rate of acceleration of his or her automobile when it was struck from the rear.

Terminology. These common injuries, which are best considered and described as *acceleration extension sprains* of the neck, are regrettably often referred to, especially in both lay and legal circles, as "whiplash injuries," a term that is both inaccurate and misleading (the head and neck are hardly comparable to the end of a whip). Moreover, the use of the emotional and dramatic term "whiplash" tends to exaggerate the seriousness of the injury and leads to unrealistic litigation. The injury should be considered for what it is, namely a *sprain* of the neck, in the full realization that some sprains are more severe than others and some even represent momentary subluxation.

Clinical Features. The patient experiences pain that is not well localized in the front of the neck, and sometimes pain radiating into the upper limbs from nerve root irritation. As with other sprains, the pain may not be particularly severe at the time of injury but becomes more severe during the ensuing few days. Neck motion, especially extension, is guarded by muscle spasm. In the majority of patients with acceleration extension sprains of the neck, the symptoms are of relatively short duration but for others with more severe sprains, the symptoms may persist for 6 months, 1 year or even longer. Those relatively few patients with particularly severe injuries may complain of symptoms that seem bizarre but are explainable, in that many different structures can be stretched at the time of injury. Thus, Macnab suggested that blurring of vision and vertigo might be explained on the basis of injury to the cervical sympathetic nerves; difficulty in swallowing could be due to hemorrhage in the wall of the oral pharynx and esophagus; nystagmus and tinnitus might be due to vertebral artery spasm.

Radiographic Features. Despite the plethora of symptoms, there is a paucity of abnormal radiographic findings. The usual radiographic examination is negative, although it is possible that stress radiography of the neck in extension might reveal evidence of occult segmental instability at one or more intervertebral disc spaces in the cervical spine.

Treatment. As with other sprains, the initial treatment of acceleration extension sprains of the neck includes splinting and analgesics. Appropriate splinting can be provided by two,

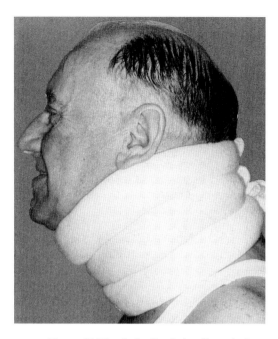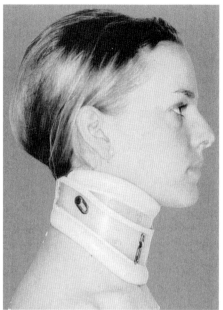

Figure 17.56. Left. Cervical ruffs made from stockinette filled with cotton wool. These three ruffs are supporting the head and providing relative immobilization of the cervical spine for this man, who had sustained an acceleration extension sprain of his neck in a rear-end collision.

Figure 17.57. Right. Adjustable and removable plastic collar for the support of stable injuries, such as an acceleration extension sprain, of the cervical spine. The collar can be adjusted to provide immobilization in a more flexed position for an extension injury.

three or even four cervical ruffs (Fig. 17.56). If symptoms persist after the acute phase, a removable plastic cervical collar usually provides adequate splinting (Fig. 17.57). When the injury has been particularly severe, the patient should lie in bed for 2 weeks or more, to take the weight of the head off the neck. Persistent neck and arm pain can be relieved temporarily by intermittent cervical traction, which can be readily applied by the patient at home (Fig. 17.58).

Patients who have sustained other significant injuries at the time of neck injury frequently complain of their neck long after symptoms have subsided from the other injuries. Thus, they should not be lightly dismissed as being "neurotic" or "litigation minded." Such patients must be reassured that their neck symptoms, although irritating and discouraging, will eventually subside. Only a very small percentage of these patients

ever require local spinal fusion for residual segmental instability.

Prevention. From your understanding of the mechanism of injury in acceleration extension injuries of the neck, you will appreciate that the most effective method of *prevention* is incorporation of head rests in the backs of all automobile seats. Such head rests prevent the sudden extension of the neck of an individual whose automobile has been struck from behind in a rear-end collision.

Fracture of the Seventh Cervical Spinous Process

The spinous process of the seventh cervical vertebra is longer than others in the cervical spine and to it are attached a multitude of muscles. As a result of sudden violent muscular contraction, this spinous process may be avulsed. The fracture is sometimes referred to as a "clay shoveler's fracture," because it is

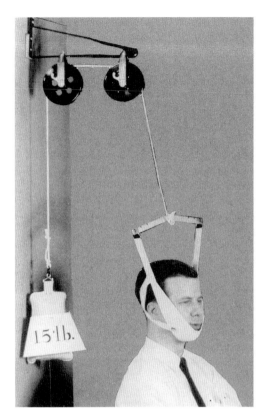

Figure 17.58. Apparatus for applying intermittent halter traction to the cervical spine. This form of treatment, which often provides temporary relief of pain, can be carried out in the patient's home.

relatively common in workmen who are shoveling wet clay that unexpectedly sticks to the shovel at the end of the backward throw. The fracture may also occur during vigorous athletics. Clinically, the patient experiences local pain and there is well-localized tenderness. The diagnosis is readily confirmed radiographically (Fig. 17.59).

Treatment. Pain can usually be relieved by cervical ruffs that prevent flexion and extension of the cervical spine (Fig.17.56), but bed rest may be necessary for a few days. Occasionally surgical excision of the avulsed spinous process is required to relieve persistent pain.

Injuries of the Thoracic and Lumbar Spine

Fractures of the thoracic and lumbar spine are relatively common, particularly in the thoracolumbar region. The most common fractures

are of the compression type, either *wedge compression* or *bursting compression,* and are stable injuries. They are usually caused by a fall from a considerable height onto the buttocks or the feet.

Less common but more serious are fracture-dislocations of the spine that are usually caused by automobile accidents. Because these are *unstable* injuries, either the spinal cord or the cauda equina is frequently damaged. The important topic of *traumatic paraplegia* is discussed in Chapter 12.

Wedge Compression Fractures

When the spine is in the flexed position, compression forces from below (as with a severe fall on the buttocks) or from above (as with a cave-in on a crouching miner) cause the spine to suddenly flex beyond its normal range. The compression is greatest on the concavity of the curve and the anterior portions of the vertebral bodies. The posterior longitudinal ligaments remain intact and one or more vertebral bodies are crushed anteriorly, the result being a *wedge compression fracture* with anterior impaction.

Clinically, the symptoms may be mild, but there is local tenderness. The impaction is seen most readily in the lateral radiograph (Fig. 17.60).

Treatment. Because wedge compression fractures are stable injuries and because the spinal cord and cauda equina are not injured, relatively little treatment is required. For the young it may be reasonable to hyperextend the spine in an attempt to correct the slight kyphosis at the fracture site and then to apply

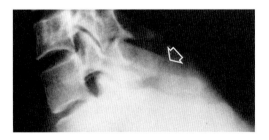

Figure 17.59. Avulsion fracture of the spinous process of C7 (so-called "clay shoveler's fracture"). The patient, a professional wrestler, sustained this fracture as he attempted to throw his reluctant opponent out of the ring.

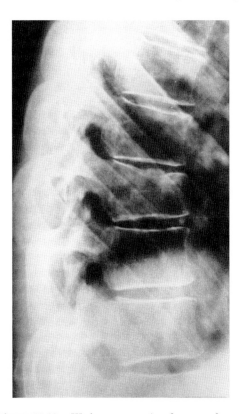

Figure 17.60. Wedge compression fracture of a vertebral body in the midthoracic region of a 35-year-old man who had slipped at the top of the stairs and bounced down one flight on his buttocks. Note that the injured vertebral body has lost height and become wedge shaped as a result of being compressed anteriorly. This is a stable injury.

a body cast. In general, however, it is wiser to allow the fracture to heal in its impacted state. If the symptoms are mild, a short period of bed rest followed by active exercises are all that are required. For more severe injuries, the patient's pain can be relieved by wearing a body cast for 4 weeks, during which time active exercises are performed. In the elderly, particularly with compression fractures through either osteoporotic bone or metastases, a spinal brace or reinforced surgical corset for the relief of pain is more practical.

Vertical Compression Burst Fractures
When the spine is relatively straight (as with a fall from a height and landing on the feet), compression forces are vertical and the result is a burst type of fracture of a vertebral body.

The intervertebral disc is driven into the cancellous bone of the vertebral body, and comminuted fracture fragments burst out in all directions. Nevertheless, the posterior spinal ligaments are intact and the spina column is relatively stable. The spinal cord and cauda equina may be injured by a bony posterior fragment that has been driven backward and encroaches on the spinal canal.

Clinically, the symptoms are more severe from a compression burst fracture than from a simple wedge compression fracture. The patient's heels should be examined both clinically and radiographically—the aforementioned mechanism of injury explains the common coexistence of a fracture of the os calcis. Radiographs reveal the bursting nature of the fracture, while both MRI and CT scans demonstrate any retropulsion of a bony fragment into the spinal canal (Fig. 17.61).

Treatment. Usually, no reduction of the fracture is required. However, if there is retropulsion of a bony fragment into the spinal canal and an associated neurological deficit, surgical excision of the fragment is required to obtain an adequate decompression of the spinal cord or cauda equina. The patient is usually most comfortable lying in bed for the first few weeks, after which he or she should wear a well-fitted plaster body cast for 8 weeks. Occasionally, residual segmental instability causes chronic low back pain of such severity that local spinal fusion is justified.

Fracture-Dislocations
Violent spinal injuries, such as may be sustained in automobile accidents, have a rotatory and sometimes a lateral force superimposed on a flexion force. The spine is literally torn apart. The posterior longitudinal ligaments are torn, the posterior facet joints may be fractured, the upper part of the involved vertebral body seems to be sheared off, and the spinal column is dislocated and completely unstable. In the thoracic region the spinal cord is almost always injured and is frequently completely transected. In the lumbar region, the cauda equina is usually damaged but not necessarily transected.

Clinical features include shock from the severity of the injury. Some degree of neurologi-

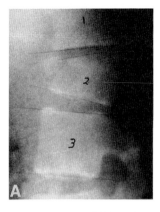
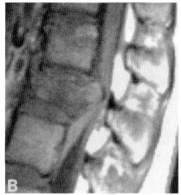
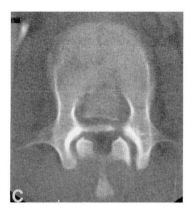

Figure 17.61.   Vertical compression burst fracture of the second lumbar vertebra of a 40-year-old man who, while attempting to escape from a prison at night with more haste than decorum, had jumped from a third-story window and landed in a vertical position on his feet. (He also sustained bilateral os calcis fractures). He had a significant neurological deficit. **A.** Note that the intervertebral disc space between the first and second lumbar vertebra is narrowed, indicating that disc material has been driven into the second lumbar vertebra. **B.** The lateral MRI reveals that bone and disc material have been driven backward to encroach on the spinal canal. **C.** The CT scan reveals significant encroachment on the spinal canal by a retropulsed fracture fragment from the burst vertebral body. Surgical excision of this fracture fragment was required to decompress this man's spinal canal, after which his neurological injury recovered.

cal deficit is usually obvious. Complete neurological examination is essential and must be repeated frequently during the first few days to detect any changes in the neurological picture. Radiographic examination depicts the gravity of the injury (Fig. 17.62).

Treatment. Management of an associated *traumatic paraplegia* (as discussed in Chapter 12), of course, takes precedence over treatment of the fracture-dislocation.

In the absence of paraplegia, the fracture-dislocation must be reduced with care and the spine stabilized to prevent subsequent neurological damage. Open reduction, rigid internal fixation, and the addition of bone grafts are indicated (Fig. 17.63).

Even in the presence of complete paraplegia, early open reduction, rigid internal fixation (including pedicle screws), and bone grafting reduce the risk of subsequent injury to nerve roots that may have been spared. Moreover, this form of treatment greatly facilitates nursing care, diminishes the incidence of decubitus ulcers, and renders the early phases of rehabilitation more effective.

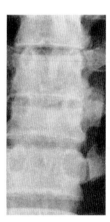
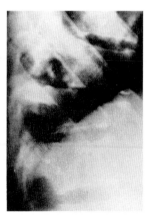

Figure 17.62.   Severe fracture-dislocation of the thoracic spine at the T9-T10 level in a 24-year-old man whose speeding sports car went out of control and hit a tree. This man was rendered completely and permanently paraplegic. Note the forward displacement of T9 and T10 and the sheared off upper part of the body of T10 in the lateral projection. The posterior longitudinal ligaments were completely disrupted and the spine was completely unstable.

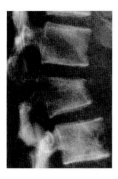 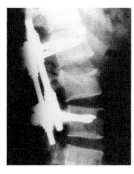

Figure 17.63. Severe fracture-dislocation between the first and second lumbar vertebrae of a 38-year-old woman who was involved in a high-speed automobile accident and who sustained a neurological injury. **Left.** Note the anterior displacement of the first lumbar vertebra and the compression of the second lumbar vertebra. **Right.** Lateral postoperative radiograph. The dislocation has been reduced and a two-level spinal fusion has been performed using an AO internal fixation device with pedicle screws. This patient's neurological injury recovered.

Thorax

Fractures of the Ribs

The ribs, being flat bones (as opposed to long bones), are composed of cancellous bone surrounded by thin cortices. As you might expect, fractured ribs heal readily despite the continued movement of breathing; nonunion is almost unknown.

Ribs are fractured by either striking or being struck by a hard object. Unless the injury is extremely severe, the fractured ends are seldom displaced because the ribs are firmly bound to one another by the intercostal muscles. Clinically there is local pain that is aggravated by deep breathing, coughing, and sneezing. Local tenderness is readily detected and the pain is increased by anteroposterior compression of the chest (which "springs" the ribs outward). The fractures are usually, but not always, readily visualized radiographically (Fig. 17.64).

Treatment

The chest wall cannot be completely immobilized. Circumferential strapping of the chest does minimize movement and provides some relief of pain, although the strapping may be irksome in itself. In the elderly, strapping of the chest is inadvisable because of the risk of hypostatic pneumonia. Injection of the regional intercostal nerves with a long-acting anesthetic agent often provides lasting comfort.

Complications of rib fractures include: 1) puncture of the pleura with a resultant hemothorax; 2) puncture of the lung with resultant pneumothorax; 3) contusion of the underlying lung (Fig. 17.65).

The Foot

Fractures of the Metatarsals

The metatarsals are most commonly fractured by either a heavy object dropping on the forefoot or a run-over injury with a metal wheel. Frequently more than one metatarsal is fractured, in which case the most significant aspects of the injury are not the fractures but the internal hemorrhage and impairment of circulation to the forefoot (Fig. 17.66).

Treatment

The metatarsal fragments should be sufficiently well aligned that no metatarsal head is left depressed into the sole (in which position it could cause a painful callus later). Pressure dressings and elastic bandages must be avoided because of the swelling and the resultant impaired circulation that may lead to compartment syndromes in the forefoot. A well-padded plaster cast is preferable. Occasionally Kirschner wire fixation is required to stabilize multiple fractures. After a period of at least 4 weeks of non-weightbearing, a walking cast can be worn for an additional 4 weeks.

Lisfranc's Fracture-Dislocations of the Tarsometatarsal Joints

A variety of uncommon fracture-dislocations of tarsometatarsal joints (with or without metatarsal fractures) are caused by a severe injury, either direct or indirect. The diagnosis is frequently missed but if an injury to the midfoot is suspected clinically, a standing "stress" radiograph helps to establish the diagnosis. The most significant dislocation or subluxation is at the cuneiform-second metatarsal joint. To achieve permanent stability of the tarsometatarsal joints (known collectively as the "Lisfranc joint"), accurate closed—or if necessary,

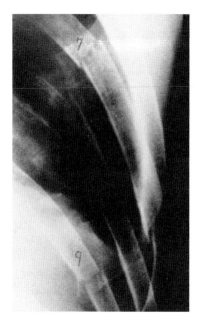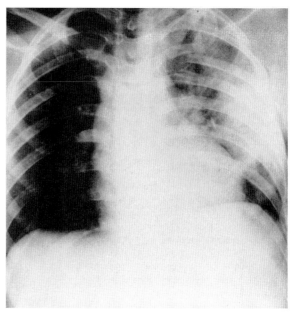

Figure 17.64.   Left. Undisplaced fractures of the 7th, 8th and 9th left ribs in a 50-year-old man who had slipped while getting out of the bathtub and struck the left side of his chest on the edge of the tub.

Figure 17.65.   Right. Contusion of the left lung in association with fractures of six ribs (second, third, fourth, fifth, sixth, and seventh) in a 54-year-old man who had been knocked down by an automobile. Note the diffuse radiographic density in the upper two thirds of the left lung.

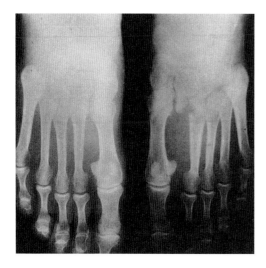

Figure 17.66. Displaced fractures at the base of the left second, third, and fourth metatarsals and an undisplaced fracture of the base of the first metatarsal in a workman whose foot had been run over by one metal wheel of a heavy trolley. The foot was grossly swollen and the circulation to the toes was temporarily impaired.

open—reduction and internal skeletal fixation with screws are required. The screws should not be removed for at least 6 months.

Fractures of the Os Calcis (Calcaneum)

The os calcis, which is composed principally of cancellous bone with a thin surrounding cortex, has a good blood supply and for these reasons fractures of this bone unite rapidly. The major problem related to these fractures is coexistent *intra-articular injury to the subtalar joint.*

The usual mechanism of injury is a fall from a considerable height onto one or both heels. Thus, both heels should always be carefully examined. Moreover, there is a high incidence of associated compression fractures of the spine that should also be examined both clinically and radiographically in every patient who has sustained a fracture of the os calcis.

In the normal os calcis, the superior surface of the tuberosity and that of the subtalar joint meet at an angle of approximately 40 de-

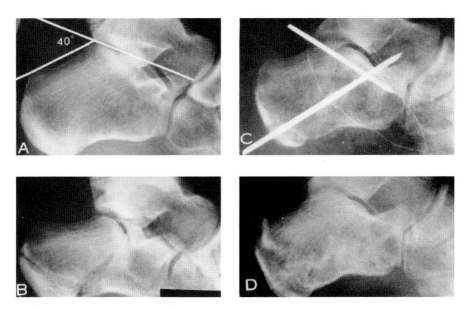

Figure 17.67. Intra-articular fracture of the os calcis in a young man who, while on a psychedelic drug "trip," took an unplanned trip from a second-story balcony to the pavement and landed on his left heel. **A.** Lateral radiograph of the patient's normal, uninjured heel showing the normal tuberosity-joint angle or salient angle of 40 degrees. **B.** Comminuted fracture of the patient's injured os calcis. The lateral portion of the subtalar joint is split off and depressed. The tuberosity-joint angle has been decreased to 20 degrees as a result of compression of the os calcis. **C.** Immediately after open reduction of the fractures, internal fixation with Kirschner wires, and packing of the resultant defect on the lateral side with cancellous bone grafts. Note that the tuberosity-joint angle has been restored. **D.** Three months after injury, the fractures have united in satisfactory position.

grees—the *tuberosity-joint angle* or *salient angle* (Fig. 17.67A). When the os calcis is crushed between the landing surface and the undersurface of the talus at the time of the fall, it is flattened somewhat and this angle is decreased or even reversed. The os calcis either splits into two or more major fragments or becomes severely comminuted into innumerable fragments. Because the subtalar joint is the most important structure in relation to fractures of the os calcis, it is best to consider such fractures in two main groups: those that do not involve the joint (*extra-articular fractures*) and those that do (*intra-articular fractures*). Special radiographic projections and CT imaging are required to visualize the os calcis in three planes.

Extra-Articular Fractures

Vertical split fractures of the tuberosity of the os calcis and horizontal "beak" fractures of the tuberosity are manifest by severe local pain and inability to bear weight. There is little swelling, however, and subtalar joint motion is not impaired.

Treatment. For *vertical split fractures,* the two major fragments should be manually compressed from side to side under anesthesia. The foot is kept elevated for 1 week, after which a well-molded plaster walking cast can be worn for 6 weeks. For the *horizontal beak type of fracture* the same period of elevation of the foot is required, but the foot is held in equinus in the walking cast to prevent further displacement. The results of treatment for extra-articular fractures are good.

Intra-Articular Fractures

Fractures in which the lateral part of the subtalar joint is split off and *severely comminuted crush fractures* both involve the subtalar joint and are much more serious than extra-articu-

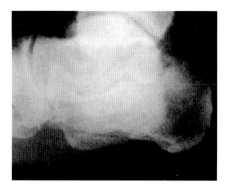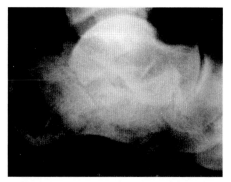

Figure 17.68.   Severely comminuted fractures of both os calci of a 41-year-old firefighter who fell 30 feet from a ladder and landed on his feet. (He also sustained a compression burst fracture of his lumbar spine.) This man's subtalar joints are irreparably damaged. After 2 weeks of elevation of both feet, delayed primary arthrodesis of both subtalar joints was performed.

lar fractures. In addition to the aforementioned symptoms, typical physical signs include significant swelling, broadening, and loss of height of the heel and painfully restricted motion in the subtalar joint. Radiographs are essential in the differentiation of these two major types of intra-articular fracture (Figs. 17.67B and 17.68). Assessment by CT imaging is very helpful.

Treatment. The only fractures of the os calcis amenable to open reduction and internal fixation are those in which *the lateral portion of the subtalar joint is split off and depressed*. Internal skeletal fixation is used to maintain the reduction. At open reduction, the depressed portion of the joint surface is elevated and bone grafts are packed into the resultant defect (Fig. 17.67C). A plaster cast is worn for 6 weeks but no weightbearing is permitted until the fracture is united.

The *severely comminuted crush fractures* of the os calcis are not amenable to reduction (Fig. 17.68). *Nonoperative* treatment of this severe injury involves elevation of the foot for at least 1 week and active exercises, followed by gradually increasing weightbearing using crutches as soon as the acute pain has subsided. The results of this form of treatment are not good in that the heel remains broad, the subtalar joint is stiff (and often painful), and there is decreased calf muscle power (as a result of elevation of the tuberosity and con-

sequent slackness in the muscle). Most patients do manage to walk about, however, with some residual symptoms within 6 months. An *operative* form of treatment for these severely comminuted crush fractures is delayed primary arthrodesis of the subtalar joint 2 or 3 weeks after injury. Weightbearing is not allowed for at least 3 months, by which time the joint is usually fused. The results of such operative treatment, particularly for persons younger than 60 years of age, would seem to be somewhat better than the results of nonoperative treatment. At least one source of residual pain, the subtalar joint, has been eliminated.

Regardless of the method of treatment, residual symptoms are likely to arise and persist from the severely damaged fat pad under the os calcis and from impingement of the broadened os calcis against the articular surface of the medial malleolus, the lateral malleolus, or both.

Fractures of the Neck of the Talus

The talus, like the carpal scaphoid, has no muscles attached to it, is largely covered by articular cartilage, and has a precarious blood supply. It is not surprising therefore, that fractures of the neck of the talus are associated with a high incidence of avascular necrosis of one fragment (the body) and nonunion.

The mechanism of injury is a severe dorsi-

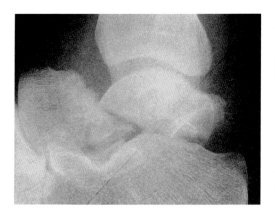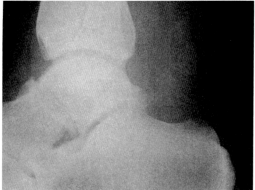

Figure 17.69.   Displaced fracture of the neck of the talus in the right foot of a young man who had his foot pressed hard on the brake pedal at the moment of a head-on collision. **Left.** Initial radiograph showing upward displacement and dorsiflexion of the foot through the fracture. **Right.** The postreduction radiograph reveals satisfactory position of the fracture fragments

flexion injury as may be incurred when the driver of an automobile has his foot pressed hard on the brake pedal at the moment of a head-on collision. If the injury is extremely severe, the body of the talus may even be dislocated posteriorly.

Treatment
Closed reduction can usually be achieved by bringing the foot, and with it the head of the talus, into equinus (Fig. 17.69). Nevertheless, internal skeletal fixation is frequently necessary to maintain the reduction. The foot and ankle are then immobilized in this position in a below-knee cast for at least 8 weeks and no weightbearing is permitted during this time.

Complications
Avascular necrosis of the body of the talus complicates approximately half of all displaced fractures of the neck of the talus. The body first becomes relatively dense radiographically and eventually becomes absolutely dense as revascularization takes place and new bone is laid down on dead trabeculae (Fig. 17.70). Despite relief of weightbearing for many months, this complication almost inevitably leads to *degenerative joint disease of both the ankle and the subtalar joints,* necessitating arthrodesis of these joints. Nonunion of the fractured neck of the talus is treated by bone

grafting, provided the body of the talus is viable.

The Ankle
The normal ankle joint moves in one plane only—the plane of plantar flexion and dorsiflexion—and thus it is not surprising that the forces of abduction, adduction, external and internal rotation to which the ankle is so frequently subjected may tear ligaments or produce intra-articular fractures. Indeed, in adults, the ankle is the most frequently injured major joint in the body.

Sprains of the Lateral Ligament
The common "sprained ankle" is nearly always the result of an inversion injury. An individual steps on an uneven surface and the foot is forcibly inverted through the subtalar joint and adducted through the ankle joint. The lateral ligament is severely stretched and a few fibers may even be torn, but the inherent stability of the ankle is not lost.

Clinically, the ankle is painful. Localized tenderness and swelling can be detected inferior and anterior to the tip of the lateral malleolus. Radiographic examination is necessary to differentiate a simple sprain from an undisplaced fracture of the fibula and, if the stability of the ankle is doubtful, stress radiography under local or general anesthesia is indicated

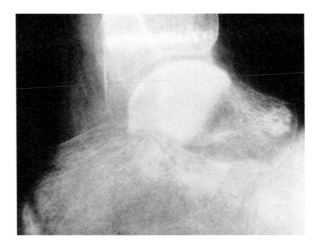

Figure 17.70.   Avascular necrosis of the body of the talus as a complication of a fracture through the neck. In this radiograph, 9 months after injury, the increased radiographic density in the body of the talus is both relative (to the surrounding living bone that has become osteoporotic from disuse) and absolute (in relation to the normal opposite talus inasmuch as, with revascularization, new bone has been laid down on dead trabeculae).

to exclude a tear of the lateral ligament (Fig. 17.71).

Treatment
Simple sprains of the lateral ligament require only adhesive strapping of the ankle to provide external support for 3 weeks, as discussed in Chapter 15 (Fig. 15.97). Weightbearing is permitted immediately and full recovery may be expected.

Tears of the Lateral Ligament
The same mechanism of injury that produces a sprain of the lateral ligament may completely tear the lateral ligament if the injury is sufficiently severe. In order for the ligament to be completely torn, the ankle joint must have been momentarily subluxated or even dislocated.

The clinical features are comparable to those of a sprain, but the swelling is greater and the joint is unstable. Radiographic examination is necessary to exclude a fracture, and stress radiography under local or general anesthesia is essential to detect the degree of ankle instability (Fig. 17.71). The uninjured ankle should be similarly assessed for comparison.

Treatment
A complete tear of the lateral ligament of the ankle is a serious injury and can be more trou-

blesome later than a fracture, because bone heals more firmly than ligaments. The foot and ankle should be immobilized in a below-knee walking cast in a position of eversion and valgus for at least 8 weeks. After the first week when the swelling has subsided, the cast should be changed to obtain a better fit and better control of the ankle.

There is no evidence that surgical repair of this ligament offers any advantage over non-operative treatment.

Complications
If healing of the torn lateral ligament is inadequate, the patient will be plagued by *recurrent subluxation or even dislocation of the ankle*, particularly when walking on uneven ground. Simple measures such as an outflared heel and outside heel and sole wedge in the shoe may control this problem but more often, a new lateral ligament must be constructed surgically by means of a tenodesis using the tendon of the peroneus brevis muscle.

Total Rupture of the Achilles' Tendon
Sudden passive dorsiflexion of the ankle that is resisted by a powerful contraction of the calf muscle in an adult may result in a complete rupture of the Achilles' tendon (tendo Achillis, calcaneal tendon). Most often the re-

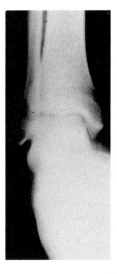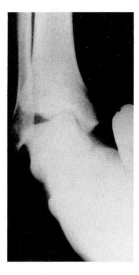

Figure 17.71.   Occult joint instability. **Left.** Anteroposterior radiograph of the ankle of a football player who, after an injury of his ankle, had pain, swelling, and local tenderness over the lateral aspect of the joint. The radiographic examination of the joint is normal but this does not exclude occult joint instability. **Right.** Anteroposterior radiograph of the same ankle while it is being stressed (stress radiograph) with the patient under general anesthesia. Note the marked opening up of the ankle joint (talar tilt) on the lateral side, indicating joint instability associated with a complete tear of the lateral ligament of the ankle. The stress simulates the original injury. (The radiopaque object medial to the medial malleolus is the thumb of the lead glove that is shielding the surgeon's hand from radiation).

sult of strenuous athletic activities, such ruptures can also occur from simple running or jumping, especially in middle-aged adults. Previous intratendinous injections of corticosteroid for tendinitis definitely cause local degenerative changes and predispose the tendon to rupture.

The patient, usually a male, experiences severe local pain and is unable to walk on his toes. Clinical examination reveals a gap in the tendon approximately 5 cm proximal to its insertion. Normally when an individual's calf is squeezed, the ankle plantar flexes but not when the tendon is ruptured (Thompson's sign).

Some years ago, nonoperative treatment consisting of prolonged immobilization of the foot in a plantar flexed (equinus) position was advocated by many but in recent years, the results of early operative repair have been proven to be definitely superior to those of nonoperative treatment.

Fractures and Fracture-Dislocations of the Ankle

In adults, the distal ends of the tibia and fibula (which are best considered as a unit) are fractured more often than any other bone, with the exception of the distal end of the radius (Colles' fracture).

Mechanism of Injury

The wide variety of injuries can be more readily understood when you appreciate that the malleoli (medial malleolus, lateral malleolus, and posterior margin of the tibia—sometimes referred to as "the third malleolus") can be either sheared off or avulsed. *Shearing injuries* fracture a malleolus at or above the joint line, the fragment having been pushed off by the talus. *Avulsion injuries* fracture a malleolus below the joint line, the fragment having been pulled off by the attached ligament. Thus, an abduction injury may produce a shearing fracture of the lateral malleolus and an avulsion fracture of the medial malleolus. A rotational injury may shear off both malleoli, tear the distal tibiofibular ligament, and even shear off "the third malleolus." If the distal tibiofibular joint is disrupted, the ankle mortice is too wide and there is always a lateral shift of the talus.

The term "*Pott's fracture-dislocation*" is often rather loosely used to include most fractures and fracture-dislocations involving the malleoli of the ankle. Thus, a *first degree injury* involves one malleolus; a *second degree injury* involves two malleoli (or one malleolus and one ligament); and a *third degree injury* includes all three malleoli (or two malleoli and one ligament).

Clinical Features

Ankle fractures and fracture-dislocations are particularly painful and the patient is unable to bear weight on the injured ankle. The swelling is variable but is often gross. The clinical deformity depends on the specific injury but, when both malleoli are fractured, the entire

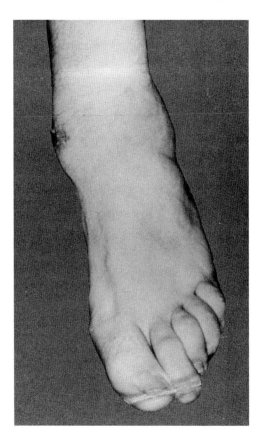

Figure 17.72.   Clinical deformity of a fracture-dislocation of the ankle. This patient had sustained a second-degree injury with fractures of both the medial and lateral malleoli. Note that the foot is displaced laterally and rotated externally in relation to the leg.

and thereby the talus, is placed in proper relationship with the distal end of the tibia by reversing the mechanism of injury, the malleoli are guided back into reasonable position. Although reduction of widely displaced fractures can usually be obtained, it may be difficult to maintain; therefore, internal fixation of both of the major fractures is usually required. Disruption of the distal tibiofibular joint must always be completely corrected, and such correction frequently necessitates internal fixation also.

Various specific fractures and fracture-dislocations are discussed below.

Isolated Fractures of the Medial Malleolus

An abduction injury may avulse the medial malleolus below the joint line, whereas an adduction injury may shear off the medial malleolus above the joint line. In either case, closed reduction is possible, but the reduction is often unstable. Unless the reduction is perfect by closed means, open reduction and screw fixation are indicated because there is frequently a flap of torn periosteum interposed between the fracture fragments (Fig. 17.73). A below-knee cast should be worn for 8 weeks

foot is displaced in relation to the leg (Fig. 17.72).

Radiographic Examination

Always include, in addition to the anteroposterior and lateral projections, two oblique projections lest the true extent of the injury escape detection.

Factors to Consider Concerning Treatment

Before discussion of the specific injuries, certain factors concerning treatment merit mention. The talus, which is still firmly attached to the foot, is the key to reduction of fractures and fracture-dislocations of the ankle, because the malleoli are attached to the talus through their ligaments. Thus, in general, if the foot,

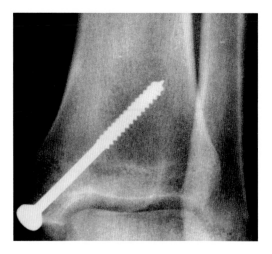

Figure 17.73.   Postreduction radiograph of the left ankle after open reduction of a displaced avulsion-type fracture of the medial malleolus and internal fixation with a lag screw (which compresses the fracture). At operation, a flap of periosteum was lifted out of the fracture site.

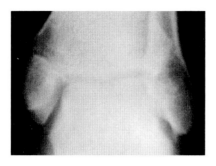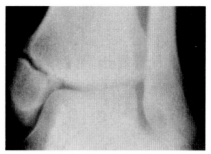

Figure 17.74.   Nonunion of a shearing-type fracture of the medial malleolus in a 30-year-old man. The nonunion is more clearly seen in the oblique projection "mortice view" (**right**) than in the anteroposterior projection (**left**).

and weightbearing may be permitted after the fourth week. A *complication* of the shearing type of medial malleolar fractures is *nonunion,* which necessitates bone grafting (Fig. 17.74).

Isolated Fractures of the Lateral Malleolus

In this, the most common injury of the ankle joint, the lateral malleolus is sheared off above the joint line by either an abduction or an external rotation injury. Closed reduction is usually satisfactory because the reduction is stable. Consequently, the only treatment required is immobilization of the ankle in a below-knee cast for 6 weeks. No weightbearing is permitted for at least 3 weeks, and often longer.

Fracture of the Lateral Malleolus and Tear of the Medial Ligament

In this common second-degree injury, which is also the result of either abduction or external rotation, the lateral malleolus is sheared off and the medial ligament of the ankle is torn so that the talus is displaced laterally. Radiographic examination reveals widening of the space between the talus and medial malleolus (Fig. 17.75). Closed reduction of the fractured malleolus and of the lateral displacement of the talus is usually satisfactory, but if the reduction is not perfect, open reduction and internal fixation of the fibula are indicated. A below-knee cast is worn for at least 6 weeks without weightbearing to allow firm healing of the ligament as well as of the fracture.

Fractures of Both Medial and Lateral Malleoli (Bimalleolar Fractures)

Severe injuries of either the abduction or external rotation type shear off the lateral malleolus above the joint line and avulse the medial malleolus below the joint line (Fig. 17.76). Although the displaced malleoli can usually be reduced by closed means, the reduction is not always stable. Under these circumstances (at least in young and middle-aged adults), stabilization requires open reduction and internal fixation of both malleoli. Immobilization in a below-knee cast is continued for at least 2 months. In elderly adults, the medial malleolar fragment may be too small and too osteoporotic for internal fixation, in which case closed reduction followed by cast immobilization is a more appropriate method of treatment.

Fractures of All Three Malleoli (Trimalleolar Fractures)

The addition of the posterior margin of the tibia as "the third malleolus" in this third-degree injury is only an indication that external rotation has been of such severity that the talus has moved posteriorly to shear off part of the posterior margin. In other respects this injury is comparable to the bimalleolar fracture and is treated in the same way (Fig. 17.77). The fracture of the posterior margin of the tibia is usually small and seldom merits open reduction unless it involves a significant part of the weightbearing surface.

Tibiofibular Separation

A severe abduction injury tears the tibiofibular ligament and either avulses the medial malleo-

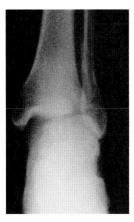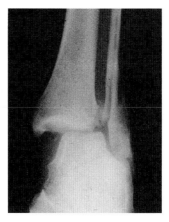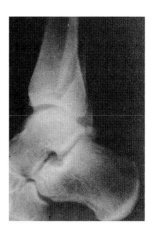

Figure 17.75.   Shearing-type fracture of the left lateral malleolus and lateral displacement of the talus in relation to the medial malleolus. **Left.** Lateral displacement of the talus is evident in the anteroposterior projection, but the fracture of the fibula is not obvious. **Center.** In this oblique projection, the fibular fracture is seen to start below the distal tibiofibular ligament, and there is no diastasis or separation of the tibiofibular syndesmosis. The lateral displacement of the talus is due to an associated tear of the medial ligament of the ankle. **Right.** In this lateral projection, what might be mistaken for a fracture of the posterior part of the tibia is the superimposed spiral fracture of the fibula.

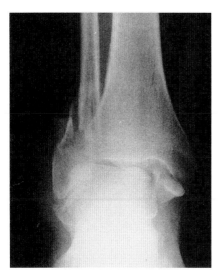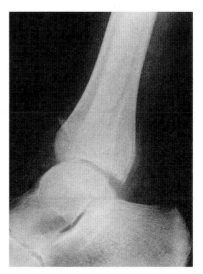

Figure 17.76.   Fracture of both medial and lateral malleoli of the right ankle (bimalleolar fracture). The combination of abduction and external rotation has avulsed the medial malleolus but has sheared off the lateral malleolus. As a result of this second-degree injury, the talus is displaced laterally in relation to the tibia. Open reduction and internal fixation are indicated for both displaced malleolar fractures, especially in young and middle-aged patients.

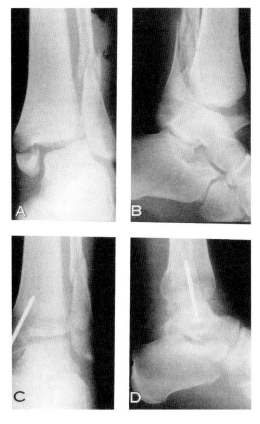

Vertical Compression Fractures of the Tibia

These so-called "pylon" fractures are caused by landing on the feet from a considerable height and may either split or shatter the distal end of the tibia with complete disruption of the ankle joint. If there are only a few main fragments, open reduction and rigid internal fixation may restore a reasonable joint surface (Fig. 17.79). The joint, however, may be irreparably damaged and the fracture too comminuted to secure by internal fixation. Under these circumstances the most reasonable form of treatment is delayed primary arthrodesis of the ankle.

Complications of Ankle Joint Injuries

Ankle *joint stiffness* is a residual problem that follows many of the above-described injuries. Active exercises help to regain motion and may have to be continued for as long as 1 year. An effective treatment of posttraumatic ankle joint stiffness is CPM with a gradually increas-

Figure 17.77. Fractures of all three malleoli (trimalleolar fracture) in the left ankle of a 36-year-old woman. **A.** Note the avulsion-type fracture of the medial malleolus, the lateral displacement of the talus, and the comminuted spiral fracture of the shaft of the fibula. **B.** In this lateral projection, the fracture of the posterior lip of the tibia ("the third malleolus") is apparent. **C and D.** Anteroposterior and lateral radiographs after open reduction of the fractured medial malleolus and internal fixation with a screw. Note that the other two fractures have been reduced and maintained in satisfactory position, although open reduction and open reduction for both medial and lateral malleoli would have been a reasonable alternative.

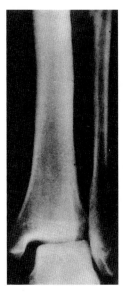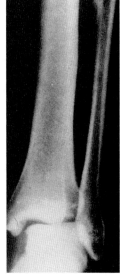

Figure 17.78. Tibiofibular separation of the left ankle in a 21-year-old skier who sustained an external rotation injury when his ankle harness failed to release. Note the lateral shift of the talus, which is more obvious in the anteroposterior projection (**left**) than in the oblique projection (**right**), and which indicates that the medial ligament of the ankle has been torn. Note also the separation or diastasis of the tibiofibular syndesmosis.

lus or tears the medial ligament (Fig. 17.78). In addition, there is usually a fracture in the shaft of the fibula proximally. The talus is shifted laterally, and reduction by closed means is usually unstable. A screw inserted across the tibiofibular syndesmosis is the most effective means of internal fixation. After immobilization in a below-knee cast for 8 weeks, the transfixion screw should be removed; otherwise it will eventually break as a result of subsequent motion at the tibiofibular joint.

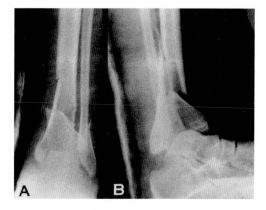

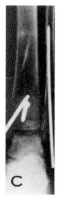
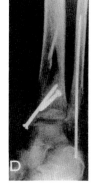
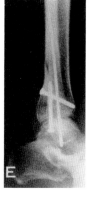

Figure 17.79.   Vertical compression fracture of the left tibia of a 30-year-old steeplejack who fell 25 feet from a scaffold. **A and B.** Initial radiographs with a temporary posterior plaster slab in place. Note the vertical fractures of the tibia and fibula with complete disruption of the ankle joint. **C, D, E.** Postoperative radiographs after open reduction and internal fixation of the tibial fractures with screws and the fibular fracture with a thin intramedullary nail. An alternative form of internal fixation would have been an AO buttress plate for the tibia and an AO plate for the fibula. Had the fractures been more comminuted, open reduction and internal fixation would not have been feasible.

The Leg
Fractures of the Shafts of the Tibia and Fibula

The shafts of the tibia and fibula are fractured more frequently than the shafts of any of the other long bones. In adults the periosteum covering the tibia is thin, especially over its subcutaneous border, and is readily torn across with the result that tibial shaft fractures are often widely displaced. Understandably, the incidence of open fractures of the subcutaneous tibia is high. Moreover, the rate of union in tibial shaft fractures is slow, particularly when there has been severe disruption of the periosteum and surrounding soft tissues. Open reduction of severely displaced fractures of the tibial shaft is fraught with complications related to additional disturbance of blood supply to the bone ends, unsatisfactory skin healing in a tensely swollen leg, and postoperative infection. Thus, in adults, fractures of the shaft of the tibia present many serious problems.

Mechanism of Injury

The leg (correctly defined as that part of the lower limb between the ankle and the knee) is particularly vulnerable to direct injury in automobile and motorcycle accidents. The forces are largely angulatory and the resultant fractures tend to be of the transverse or short oblique type—often with some comminution—the tibia and fibula being fractured at the same level. Rotational injuries of the tibia, which are common in skiers, tend to be oblique or spiral and may also be comminuted, but the periosteum is usually intact.

Clinical Features

Swelling is a prominent feature of combined tibial and fibular fractures and, because the fascial compartments of the leg are relatively closed spaces, internal swelling frequently causes one, or more, compartment syndromes that compromise the circulation to the intracompartmental muscles. The skin may become so stretched by the swelling that areas of the epidermis lose their nutrition and become lifted up from the dermis to form fracture blisters, as discussed in Chapter 15 (Fig. 15.58).

ing range of motion over a period of several weeks. Residual *swelling* of the soft tissues is almost inevitable and is difficult to prevent. After the period of immobilization, chronic swelling can be decreased, at least to some extent, by active exercises and by wearing an elastic stocking. *Nonunion* is rare (except for the medial malleolus), but *malunion* is relatively common, usually as a result of loss of position of fragments after closed reduction. *Degenerative joint disease* of the ankle is an almost inevitable sequela to malunion.

Radiographic Features

Unstable fractures of the tibia and fibula should always be temporarily splinted before the radiographic examination is conducted to prevent unnecessary pain and further damage to the soft tissues (Fig. 17.80). Four projections—anteroposterior, lateral and two obliques—are sometimes necessary to provide the best indication of the extent of the injury and the relationship of the fracture fragments to one another.

Treatment

When both the tibia and fibula are fractured, treatment is aimed at reduction of the tibia. Even a slight amount of residual angulation or slight rotation at the fracture site results in obvious deformities and should not be allowed to develop during treatment. Shortening of less than 2 cm is less serious as it can be well compensated by the patient while walking (with or without a lift in the heel of the shoe). The treatment of open fractures has been discussed in Chapter 15.

   Stable transverse, oblique, and spiral fractures of the shaft of the tibia can usually be well managed by closed means using the principle of the intact periosteal hinge (Fig. 17.81). When the mechanism of injury has been reversed and the fracture reduced, the intact periosteal hinge renders the reduction stable and prevents overreduction. The plaster cast must be applied in such a way that it holds the reduced fracture in the most stable position—just as the surgeon's hands were holding it. Therefore the cast should be applied first up to the knee (with the patient's leg

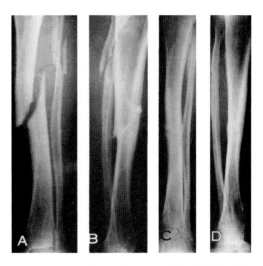

Figure 17.81.   Oblique fracture of the midshaft of the tibia and a comminuted fracture of the fibula at a higher level, the result of a rotational injury. **A and B.** Initial radiographs. Note the overriding of the tibial fragments. **C and D.** Four months after closed reduction and immobilization of the lower limb in a long leg cast. Both fractures are united in satisfactory position.

hanging over the edge of a table) and then carefully molded before it is extended to the top of the thigh with the knee flexed at least 30 degrees. Inclusion of the partially flexed knee in the long leg cast helps to control rotation at the fracture site. Union is usually well advanced within 3 to 4 months (Fig.17.81). An alternative form of treatment (for other than spiral fractures) involves the use of a close fitting long leg walking cast in which the patient is encouraged to bear weight within a few days or more when the acute soreness has subsided. Even comminuted fractures of the tibia treated with early weightbearing heal well, although there may be slight residual shortening (Fig. 17.82).

   Incomplete correction of an angulatory deformity or subsequent loss of alignment in a cast after swelling has subsided can be corrected by appropriate wedging of the cast. Sometimes it is preferable to remove the cast completely, correct the residual deformity, and apply a new, closely fitted cast.

   For many fractures of the shaft of the tibia an acceptable alternative method of treatment is *functional fracture-bracing* after an initial period of 3 to 4 weeks of cast immobilization

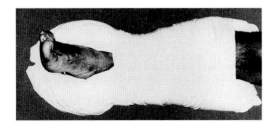

Figure 17.80.   Pillow splint for a fractured leg or ankle. There is less risk of circulatory disturbance and skin maceration with this type of splint than with an air splint.

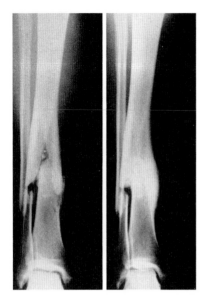

Figure 17.82. Comminuted fractures of the shafts of the tibia and fibula of a 22-year-old man who had been struck by an automobile while on his motorcycle. **Left.** The initial radiograph reveals shortening but satisfactory alignment. **Right.** The radiograph 6 months after closed treatment and early weightbearing in a long leg cast reveals firm union of the fractures with residual shortening of 2 cm. This amount of shortening is acceptable.

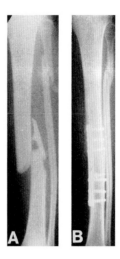

Figure 17.83.   A and B. Initial radiograph and radiograph 6 months after a comminuted fracture of the midshaft of the tibia and the fibula. Note the large "butterfly" fragment. The tibial fracture has been treated by open reduction and internal fixation using a plate and screws. The result is satisfactory but could have been achieved equally well by a locked intramedullary nail.

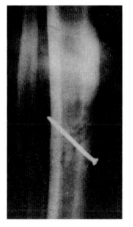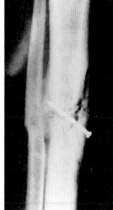

Figure 17.84. Closed oblique fracture of the tibia in a young adult. This simple fracture was treated by open reduction and inadequate internal fixation. **Left.** After operation a satisfactory reduction of the fracture. **Right.** Four months later, there is clear evidence of osteomyelitis, sequestra, and an infected nonunion.

including the knee joint temporarily as discussed in Chapter 15 (Fig. 15.41).

Unstable oblique and spiral fractures of the tibia are prone to angulate and shorten after closed reduction. For this reason open reduction has often been performed using the AO system of internal fixation. Although used less frequently now than in the past for fractures of the tibia, this is still a reasonable method of treatment, provided it is restricted to carefully selected patients and their fractures. (Fig. 17.83). As mentioned above, open reduction of tibial shaft fractures is fraught with *complications,* one of the most serious of which is postoperative infection with a resultant *infected nonunion* (Fig. 17.84).

Unstable transverse and markedly comminuted fractures of the tibial shaft are severe injuries that are associated with extensive soft tissue disruption. The latter accounts for their gross instability. Although these fractures could certainly benefit from being stabilized,

the risks of open reduction and internal fixation are particularly serious. These, the most serious of all fractures, should be treated with the least possible disturbance of the fracture site. Under primitive circumstances in which

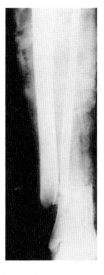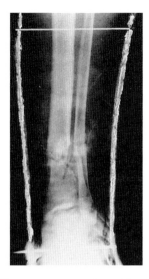

duced fracture site under radiographic control with an image intensifier.

Unstable segmental fractures of the tibial shaft are especially serious and can be difficult to control. Understandably these are often open fractures and are the result of an extremely severe injury. By means of external skeletal fixation "at a distance," these fractures can be stabilized; at the same time the associated soft tissue injuries are available for frequent inspections and are afforded the optimum opportunity to heal (Fig. 17.86).

Complications

Fractures of the shafts of both the tibia and fibula are frequently complicated. The most

Figure 17.85.   Unstable transverse comminuted fracture of the left tibia and fibula in a 30-year-old tree surgeon who, while treating a large tree, fell out of his patient! The 25-foot fall resulted in a severe fracture that was open from within. **Left.** This initial radiograph was obtained with a temporary posterior plaster splint in place. Note the comminution and that the proximal fragment must be protruding through the skin on the medial aspect of the leg. The periosteum had been severely torn and consequently the fracture was extremely unstable. **Right.** After complete cleansing and debridement of the open wound, reduction of the fractures, wound closure, and the insertion of two transfixation pins—one in the os calcis, the other in the proximal part of the tibia. The wound was managed by repeated debridements and delayed closure. Both pins have been incorporated in a light plaster cast to maintain the reduction by fixation "at a distance." An external fixator would have been a preferable method of treatment.

open reduction and internal fixation are not available, the fracture can usually be aligned by light skeletal traction through a pin in the os calcis and countertraction through a pin in the proximal end of the tibia, both pins being incorporated in a light plaster cast (Fig. 17.85). After 6 weeks, by which time the fracture is usually "sticky" (stable but still mobile), a long leg cast is applied.

An alternative method of treating completely unstable closed fractures of the midshaft of the tibia is closed ("blind") intramedullary nailing (with locked nails) from the upper end of the tibia. The fracture site is not opened and the nail is driven across the re-

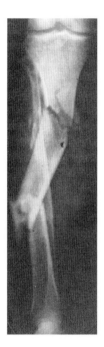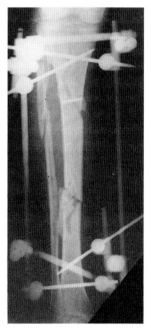

Figure 17.86.   Unstable segmental fracture of the right tibia and fracture of the fibula in a 24-year-old man who had been involved in a motorcycle accident. The fracture was open from without. There was considerable skin loss and an associated arterial injury. **Left.** Initial radiograph showing the large middle segment. Did you notice that this is an anteroposterior projection of the knee but a lateral projection of the ankle? This indicates a 90-degree external deformity through the fractures. **Right.** After complete cleansing and debridement of the open wound, reduction of the fractures, delayed wound closure (which necessitated skin grafts), and the application of an external skeletal fixator. No cast was necessary and the fixation "at a distance" facilitated subsequent care of the soft tissues.

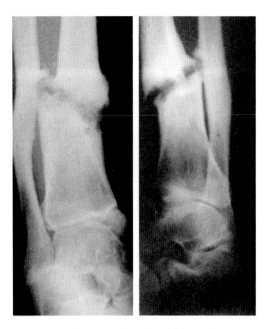

Figure 17.87. Nonunion of an oblique fracture in the distal third of the right tibia. Note the broadening and sclerosis of the fracture ends, the varus deformity at the fracture site, and the healed fracture of the fibula. Did you also notice the nonunion of the medial malleolus?

serious complication is osteomyelitis after an open fracture or open reduction of a closed fracture, the treatment of which is discussed in Chapter 15. *Ankle stiffness* is common and may require vigorous exercises for 1 year or longer. An alternative is the use of CPM, as described above for ankle stiffness after ankle fractures. *Arterial injury,* a serious complication of high tibial fractures, must be recognized early and treated adequately to avoid gangrene. Compartment syndromes are serious but preventable as discussed in Chapter 15. *Nerve injury* is common, particularly to the lateral popliteal nerve, with high fractures of the fibula, and occasionally from the local pressure of a plaster cast. *Persistent swelling* is almost inevitable but usually responds to active exercises and the use of an elastic stocking. *Delayed union* and *nonunion* are common, particularly in severely displaced fractures. If a tibial fracture is still mobile 4 months after injury, grafting with autogenous cancellous bone is indicated (Fig. 17.87). *Malunion,* which is nearly always preventable, produces

not only an obvious deformity but may lead to degenerative joint disease in the malaligned knee or ankle joint as described in Chapter 15 (Fig. 15.74).

Fractures of the tibia alone are not common. Being stabilized to some extent by the intact fibula, they are not severely displaced. Provided the fracture is reduced—by correcting angulation and rotation at the fracture site—the fibula does not hold the fragments apart. These fractures should be treated in the manner described above for stable transverse and oblique fractures.

Fractures of the fibula alone are relatively rare and you should always look for an associated fracture in the tibia or a fracture dislocation at the ankle with disruption of the tibiofibular joint. Because the fibula is not a weightbearing bone, isolated fibular shaft fractures require no immobilization and no restriction of weightbearing.

The Knee

Fractures of the Proximal End of the Tibia (Tibial Plateau Fractures)

The proximal end of the tibia, being composed almost entirely of cancellous bone and surrounded by a thin cortex, is susceptible to crushing injuries, particularly in individuals older than age 60 in whom the cancellous bone tends to be relatively osteoporotic.

Mechanism of Injury

A severe abduction injury, usually a direct blow on the lateral aspect of the limb with the foot fixed on the ground, forces the knee into valgus and drives the femoral condyle into the lateral tibial plateau. The osteoporotic bone fractures before the medial ligament of the knee tears. The joint surface of the lateral tibial plateau may be crushed and depressed, the medial or lateral condyles, or both, may be split off and associated with a transverse fracture. Frequently, the fractures are exceedingly comminuted. Clinically, the knee is acutely painful, and, because the fractures are intraarticular, there is always a tense hemarthrosis. Radiographic examination with at least four projections helps to assess the extent of the comminution (Fig. 17.88).

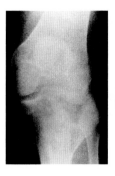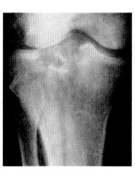

Figure 17.88.   Fractures of the lateral plateau of the tibia. **Left.** Severely comminuted fracture of the lateral plateau of the left tibia in a 75-year-old woman. The outer portion of the plateau has been split off and the lateral femoral condyle has been driven into the metaphysis of the tibia. Note the resultant valgus deformity of the knee. This elderly woman's fracture was treated by continuous traction through a pin in the tibia. Her knee was kept mobile. **Right.** Fracture of the lateral plateau of the right tibia in a 34-year-old man with depression of the joint surface. Note the lateral displacement of the lateral plateau in relation to the lateral femoral condyle. This young man's fracture was treated by open reduction and internal fixation of the vertical fracture, elevation of the joint surface through a "window" in the anterior cortex, and packing of the resultant defect with cancellous bone grafts.

Treatment

Although the knee joint may seem to be irreparably damaged, particularly with depressed lateral tibial plateau fractures, the intact lateral meniscus (which covers much of the articular surface of the lateral tibial plateau) provides a better gliding surface for the lateral femoral condyle than would be imagined from studying only the radiographs. This is fortunate because complete restoration of the tibial joint surface is often impossible by any means. Whatever form of treatment is used, the knee should be kept moving because residual knee joint stiffness is more disabling than residual deformity. In general, open reduction and internal fixation are more appropriate in relatively young adults than in the elderly. Treatment is best considered in relation to the various types of fractures.

Fractures of the lateral plateau with depression of the joint surface are usually severely comminuted (Fig. 17.88). In the elderly, the most suitable form of treatment is closed re-

duction to shift the tibial plateau back into place, followed by continuous balanced traction through a pin in the tibial shaft, the limb resting on the Pearson knee attachment of a Thomas splint. By this means, active motion can be initiated almost at once. The contour of the joint surface is disregarded, but a valgus deformity is assiduously avoided. The traction is continued until the fracture is united, by which time the patient has a useful range of knee motion. In younger persons, the lateral condyle can be reduced at open operation and bolted to the medial condyle. At the same time the articular surface is elevated and the underlying defect is filled with autogenous cancellous bone grafts. The AO system of rigid internal fixation is particularly helpful in managing these fractures. After 4 weeks of immobilization in an above-knee cast, the patient is encouraged to move the knee by active exercises, but weightbearing is not permitted until the fracture is united.

Fractures of both tibial plateaus with marked comminution are best treated by means of continuous balanced traction and early knee motion as described above. Even these fractures, which occur mostly in the elderly, can be treated by open reduction and internal fixation.

Fractures of the tibial plateaus with little comminution are seen more frequently in middle-aged adults and are grossly unstable. The most suitable form of treatment is frequently open reduction and internal fixation of the condyles (Fig. 17.89). The transverse element of the fracture can then be treated by immobilization in an above-knee cast or by more extensive internal fixation.

Even the most severely comminuted fractures of the proximal end of the tibia can be successfully treated in young persons by the AO type of open reduction and internal fixation combined with the immediate application of CPM (Fig. 17.90 A to G).

Complications

The most serious complication of tibial plateau fractures is residual *knee stiffness* from both intra-articular and periarticular adhesions. Residual stiffness 6 months after injury is an indication for a gentle manipulation of

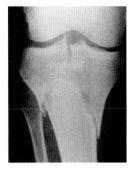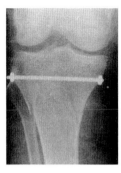

Figure 17.89.   Fractures of both tibial condyles with little comminution in a 44-year-old woman. **Left.** Initial radiograph reveals separation of the two tibial plateaus. **Right.** After open reduction of the intra-articular part of the fracture and internal fixation with a transfixion bolt. Plaster immobilization was used to control the transverse element of the fracture.

the knee under anesthesia followed by continuous passive motion (CPM). *Injury to the lateral popliteal nerve* is common as a result of a local direct injury but can also be caused by local pressure from a plaster cast. *Degenerative joint disease* is less common than might be expected, partly because the most severely comminuted injuries occur in the elderly whose limited use of the knee and limited number of years in which to use it are such that significant degenerative changes may not develop. In younger persons, posttraumatic osteochondral defects limited to either the medial or the lateral compartment of the knee can be effectively treated by means of an osteochondral allograft as described by Gross.

Injuries of the Semilunar Cartilages (Menisci)

The fibrocartilaginous menisci of the knee joint, although firmly attached to the tibia at their anterior and posterior ends, are only loosely attached peripherally and have a free-tapered margin centrally. Thus, they are free to move slightly inward and outward during normal knee function. Of importance to the feasibility of surgical repair of torn menisci is the fact that the peripheral part of each meniscus is vascular, but the central part is avascular. Under certain conditions described below, a meniscus may be ground between the joint surfaces with resultant splitting or tearing.

The medial meniscus is much more vulnerable to such injuries than the lateral meniscus; much of the discussion that follows pertains to tears of the medial meniscus.

Tears of the Medial Meniscus

The common injury of a torn medial meniscus occurs predominantly in young men, particularly those who engage in such sports as rugger, soccer, football, and hockey as well as those who work in a squatting position. Tears of the rather mobile medial meniscus are at least six times more common than those of the less mobile lateral meniscus. The difference in incidence may also be explained in part by their mechanism of injury.

Mechanism of Injury. When an individual takes weight on the partially flexed knee and the tibia is externally rotated in relation to the femur, the medial meniscus is drawn toward the center of the joint. An abduction strain draws it in even more. If at that moment, the normal ranges of external rotation and abduction are exceeded, as a result of either a fall or a blow on the lateral side of the knee, the medial meniscus may be trapped and then ground between the femoral condyle and the tibial plateau. It is then split along its long axis. In the aforementioned sports, the lateral side of the lower limb is struck much more frequently than the medial side, and knee abduction injuries are more common than adduction injuries. This may explain the much higher incidence of tears of the medial meniscus.

Types of Tears of the Medial Meniscus. The most common injury to a medial meniscus is the *bucket handle tear* (Fig. 17.91). Less common are the *posterior horn* and *anterior horn tears* (Fig. 17.92). Occasionally the peripheral soft tissue attachment of the meniscus is torn.

Clinical Features. The patient, who is often able to relate a history of the typical injury, is usually unable to bear weight on the affected limb. If the tear has been of the bucket handle type with the inner portion dislocated into the intercondylar notch, the patient cannot fully extend the knee because of a mechanical block anteriorly. The term "locked knee" is often used to describe this phenomenon, but the knee is still free to flex and is more precisely

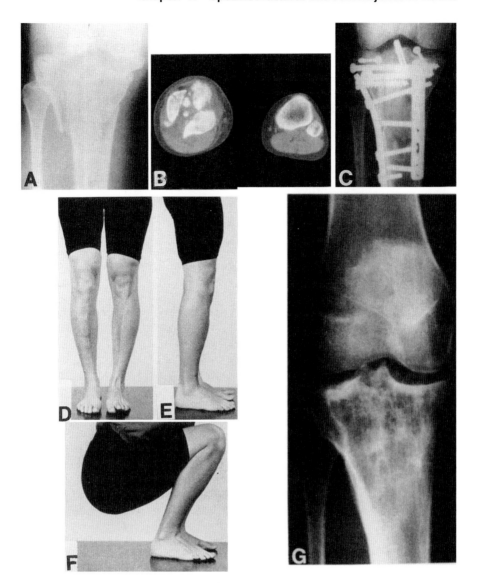

Figure 17.90. An extremely comminuted intra-articular fracture of the proximal end of the right tibia in a 23-year-old female Olympic skier who was injured in a high-velocity downhill accident. **A.** Note the extreme comminution in this anteroposterior radiograph. **B.** The swelling and comminution are more dramatically revealed in a CT scan comparing the two lower limbs. **C.** An anteroposterior radiograph after meticulous open reduction and rigid internal fixation using two AO plates and multiple screws (by Dr. J. Schatzker). The patient's injured limb was treated immediately postoperatively by CPM, which was continued for 21 days. **D.** Five years later, there is no deformity. **E and F.** A full range of knee motion has been maintained. **G.** Even after 5 years, there is no radiographic evidence of posttraumatic arthritis. The patient had returned to all of her preinjury sports, including skiing.

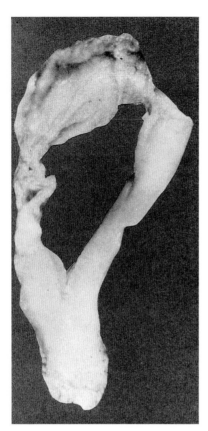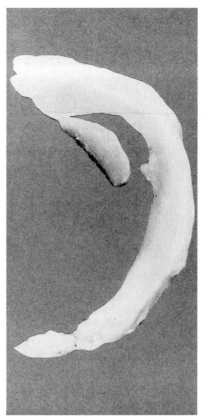

Figure 17.91. **Left.** A "bucket handle tear" of the left medial meniscus. The excised meniscus is seen from above. The inner portion of the meniscus had been displaced into the intercondylar notch.

Figure 17.92. **Right.** A tear of the posterior horn of the right medial meniscus. The excised meniscus is seen from above.

spoken of as being "blocked" rather than "locked." Attempts to completely extend the knee passively are blocked by a springy resistance. Because the fibrocartilaginous menisci are avascular, there may not be any hemorrhage into the joint, but a synovial effusion gradually develops over a few days. Even without treatment, the inner portion of the meniscus may slip back into place during the ensuing week or more, only to be displaced again as the result of a minor injury. In the patient's words, he or she has "a trick knee." In between such episodes, there may be little to find clinically other than measurable wasting of the quadriceps muscle.

A tear of the *posterior* or the *anterior horn* does not cause a block to extension, although it may cause a "catching" sensation. The patient feels that his or her knee is unstable and likely to "give way" but has difficulty localizing the problem to one side of the joint or the other. The patient experiences intermittent episodes of joint effusion and gradually the quadriceps muscle becomes atrophied.

Of considerable value in the clinical diagnosis of *posterior* or *anterior horn tears* is the McMurray test, which is conducted in this way: with the patient's knee acutely flexed and one of the examiner's hands holding the foot, the tibia is alternately internally and externally rotated and then abducted and adducted. The free end of a posterior horn tear is thereby made to slip in and out between the joint surfaces with a palpable, and sometimes audible,

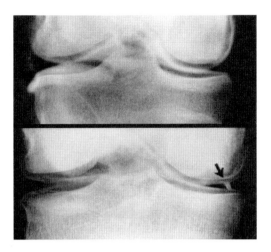

Figure 17.93.   Arthrograms of the knee using a radio-paque dye. **Top.** Normal arthrogram of the right knee. Note the smooth wedge-shaped medial and lateral menisci clearly outlined by the dye in the joint. **Bottom.** Arthrogram of the right knee revealing penetration of the dye into a vertical tear in the medial meniscus (*arrow*). By means of several oblique projections, the location and extent of the tear can be determined.

click. If no such sign is detected with the knee in acute flexion, the test is repeated in gradually increasing extension, because it is only as the knee is partially extended that the click from the free end of an anterior horn tear will be palpated. The greater the extension of the knee at the time of the click, the farther forward is the tear in the anterior horn.

Arthroscopy of the knee joint has proven to be of much value in the accurate diagnosis of tears of the menisci, both medial and lateral.

Radiographic Features. Plain radiographs provide no information concerning the state of the radiolucent menisci. Arthrography, by contrast, may prove extremely informative, particularly when the clinical signs are equivocal (Fig. 17.93). Magnetic resonance imaging of the knee is a valuable noninvasive method of assessing the menisci.

Treatment. When the diagnosis of a torn medial meniscus is established, only the torn part of the meniscus should be surgically excised (partial meniscectomy). Repeated episodes of displacement of the torn part of the meniscus are troublesome and temporarily disabling and they lead inevitably to degenerative disease of the knee joint. If the tear is in

the peripheral vascular part of the meniscus, it should be surgically repaired. Total meniscectomy should be avoided because it eventually leads to degenerative disease of the involved compartment of the knee.

Therefore, for either bucket handle tears or flap tears of the central part of a meniscus, it is appropriate to excise only the "handle" or the "flap," that is, to perform only a partial meniscectomy, which can be done either through an open arthrotomy or through the arthroscope (arthroscopic surgery).

Whenever it is feasible, surgical repair of peripheral tears of menisci is preferable to partial meniscectomy. Such a repair can be performed either at arthrotomy or by arthroscopic surgery.

Tears of the Lateral Meniscus

Because both the history and the physical signs are less definite, the relatively uncommon tears of the lateral meniscus are usually more difficult to diagnose clinically than those of the medial meniscus. The McMurray test may elicit a click from a torn posterior horn of the lateral meniscus when the flexed knee is gradually extended with the tibia adducted and internally rotated. Arthrography and MRI are both helpful in establishing the diagnosis, as well as in detecting the presence of a congenital discoid lateral meniscus, which is more prone to tear than a normal lateral meniscus (as discussed in Chapter 8).

Treatment. The only reasonable forms of treatment for tears of the lateral meniscus are partial meniscectomy and surgical repair of the tear.

Ligamentous Injuries of the Knee

The knee is basically a hinge joint through which occur flexion, extension, and minor degrees of rotation. Its medial and lateral stability is provided by the strong medial and lateral collateral ligaments, whereas its anterior and posterior stability is provided by the anterior and posterior cruciate ligaments. Thus, these ligaments are vulnerable to any severe injury that forces the knee to move in an abnormal plane or beyond the normal range of motion. Such injuries are common in sports such as football and hockey. A given ligament may be merely *sprained* (stretched with resultant tearing of a few fibers) or it may be *torn across,* either partially or completely.

Tears of the Medial Collateral Ligament

Because the outer side of the knee is more exposed and more often struck than the inner aspect, the medial ligament is more often torn than any other ligament of the knee. A fierce football or rugger tackle from the lateral side, for example, forces the ball carrier's knee into valgus and tends to open the knee joint on the medial side, thereby spraining or even tearing the medial ligament. If the injury is particularly severe, it may cause a tear of both portions (superficial and deep) of the medial ligament and also a tear of the medial meniscus and the anterior cruciate ligament, "the unhappy triad" described by O'Donoghue.

Clinical Features. The patient usually feels "something give" in his or her knee at the moment of injury. The joint rapidly fills with blood and becomes acutely painful. Local tenderness is most significant over the course of the medial ligament, usually near its proximal attachment, and even gentle attempts to abduct the knee aggravate the pain. When a complete tear is suspected, examination should be repeated with the patient under general anesthesia to assess the stability of the knee.

Radiographic Features. Plain radiographs may show nothing more than soft tissue swelling. Stress radiographs, taken with the patient anesthetized, are extremely valuable in detecting occult joint instability (Fig. 17.94).

Treatment. With *partial tears* of the medial ligament, the knee joint is stable even under anesthesia. The only treatment required is aspiration of the hemarthrosis and immobilization of the extended knee in a cylindrical plaster cast for 6 weeks, during which time the patient is allowed to walk and is encouraged to do isometric quadriceps exercises. With *complete tears* of the medial ligament, especially with associated tears of the anterior cruciate ligament, the knee joint is unstable. For middle-aged and elderly persons, nonoperative treatment by immobilization may be acceptable; but for young persons, especially athletes, the ideal form of treatment is imme-

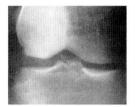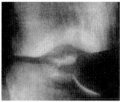

Figure 17.94. Occult joint instability of the right knee in a 21-year-old football player who had been tackled from the lateral side. **Left.** Anteroposterior radiograph showing a normal relationship between the femur and tibia. This does not, however, exclude occult joint instability. Note the undisplaced fracture of the tibial spine. **Right.** Anteroposterior radiograph of the same knee while it is being stressed in abduction with the patient under anesthesia. Note the marked opening up of the knee joint on the medial side, which indicates a complete tear of both the superficial and deep portions of the medial ligament. Note also the upward displacement of the tibial spine fracture, which indicates that the anterior cruciate ligament has been avulsed with its bony insertion.

diate exploration of the joint, surgical repair of the torn ligament or ligaments and capsule, and (if it is torn) partial excision or repair of the medial meniscus. A delay of even a few days renders surgical repair much less satisfactory, as the torn ends of the ligament become progressively more friable. Postoperative immobilization of the knee in a cylindrical cast for 6 weeks is often used to permit sound healing of the ligament. Nevertheless, some orthopaedic surgeons have applied CPM during the first 3 postoperative weeks with excellent results.

Tears of the Lateral Ligament

For reasons already mentioned, tears of the lateral ligament are less common than those of the medial ligament. The clinical and radiographic features as well as the treatment of lateral ligament tears are comparable to those of medial ligamentous tears with the sides reversed (Fig. 17.95). A traction injury of the lateral popliteal (peroneal) nerve is a frequent complication of tears of the lateral ligament and may even be irrecoverable.

Tears of the Cruciate Ligaments

The cruciate ligaments may be torn in association with tears of the medial or lateral liga-

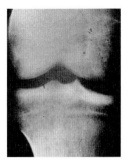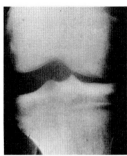

Figure 17.95. Occult joint instability of the right knee of a 20-year-old man who was knocked down by an automobile. **Left.** Anteroposterior radiograph showing a normal relationship between the femur and the tibia. This does not, however, exclude joint instability. **Right.** Anteroposterior radiograph of the same knee while it is being stressed in adduction with the patient under anesthesia. Note the marked opening up of the knee joint on the lateral side, which indicates a complete tear of the lateral ligament. This patient also had a traction injury of his lateral popliteal (peroneal) nerve.

ments but isolated tears of the cruciate ligament may also occur. Thus, if the tibia is driven forward on the femur (or the femur is driven backward on the tibia), or if the knee joint is suddenly hyperextended, the *anterior* cruciate ligament may be torn. Examination reveals that the flexed knee is unstable when the tibia is pulled forward, the "*anterior drawer sign.*"

Another sign of anterior cruciate ligament insufficiency is the "lateral pivot shift" phenomenon described by Galway and MacIntosh. When the patient is completely relaxed, the involved flexed knee is passively extended and the tibia is internally rotated by the examiner; the lateral tibial plateau subluxates anteriorly in relation to the lateral femoral condyle. If a valgus strain is then applied to the knee and the joint is passively flexed, the subluxation is dramatically reduced as can be readily appreciated by both the examiner and the patient.

The reverse mechanism of injury may produce a tear of the *posterior* cruciate ligament, in which case examination reveals that the flexed knee is unstable when the tibia is pushed backward—the "*posterior drawer sign.*"

Treatment. Provided the medial and lateral ligaments of the knee are intact, strong quadriceps and hamstring muscles may effectively stabilize the knee even when one or other cruciate ligaments are torn. Operative repair is difficult and the most reasonable form of treatment for nonathletes is immobilization of the knee in a cylindrical cast. The patient is allowed to walk in the cast for 6 weeks and is encouraged to do quadriceps exercises during the period of immobilization and after as well.

For active athletic individuals who require good stability of the knee, however currently available intra-articular or extra-articular methods of surgical repair, which are reasonably effective, are definitely indicated. A reasonable alternative to postoperative cast immobilization is postoperative CPM for 3 weeks.

Complications of Ligamentous Injuries of the Knee

The most troublesome complication of these injuries, especially for athletes, is residual *instability of the knee joint.* A knee brace is inadequate to provide stability and leads to disuse atrophy of surrounding muscles, which aggravates the instability. Active exercises are indicated and help to develop strength in the muscles, particularly the quadriceps. Late repair of neglected ligamentous injuries may necessitate extensive reconstructive operations. Less frequently, residual *knee stiffness* is resistant to physiotherapy and requires manipulation under an anesthetic. (This complication can be prevented by the postoperative use of CPM). Occasionally *calcification* is seen at the site of avulsion of the proximal end of the medial ligament from the femoral condyle. This radiographic indication of a former injury at this site is sometimes referred to as *Pellegrini-Stieda's "disease."*

Traumatic Dislocation of the Knee

Extremely severe injuries to the knee, such as may be sustained in an automobile accident, tear all four major ligaments and result in a complete dislocation of the joint, an uncommon injury with understandably dramatic clinical and radiographic features (Fig. 17.96). The most serious immediate *complication* is a *severe injury to the popliteal artery,* which car-

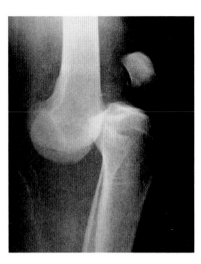

Figure 17.96.   Traumatic anterior dislocation of the knee in a 28-year-old man who had sustained multiple injuries in an automobile accident. This amount of displacement indicates that all four major ligaments have been completely disrupted. The dislocation was complicated by an avulsion injury of the popliteal artery that necessitated surgical reconstruction with an arterial prosthesis. It was also complicated by a severe traction injury of the lateral popliteal (peroneal) nerve.

ries the risk of distal gangrene. The *medial or lateral popliteal nerves* may also suffer a serious injury. Treatment demands urgent reduction of the dislocation in the hope of minimizing the arterial and nerve injury, after which the popliteal artery should be dealt with and the major ligaments surgically repaired.

Fractures of the Patella

The patella is a sesamoid bone firmly embedded in the broad quadriceps expansion, and the pull of the quadriceps muscle is not so much through the patella as around it—through the aponeurotic expansion on the two sides and to a lesser extent in front. Thus, the patella is vulnerable to two entirely different types of injury. In the *indirect type*, tears of the quadriceps expansion at the level of the patella produce a transverse *avulsion fracture* of the patella, whereas in the *direct type* (from a local blow), the patella is forcibly jammed against the lower end of the femur and sustains a *crush fracture* that is usually stellate and may be severely comminuted.

Avulsion Fractures

A sudden powerful contraction of the quadriceps muscle with the knee flexed, as may occur when an individual stubs a foot against something and tries to keep from falling, may literally rip the entire quadriceps expansion transversely. Included in the tear is a transverse avulsion "tear" or fracture of the patella, the fragments of which are pulled far apart.

Clinically, the patient cannot actively extend the knee and because the fracture is intra-articular, a hemarthrosis is inevitable. The lateral radiographic projection depicts the nature of the fracture most clearly (Fig. 17.97).

Treatment.   Avulsion fractures of the patella, at least in young individuals, require open reduction and internal fixation of the patella and repair of the medial and lateral quadriceps expansion. Kirschner wires crossing the fractures and a figure-eight wire (which passes around the ends of the Kirschner wires) provide the most effective type of internal fixation. A cylindrical walking cast is worn for 3 weeks, after which active exercises are encouraged. Full flexion of the knee is avoided for 10 weeks. For the elderly, excision of the patella and repair of the expansion may be preferable.

Comminuted Crush Fractures

A direct fall on the flexed knee or a blow on the flexed knee from an object (such as the dashboard of an automobile at the time of a head-on collision) may produce a minor undisplaced crack of the patella or may crush the patella so severely that it is literally shattered into many fragments.

Clinically, the patient is able to extend the knee because the medial and lateral quadriceps expansions are intact. A hemarthrosis is inevitable and often excessive. The lateral radiographic projection is most useful in assessing the extent of the comminution (Fig. 17.98).

Treatment.   Undisplaced crush fractures require aspiration of the hemarthrosis followed by 3 weeks of immobilization in a cylindrical walking cast. The fracture, if not displaced at the time of injury, will not become displaced subsequently. For the severely comminuted stellate fractures of the patella, it is clearly impossible to restore a smooth articular surface. The most appropriate method of treatment is total excision of all the patellar fragments and reconstruction of the quadriceps expansion. The functional results of such treatment are reasonably good, provided the quadriceps muscle is actively exercised. Even so, the patient may lose the ability to actively extend the knee through the last 5 degrees or so ("extensor lag").

Complications of patellar fractures include *chondromalacia of the patella* and also *post-traumatic degenerative joint disease* of the patellofemoral component of the knee.

Traumatic Dislocation of the Patella

The mechanism of injury, clinical features, and treatment of this injury in adults are comparable to those in older children and adolescents. They are discussed in Chapter 16.

Intercondylar Fractures of the Femur

The intercondylar type of fracture of the distal end of femur is comparable in many ways to that of the distal end of the humerus. Relatively uncommon, this severe fracture is usually the result of a fall on the flexed knee from a considerable height. The wedge-shaped ar-

ticular surface of the patella is driven like a wedge between the two condyles and splits one or both from the shaft. Thus, the vertical component of the fracture is always intra-articular. Proximally there may be a transverse component, in which case the comminuted fracture lines are T-shaped.

Clinically, the knee joint is grossly swollen by a tense hemarthrosis and there is usually evidence of abrasions or bruising over the front of the knee indicating the mechanism of injury. The patella may also be fractured. Radiographic examination may require several projections to reveal the true extent of the injury inasmuch as the comminution may be extreme (Fig. 17.99).

Treatment

The form of treatment depends primarily on the degree of comminution of the fracture. Of course, the most important fracture to be completely reduced is the vertical fracture that extends into the knee joint. *Single fractures* that have split off only one condyle are best treated by open reduction and internal fixation with screws to restore the joint line. Widely displaced *double fractures* with a trans-

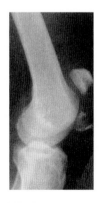 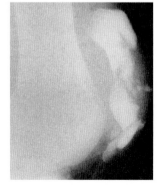

Figure 17.97.   Left. Avulsion fracture of the patella in a 40-year-old man who, while running across a field, caught his foot in a groundhog hole. Note the wide separation of the fragments, indicating a complete transverse tear of the entire quadriceps expansion. The patient was treated by internal fixation of the fractured patella and repair of the quadriceps expansion.

Figure 17.98.   Right. Comminuted crush fracture of the patella in a 42-year-old woman who was a passenger in the front seat of an automobile at the time of an accident. As she shot forward at the moment of impact, her patella was crushed and shattered by the dashboard. She was not wearing a seat belt! Treatment consisted of excision of the fragmented patella and reconstruction of the quadriceps expansion.

verse component may also be treated by open reduction and internal fixation of both the transverse and the vertical components using either a blade plate or plates and screws. Provided the internal fixation is rigid, the knee joint can be treated immediately postoperatively by CPM for 3 weeks, followed by intermittent active motion without weightbearing until the fractures are united. Severely *comminuted fractures*—the "bag of bone fragments" type of fracture in the intercondylar region—defy internal fixation and are best treated by continuous skeletal traction, which permits some knee motion as soon as the acute pain has subsided (Fig. 17.100). Such motion sometimes helps to guide the articular fragments into acceptable position and diminishes the risk of permanent knee stiffness. In the elderly, most intercondylar fractures of the femur are better treated by continuous skeletal traction than by open reduction.

Complications of these fractures include persistent *knee joint stiffness* (if the knee joint has been immobilized postoperatively) and

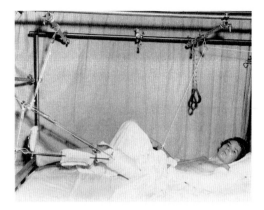

Figure 17.100. Continuous skeletal traction through a pin in the tibia for a severely comminuted supracondylar fracture of the femur. The thigh is resting in a Thomas splint and the leg is resting in a hinged Pearson knee attachment, which permits knee motion.

the late development of posttraumatic *degenerative joint disease of the knee.*

The Thigh

Fractures of the Femoral Shaft

The femur is the largest bone in the body and its shaft is particularly strong in adults. A violent direct injury, such as may be sustained in an automobile accident, is required to produce a fracture of the femoral shaft. There is often extensive tearing of the periosteum and some degree of comminution with resultant instability of the fracture. Massive internal hemorrhage may lead to profound shock. Although union of the fracture can usually be achieved by closed treatment, it normally requires 20 weeks, and sometimes much longer.

Clinical Features

The patient's thigh is grossly swollen from internal hemorrhage. It is usually markedly deformed and completely unstable. The diagnosis is so obvious clinically that radiographic examination is best deferred until splinting of the fracture and resuscitative measures have been carried out.

Treatment

During the *emergency treatment* of patients who have sustained a displaced fracture of the femoral shaft, the limb should be immobilized

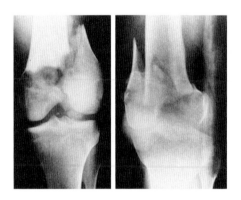

Figure 17.99. Severely comminuted intercondylar fracture of the left femur in a 20-year-old workman who fell 25 feet from a ladder and landed on his left knee. **Left.** Anteroposterior radiograph revealing a T-shaped fracture, the vertical limb of which extends into the knee joint. Note the marked comminution. Did you also notice the undisplaced fracture of the patella? This is in keeping with the mechanism of injury, namely a fall on the flexed knee. **Right.** Oblique radiograph revealing additional data concerning the displacement of the fragments and the extent of the comminution. This young man's fracture was treated by continuous skeletal traction through a pin in the tibia (Fig. 17.100).

in a temporary splint to relieve pain and to prevent further injury to the soft tissues (Fig. 17.101). Associated shock must be treated immediately.

Nonoperative treatment carries fewer risks than operative treatment and is suitable for the majority of femoral shaft fractures. It does, however, require a considerably longer period in the hospital and a longer period of protection from the stresses of weightbearing. For these reasons, nonoperative treatment is currently used primarily in situations in which there are no adequate facilities for open reduction and internal fixation. Continuous traction of either the fixed or balanced type is applied using a Thomas splint. Whereas oblique, spiral, and comminuted fractures require no prior reduction, transverse fractures in adults should first be reduced under general anesthesia and the traction device applied to maintain the reduction. Frequent radiographs are obtained to monitor the position of the fragments. Traction is continued for approximately 12 weeks, during which time the patient is encouraged to exercise all muscles in the injured limb. When *clinical union* has been achieved, as evidenced by absence of local tenderness at the fracture site and absence of pain on applying angulatory forces, the traction device may be discarded (Fig. 17.102). Active exercises are continued but no weightbearing is permitted until there is evidence of *radiographic consolidation*. Understandably, this nonoperative method of treatment is no longer feasible in developed countries because of socioeconomic factors.

An alternative method of treatment for fractures of the distal third of the femur is

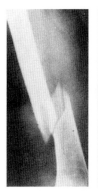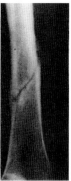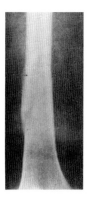

Figure 17.102.   Spiral comminuted fracture of the distal third of the femur in a 45-year-old woman. **Left.** Initial radiograph revealing displacement and comminution. **Center.** The position of the fragments obtained by continuous skeletal traction. **Right.** Three months after injury, union is progressing satisfactorily.

functional fracture-bracing after a period of approximately 5 weeks of traction (as discussed in Chapter 15).

Operative treatment including internal fixation with a large intramedullary nail is best suited for most fractures of the femoral shaft and is currently the favored method for such fractures. Although union of the fracture is not accelerated, the fracture is prevented from angulating or shortening pending consolidation (Fig. 17.103). Because there are considerable risks, especially of infection, intramedullary nailing should not be undertaken lightly or merely for the "convenience" of either the patient or the surgeon. The following circumstances represent clear-cut indications for intramedullary nailing of femoral shaft fractures: 1) failure to achieve an acceptable reduction by closed means; 2) associated multiple injuries (including head injury); 3) coexistent femoral artery injury requiring repair; 4) the elderly for whom prolonged bed rest is deleterious; and 5) pathological fractures. The ideal method of intramedullary nailing is the closed or "blind" technique, in which the fracture site is not opened, the nail being inserted across the fracture site under radiographic control using an image intensifier. The nail can be "locked" both proximally and distally by transverse screws that penetrate both the bone and the intramedullary nail (through holes in the latter) (Fig. 17.104).

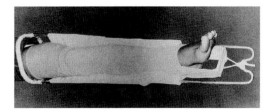

Figure 17.101.   Thomas splint used for temporary immobilization of a displaced fracture of the femoral shaft during the emergency care of the patient.

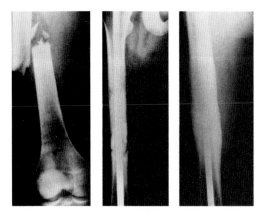

Figure 17.103. Comminuted transverse fracture of the middle third of the right femur in a 37-year-old physician who was injured in an automobile accident. **Left.** Initial radiograph reveals varus angulation and significant overriding of the fragments. Note also the comminution. **Center.** Two months after closed reduction and closed ("blind") intramedullary nailing. Union is progressing at the usual rate. **Right.** One year after injury, complete radiographic consolidation of the fracture. An alternative fixation for this fracture would have been a "locked" femoral intramedullary nail as depicted in Fig. 17.104.

Complications

Shock and *fat embolism* (both of which are discussed in Chapter 15) are early complications of fractured femoral shafts. The most troublesome late complication is *persistent knee stiffness* (which is to a large extent preventable through early and continued active exercises). Either the quadriceps muscle or the patella may become adherent to the distal end of the femur, requiring surgical release followed by CPM. *Nonunion* in the absence of infection is rare, but *delayed union* is an indication for autogenous cancellous bone grafting.

The Hip

Intertrochanteric Fractures of the Femur

Fractures *between* the lesser and greater trochanters (*intertrochanteric fractures*), as well as those *through* the trochanters (*peritrochanteric fractures*) are best considered together as extracapsular or *intertrochanteric fractures,* because their clinical manifestations and treatment are similar.

Intertrochanteric fractures are especially common in adults older than age 60 and occur more frequently in women than men. Thus, these extracapsular fractures have the same age and sex incidence as intracapsular fractures of the neck of the femur and Colles' fractures of the distal end of the radius. They also occur for the same reason, that is, through bone that has become markedly weakened by a combination of senile and postmenopausal osteoporosis. Intertrochanteric fractures are often severely comminuted.

Clinical Features

The patient, usually an elderly woman, is either knocked down or falls down, lands on the outer aspect of the hip, and is unable to get up because of pain and complete instability at the fracture site. Examination reveals that

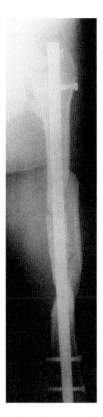

Figure 17.104. A locked intramedullary nail for the treatment of a comminuted segmental fracture of the shaft of the left femur of a 40-year-old woman who, as a pedestrian, was struck by a speeding automobile. She suffered multiple serious injuries. The system of locking the intramedullary nail both proximally and distally prevents both rotation and shortening at the fracture site.

the entire lower limb lies in complete external rotation (Fig. 17.105). The limb usually appears short and the upper part of the thigh is swollen as a result of extracapsular bleeding into the soft tissues. Ecchymosis may appear in a few days. With intracapsular fractures of the femoral neck, the bleeding is into the joint rather than into the groin or thigh. *Radiographic examination* clearly depicts the extent of the fracture (Fig. 17.106).

Treatment

The blood supply in the cancellous bone of the trochanteric region is abundant, and intertrochanteric fractures virtually all unite. Thus, union can almost always be obtained by closed treatment using continuous traction. Nevertheless, union requires from 12 to 16 weeks

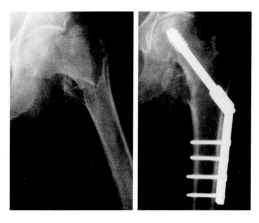

Figure 17.106. An unstable comminuted intertrochanteric fracture of the left femur of a 74-year-old lady who had fallen and landed on the outer aspect of her left hip. **A.** In the anteroposterior radiograph, note the comminution and shortening. **B.** The postoperative radiograph reveals an excellent reduction of the fracture and internal fixation with a compression-screw plate [dynamic hip screw (DHS)].

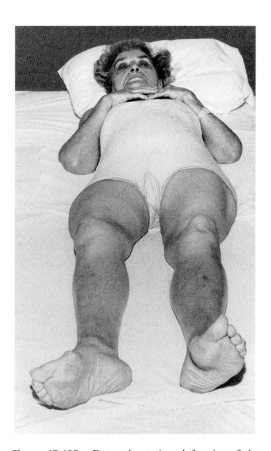

Figure 17.105. External rotation deformity of the entire right lower limb of an elderly woman. This deformity is seen with either a displaced intertrochanteric fracture or a displaced fracture of the femoral neck. It is usually more marked in the former.

and many elderly persons cannot tolerate such a prolonged period of bed rest even with the best possible nursing care. For this reason, the preferred method of treatment is open reduction of the fracture and internal fixation with a compression screw-plate (dynamic hip screw—DHS) (Fig. 17.106). The distinct advantage of such internal fixation, particularly for the elderly, is that the patient is free to move about in bed immediately after operation, may be out of bed in a chair within a few days, and may be allowed to walk bearing partial weight on the injured limb with the help of crutches or a walker within a few weeks. For younger, more vigorous and more active persons who occasionally sustain an intertrochanteric fracture, it is safer to defer weightbearing until the fracture has clinically united, because the fixation device may break due to metal failure if subjected to excessive stresses before the fracture is united.

In recent years, an alternative method of treatment for intertrochanteric fractures is the insertion, under radiographic control, of severed curved Enders nails from the medial side of the distal end of the femur. The nails are driven proximally to cross the fracture site.

Complications

Extracapsular or intertrochanteric fractures of the femur have relatively few complications in comparison with intracapsular fractures of the neck of the femur. Nonunion and avascular necrosis almost never complicate intertrochanteric fractures; malunion in the form of coxa vara is not uncommon, but the resultant shortening seldom exceeds 2 cm. This complication is of little significance in the elderly but should be avoided in younger patients by protecting the hip from weightbearing until the fracture is clinically united.

In the elderly, the mortality rate from intertrochanteric fractures of the femur is high—20% or higher.

Fractures of the Femoral Neck

Femoral neck fractures, whether they be *subcapital, transcervical* (midcervical), or *basilar* (base of the neck), may be considered together. They are all within the capsule of the hip joint (*intracapsular*) and both their clinical manifestations and their treatment are similar. Fraught with complications, femoral neck fractures are among the most troublesome and problematical of all fractures.

Garden's classification of intracapsular fractures of the femoral neck includes the following four types: type I—incomplete; type II—complete but undisplaced; type III—partially displaced; type IV—completely displaced. As you might expect, types III and IV have a high incidence of avascular necrosis of the femoral head (because of the precarious blood supply) and nonunion (because of the thin periosteum surrounding the neck).

Fractures of the femoral neck, like intertrochanteric fractures and Colles' fractures of the distal end of the radius, are especially common in adults older than age 60 and occur more frequently in women than men. The explanation is that these fractures occur through bone that has become markedly weakened by a combination of senile and postmenopausal osteoporosis.

Clinical Features of Displaced Fractures

The patient, most commonly an elderly woman, has a trivial mishap such as losing her footing on a slippery surface or tripping over an object. As she tries to "catch herself," she may suddenly put a torsional force on one hip that fractures the neck of the femur and *then* she falls—so fragile is the femoral neck in the elderly. Under these circumstances, the fracture is the *cause* of the fall rather than the *result* of it. If the fracture is displaced, as 95% are, the patient is unable to get up because of pain and complete instability at the fracture site. Examination reveals that the entire lower limb lies in external rotation, although not usually so complete as that seen in patients with an intertrochanteric fracture (Fig. 17.105). The limb usually appears short but there is no obvious swelling because the hemorrhage from an intracapsular fracture is into the joint rather than into the soft tissues of the groin or thigh.

Radiographic Features

Because the distal fragment is always externally rotated and shifted proximally, the femoral neck appears short. Upward displacement of an intracapsular fracture is somewhat limited by the hip joint capsule (Figs. 17.107 and 108). Two projections at right angles to each other—an anteroposterior and a "cross-table lateral" projection—are essential to determine the relationship of the fragments to one another. In general, the more nearly vertical the fracture line, the greater the shearing forces across it and the poorer the prognosis for healing. In 5% of femoral neck fractures, the fragments, rather than being completely displaced, are *impacted* (as seen in both radiographic projections), and the fracture is therefore relatively stable (see Fig. 17.114).

Special Problems Related to Femoral Neck Fractures

The gross instability of the fracture site is aggravated by the long lever arm (the full length of the lower limb) distal to the fracture. Inability to control the proximal fragment necessitates internal fixation of the fracture, yet the osteoporotic bone is not well suited to holding metallic devices. Furthermore, the periosteum covering the intracapsular neck of the femur is exceedingly thin and has limited powers of osteogenesis. Fracture healing in the femoral neck is therefore almost entirely dependent on endosteal callus formation. Added

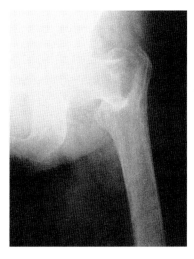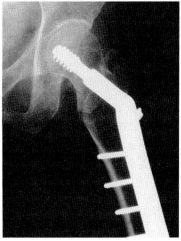

Figure 17.107. A basilar (base of neck) fracture of the femoral neck in a 78-year-old lady. **A.** In the anteroposterior radiograph, note the shortening of the femur. **B.** The fracture has been reduced and fixed with a compression-screw plate [dynamic hip screw (DHS)].

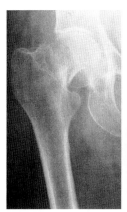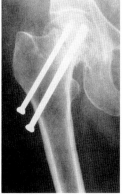

Figure 17.108. A subcapital fracture through the proximal part of the neck of the femur in an 80-year-old lady who slipped on a waxed floor, tried to "catch herself," and experienced severe pain in her right hip immediately before she fell to the floor. **A.** In the anteroposterior radiograph, note the shortening of the femoral neck through the fracture. **B.** The fracture has been reduced and pinned by three cannulated threaded screws under image intensification. (The third screw is hidden behind the inferior screw laterally, but only partly hidden proximally.)

to all of these unfavorable conditions is the precarious blood supply to the femoral head through vessels that course along the femoral neck, which are vulnerable to disruption at the moment of fracture. The development of a

tense hemarthrosis may compress any uninjured vessels and further compromise circulation to the femoral head. Thus, a displaced fracture of the femoral neck poses many serious problems, most of which are difficult to solve. Indeed, it is often referred to as "*the unsolved fracture.*"

Treatment of Displaced Fractures
In the years before the development of internal fixation, a fractured femoral neck in an elderly person usually triggered a series of deleterious events that led to the unfortunate victim's painful demise. From a humanitarian point of view alone, internal fixation of displaced fractures of the femoral neck is indicated. The elderly merit relief of pain no less than the young. Improvements in general anesthesia and general supportive measures for the frail and elderly have made early operation reasonably safe. Such patients are usually much more likely to survive if they have an operation for their fractured femoral neck than if they do not.

Closed reduction and internal fixation of the fracture should be performed as soon as possible. Aspiration of the hemarthrosis at this time may minimize the risk of avascular necrosis. Reduction can usually be obtained by flexing, adducting, then internally rotating and

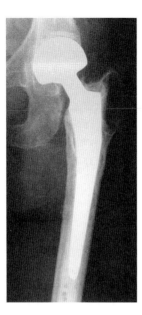

Figure 17.109. A bipolar type of endoprosthesis that provides a hemiarthroplasty after surgical excision of the head and fractured neck of the femur as an alternative form of treatment in very elderly and frail patients for whom internal fixation would be deemed to be less satisfactory. (In this type of endoprosthesis, movement takes place at two interfaces: between the cup of the prosthesis and the patient's acetabulum, and between the head and the cup of the prosthesis.)

extending the injured hip. Radiographic examination in two projections is used to assess the reduction (which must be excellent). Internal fixation of the reduced fracture can be obtained either by a DHS (also known as a compression screw plate) (Fig. 17.107) or by three parallel cannulated screws (Fig. 17.108). After satisfactory nailing of the fracture, the patient may be out of bed in a chair within a few days and allowed to walk bearing partial weight on the injured limb with the help of crutches or a walker within a few weeks.

Various techniques including the use of radio-opaque dyes and radioactive isotopes scintigraphy have been developed to assess the circulation of the femoral head at the time of operation. The results of these techniques serve as a useful guide to treatment, because, if the femoral head of a middle-aged or elderly patient is completely avascular, it is better excised and replaced by a hemiarthroplasty using a bipolar endoprosthesis rather than reduced and nailed (Fig. 17.109). Prosthetic hemi-

arthroplasty is also indicated if the patient is very elderly, if a satisfactory closed reduction cannot be obtained, or if the fracture is pathological due to a skeletal metastasis. The postoperative regimen of immediate mobilization and early walking is as applicable after this type of treatment in the elderly as after nailing of the fracture.

Complications of Displaced Fractures

Only 50% of patients who have sustained a displaced femoral neck fracture obtain a satisfactory result from simple nailing. The explanation for the unsatisfactory results in the remaining 50% of patients lies in the aforementioned inherent problems related to these fractures and in the extremely high incidence of serious complications—by far the highest incidence of complications of any fracture in the body. The most significant of these complications are *avascular necrosis of the femoral head, nonunion,* and *degenerative joint disease of the hip.*

Avascular necrosis is a common complication of femoral neck fractures because of the precarious blood supply to the femoral head. Radiographic evidence of this complication is not apparent immediately and may not become apparent for several months or longer. You may find it helpful at this time to review the pathogenesis of avascular necrosis of the adult femoral head, both the idiopathic and the posttraumatic type, in Chapter 13 (Fig. 13.27). Union of the fracture is delayed but not necessarily prevented. If the fracture unites, revascularization proceeds slowly up the neck. However, disintegration and collapse of the femoral head ensue before revascularization is complete and subsequent degenerative joint disease is inevitable (Fig. 17.110). The fracture may fail to unite, in which case revascularization of the femoral head cannot occur (Fig. 17.111). The treatment of avascular necrosis of the femoral head complicating femoral neck fractures, with or without nonunion, is excision of the head and neck and hemiarthroplasty with a bipolar endoprosthesis.

Nonunion develops in more than 30% of displaced fractures of the femoral neck and may be due in part to avascular necrosis. It can also occur as the result of continued move-

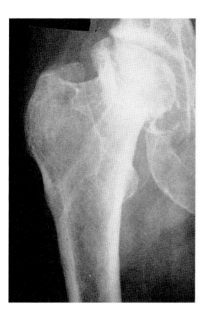

Figure 17.110. Posttraumatic avascular necrosis of the femoral head in a 70-year-old woman as a complication of a fractured femoral neck. This radiograph 2 years after fracture reveals evidence of extensive avascular necrosis of the femoral head. The fracture of the neck of the femur has healed and the fixation device has been removed. Proximal to the original fracture site, however, is a larger segment of avascular necrosis. This triangular-shaped segment containing the weightbearing surface has collapsed, resulting in significant joint incongruity. Note the evidence of bone deposition and bone resorption in the femoral head demarcating the necrotic fragment from the remainder of the head. Note also that this patient's hip is adducted due to an adduction contracture. This patient's hip is irreparably destroyed.

avascular necrosis with subsequent femoral head deformity or damage to the articular cartilage from the original injury or its treatment. In the elderly patient with a short life expectancy, there may not be time for this complication to develop. In younger persons, posttrau-

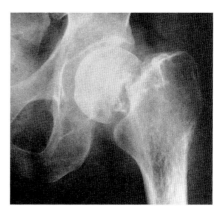

Figure 17.111. Avascular necrosis of the femoral head complicating a fracture of the femoral neck in a 40-year-old woman. The femoral head exhibits a relative increase in radiographic density (relative to the osteoporotic viable bone in the area). The fracture has failed to unite. Consequently, the femoral head has not been revascularized.

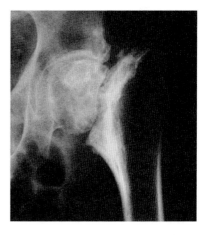

Figure 17.112. Nonunion of a fracture of the femoral neck in an 85-year-old woman. The fracture had occurred 5 years previously and although there was no bony union, there was a firm fibrous union and the patient did not have pain. If pain had been a problem in this very elderly woman, a reasonable form of treatment would have been replacement of the proximal fragment with a metallic endoprosthesis.

ment at the site of the fracture that has not been rigidly immobilized by the internal fixation device (Fig. 17.112). In the elderly and in all patients with nonunion combined with avascular necrosis, the most reasonable form of treatment is excision of the ununited femoral head and neck and replacement hemiarthroplasty with a metallic endoprosthesis. For younger patients whose femoral head is viable, reconstructive operations such as subtrochanteric femoral osteotomy or bone grafting are indicated because a united fracture and a viable femoral head are always superior to a metallic prosthesis (Fig. 17.113).

Posttraumatic degenerative joint disease develops slowly over the years as a result of either

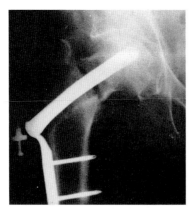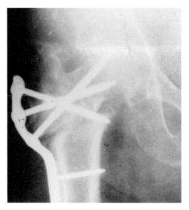

Figure 17.113.   Nonunion of a basilar fracture of the neck of the right femur in a 50-year-old man. The femoral head is viable. **Left.** One year after the fracture. Note that the fracture is ununited and the nail is beginning to bend (and soon would break from metal failure). The bolt of the nail plate junction has come loose and the rarefied area above and below the nail indicates that the nail has been moving up and down in the distal fragment. **Right.** Three months after removal of the previous metal and subtrochanteric osteotomy of the femur with medial displacement of the femoral shaft. Both the fracture and the osteotomy are uniting satisfactorily.

matic degenerative joint disease of the hip is a serious complication that requires treatment by one or more methods, as discussed in Chapter 11.

Impacted Fractures

The femoral neck fracture is truly impacted in only 5% of patients and is therefore reasonably stable. Such a patient may actually walk around for several days on the impacted fracture before seeking medical attention. Physical signs are minimal and the involved hip may be passively moved without causing pain. Radiographic examination in two planes reveals the impaction, the distal fragment nearly always being in abduction, hence the term *impacted abduction fracture.*

Treatment of impacted femoral neck fractures is somewhat controversial. If the fracture remains impacted, it can be expected to heal within 3 months without operation. Impacted fractures, with or without a subsequent fall, may become *disimpacted* and are therefore unstable. They then present all the serious problems associated with displaced fractures of the femoral neck. For completely cooperative and dependable patients in whom there is good clinical and radiographic evidence of

firm impaction, nonoperative treatment is reasonable. The patient is kept in bed for 4 weeks, then allowed up on crutches with no weightbearing on the involved limb for at least 8 weeks from the time of fracture. For less cooperative and less dependable patients, and for those in whom the clinical and radiographic findings suggest that the fracture is not firmly impacted, the safest form of treatment is a simple form of internal fixation using cannulated screws without disturbing the impaction (Fig. 17.114).

Traumatic Dislocations and Fracture-Dislocations of the Hip

The normal adult hip is one of the most stable joints in the body. Being a ball-and-socket joint, its stability depends largely on the shape of its articulating surfaces. Thus, severe violence is required to dislocate the hip. The hip may be dislocated *posteriorly* or *anteriorly* (with or without an associated fracture) or it may be dislocated *centrally* (in which case there is always an associated fracture).

Posterior Dislocations and Fracture-Dislocations

The normal hip joint is most vulnerable to dislocation when it is in a position of flexion

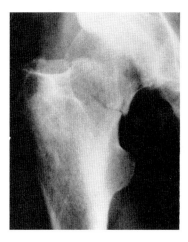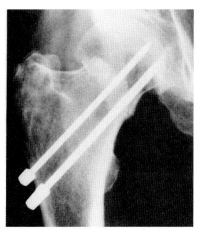

Figure 17.114.   Impacted abduction fracture of the femoral neck in a 71-year-old woman who was an alcoholic. The clinical findings were minimal. **Left.** Initial radiograph reveals impaction of the femoral neck into the head on the lateral side but no impaction on the medial side. There is a resultant abduction deformity at the fracture site. **Right.** The same hip after closed ("blind") pinning of the fracture with three threaded pins. Do you see only two pins? (The third pin is posterior to the inferior pin and superimposed upon it in this anteroposterior radiograph.)

and adduction. In this position, a force transmitted along the shaft of the femur (as may occur from a dashboard injury or a fall on the flexed knee) may drive the femoral head posteriorly over the lip of the acetabulum to produce a posterior dislocation—much the most common type. Because the femoral head escapes through a rent in the capsule, it is an extra-articular type of dislocation.

Clinical and Radiographic Features. The patient invariably lies with the injured hip in a position of flexion, adduction, and internal rotation and the limb appears short. There is usually painful muscle spasm about the hip. Radiographic examination reveals that the femoral head lies well above the acetabulum (Fig. 17.115). Oblique projections reveal that it is also posterior.

Treatment. As long as the hip is dislocated, the torn capsule and surrounding structures constrict the femoral neck vessels and jeopardize the blood supply to the femoral head. For this reason, posterior traumatic dislocation of the hip represents an emergency. The dislocation should be reduced as soon as possible to prevent the serious complication of avascular necrosis of the femoral head. Indeed, in adults whose hips are reduced within 8 hours from

the time of injury, the incidence of avascular necrosis is relatively low, whereas in those whose hips have remained unreduced for longer than 8 hours, the incidence of this complication is high (approximately 40%).

Closed reduction is accomplished by applying upward traction on the flexed thigh in external rotation and by forward pressure on the femoral head from behind. After reduction, which must be perfect both clinically and radiographically, the patient may be kept in bed with the limb in traction for 3 weeks, but a more practical form of treatment is immobilization of the reduced hip in a hip spica cast in its most stable position (extension, abduction, and external rotation) for 3 weeks to allow strong healing of the torn capsule.

Posterior Fracture-Dislocations

In approximately 50% of patients with posterior dislocations of the hip, a portion of the posterior lip (labrum) of the acetabulum is pushed off at the moment of the dislocation. Occasionally, this portion of detached labrum is displaced into the joint by the femoral head during closed reduction, in which case the reduction is incomplete, that is, not concentric, as evidenced by a widened joint space medi-

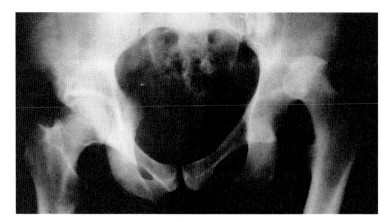

Figure 17.115.   Traumatic posterior dislocation of the left hip in a 44-year-old man who had been involved in a head-on collision. Note that the femoral head is lying well above the acetabulum and that the femur is adducted.

ally. This situation requires an open reduction to remove the entrapped portion of the labrum. A major fracture of the posterior bony margin of the acetabulum creates a significant defect in the acetabulum with resultant instability of the hip and may be driven posteriorly to damage the sciatic nerve. If the fragment is small, it is usually pulled into place at the time of closed reduction. If it is large, particularly if there is an associated sciatic nerve injury, the hip should be explored from behind, the fragment replaced and held with screws (Fig. 17.116). Less often, a tangential fragment of the anterior aspect of the femoral head is sheared off and needs to be removed.

Complications. Posterior dislocations and fracture-dislocations of the hip may be complicated by *avascular necrosis of the femoral head,* especially when there has been a delay in reduction, as previously mentioned. A *sciatic nerve lesion,* usually a neuropraxia only, may complicate posterior fracture-dislocations.

Posttraumatic degenerative joint disease of the hip is an inevitable sequela to either avascular necrosis of the hip or residual incongruity of the joint surface at the site of a fracture-dislocation (Fig. 17.116).

Anterior Dislocations and Fracture-Dislocations

Much less common than posterior dislocation, anterior dislocations are caused by a vio-

lent injury that forces the hip into extension, abduction, and external rotation—the position in which the hip is still lying when the patient is first seen. Radiographic examination depicts the femoral head below the acetabulum in the region of the obturator foramen. Oblique projections reveal that it is anterior (Fig. 17.117).

Treatment. Closed reduction, which should be performed as soon as possible for reasons already mentioned, can be obtained by applying traction on the flexed thigh and then internally rotating and adducting the hip. After reduction, which must be perfect both clinically and radiographically, the patient's hip should be immobilized in a hip spica cast in its most stable position (flexion, adduction, and internal rotation) for 3 weeks. Anterior fracture-dislocations are rare, the fracture component usually being of the femoral head rather than of the acetabulum.

Complications. Anterior dislocations and fracture-dislocations of the hip are seldom complicated by avascular necrosis of the femoral head or by nerve injuries. *Posttraumatic degenerative joint disease* of the hip may develop, particularly as a complication of a fracture-dislocation.

Central Fracture-Dislocations

A severe blow to the lateral aspect of the hip, especially when it is abducted (as may be sus-

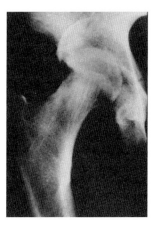
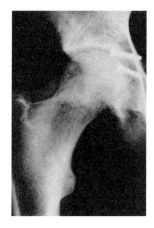
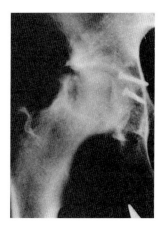

Figure 17.116.   Posterior fracture-dislocation of the right hip in a 23-year-old bush pilot whose small aircraft had crashed. **Left.** Initial radiograph revealing that the femoral head is lying above its normal position. Note the area of increased radiographic density above the lateral portion of the femoral head. This represents a widely displaced fracture of the posteromedial margin of the acetabulum. **Center.** Complete reduction of the femoral head. The screws are holding the reduced posteromedial margin of the acetabulum in place. **Right.** One year later, there is clear evidence of degenerative joint disease of the hip secondary to avascular necrosis of the femoral head.

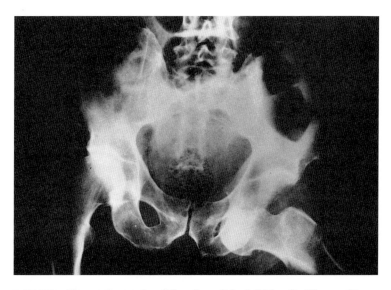

Figure 17.117.   Traumatic anterior dislocation of the left hip of a 30-year-old man who was struck by a truck. Note that the femoral head is below the acetabulum and medial to it and that the femur is abducted. (Compare with Fig. 17.115.)

tained when an individual is struck from the side by an automobile or falls from a great height and lands on the hip), may drive the femoral head centrally through a comminuted fracture in the medial wall of the acetabulum. The amount of medial penetration of the fem-

oral head into the pelvis varies from slight to extreme, depending on the violence of the injury. The radiographic appearance is often striking (Fig. 17.118, left).

Treatment. Slight medial displacement of the femoral head can usually be reduced by

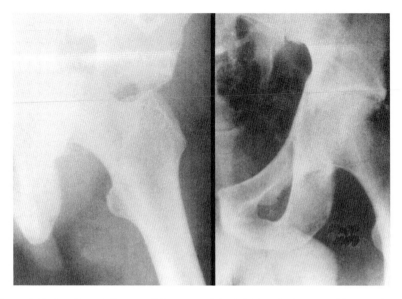

Figure 17.118. Central fracture-dislocation of the left hip of a 27-year-old man who was struck on the left side and then run over by a car. **Left.** The femoral head has been driven into the pelvis along with the medial wall of the acetabulum. The acetabular roof, however, is intact. **Right.** Two years after closed reduction, which had been accomplished by combined skeletal traction distally through the femoral shaft and laterally through the greater trochanter. The results are not always so satisfactory.

longitudinal traction through a pin in the lower end of the femur combined with lateral traction through a pin in the greater trochanter. Continuous traction is maintained for 8 weeks to allow healing of the fractures. Even extreme central dislocation of the femoral head can sometimes be reduced by such means (Fig. 17.118, right). If the comminution of the medial acetabular wall is not extensive, open reduction of the fracture-dislocation and internal fixation of the fractures are indicated. However, if the comminution is extreme and there is no possibility of obtaining a stable joint, the central fracture-dislocation is sometimes left as it is, in the realization that the hip is irreparably damaged. Joint motion is restricted but function is often better than might be expected. Late reconstruction may involve arthrodesis of the hip for young adults or total joint replacement for middle-aged or elderly patients.

Complications. An understandably common complication of central fracture-dislocation of the hip is *posttraumatic degenerative joint disease,* the severity of which depends on the amount of articular cartilage damage initially and the amount of residual incongruity of the joint surfaces.

The Pelvis

Fractures of the Pelvis

The adult pelvis, which includes the sacrum and the two innominate bones, is a strong, rather unyielding ring surrounding and surrounded by vital soft tissue structures, including the pelvic viscera as well as the major blood vessels and nerves.

Violent injuries are required to fracture the adult pelvis, the most common being serious automobile accidents (accounting for two thirds of all pelvic fractures), falls from great heights, cave-ins, and crushes. Thus, it is not surprising that more than half the patients who have sustained a major pelvic fracture have sustained multiple injuries to other structures, some of which prove fatal, and many have significant complicating soft tissue injuries in the pelvic region. The most important aspects of fractures of the pelvis are not the fractures themselves but rather the associated *complications*—extensive internal hemorrhage from torn vessels and extravasation of urine from rupture of the bladder or urethra.

Clinical Features

The history of injury often provides a clue concerning the type of pelvic fracture and the complicating injuries that are likely to have been sustained. Shock, which may be profound, is a prominent feature in most patients because of the extensive internal hemorrhage. Physical examination reveals local swelling and tenderness. In unstable fractures, there may also be deformity of the hips as well as instability of the pelvic ring.

Radiographic Features

Special radiographic projections are required to assess the precise nature of a pelvic fracture. The anteroposterior projection provides only a two-dimensional concept of the injury, and the lateral projection, which would normally provide the third dimension, is unsatisfactory because of the overlap of the two innominate bones. Thus, to obtain a three-dimensional concept of the disturbed anatomy of the injury it is necessary to obtain: 1) an anteroposterior projection; 2) a tangential projection in the plane of the pelvic ring (with the tube directed upward 50 degrees); 3) an inlet projection looking down into the pelvic ring (with the tube directed downward 60 degrees); and 4) right and left oblique projections.

In complex fractures of the pelvis, computed tomography is useful in detecting the precise site of the fracture(s) and the relationship between the fragments.

Emergency Treatment

A patient with a fractured pelvis requires emergency care centered on the two major *complications*—internal hemorrhage and extravasation of urine.

The pelvis is a particularly vascular anatomical area. Consequently, displaced fractures of the pelvis may tear vessels (such as the large superior gluteal artery), resulting in major internal hemorrhage and subsequent profound hemorrhagic shock.

While the patient's shock is being treated, a catheter should be inserted into the bladder

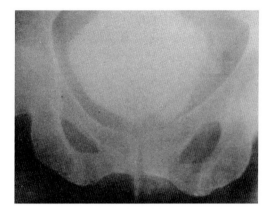

Figure 17.119. Cystogram in a 31-year-old man who had sustained an apparently undisplaced fracture of the left inferior and superior pubic rami. There must, however, have been some displacement of the fractures at the moment of impact, because the left lateral wall of the bladder has been ruptured. Note the radiopaque dye lying outside the bladder wall in the extraperitoneal tissues.

to investigate the possibility of associated injury to the bladder or urethra. If there is blood in the urethra and a catheter cannot be passed, the urethra is almost certainly torn. A suprapubic cystotomy should be performed pending surgical repair of the urethra. If the catheter can be passed into the bladder and the urine contains blood, a cystogram should be carried out immediately to determine if the bladder has been ruptured. If so, it should be repaired as soon as possible (Fig. 17.119).

Treatment of Pelvic Fractures

Because the bone of the pelvis is principally of the cancellous type and its blood supply is abundant, fractures of the pelvis unite rapidly. Treatment of the various types of fractures is aimed at correcting significant fracture deformities to prevent malunion and resultant disturbance of function.

Types of Fractures

The wide variety of fracture patterns results from the equally wide variety of mechanisms of injury. Two major groups merit separate consideration—those that are *stable* and those that are *unstable*. In each group there are individual fracture patterns, each with its specific

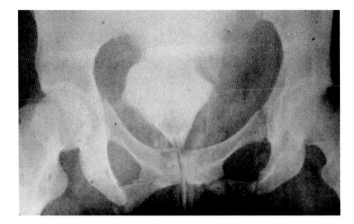

Figure 17.120.   Cystogram in a 40-year-old woman who had sustained relatively undisplaced fractures of both pubic rami on both sides. The bladder (which was full at the time of injury) has ruptured through the dome, as indicated by the dye that has extravasated into the peritoneal cavity. This type of rupture of the bladder is not due to a tear in the bladder wall from a sharp fracture fragment but is caused by a compressive blow on a full bladder—the same blow that fractures the pelvis.

mechanism of injury and method of treatment.

Stable Fractures of the Pelvis. Isolated fractures that do not transgress the pelvic ring do not interfere with stability of the pelvis in relation to weightbearing and do not require reduction.

Isolated fractures of the ilium from a direct injury, although painful, are of little significance and require only relief from weightbearing on the affected side until pain subsides within a few weeks.

Isolated fractures of the pubic rami result from a fall or a "straddle" type of injury. When both pubic rami are fractured, the most significant aspect of the injury is an associated tear of the urethra or rupture of the bladder (Fig. 17.120).

Unstable Fractures of the Pelvis. Fractures that transgress and therefore disrupt the pelvic ring are serious injuries that interfere with stability of the pelvis and are potentially lethal! Disruption at one fracture site in the pelvic ring can occur only if the ring is also disrupted (fractured, subluxated, or dislocated) at a second site. Thus, both sites of disruption must be detected to appreciate what has happened as well as to determine what must be done to correct it. The lower limbs, through their

capsular attachment to the pelvis, can be used to correct fracture deformities. The major types of unstable pelvic fractures are best considered individually.

Anteroposterior compression fractures are the result of a severe crushing injury from front to back. The two innominate bones are forced apart anteriorly at the symphysis pubis (in a sense externally rotated), and both sacroiliac joints are spread open, although the sacroiliac disruption is difficult to detect radiographically (Fig. 17.121). The gap at the symphysis pubis can be closed by completely internally rotating both lower limbs (and in a sense internally rotating the two innominate bones); in addition, side-to-side compression is used to close the gap. A full hip spica cast is then applied, with both lower limbs internally rotated and with side-to-side molding compression over the padded iliac crests. This is much more effective than a pelvic sling.

Lateral compression fractures are the result of a severe blow on one side or a crushing injury from side to side. The pubic rami are fractured and displaced on the *side* of impact and the second site of disruption is either through the sacrum or the sacroiliac joint on the *same* side. The mobile segment of the pelvic ring is hinged at its upper end and driven

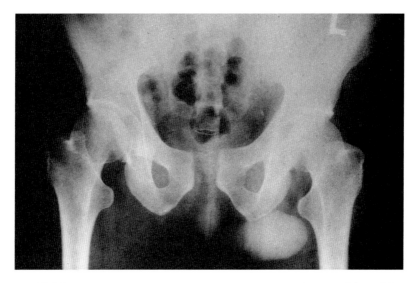

Figure 17.121.   Anteroposterior compression type of unstable fracture of the pelvis in a 30-year-old auto mechanic who was pinned to the wall by a rolling automobile. Note the separation of the two innominate bones at the symphysis pubis. The innominate bones have swung outward through the sacroiliac joints, but this is not apparent radiographically.

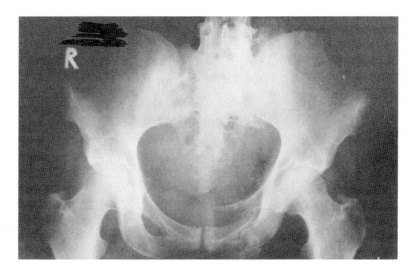

Figure 17.122.   Lateral compression type of unstable fracture of the pelvis in a 21-year-old racing car driver whose car was sideswiped by another as he "spun out" on a tight corner. Note the displaced fractures of the left inferior and superior rami and the disruption in the region of the sacroiliac joint on the same side (the site of the second break in the pelvic ring). The lower end of the mobile segment has been driven medially.

medially at its lower end (Fig. 17.122). This fracture is more likely than any other to rupture the bladder. A pelvic sling or binder would increase the displacement at the fracture site and should be avoided. The fracture may reduce spontaneously when the patient is lying on a firm surface; for this reason, an orthopaedic turning bed is useful in treatment, because the patient can be turned over without risk of lateral compression. Occasion-

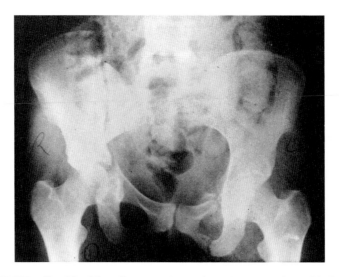

Figure 17.123.   Combined lateral compression and rotation type of unstable fracture of the pelvis (bucket handle type) in a 44-year-old woman whose automobile had gone out of control and had rolled several times. Note the vertical fracture line lateral to the sacroiliac joint on the right side and the fractures of both pubic rami on the opposite side. There is also an undisplaced fracture of the acetabulum on the right side. The mobile segment, which in this patient has shifted upward, is also free to swing forward and inward like a bucket handle.

ally continuous traction on the abducted lower limb is required to obtain and maintain reduction.

Combined lateral compression and rotation fractures resemble a bucket handle in that the pubic rami are fractured on the side *opposite* the impact while either the sacrum or iliac wing is crushed and split on the *same* side as the impact. When the fracture is through the sacrum, the sacral plexus of nerves may be injured. The mobile segment, hinged above on one side and below on the other, is usually forced upward, inward, and over (in a sense internally rotated) (Fig. 17.123). The fracture deformity can usually be corrected by applying traction on the lower limb on the side of the displaced segment and then externally rotating the limb. A full hip spica cast is then applied with the lower limb in complete external rotation.

Vertical shear fractures occur as a result of falls from a great height or from certain types of industrial accidents. The pubic rami and either the ilium or sacrum in the region of the sacroiliac joint are fractured on the *same* side by the upward thrust. Occasionally the upper site of disruption is through the sacroiliac joint. The mobile segment, which is confined to one half the pelvis, is driven proximally and its lower end may be swung either forward or backward. The nerves of the sacral plexus are likely to be seriously injured. Vertical shear fractures are exceedingly unstable and require strong continuous skeletal traction through a pin in the femur to obtain as well as to maintain reduction. If the lower end is swung forward, the traction is applied with the hip extended. If the distal end is swung backward, the traction is applied with the hip flexed. Because of the risk of recurrent proximal displacement of the mobile segment in shear fractures, the traction must be maintained for approximately 2 months.

Under certain circumstances, such as an associated bladder injury or multiple injuries, an effective form of treatment for completely unstable fractures of the pelvis is open reduction combined with external skeletal fixation (Fig. 17.124). For complex and grossly unstable fractures of the pelvis and the acetabulum, open reduction and internal fixation with plates and screws may be required.

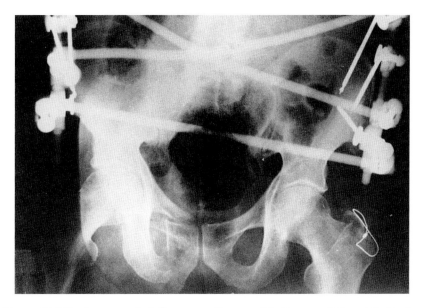

Figure 17.124.   Severe vertical shear type of an unstable fracture of the pelvis that has been treated by open reduction and external skeletal fixation. The patient had sustained multiple serious injuries, including a ruptured bladder, in a mine accident. The firm fixation "at a distance" facilitated his nursing care. The pubic rami are not completely reduced but the right sacroiliac joint, which had been dislocated, is in good position. Note also the wire loop in the region of the greater trochanter, which had been avulsed at the time of injury to the pelvis.

Aftercare for unstable pelvic fractures involves relief of weightbearing until the mobile segment is firmly stabilized by bony union. For most unstable fractures, firm clinical union is usually achieved after 2 months. The shear-type fracture, however, is subjected to further shearing forces with weightbearing, and as mentioned above, should be protected for 3 months.

Complications of Pelvic Fractures. *Internal hemorrhage* and resultant *shock* are the most common complications of unstable fractures. Either the *bladder* or the *urethra* is injured in approximately 15% of patients who have sustained a fracture of the pelvis. The bladder, which is particularly vulnerable when it is full, is injured almost twice as often as the urethra (Figs. 17.119 and 120).

Injury to the sacral plexus of nerves is a typical and serious complication in association with fractures of the bucket handle and vertical shear type.

Acetabular fractures and fracture-dislocations vary widely in their degree of severity and displacement. Being either intra-articular fractures or dislocations, the basic principles concerning all such injuries include precise diagnosis and three-dimensional assessment (which may require CT scans and three-dimensional reconstruction), plus accurate reduction and internal fixation followed by CPM to minimize posttraumatic arthritis of the hip (Fig. 17.125).

THE CARE OF ATHLETES

From the beginning of time, athletes have felt the need to excel in some type of physical activity, to compete in such activities against others, and to challenge their own previous performances. Sports have become highly organized and have come to involve a large percentage of the young and not-so-young throughout the world.

For some, sports represent a pleasant recreational activity, whereas for others, sports represent a fiercely competitive vocation. Indeed, for the professional athlete, sport is synonymous with livelihood. Because all competitive

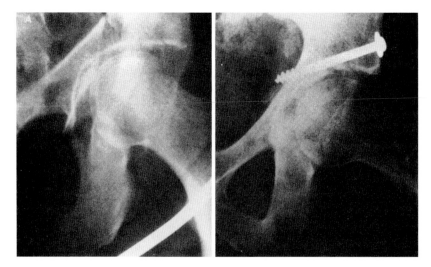

Figure 17.125. An intra-articular fracture of the left acetabulum in a 28-year-old motorcyclist who was struck by an automobile and sustained multiple injuries. **Left.** Note the fractures that involve the inner wall of the pelvis, the sciatic notch, and the inferior pubic ramus. The acetabular fractures were treated by open reduction and internal fixation with a single lag screw. Continuous passive motion of the hip was initiated immediately postoperatively and continued for 16 days. **Right.** Ten weeks postoperatively, the anteroposterior radiograph reveals satisfactory reduction and healing of the fractures. Thirty months later, the patient still had a full range of painless motion of the injured hip with no radiographic evidence of posttraumatic arthritis.

athletic endeavors involve feats of strength, speed, endurance, skill, and agility in varying proportions, it is understandable that physical injuries must be considered an inevitable part of the game for all who participate—nothing ventured, nothing sprained.

Physicians and surgeons have always had a responsibility for the care of injuries in athletes. Such care is now well organized in that physicians or surgeons are provided for professional athletic teams and also for amateur teams in colleges and universities. There is a need to extend this care to the young athletes in secondary schools as well. Indeed, a relatively new specialty, *Sports Medicine*, has evolved. It is concerned with the etiology, diagnosis, treatment, and prevention of disorders and injuries of athletes, as well as with the ideal methods of athletic training. It involves a knowledge of optimum cardiorespiratory and muscle physiology as well as psychology of serious competition.

The establishment of sports medicine clinics in many centers has helped to improve the standard of orthopaedic care for both amateur and professional athletes.

The Etiology of Athletic Injuries and Their Prevention

With the increasing emphasis on physical fitness for all ages, it has been estimated that there are currently some 30 million recreational runners or "joggers" in North America alone. Of the serious runners, at least half will at some time develop one or more "overuse syndromes" that include (in order of decreasing frequency): painful chondromalacia of the patella ("patellofemoral pain syndrome"), tibial stress syndrome, Achilles peritendinitis, plantar fasciitis, patellar tendinitis, iliotibial band friction syndrome, tibial stress fracture, tibialis posterior tendinitis, and peroneal tendinitis. The majority of these injuries or syndromes can be managed by the combination of reduction in running mileage, better training, local heat, and nonsteroidal anti-inflammatory drugs (NSAIDS).

Athletic injuries are either *intrinsic* or *ex-*

trinsic in origin. *Intrinsic injuries* arise from the athlete's own physical activity, such as a violent muscular exertion or an awkward motion; the athlete "hurts himself or herself." Such injuries are frequently due to inadequate physical condition or inadequate skill, both of which reflect inadequate athletic conditioning and training for the particular sport. Athletic conditioning and training, of course, are hard work but all play and no work makes the athlete a dull and vulnerable participant. Thus, the majority of intrinsic injuries are "overuse syndromes" and are to a large extent *preventable* through appropriate conditioning and training.

Extrinsic injuries are incurred by falls or blows from external forces; the athlete "gets hurt" by something or somebody other than himself or herself. These injuries, which are especially common in body-contact sports, are also to some extent *preventable* through adequate conditioning and training. They are also at least partly preventable through the design and use of appropriate protective gear such as eye shields, helmets, and shoulder pads. Some extrinsic injuries can be prevented by the formulation and enforcement of safer rules and regulations in a particular sport. An analysis of the etiology and pathogenesis of athletic injuries by means of a review of movies taken during a game has already led to a better understanding of the specific activities that are especially dangerous in a given sport (such as "clipping" and "spearing" in North American football). Such activities can then be reasonably made illegal. Many serious injuries have been prevented by altering the surface on which the sport is performed; for example, artificial turf for football and the padded canvas "floor" for boxing.

Thus, physicians and surgeons share with athletes, trainers, coaches, referees, and officials of athletic associations the important responsibility and obligation to prevent athletic injuries as much as possible.

Terminology of Athletic Injuries

Musculoskeletal injuries incurred in sports are comparable to those incurred in other physical activities. Many athletic injuries are quite un-derstandably described by trainers, coaches, and the athletes themselves in colorful athletic jargon. Consequently, the following *glossary* of laymen's "locker-room terms" may be helpful in putting these injuries into professional perspective.

Baseball (or cricket) finger: avulsion of the extensor tendon of the distal interphalangeal joint. The injury may occur either through tendon or bone.

Blocker's arm (disease): either posttraumatic subperiosteal bone formation or myositis ossificans on the lateral aspect of the arm.

Bone bruise: a subperiosteal hematoma, usually over the subcutaneous portion of either the tibia or the ulna.

Boxer's fracture: fracture of the neck of the fifth metacarpal.

Charley horse: a contusion and tearing of muscle fibers with resultant hematoma. The muscle most frequently injured is the quadriceps.

Footballer's (soccer player's) ankle: bony outgrowth from the anterior aspect of the distal end of the tibia and the superior surface of the neck of the talus, from repeated passive plantar flexion associated with kicking a ball.

Hip pointer: a contusion over the bony prominence of the iliac crest.

Jammed neck: a sprain of the joints of the cervical spine, usually from a lateral flexion injury.

Jumper's knee: patellar tendinosis.

Muscle cramp: sudden and severe pain associated with persistent spasm of a muscle, usually the gastrocnemius.

Pitcher's arm: medial epicondylitis of the elbow from chronic irritation of the common flexor origin.

Pulled groin: a strain of the adductor muscle origin.

Pulled hamstrings: a strain of the hamstring muscle origin.

Runner's knee: iliotibial band tendinosis.

Separated shoulder: either subluxation or dislocation of the acromioclavicular joint.

Shin splints: a painful condition in the region of the anterior tibial compartment of the leg from repetitive running on hard surfaces. There is inflammation and swelling in the musculotendinous portion of the muscles.

Shoulder pointer: a contusion over the bony prominence of the acromion.

Tennis elbow: lateral epicondylitis of the elbow from chronic irritation of the common extensor origin.

Tennis leg: partial rupture of the musculotendinous junction of the gastrocnemius muscle with or without rupture of the plantaris muscle.

Torn cartilage: torn meniscus of the knee joint.

The Athlete's Response to Injury

Athletes as a group are in a state of excellent physical health and are strongly motivated to make a speedy recovery from their injuries so that they may return to unrestrained athletic activity as soon as possible. To serious athletes, particularly professionals, who have trained themselves to compete in feats of strength, speed, endurance, skill, and agility, even a relatively minor injury may make the dramatic difference between victory and defeat. More serious injuries may even threaten their entire athletic career and livelihood.

It is not surprising that, although athletes are perfectly willing to risk injury during every competition, their psychological reaction to injury may *seem* to be unduly marked. It is hardly different, however, from the psychological reaction of a concert pianist or a surgeon who has injured his or her hand or an opera singer who has injured his or her vocal cords. Athletes, as a group, are sometimes considered to be "neurotic," but this is not really so. An athlete may become neurotic, though, if either the injury, or the concern about it, is not taken seriously by the treating physician or surgeon.

Aims of Treatment of Athletic Injuries

In addition to the aforementioned responsibility of *preventing* athletic injuries, the sports physician or surgeon must accept responsibility for the *treatment* of such injuries. The *principles* of musculoskeletal treatment discussed in Chapters 6 and 15 are as applicable to athletes as they are to any other individual. The following *aims* of treatment are particularly pertinent to athletes.

1. To base treatment on an accurate diagnosis of the precise nature and extent of the injury.
2. To initiate treatment immediately, at least within minutes of the injury.
3. To provide optimum definitive treatment that will restore function as completely as possible.
4. To minimize the inflammatory reaction to the injury. The repeated local injection of corticosteroids into a given site, however, should be avoided because of its deleterious effect on the tissues.
5. To accelerate the phases of tissue regeneration and repair.
6. To maintain and improve the function of surrounding muscles.
7. To advise the injured athlete (as well as the coaches and managers) concerning the most appropriate time for return to unrestrained athletic activity. It is usually unwise to inject local anesthetic into a recently injured structure for the purpose of allowing the athlete to participate. The unhealed structure so injected, having lost the protection of pain, is particularly vulnerable to further injury. The interval of restraint should be as short as possible, but as long as necessary, to protect the athlete from further injury during the healing phase.
8. To meet the psychological as well as the physical needs of the injured athlete.

Medical Aspects of Athletic Conditioning and Training

Until relatively recently, the conditioning and training of athletes has been based on empiricism rather than scientific knowledge. Through the application of a rapidly increasing body of pertinent scientific knowledge, sports physicians and surgeons have in recent years made many valuable contributions to these important aspects of an athlete's life.

Knowledge of muscle physiology has helped to develop the most effective methods for improving muscle strength and endurance. Likewise, recent advances in cardiorespiratory physiology have contributed greatly to improvements in athletic performance and stamina. Certain conditioning exercises, once used extensively on an empirical basis, are now known to have harmful effects and are no longer recommended. For example, "deep knee bends," which stretch the ligaments of the knee joint and "sit ups," which frequently lead to troublesome low back pain.

Athletes will continue to break records in the pursuit of athletic excellence. The medical profession must strive to do likewise in relation to the care and prevention of athletic injuries.

THE CARE OF THE ELDERLY AND THEIR FRACTURES

As a result of our increasing life span, more people are now reaching "old age," at which time decreasing coordination causes more frequent falls. Furthermore, weakening of the bones from a combination of senile and postmenopausal osteoporosis renders elderly individuals more susceptible to even minor injury. In this elderly age group, musculoskeletal injuries, particularly if treated by prolonged bed rest, may initiate a cascade of pathological processes that lead to the patient's progressive deterioration, even to death.

In recent decades medical science, through the development of improved diagnostic, therapeutic, and monitoring methods, has produced a significant increase in the *duration* or *quantity* of human life. More emphasis is required on methods of improving the *quality* of human life during these added years.

The Response of the Elderly to Injury

A significant musculoskeletal injury in an elderly person elicits a response that is influenced by that patient's pre-existing physical and mental condition. In this age group, pre-existing degenerative and nutritional disturbances are common. It has been estimated that at least 10% of elderly persons have some disturbance of their glucose metabolism alone. Thus, it is a combination of pre-existing complications and frequent superimposed posttraumatic complications that account for *the high incidence of morbidity and mortality* after a significant fracture in the elderly.

Added to the purely *physical problems* of old age are the common *psychological problems* of loneliness, insecurity, and feelings of being "no longer useful" or "no longer needed." Such psychological problems are accentuated by accidents. Others, such as fear, confusion, and desperation, may be initiated by the unfamiliar setting of a hospital.

For all of these reasons the elderly person who has sustained a fracture needs and deserves alert medical care, realistic fracture treatment, and kindly consideration. It is important to minimize both *mortality* and *morbidity*—both physical and mental. The specialty of geriatrics, concerned as it is with the care of the elderly, has contributed greatly to our understanding of the many problems associated with the care of musculoskeletal injuries in these patients.

Aims of Treatment for the Elderly

The *principles* of fracture treatment discussed in Chapters 6 and 15 are as applicable to the elderly as to the young. The *aims* of fracture treatment, however, are modified as necessary to fit the general needs of this group, as well as the specific needs of each individual patient. General modifications of these aims merit consideration.

1. *To relieve pain.* The elderly withstand pain badly but they also tolerate usual adult doses of narcotics and sedatives badly, particularly if they have some degree of preexisting cerebral arteriosclerosis. Immobilization of the fracture is still the most effective method of relieving pain arising from the soft tissues surrounding the fracture site.

2. *To obtain and maintain satisfactory position of the fracture fragments.* There is less need for perfect anatomical reduction of fractures in the elderly than in the young. For example, what might be considered satisfactory position after reduction of a Colles' fracture in an elderly person might not be at all satisfactory for a younger per-

son, who must use the healed wrist more and for many more years and who is more concerned about its appearance. Incomplete reduction of an intra-articular fracture can sometimes be considered satisfactory for an elderly person who is unlikely to develop degenerative joint disease during the relatively few remaining years of life. Fractures such as those of the femoral neck that require internal fixation, however, must be just as accurately reduced in the elderly as in the young.

3. *To allow, and if necessary, encourage union.* During adult life, increasing age does not significantly affect the rate of fracture healing. Indeed, the period of immobilization of a given fracture can be somewhat reduced in the elderly who are unlikely to apply as much stress to their healing fractures as a younger person. Moreover, persistent joint stiffness is much more frequent in the elderly than in the young and for this reason the period of immobilization should be as short as necessary to achieve clinical union.

4. *To restore optimum function.* Rehabilitation of the elderly must begin from the time of initial treatment, but the goals must be realistic. Rehabilitation of the elderly does not mean rejuvenation, but the elderly person who has sustained a fracture should be rehabilitated to at least the preinjury state of physical and mental function.

The Treatment of Fractures in the Elderly

The treatment of specific fractures, dislocations, and joint injuries is discussed in an earlier section of this chapter and need not be reiterated. Much clinical judgment, both medical and surgical, is required in determining the optimum form of treatment for a given elderly patient. Consultation between physician and surgeon is essential.

Under some circumstances, the risk of operation for a fracture in an elderly person is less than the risk of withholding operation. This is particularly true if the nonoperative alternative involves a long period of enforced bed rest as it would, for example, with a displaced intertrochanteric fracture of the femur.

The Prevention of Fractures in the Elderly

The most important predisposing factor in the high incidence of fractures among the elderly is the previously mentioned combination of *senile* and *postmenopausal osteoporosis*. The bones become slowly but progressively weaker and may fracture as a result of even a trivial injury. In a sense, many fractures in the elderly are pathological fractures, in that they occur through abnormal (osteoporotic) bone—bone that is pathological, weaker, and more susceptible to fracture than normal bone.

One approach to *prevention* of the increasing problem of fractures in the elderly is the prevention of the predisposing osteoporosis. You will recall from Chapter 3 and Chapter 11 that in *osteoporosis (osteopenia, too little bone)*, bone deposition is decreased because of decreased osteoblastic formation of matrix and bone resorption is increased, with the result that there is a marked diminution in the total amount of bone. This imbalance between bone deposition and bone resorption, an imbalance faced by astronauts in a weightless state and moon walkers who are subjected to only one sixth of the earth's force of gravity, is, at least under certain circumstances, reversible.

In the present era of scientific achievement, exemplified by man's conquest of space, the moon, and beyond, the *prevention* of osteoporosis in the elderly *through scientific investigation* would seem a realistic goal. Science, like truth, is stranger than science fiction—and more exciting!

SUGGESTED ADDITIONAL READING

Aaron AD. Bone grafting and healing. In: Kasser JR, ed. Orthopaedic update knowledge 5. Rosemont, IL: American Academy of Orthopaedic Surgeons, 1996:21, 28.

Adams JC, Hamblen DL. Outline of fractures. 10th ed. Edinburgh: Churchill Livingstone, 1992.

Adams BD. Wrist and head: trauma. In: Kasser JR, ed. Orthopaedic knowledge update 5. Rosemont, IL: American Academy of Orthopaedic Surgeons, 1996;311–328.

Allgower M, Spiegel PG. Internal fixation of fractures. Evolution of concepts. Clin Orthop 1979; 138:26–29.

An HS, Vaccaro A, Cotler JM, et al. Low lumbar burst fractures: comparison among body cast, Harrington, Rod, Luque, Rod and Steffee plate. Spine 1991;16:440–444.

Apley AG, Solomon L. Principles of fracture treatment. Apley's system of orthopaedics and fractures. Oxford: Butterworth Heinemann, 1993; 515–565.

Apley AG, Solomon L. Fracture pathology and diagnosis. Concise system of orthopaedics and fractures. 2nd ed. London: Butterworth's, 1994; 211–230.

Behrens F, Shepard N, Mitchell N. Alteration of articular cartilage by intra-articular injections of glucocorticoids. J Bone Joint Surg 1975;57A: 70–76.

Bone LB. Emergency treatment of the injured patient. In: Browner BD, Jupiter JB, Trafton PG, eds. Skeletal trauma: fractures, dislocations, ligamentous injuries. Vol. 1. Philadelphia: WB Saunders, 1992;127–156.

Bone LB, Babikian G, Border JR, et al. Multiple trauma: pathophysiology and management. In: Frymoyer JW, ed. Orthopaedic knowledge update 4. Rosemont, IL: American Academy of Orthopaedic Surgeons, 1993;141–153.

Bone LB, McNamara K, Shine B, et al. Mortality in multiple trauma patients and fractures. J Trauma 1994;37:262–264.

Browner BD, Jupiter JB, Levine AM, et al. Skeletal trauma: fractures, dislocations, ligamentous injuries. Vol. 1. Philadelphia: WB Saunders, 1992.

Browner BD, Jupiter JB, Levine AM, et al. Skeletal trauma: fractures, dislocations, ligamentous injuries, Vol. 2. Philadelphia: WB Saunders, 1992.

Buckwalter JA. Pharmacologic treatment of soft-tissue injuries (current concepts review) J Bone Joint Surg 1995;77A(12):1902–1914.

Bullough PG. Bullough and Vigorita's orthopaedic pathology. 3rd ed. London: Mosby-Wolfe, 1997.

Cameron CD, Meek RN, Blachut PA, et al. Intramedullary nailing of the femoral shaft: a prospective randomized study. J Orthop Trauma 1992; 6:448–451.

Carter DR, Blenman PR, Beaupre GS. Correlation between mechanical stress history and tissue differentiation in initial fracture healing. J Orthop Res 1988;6:736.

Charnley J. The closed treatment of common fractures. 3rd ed. Edinburgh: Churchill Livingstone, 1961.

Clark CR, Bonfiglio M, eds. Orthopaedics: essentials of diagnosis and treatment. Edinburgh: Churchill Livingstone, 1994.

Connolly JF, Guse R, Tiedeman J, Dehne R. Autologous marrow injection for delayed unions of the tibia: a preliminary report. J Orthop Trauma 1989;3(4):276–282.

Connolly JF, Mendes M, Browner BD. Principles of closed management of common fractures. In: Browner BD, Jupiter JB, Levine AM, et al, eds. Skeletal trauma: fractures, dislocations, ligamentous injuries. Vol. 1. Philadelphia: WB Saunders, 1992;211–230.

Court-Brown CM, McQueen MM, Quaba AA, eds. Management of open fractures. London: Martin Dunitz, 1996.

Cuomo F, Goss TP. Shoulder trauma: bone. In: Kasser JR, ed. Orthopaedic knowledge update 5. Rosemont, IL: American Academy of Orthopaedic Surgeons, 1996;217–232.

Dandy DJ. Essential orthopaedics and trauma. 2nd ed. Edinburgh: Churchill Livingstone, 1993.

deHaas WG, Watson J, Morrision DM. Noninvasive treatment of ununited fractures of the tibia using electrical stimulation. J Bone Joint Surg 1980;62B:465–470.

Einhorn TA. Enhancement of fracture-healing (current concepts review). J Bone Joint Surg 1995;77A:940–956.

Filan SL, Herbert TJ. Herbert screw fixation of scaphoid fractures. J Bone Joint Surg 1996;78B: 519–529.

Frank CB. Ligament healing: current knowledge and clinical applications. J Am Acad Orthop Surg 1996;4:75–83.

Frank CB, Jackson DW. The science of reconstruction of the anterior cruciate ligament. Current concepts review. J Bone Joint Surg 1997;79A: 1556–1576.

Frymoyer JW, ed. Orthopaedic knowledge update 4. Home study syllabus. Rosemont, IL: American Academy of Orthopaedic Surgeons, 1993.

Galway HR, MacIntosh DL. The lateral pivot shift: a symptom and sign of anterior cruciate ligament insufficiency. Clin Orthop 1980;147:45–50.

Garrett WE Jr. Muscle strain injuries: clinical and basic aspects. Med Sci Sports Exerc 1990;22: 436–443.

Ghazavi MT, Pritzker KT, Davis AM, et al. Fresh osteochondral allografts for post-traumatic osteochondral defects of the knee. J Bone Joint Surg 1997;79B:1008–1013.

Goodship AE, Kenwright J. The influence of induced micromovement upon the healing of experimental tibial fractures. J Bone Joint Surg 1985;65B:650.

Goodship AE, Lawes TJ, Harrison L. The biology of fracture repair. In: Hughes SPF, McCarthy ID, eds. Sciences basic to orthopaedics. London: Mosby-Wolfe, 1997:128–143.

Gossling HR, Polsburg SL, eds. Complications of fracture management. Philadelphia: JB Lippincott, 1984.

Gruen GS, Routt CMH. Pelvis and acetabulum: trauma. In: Kasser JR, ed. Orthopaedic knowledge update 5. Rosemont, IL: American Academy of Orthopaedic Surgeons, 1996;365–378.

Gustilo RB, Anderson JT. Prevention of infection in the treatment of one thousand and twenty-five open fractures of long bones. J Bone Joint Surg 1976;58A:453–458.

Gustilo RB, Merkow RL, Templeman D. The management of open fractures (current concepts review). J Bone Joint Surg 1990;72A:299–304.

Hamilton HW, Morris JS. Continuous passive motion in postoperative knee rehabilitation. In: Feagin JA Jr, ed. Crucial ligaments: diagnosis and treatment of ligamentous injuries about the knee. 2nd ed. New York: Churchill Livingstone, 1994;751–757.

Hanley EN, Jr, Simpkins A Jr. Operative treatment of spinal injuries: surgical management. In: Browner BD, Jupiter JB, Levine AM, et al, eds. Skeletal trauma: fractures, dislocations, ligamentous injuries. Vol. 1. Philadelphia: WB Saunders, 1992;645–664.

Hansen ST Jr, Swiontkowski MF, eds. Orthopaedic trauma protocols. New York: Raven Press, 1993.

Heckman JD, ed. Emergency care and transportation of the sick and injured. 5th ed. Park Ridge, IL: American Academy of Orthopaedic Surgeons, 1992.

Jackson WJ, ed. Instructional course lectures. Vol. 44. Park Ridge, IL: American Academy of Orthopaedic Surgeons, 1995.

Jackson RW. The painful knee: Arthroscopy or MR imaging. J Am Acad Orthop Surg 1996;4:93–99.

Johnson KD. Hard-tissue trauma. In: Poss R, ed. Orthopaedic knowledge update 3. Park Ridge, IL: American Academy of Orthopaedic Surgeons, 1990;75–80.

Johnson EE, Urist MR, Finerman AM. Resistent non-unions and partial or complete segmental defects of long bones. Treatment with implants of a composite of human bone morphogenetic protein (1 BMP) and autolyzed, antigen-extracted, allogeneic (AAA) bone. Clin Orthop 1992;277:229–237.

Johnson RJ, Lombardo J, eds. Current review of sports medicine. Philadelphia: Current Medicine, 1994.

Kasser JR, ed. Orthopaedic knowledge update 5. Home study syllabus. Rosemont, IL: American Academy of Orthopaedic Surgeons, 1996.

Koval KJ. Hip trauma. In: Kasser JR, ed. Orthopaedic knowledge update 5. Rosemont, IL: American Academy of Orthopaedic Surgeons, 1996; 379–388.

Lane JM, ed. Fracture healing. Edinburgh: Churchill, Livingstone, 1987.

Marsh JL. Elbow and forearm: trauma. In: Kasser JR, ed. Orthopaedic knowledge update 5. Rosemont, IL: American Academy of Orthopaedic Surgeons, 1996;269–281.

McGinty JB, Caspari RB, Jackson RW, et al. Operative arthroscopy. 2nd ed. Hagerstown: Lippincott-Raven, 1996.

McRae R. Practical fracture treatment. 3rd ed. Edinburgh: Churchill, Livingstone, 1994.

Michelson JD. Fractures about the ankle. Current concepts review. J Bone Joint Surg 1995;77: 142–152.

Miller MD. Review of orthopaedics. 2nd ed. Philadelphia: WB Saunders, 1996.

Moed BR. Femur: trauma. In: Kasser JR, ed. Orthopaedic knowledge update 5. Rosemont, IL: American Academy of Orthpaedic Surgeons, 1996;427–436.

Morrey BJ. Current concepts in the treatment of fractures of the radial head, the olecranon and the coronoid. In: Instructional course lectures. Vol. 44. Rosemont, IL: American Academy of Orthopaedic Surgeons, 1995.

Muëller ME, Allgower M, Schneider R, et al; Schatzker J, trans. Manual of internal fixation—techniques recommended by the AO group. 2nd ed. Berlin: Springer-Verlag, 1979.

Pan WT, Einhorn TA. The biochemistry of fracture healing. Current orthopaedics. London: Longman Group, UK Ltd, 1992;207–213.

Perry CR. Knee and leg: bone trauma. In: Kasser JR, ed. Orthopaedic knowledge update 5. Rosemont, IL: American Academy of Orthopaedic Surgeons, 1996;453–462.

Peterson L, Renström P. Sports injuries: their prevention and treatment (English language edition.) London: Martin Dunitz, 1986.

Poss R, ed. Orthopaedic knowledge update 3. Home study syllabus. Rosemont, IL: American Academy of Orthopaedic Surgeons, 1990.

Rockwood CA, Green DP, Bucholz RW, Heckman JD, eds. Rockwood and Green's fractures in adults. Vols. 1 and 2. 4th ed. Philadelphia: Lippincott Raven, 1996.

Rodgrigo JJ. Orthopaedic surgery, basic science and clinical science. Boston: Little Brown, 1986.

Rorabeck CH. Compartment syndromes. In: Browner BD, Jupiter JB, Levine AM, et al, eds. Skeletal trauma: fractures, dislocations; ligamentous injuries. Vol. 1. Philadelphia: WB Saunders, 1992:285–309.

Salter RB, Gross A, Hall JH. Hydrocortisone arthropathy—an experimental investigation. Can Med Assoc J 1967;97:374–377.

Salter RB, Harris DJ. The healing of intra-articular fractures with continuous passive motion. In: American Academy of Orthopaedic Surgeons instructional course lecture series. St. Louis: CV Mosby, 1979;102–117.

Salter RB, Hamilton HW, Wedge JH, et al. Clinical application of basic research on continuous passive motion for disorders and injuries of synovial joints: a preliminary report of a feasibility study. J Orthop Res 1984;1:325–342.

Salter RB. Continuous passive motion (CPM): a biological concept for the healing and regeneration of articular cartilage, ligaments and tendons: from origination to research to clinical application. Baltimore: Williams & Wilkins, 1993.

Sarmiento A, Mullis DL, Latta LL, et al. A quantitative comparative analysis of fracture healing under the influence of compression plating vs. closed weight bearing treatment. Clin Orthop 1980;149:232–239.

Sarmiento A, Latta LL. Closed functional treatment of fractures. Berlin: Springer-Verlag, 1981.

Sarmiento A, Latta LL. Functional fracture bracing: tibia, humerus, and ulna. Berlin: Springer-Verlag, 1995.

Sarmiento A, Sharpe FE, Ebramzadth E, et al. Factors influencing the outcome of closed tibial fractures treated with functional bracing. Clin Orthop 1995;315:8–24.

Schatzker J, Tile M. The rationale of operative fracture care. 2nd ed. Berlin: Springer-Verlag, 1996.

Schemitsch EH, Richards RR. The effect of malunion on functional outcome after plate fixation of fractures of both bones of the forearm in adults. J Bone Joint Surg 1992;74A: 1068–1078.

Schenk RK. Biology of fracture repair. In: Browner BD, Jupiter JB, Levine AM, et al, eds. Skeletal trauma: fractures, distortions, ligamentous injuries. Vol. 1. Philadelphia: WB Saunders, 1992: 31–75.

Shuler TE. Trauma. Section 1: adult trauma. In: Miller MD, ed. Review of orthopaedics. 2nd ed. Philadelphia: WB Saunders, 1996;350–392.

Schultz RJ. The language of fractures. 2nd ed. Baltimore: Williams & Wilkins, 1990.

Schutzer SF, Gossling HR. The treatment of reflex sympathetic dystrophy syndrome (current concepts review). J Bone Joint Surg 1994;66A: 625–629.

Snider RK, ed. Essentials of musculoskeletal care. Rosemont, IL: American Academy of Orthopaedic Surgeons, 1997.

Swiontkowski MF. Intracapsular hip fractures. In: Browner BD, Jupiter JB, Levine AM, et al, eds. Skeletal trauma: fractures, dislocations, ligamentous injuries. Vol. 2. Philadelphia: WB Saunders, 1992:1369–1442.

Teitz CC, Garrett WE Jr, Miniaci A, et al. Tendon problems in athletic individuals. An instructional course lecture, The American Academy of Orthopaedic Surgeons. J Bone Joint Surg 1997; 79A:138–152.

Tile M. Fractures of the pelvis and acetabulum. 2nd ed. Baltimore: Williams & Wilkins, 1995.

Tornetta P III, Mostafvi HR. Hip dislocation: current treatment regimens. J Am Acad Orthop Surg 1997;5:27–36.

Uhthoff H, ed. Current concepts of external fixation of fractures. Berlin: Springer-Verlag, 1982.

Urist MR. Bone-formation by osteoinduction. Science 1965;150:893–899.

Urist MR, Silvermann BF, Büring K, et al. The bone induction principle. Clin Orthop 1967;53: 243–283.

Urist MR. Bone morphogenetic protein with special reference to bone transplants, implants and the bone—bone marrow consortium. In: Peck IVA, ed. Bone and mineral research. Vol. 6. New York: Elsevier Science Publishers, 1989.

Wiss DA, Kull DM, Perry J. Lisfranc fracture-dislocations of the foot: a clinico-kinescological study. J Orthop Trauma 1988;1:267–274.

Zuckerman JD. Hip fracture. Review article, current concepts. New Engl J Med 1996;334: 1519–1525.

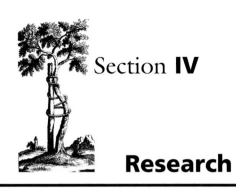

Section **IV**

Research

18 The Philosophy and Nature of Medical Research with One Example

"The practice of Medicine is an art—based on science."

—Sir William Osler

Although a discussion of medical research may be considered by some to be "beyond undergraduate core curriculum," I am directing this chapter to you as a student because you have the *potential* to become a scientist or clinician-scientist—either part-time or full-time—and also because of my own personal conviction that research is essential to the continuing progress of all medical and surgical specialties as well as other health care professions.

My purpose is threefold: first to help you to appreciate the importance and philosophy of medical research; second, to stimulate you to contemplate the possibility of your own personal involvement; and third, to share with you some thoughts concerning the *nature* of such research as well as some guidelines concerning the scientific method—thoughts and guidelines that I have found especially helpful during 43 years of consistent involvement in this fascinating and exciting facet of academic medicine.

For these purposes, the terms "medical" and "medicine" are used in their broadest context in that they are meant to include all medical and surgical specialties and other

health care professions, even though I write from my perspective as an orthopaedic surgeon-scientist.

A DEFINITION OF RESEARCH

The English noun *research* is derived from the French verb *rechercher*, which means simply to look again or to take a second look—in contradistinction to being satisfied with one superficial look. Thus, research involves taking a fresh and concentrated look at a given problem in an attempt to find a solution.

As the philosopher and critic John Ruskin wrote in 1853, "The work of science is to substitute facts for appearances and demonstrations for impressions."

From a distillation of definitions in various dictionaries, research could be defined as "an investigation or experimental study of some phenomenon directed to the discovery and interpretation of new data through the critical approach of the scientific method."

In Chapter 5, I referred to solving the mystery of a diagnosis as "the detective work of *clinical* medicine." In this sense, medical research is the detective work of *scientific* medicine. Thus, the modern day medical investigator who is striving to solve a biological mystery must bring to bear on the problem the same powers of astute observation, the same gathering of clues or data, and the same processes of inductive and deductive reasoning used by the modern day detective or criminal investigator. As in detective work, so also in research, the magnifying glass of Sherlock Holmes has been replaced by the light microscope and even more sophisticated equipment such as transmission and scanning electron microscopes.

THE VARIOUS TYPES OF RESEARCH

Medical research is usually divided, somewhat arbitrarily, into two major categories: basic research and applied research. Although these two categories of medical research share the same demanding discipline of the scientific method, they differ in some respects.

Basic research, which is also called "pure research" or "fundamental research," is usually pursued for the sake of acquiring knowledge and understanding for their own sake, albeit with the hope that such acquisitions may prove eventually to be relevant to health, even if indirectly. As the Nobel laureate, John Polanyi, has written, "The prime objective of basic science is to foster the discovery of new ideas and the applications will flow naturally from these discoveries."

Applied research, which is also known as "clinically oriented research," "mission-oriented research," or "targeted research," is usually pursued for the sake of solving a specific clinical problem in man so that the resultant solution may be applied directly and immediately. Such research may be conducted through experimental investigations in animals or through clinical investigations in human patients. Nevertheless, through applied or mission-oriented research, basic or fundamental concepts may be discovered and, just as through basic research, practical applications of the research may be forthcoming. These two types of research represent a continuum of investigation and they share the focus of excellence.

Although basic research and applied research are of equal importance and often interdependent, it is understandable that in medical research the emphasis is on applied or clinically oriented research, that is, as applied to the care of patients. However, the great French scientist Louis Pasteur wisely said, "There are really no *applied* sciences—only the *application* of science, a very different matter."

THE IMAGE OF MEDICAL RESEARCH

As an undergraduate student of today, you may have been negatively influenced by the current trend among some of the young to harbor anti-establishment and antiscience feelings. Also, much has been said discussed about budgetary constraints on research funding through governments, resulting in few opportunities for full-time or part-time positions in medical research. Although such negative attitudes have often been exaggerated, they may explain—at least in part—why only approximately 5% of undergraduate medical students in North America are currently attracted to careers in medical research.

This negative image of research, although unjustified, is not new, for as the nineteenth century philosopher and critic John Ruskin wrote, "Science lives only in quiet places, and with odd people, mostly poor." But all of that has changed! Visit the medical or surgical research laboratories in your own university and you will find them to be not "quiet places," but rather hives of intellectual and physical activity. You may find the medical or surgical scientists unusual or uncommon individuals, perhaps, but not "odd," and they are no longer "mostly poor."

THE GOALS AND IMPORTANCE OF RESEARCH

In the broad fields of medicine and surgery and their related basic sciences, the primary goal of the various types of research is to achieve a more complete understanding of biological processes, both normal and abnormal. Achieving these goals permits significant advances in the treatment of disorders and injuries in humans through the development of more effective methods of prevention, detection, or treatment. In this sense, all medical research has a bearing on health—either directly or indirectly, either immediately or eventually.

In an academic setting, research has an additional goal, namely the enrichment of the *education*—as opposed to the mere *training*—of a clinician. In this context, the term "education" implies the intelligent understanding of clinical teaching, whereas the term "training" implies uncritical acceptance of such teaching.

Research enhances the quality of medical education, both undergraduate and postgraduate, because the scientific atmosphere has a beneficial impact on all aspects of the educational program, and such an atmosphere is testimony to the fact that medicine as a science is dynamic—growing and constantly changing for the better. Furthermore, a lively and exciting program of medical research in a given university attracts the brightest young people as postgraduate students and new faculty members to that university.

Through your personal involvement in scientific investigations as an undergraduate or postgraduate student, you should acquire qualities such as intellectual curiosity, critical thinking, logic, and discrimination that can be applied to your own work and to the work of your colleagues. In any postgraduate surgical training program that does not include a significant amount of research activity, the potential clinician will receive more of a technical or trade school training than a true medical education in both the art and science of medicine.

In any university, the importance of medical research varies directly with the degree to which these two major goals are being achieved. Although much more emphasis on medical research is required worldwide, such research has already gained a position of importance in many major universities because of its contribution to new knowledge and medical education.

First-rate medical research within a university medical school invariably improves the quality of patient care, first in the affiliated teaching hospitals of that university and then in hospitals throughout the world, because new scientific knowledge is soon shared with fellow clinicians and scientists internationally through the media of scientific meetings and publications.

THE MOTIVATION FOR SEARCH AND RESEARCH

Search for knowledge that is both true and new has always challenged and motivated intelligent humans. In his famous 12th century prayer, the physician-philosopher Maimonides expressed such motivation this way: "Let the thought never arise that I have attained enough knowledge."

The acknowledged "father" of surgical research is the 18th century surgeon, John Hunter, whose insatiable curiosity concerning all biological phenomena combined with his brilliant logic led to innumerable experiments with highly significant results that changed the course of surgical practice. He became one of the first surgeons in the world to apply the scientific method to surgical problems and to put surgery on a scientific, as opposed to an empirical, basis.

In a letter to Jenner concerning smallpox, Hunter wrote: "I think your solution is just; but why only think? Why not try the experiment?" The underlying motivation of the scientist to become engaged in research—in fact wedded to it—is a combination of intellectual curiosity and dissatisfaction with the current state of knowledge and understanding. As Voltaire said: "Without the spirit of constructive discontent we would still be eating acorns and sleeping under the stars."

PERSONAL QUALITIES OF THE MEDICAL SCIENTIST

As a potential medical scientist, you should consider the following eight personal qualities as among the most important for research. You must *have* integrity, intelligence, ingenuity, and initiative, and you must *be* inquisitive, innovative, industrious, and incisive.

THE PHILOSOPHY OF MEDICAL RESEARCH

Inherent in the philosophy of research is the idea of "constructive discontent" with existing knowledge and traditionally accepted—but unproven—concepts. As an undergraduate student, you will have acquired an incredible amount of cognitive information, at least some of which needs to be challenged. George Perkins, a distinguished British orthopaedic surgeon who dared to differ with his more traditional-minded contemporaries, once stated that, "The training of a medical doctor is such that it is difficult for him (or her) to break with tradition"—a sad commentary relevant to the difference between "training" and "education."

Although the success of research depends upon many factors, the pivotal and initiating factor is the scientific curiosity of the investigator, a curiosity that compels him or her to discover—or uncover—new data and new concepts through the application of the scientific method.

Understandably, the life of the clinician-scientist is not easy, but it can be very rewarding in terms of the quiet satisfaction that comes from achieving a scientific goal. In a sense, the clinician-scientist is a bridge builder who constantly strives to close the gap between the practical art and theoretical science of medicine. To be effective in this role, the medical scientist must merit the respect of both fellow clinicians and scientists, an effort that calls for exemplary performance in both fields. This important concept is epitomized by the motto of the Royal College of Physicians and Surgeons of Canada: *Mente Perspicua Manuque Apta*—"A keen mind and skillful hands."

THE NATURE OF MEDICAL RESEARCH—A CYCLE

Even the most inspired and idealistic of potential scientists must accept and work within the rigorous discipline of the scientific method, the essence of all research. Seemingly complex and formidable at first to the uninitiated or inexperienced, the scientific method is best understood if presented as a series of well-planned phases or steps.

During many years of teaching and supervising both undergraduate and postgraduate research fellows, I have found the concept of what I call the "cycle of medical research" to be most helpful in outlining and explaining the multiple phases of the time-honored scientific method (Fig. 18.1). The cycle consists of a series of guidelines that starts with patients and returns to patients, because medical research of the mission-oriented or targeted type is designed to find the solution to a clinical problem. In due course, whenever appropriate, the newly found knowledge is applied to that problem.

In this cycle of medical research, there are 16 phases, each of which merits attention.

1. Recognize an Unsolved Clinical Problem

To find a solution to an unsolved *clinical* problem, it is essential that as a clinician-scientist, you first *recognize* the problem, or a component of it, and this involves being a keen and alert observer—a human biology watcher. Unfortunately, a pure clinician may "have eyes but see not" and may miss the critical observation that would lead to recognizing an unsolved clinical problem and to its investigation. "In the field of observation," wrote Louis Pasteur, "chance favors the prepared mind."

2. Think

To *think* deeply, contemplatively, and speculatively about an unsolved problem requires determination and self-discipline, because there are so many interruptions in the daily—and nightly—life of a physician or surgeon. Furthermore, such thinking is more difficult and taxing than, for instance, making a fairly obvious diagnosis, prescribing a routine medical regimen, or performing a routine surgical operation. It may, however, bring its own rewards, such as the intellectual exhilaration that results from successful problem-solving.

Nobel laureate, Albert Szent-Gyorgi, has stated, "Discovery consists of seeing what everybody else has seen—but thinking what nobody else has thought."

3. Review the Scientific Literature

Before embarking on any research project, you will need to review the scientific background against which your work will stand. In medical research as in other forms of research,

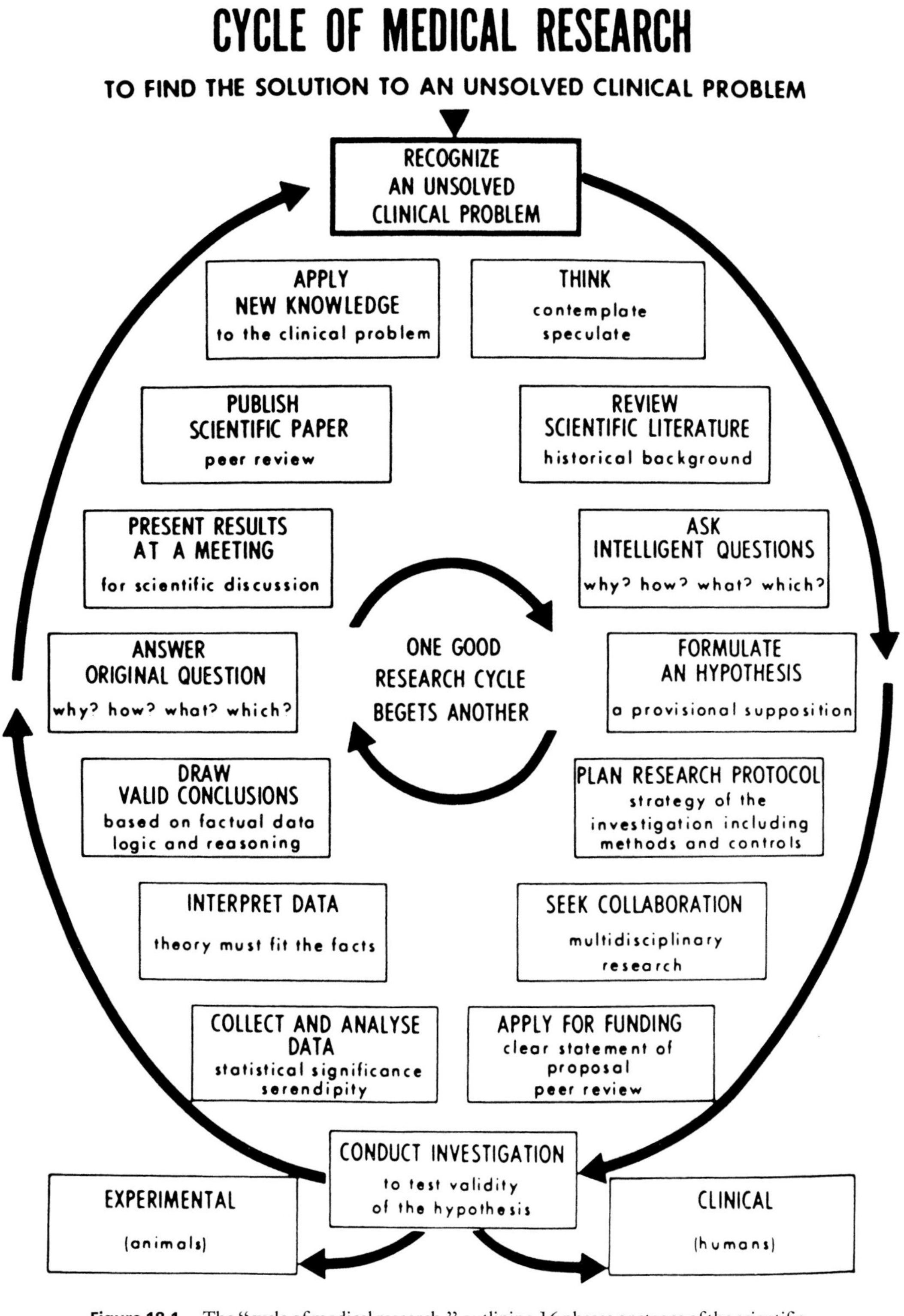

CYCLE OF MEDICAL RESEARCH

TO FIND THE SOLUTION TO AN UNSOLVED CLINICAL PROBLEM

Figure 18.1.   The "cycle of medical research," outlining 16 phases or stages of the scientific method relevant to applied research.

there have been many examples of "rediscovering the round wheel," which could have been avoided had the investigator been aware of the historical background of the subject. Santayana expressed the thought that those who do not read history are doomed to repeat the errors (and one might add, the experiments) of the past. Fortunately, literature surveys have been tremendously facilitated by modern computerized library science. As you review the scientific literature relevant to the recognized problem, you will benefit from the labors of fellow scientists and be stimulated to build upon such labors through original thinking and questioning.

4. Ask an Intelligent Question

Having read the historical background of the problem, you need to ask an intelligent question, and one that can be reasonably answered through research. Regarding a specific phenomenon under investigation, that question frequently begins with, Why? How? What? or Which? Much time, effort, and money will be wasted if an inappropriate question forms the underlying basis for a research project, for as the scientist Sir Henry Tizard has emphasized, "The secret of success in science is to ask the right question."

5. Formulate a Hypothesis

As the first step toward answering your own question, you should formulate a hypothesis—literally a subordinate thesis or a theoretical and provisional supposition that serves as a starting point for further investigation by which it may be proved or disproved. The working hypothesis is a carefully reasoned, but as yet unproven answer to the question. Its validity must be tested through the planned research project.

6. Plan the Research Protocol

The next step in the cycle of medical research is to plan in detail the *protocol* of the investigation, that is, the experimental design, including the subjects of the investigation (either animals or human patients), the investigational methods, the equipment, the controls to deal with all possible variables, and the proposed methods of analysis of the data, including the determination of statistical significance. The protocol should be planned with the purpose of the investigation in mind, namely the testing of the validity of your hypothesis.

Understandably, it may be tempting for a scientist to become so personally invested in a cherished hypothesis that, throughout the scientific investigations, he or she persistently tries to prove that the hypothesis is correct, even in the face of contradictory research data. Thus, as relevant and proven scientific data, both positive and negative, become apparent, the scientist who conceived the original hypothesis must be willing and prepared either to modify it or replace it completely and to use the modified or new hypothesis as a starting point for further research.

7. Seek Collaboration

As biomedical research becomes increasingly complex and sophisticated, you must be prepared to collaborate with scientists of other disciplines, such as physiology, biochemistry, microbiology, molecular biology, genetics, immunology, biophysics, and biomedical engineering, in multidisciplinary research. Through such collaborative research, one mind fertilizes another, and the scientific investigation grows in both depth and breadth. It was the importance of collaboration in research that Claude Bernard was extolling when he wrote, "Art is I; Science is We."

8. Apply for Funding

This enlightened era of science is intermittently darkened by the clouds of antiscience and the constraints of research budgets from governments and other agencies. It should be encouraging for you, as a potential clinician-scientist, to realize that there is still money available to support well-planned, clearly stated, exciting, significant, and original research. The peer review system would still seem to be the most appropriate mechanism through which your grant application may receive the fairest consideration and the highest possible standards of research may be maintained. Two of the criteria by which your fellow scientists in the peer review system judge a given proposal are the scientific significance of the project in terms of new knowledge or understanding and the likelihood of its success.

9. Conduct the Investigation

Throughout the scientific investigation, your objective is neither to prove nor disprove your hypothesis, but rather to test its validity with complete objectivity. As a clinical physician or surgeon, your inherent reverence for human life and human comfort will compel you to confine experimental investigations to animals. An investigator must also understand that any proposed clinical investigations in humans must be morally and ethically acceptable to the review mechanisms of a university-based "human clinical investigation (or experimentation) committee," which includes clinician-scientists and members of other professions. Experimental investigations in animals must also be acceptable, in that they must meet established government regulations to protect the comfort of the animals.

10. Collect and Analyze the Data

As you make observations and collect data during the progress of your investigation, you should be alert to the possibility that an unexpected finding may have much significance—a phenomenon called *serendipity* (a word coined by Sir Horace Walpole in 1754 based on a Persian fable, "The Three Princes of Serendip." At that time, Serendip was the Arabic name for Ceylon, which is now known as Sri Lanka. Every time the three princes went on a journey, they found, quite by chance, valuable things they were not even looking for; hence the origin of serendipity). Winston Churchill has written, "Men occasionally stumble over the truth, but most of them pick themselves up and hurry off as though nothing had happened." Nevertheless, through serendipity many important discoveries have been made, including the following: the discovery of North America by Christopher Columbus, the invention of the phonograph by Thomas Edison, the invention of the telephone by Alexander Graham Bell, and the discovery of penicillin by Sir Alexander Fleming. Provided that the protocol of your investiga-

tion has been well planned, it should be possible for you to analyze your data accurately and determine its statistical significance.

11. Interpret the Data

This is one of the most important phases of the medical research cycle because, although you may have collected important data, unless the interpretation of these data is correct, you may find yourself off the cycle and into the ditch of delusion. In the interpretation of the data, you must consider all the data, not just those parts that seem to "fit" the hypothesis. Doing the latter deludes yourself and others, making the facts fit the theory rather than making the theory fit the facts. It may have been this type of intellectual delusion that George Bernard Shaw was contemplating when he wrote, "Beware of false knowledge—it is more dangerous than ignorance."

12. Draw Valid Conclusions

Through the application of sound logic and scientific reasoning, you should draw valid conclusions, insofar as that is possible, on the basis of the factual data. This is another difficult phase of the cycle of medical research because the clinician-scientist may be tempted, subconsciously and unwittingly, to draw conclusions that are not justified by the factual data. When more than one interpretation of the data seems reasonable, it may be necessary to initiate another cycle of research to clarify the matter.

13. Answer the Original Question

By the time you have reached this phase of the cycle, you may well be able to answer the original question. One of the world's leaders in the philosophy of science, Sir Karl Popper, has stated that, "Knowledge advances by refutation of false doctrines, not by verification of true ones," and that "It is not the possession of knowledge, or irrefutable truths, that constitute the man of science but rather, the incessant search for truth." The search for truth, however, is never-ending, because the more questions you answer, the more questions you will raise to take their place. Each of these questions, in turn, will serve as the catalyst for the creation of another research cycle.

14. Present Results at a Meeting

Having completed the investigation, it is important for you to present the results at a scientific meeting to gain the benefits of the peer review that comes with the resultant discussion, both positive and negative. Indeed, constructive criticism of a given scientific investigation can only help to improve its final presentation. It would be considered unprofessional for a medical scientist to share the results of research with the general public through the lay media—press, radio, or television—before these results have been either presented at a major scientific meeting or published in the scientific literature.

15. Publish a Scientific Paper

If your investigation has been worth doing, it is worth publishing, and you should seek publication in a reputable scientific journal that is critically refereed, that is, peer reviewed. Indeed, you have a moral obligation to publish a significant scientific investigation because, as Richard Bach has written in his book entitled *Jonathan Livingston Seagull,* "It is good to be a seeker but sooner or later you have to be a finder, and then it is well to give what you have found, a gift unto the world for whoever will accept it."

16. Apply the New Knowledge

As implied in the adjective "applied," this type of mission-oriented or targeted research frequently leads to new knowledge that can be applied to the unsolved clinical problem that initiated the cycle of medical research. The application may be relevant to an improved understanding of the etiology, pathology, pathogenesis, detection, treatment, or even prevention of the clinical problem under investigation. Such application is in keeping with Booker's law, which states that "an ounce of application is worth a ton of abstraction."

Thus the cycle of medical research is complete, and you will have progressed from realistic research to clinical reality—"from the laboratory bench to the patient's bedside." It

is hoped that you will have come to appreciate that it is better to move in the best circles of research than to walk the straight and narrow path of empiricism.

No matter how successful a scientist may be in solving problems, his or her "spirit of constructive discontent," of which Voltaire wrote, is self-perpetuating, because one good idea begets another and one discovery leads to another.

In the final analysis, the success of any given medical research project will depend on the intelligence and inquisitiveness of the individual scientist whose goal should not be to follow the established path of clinical empiricism but rather, through research, to explore where there is no path and leave a trail that leads into the future!

ONE EXAMPLE OF MEDICAL RESEARCH

As stated in "An Open Letter to a Medical Student" in the preliminary pages of this 3rd edition, "I have broadened the title of this chapter, which becomes 'The Philosophy and Nature of Medical Research with One Example.'" The example I have chosen is the basic and applied research that several of my research fellows and I have conducted during the past 28 years on the biological concept of continuous passive motion (CPM) for the healing and regeneration of articular cartilage, ligaments, and tendons. I have summarized the evolution of this concept from its origination, to research, to clinical applications. I trust this example will help you to appreciate more fully the intellectual excitement and exhilaration of medical research.

An Overview of Continuous Passive Motion (CPM)[1]
Historical Background
The Limited Potential of Articular Cartilage to Heal or to Regenerate

Articular cartilage can heal only by a scar (for example, by fibrous tissue or at best by fibro-

---

Footnote 1.1. This overview of continuous passive motion is largely taken from Chapter 32 of the author's monograph entitled "Continuous Passive Motion (CPM): A Biological Concept for the Healing and Regeneration of Articular Cartilage, Ligaments and Tendons: From Origination to Research to Clinical Applications," published by Williams & Wilkins, Baltimore (1993) with the kind permission of the publisher.

cartilage) and, under ordinary circumstances, is incapable of regeneration. The limited potential of articular cartilage either to heal after injury or to regenerate after destruction was recognized by Hippocrates and has been demonstrated by many scientific investigators during the past six decades (15, 27). Once articular cartilage is damaged either by disease or by injury, its inability either to heal or to regenerate means that it is destined to degenerate with subsequent use of the involved joint and that late degenerative arthritis (osteoarthritis) is the inevitable outcome.

Rest and Motion in Orthopaedics

Despite the fact that rest and motion have always been two of the most commonly prescribed methods of management of diseased and injured musculoskeletal tissues, their indications, duration, and therapeutic value remain controversial.

The history of rest and motion in the management of musculoskeletal disorders and injuries from Hippocrates to the present time also provides relevant background data (14). On the basis of clinical empiricism throughout the past 25 centuries, at least up to the last 3 decades, the vast majority of physicians and surgeons throughout the world have advocated rest rather than motion. They have embraced the time-honored but unproven principle that diseased and injured tissues need rest to heal. During the past 3 decades, however, although still on an empirical basis, some clinicians have joined the ranks of those who advocate motion.

By contrast, on the basis of scientific investigation, the deleterious effects of prolonged immobilization of synovial joints in animals have been demonstrated by numerous orthopaedic clinician-scientists, including the author. Several clinical investigators have also demonstrated similar deleterious effects of prolonged immobilization (Imm) of synovial joints in humans. Furthermore, the beneficial effects on articular cartilage of intermittent active motion (IAM) of joints (as compared to Imm) have been reported. Thus, the relative value of rest and motion in managing musculoskeletal disorders and injuries is much less controversial on the basis of scientific investigation than on the basis of clinical empiricism.

Preliminary Thinking Behind the Concept of CPM, the Impossible Dream, and the Challenge of Arthritis

The Arthritis Society has estimated that approximately 3.4% (8.5 million people) of the population of North America suffer from pain and limitation of motion of one or more joints due to some form of arthritis.

The development of total joint excision and prosthetic joint replacement for irreversibly destroyed arthritic joints in older individuals has been, without question, the most important technological and biomechanical advance in orthopaedic surgery of the twentieth century. Nevertheless, because of the inherent problems of artificial joints, such as subsequent prosthetic loosening, migration, wear, and even breakage, prosthetic joint replacement is inappropriate for children, adolescents, and active young adults.

For centuries, the "impossible dream" of both clinicians and scientists has been the development of a method of stimulating healing and regeneration of articular cartilage.

Given the notoriously limited capacity of articular cartilage either to heal or regenerate and the age- and stress-related limitations of prosthetic joints, the greatest challenge facing orthopaedic surgeon-scientists in relation to arthritis is to develop biological alternatives to prosthetic and biomechanical methods of treatment, especially for physically active children, adolescents, and young adults.

In 1971, in an editorial on cartilage repair, Cruess expressed this philosophy: "It seems necessary to provide the best conditions for cartilage repair in the hope that natural processes may be enhanced and so-called reconstructive procedures may be avoided (1)." By "so-called reconstructed procedures," he was referring to prosthetic joint replacements.

The author shares this philosophy, and during the past 28 years, has tried to stimulate the natural recuperative powers of the body and to provide the best conditions for cartilage repair through the use of CPM of synovial joints for the healing and regeneration of articular cartilage, ligaments, and tendons.

The Reasoning That Led to CPM

The reasoning that led to the biological concept of CPM of synovial joints was based on the author's numerous observations and deductions, including the following:

First, clinical observations revealed the following deleterious effects of prolonged Imm of synovial joints in patients: persistent stiffness and pain, muscle atrophy, disuse osteoporosis, and late degenerative arthritis with subsequent use of the involved joints.

Second, clinical observations showed the beneficial local effects of early active motion as opposed to prolonged Imm of diseased and injured joints.

Third, original basic research had shown the harmful effects of Imm of rabbit knee joints under compression produced either by compression clamp or by Imm of joints in a forced position. The author demonstrated a lesion of "pressure necrosis" of articular cartilage in the compressed area in 6 days (17). Subsequent use of a joint with this lesion led to degenerative arthritis.

Fourth, original basic research had also shown the harmful effects of prolonged Imm (6 to 12 weeks) of the flexed knee joint of the rabbit without compression. The author demonstrated a lesion of "obliterative degeneration" of articular cartilage in the noncontact areas resulting from the adherence of the synovial membrane to the joint surface. Subsequent use of such immobilized joints also led to degenerative arthritis (22).

Finally, lessons from cardiac surgery (especially open heart operations), peripheral vascular surgery, and thoracic surgery showed that injured tissues do not need to be put to rest to heal.

Having noted both clinically and experimentally that intermittent motion of synovial joints was better for articular cartilage and other articular tissues than Imm, the author asked the pivotal question, "If intermittent motion is good for articular cartilage, would continuous motion be even better?" Because of the fatigability of skeletal muscle, continuous motion would have to be passive rather than active. Thus, in 1970 the author originated the biological concept of CPM of synovial joints as a possible means of stimulating the healing and regeneration of articular cartilage, as well as other articular tissues, and of either preventing or overcoming joint stiffness.

This concept clearly represents the complete antithesis of the traditional and time-honored principle of immobilization of diseased and injured joints and related tissues.

Basic Premises and Hypotheses of CPM

The biological concept of CPM of synovial joints is based on the following basic premises:

- Synovial joints are designed to move and are meant to do so. Indeed, the 24 costovertebral joints move continuously with every cycle of breathing in and breathing out throughout our entire lives.
- The nutrition of articular cartilage by synovial fluid is enhanced by joint motion.
- Prolonged Imm of synovial joints and persistent limitation of joint motion are deleterious to the articular cartilage and related tissues, including synovial membrane, ligaments, tendons, and muscles.

The three hypotheses of CPM of synovial joints are that it should have the following beneficial effects:

1. Enhance the nutrition and metabolic activity of articular cartilage.
2. Stimulate pluripotential mesenchymal cells to differentiate into articular cartilage, as opposed to either fibrous tissue or bone, and thereby lead to regeneration of cartilage (and achieve the "impossible dream").
3. Accelerate healing of both articular cartilage and periarticular tissues, such as tendons and ligaments.

The purpose of the numerous experimental investigations undertaken over the past 28 years has been to test the validity of these hypotheses in a variety of experimental models.

Basic Research on CPM

During the past 28 years, the author and a succession of basic research fellows have investigated the effects of CPM on a variety of experimental models of disorders and injuries of articular cartilage and periarticular tissues in the knee joints of both adolescent and adult rabbits. These experimental investigations have included the following topics:

- Full-thickness defects in a joint surface, short- and long-term (1 year)
- Partial-thickness defects in a joint surface
- Intra-articular fractures, short- and long-term (6 months)
- Acute septic arthritis
- Intra-articular fluid pressures
- Clearance of a hemarthrosis
- Wound healing
- Muscle atrophy
- Tendon healing in partial-thickness and full-thickness lacerations
- Ligament healing in a tenodesis model and a carbon fiber model
- Free intra-articular periosteal autografts
- Autogenous osteoperiosteal grafts for biological resurfacing of defects in a joint surface
- Autogenous periosteal grafts for biological resurfacing of patellar groove defects
- Durability of regenerated cartilage from periosteal autografts at 1 year
- Cellular origin of regenerated cartilage from periosteal autografts and allografts
- Biological resurfacing of patellar cartilage defects with autogenous periosteal grafts
- Chondrogenic potential of autogenous and allogeneic periosteal grafts
- Cryopreservation of periosteum and the chondrogenic potential of cryopreserved periosteal allografts
- Joint surface debridement: chondral shaving and subchondral abrasion

In each of these experimental models, CPM of the involved knee joint of each rabbit was provided by a specially designed, electrically powered apparatus. Continuous passive motion has consistently been initiated immediately after the operation while the animal is still under general anesthesia. It is continued nonstop for periods ranging from 1 to 4 weeks, with one complete cycle occurring every 45 seconds (an arbitrary frequency that has subsequently been proven to be more effective than either a faster or slower frequency). The effects of CPM have been compared to those of Imm and IAM (cage activity).

The Results of Basic Research

A brief summary of our published results to date (1998) of some of these scientific investigations (with relevant references) will serve to document the following beneficial biological effects of CPM:

1. Regeneration of hyaline articular cartilage occurred in 52% of full-thickness defects with CPM, compared with only 18% in immobilized (Imm) joints and 9% in joints allowed IAM (26, 27). The superiority of the repair tissue stimulated by CPM is maintained up to 1 year postoperatively (23).
2. The potential for healing or regeneration of partial-thickness defects is so limited that even CPM did not have a significantly beneficial effect on such healing or regeneration (24).
3. Healing of the fracture in the articular cartilage in intra-articular fractures occurred in 80% of animals with CPM, compared with only 20% with either Imm or IAM. Also noted was prevention of posttraumatic arthritis secondary to intra-articular fractures with CPM, at 6 months after fracture (19).
4. A significant protective effect of CPM on articular cartilage was noted in an experimental model of septic arthritis (20).
5. Increasing degrees of flexion of the rabbit knee produced significantly higher intra-articular fluid pressures. A sinusoidal oscillation in fluid pressure was observed during CPM (10).
6. The rate of clearance of an experimental hemarthrosis of the knee joint was twice as fast with CPM as with Imm (11).
7. Wound healing of parapatellar arthrotomy incisions was significantly enhanced by CPM compared with Imm (28).
8. Compared with the results in the rabbits treated by immobilization, CPM significantly reduced muscle atrophy in the gastrocnemius muscle as determined from the dry and wet weights (2).
9. Significantly thicker tendon callus forma-

tion, better alignment of tendon fibers, and increased breaking strength occurred in CPM-treated animals with a partial-thickness laceration of the patellar tendon (16).

10. In an experimental model of a semitendinosus tenodesis to replace the medial collateral ligament of the knee joints, the CPM-treated animals exhibited significantly stronger healing of the tenodesis (a return to 86% of the normal strength at 12 weeks, compared with that in the Imm- and IAM-treated animals [18]). Similar beneficial effects of CPM were seen in an experimental model of medial collateral ligament reconstruction using carbon fiber (32).

11. The chondrogenic potential of free intra-articular periosteal autografts is significantly enhanced by the postoperative use of CPM (8).

12. In an investigation of the chondrogenic potential of autogenous osteoperiosteal grafts in a full-thickness defect in a joint surface, it was found that after 5 weeks, hyaline cartilage was the predominant tissue in only 10% of the defects in the Imm and IAM groups, compared with 70% in the CPM group (9).

13. Under the influence of CPM, free autogenous periosteal grafts glued into a full-thickness patellar groove defect provide a biological resurfacing of the defect by tissue that resembled articular cartilage grossly, histologically, and biochemically, and that contained predominantly type II collagen. This means that osteoprogenitor cells of the periosteum changed their phenotype expression under the influence of CPM (12).

14. The hyaline cartilage that is produced by autogenous periosteal grafts in full-thickness osteochondral defects under the influence of CPM is capable of withstanding a full year of articular function without marked deterioration (13).

15. The cellular origin of the neochondrogenesis in full-thickness defects under the influence of CPM was studied using tritiated thymidine and was found to be primarily the progenitor cells of the autogenous periosteal graft (31). With allografts of periosteum, however, the cellular origin of the new tissue was from both the periosteal graft and the subchondral tissues (30).

16. The quality of the neochondrogenesis produced by autogenous periosteal grafts in full-thickness defects in the patella was significantly better in the CPM-treated animals than in those treated by either Imm or IAM (7).

17. Autogenous and allogeneic periosteal grafts were almost equally effective in producing neochondrogenesis as a biological resurfacing of a full-thickness defect in a joint surface at 6 weeks or 12 weeks (25).

18. Periosteal grafts harvested from the tibiae of rabbits may be cryopreserved successfully for at least 4 months using the cryopreservative DMSO and a controlled rate of freezing of 1.0° C/min (5). We found no significant difference in chondrogenic potential between fresh and cryopreserved periosteal allografts. Grafts obtained from young rabbits were more chondrogenic than those obtained from adult rabbits. We found no evidence of rejection in any of the allografts up to 6 weeks after the transplantation (6).

19. In an experimental investigation of joint surface debridement, it was found that partial-thickness defects created by chondral shaving did not heal; rather, the remaining articular cartilage degenerated. By contrast, full-thickness defects created by subchondral abrasion do heal by regeneration of hyaline-like cartilage under the influence of CPM (4).

Summary and Conclusions from Basic Research

The results of these various experimental investigations to date have demonstrated that CPM is significantly superior to either Imm or IAM in stimulating the healing and regeneration of articular tissues as well as in preventing joint stiffness. Of considerable clinical significance is the consistent observation that the rabbits seem to have been comfortable while their operated knees were being moved continuously, in that they ate and drank well and slept well during the 1- to 4-week period of CPM. At the completion of the CPM period, the involved knee joints were completely mobile and the parapatellar skin incisions were well healed.

From the author's first 28 years of basic research on the biological concept of CPM, the following conclusions have been reached:

- CPM is well tolerated by both adolescent and adult rabbits and would seem to be relatively painless.
- CPM has a significant stimulating effect on the healing of articular tissues, including cartilage, tendons, and ligaments.
- CPM prevents adhesions and joint stiffness.
- CPM does not interfere with the healing of incisions over the moving joint and, indeed, enhances such healing.
- The time-honored principle that healing tissue must be put to rest is incorrect; indeed, it is this principle that must be put to rest rather than the healing soft tissues.
- Regeneration of articular cartilage through neochondrogenesis, both with and without periosteal grafts, is possible under the influence of CPM, which represents a turnabout of traditional thought.

Clinical Applications

Clinical Applications of the Basic Research—A Feasibility Study. In 1978, after the first 8 years of basic research on the effects of CPM on the healing and regeneration of articular cartilage and periarticular tissues had revealed that CPM was both safe and effective, the author deemed it justifiable on ethical grounds to proceed from realistic research to clinical reality, that is, to begin the clinical application of CPM to the care of orthopaedic patients for specific indications. Consequently, a project was initiated to design and develop CPM devices for humans in collaboration with a professional engineer, John H. Saringer and his associates in the Department of Mechanical Engineering at the University of Toronto.

These CPM devices for humans are currently being produced by Mr. Saringer at an independent company, Toronto Medical Corp.; they include devices for the ankle, ankle-knee-hip, the finger(s), the wrist, the elbow, and the shoulder. The author has no vested interest in this company, holds no patents, and receives no royalties from the sales of these devices; consequently, he has no conflict of interest.

In both animal studies and in patients, CPM has been instituted immediately after operation while the patient is still under general anesthesia and has been continued nonstop, day and night, for a minimum period of 1 week, after which active exercises of the involved joint are encouraged. The rate of motion of the various CPM devices has been one complete cycle every 45 seconds, although in some of the more recent models the rate can be varied (21).

Indications for CPM in Patients. Since 1978, the clinical indications for the use of CPM for patients have been the immediate and continuing postoperative management after the following operative procedures:

- Open reduction and rigid internal fixation of displaced intra-articular fractures
- Open reduction and rigid internal fixation of displaced metaphyseal and diaphyseal fractures
- Arthrotomy, capsulotomy, arthrolysis and debridement for posttraumatic arthritis with persistent limitation of joint motion (3)
- Surgical release of extra-articular contractures of joints (e.g., quadricepsplasty)
- Arthrotomy and drainage (combined with appropriate antibiotics) for acute septic arthritis
- Incision and drainage (combined with appropriate antibiotics) for acute tenosynovitis
- Synovectomy for rheumatoid arthritis and hemophilic arthropathy
- Biological resurfacing (with a periosteal graft) for a major defect in a joint surface
- Surgical repair of an acute ligamentous tear
- Reconstruction of a chronic ligamentous tear using a tendon graft
- Surgical repair of a complete laceration of a tendon (especially in the hand)
- Rigid internal fixation of a metaphyseal osteotomy (e.g., for arthritis of the knee)
- Total prosthetic joint replacement

As may be concluded, most of these indications are related to disorders and injuries that we have already investigated scientifically in our research laboratory.

Results of These Clinical Applications.
- Relative freedom from pain
- Maintenance of an increased range of joint motion
- Normal wound healing
- Absence of complications
- Short period of hospitalization
- Short period of rehabilitation
- Results are better than those of historical controls

Freedom from Pain

The relative freedom from pain experienced by patients treated with CPM immediately postoperatively confirms the observation of the same phenomenon in experimental investigations in rabbits. A hypothetical explanation for this fortuitous phenomenon may be related to the "gate control theory" of pain as proposed by Wall and Melzack (29). Thus, with CPM it is possible that the continuous generation of proprioceptive impulses from the continuously moving joint and their transmission to the spinal cord or brain may block the transmission of pain impulses to the brain (Melzack, personal communication). Further investigation, both clinical and experimental, will be required to test the validity of this hypothesis.

Acknowledgments

The author acknowledges with gratitude the valuable assistance of the following series of 20 basic research fellows from the University of Toronto Postgraduate Training Programme in Orthopaedic Surgery: Drs. D.F. Simmonds, B.W. Malcolm, E.J. Rumble, D. MacMichael, N.D. Clements, D. Ogilvie-Harris, E.R. Bogoch, D.A. Wong, R.S. Bell, R.R. Minster, S.W. O'Driscoll, J.J. Murnaghan, J.P. Delaney, R. Zarnett, R.M. Rodger, H. Kreder, M.E. Moran, H. Kim, S.J. Lewis and A. Khachatrian.

The author is also grateful to F.W. Keeley, Ph.D. for his expert advice concerning the many biochemical determinations and to Nomi Pittel for her splendid preparation of the histological sections.

Grateful thanks are extended to the Medical Research Council of Canada for its continuing support of the experimental investigations.

John H. Saringer, P.Eng. deserves special thanks for his ingenuity and resourcefulness in his collaboration in the design and development of CPM devices for patients.

REFERENCES

1. Cruess RL. Cartilage repair. J Bone Joint Surg 1971;53B:365. Editorial.
2. Dhert WJA, O'Driscoll SW, van Royen B. Effects of immobilization and continuous passive motion on post-operative muscle atrophy in mature rabbits. Can J Surg 1988;31(3):185–188.
3. Graham KR, Salter RB. The efficacy of continuous passive motion instituted after surgical release of the post-traumatic persistent stiff elbow. A clinical investigation. J Trauma 1989;29:1301. Abstract.
4. Kim HKW, Moran ME, Salter RB. The potential for regeneration of articular cartilage in defects caused by chondral shaving and subchondral abrasion. An experimental investigation in rabbits. J Bone Joint Surg 1991;73A:1301–1315.
5. Kreder HJ, Salter RB, Keeley FW. Cryopreservation of rabbit periosteum for transplantation. Trans 34th Annual Meeting Orthop Res Soc 1988:113. Abstract.
6. Kreder HJ, Salter RB, Moran ME, et al. Biological resurfacing of joint defects and cryopreserved allogeneic periosteum stimulated by continuous passive motion. Clin Orthop 1994;300:288–296.
7. Moran ME, Kim HKW, Salter RB. Biological resurfacing of a major defect in the articular cartilage of the patella with an autogenous periosteal graft subjected to continuous passive motion. J Bone Joint Surg 1992;74B:659–667.
8. O'Driscoll SW, Salter RB. The induction of neochondrogenesis in free periosteal autografts under the influence of continuous passive motion: an experimental investigation in the rabbit. J Bone Joint Surg 1984;66A:1248–1257.
9. O'Driscoll SW, Salter RB. The repair of major osteochondral defects in joint surfaces by neochondrogenesis with autogenous osteoperiosteal grafts stimulated by continuous passive motion: an experimental investigation in the rabbit. Clin Orthop 1986;208:131–140.
10. O'Driscoll SW, Kumar A, Salter RB. The effect of the volume of effusion, joint position and continuous passive motion on intra-articular

pressure in the rabbit knee. J Rheumatol 1983; 10:360–363.

11. O'Driscoll SW, Kumar A, Salter RB. The effect of continuous passive motion on the clearance of a hemarthrosis from a synovial joint: an experimental investigation in the rabbit. Clin Orthop 1983;176:305–311.

12. O'Driscoll SW, Salter RB, Keeley FW. The chondrogenic potential of free autogenous periosteal grafts for biological resurfacing of major full-thickness defects in joint surfaces under the influence of continuous passive motion: an experimental investigation in the rabbit. J Bone Joint Surg 1986;68A:1017–1035.

13. O'Driscoll SW, Salter RB, Keeley FW. Durability of regenerated articular cartilage produced by free autogenous periosteal grafts in major full-thickness defects in joint surfaces under the influence of continuous passive motion: a follow-up report at one year. J Bone Joint Surg 1988;70A:595–606.

14. Salter RB. Motion vs. rest: why immobilize joints? J Bone Joint Surg 1982;64B:251–254.

15. Salter RB. Regeneration of articular cartilage through continuous passive motion past, present and future. In: Straub R, Wilson PD, eds. Clinical trends in orthopaedics. New York: Thieme-Stratton, 1982.

16. Salter RB, Bell RS. The effect of continuous passive motion on the healing of partial thickness lacerations of the patellar tendon in the rabbit. Ann Coll Phys Surg Can 1981;14:209. Abstract.

17. Salter RB, Field P. The effects of continuous compression on living articular cartilage. An experimental investigation. J Bone Joint Surg 1960;42A:31–39.

18. Salter RB, Minster RR. The effect of continuous passive motion on a semitendinosus tenodesis in the rabbit knee. Orthop Trans 1982; 6:292. Abstract.

19. Salter RB, Ogilvie-Harris DJ. The healing of intra-articular fractures with continuous passive motion. In: Cooper R, ed. AAOS instructional course lectures. St. Louis: CV Mosby, 1979:102–117.

20. Salter RB, Bell RS, Keeley FW. The protective effect of continuous passive motion on living articular cartilage in acute septic arthritis: an experimental investigation in the rabbit. Clin Orthop 1981;159:223–247.

21. Salter RB, Hamilton HW, Wedge JH, et al. The clinical application of basic research on continuous passive motion (CPM) for disorders and injuries of synovial joints: a preliminary report. J Orthop Res 1983;1:325.

22. Salter RB, McNeill OR, Carbin R. The pathological changes in articular cartilage associated with persistent joint deformity: an experimental investigation. In: Gordon D, ed. Studies of rheumatoid disease: proceedings of the Third Canadian Conference on Research in the Rheumatic Diseases. Toronto: University of Toronto Press, 1965:33–37.

23. Salter RB, Minster RR, Clements N, et al. Continuous passive motion and the repair of full-thickness defects: a one-year follow-up. Orthop Trans 1982;6:266. Abstract.

24. Salter RB, Ogilvie-Harris DJ, Bogoch ER. Further studies in continuous passive motion. Orthop Trans 1978;2:292. Abstract.

25. Salter RB, Rodger RM, Wilson D, et al. The fate of allogeneic periosteum transplanted into an osteochondral defect and subjected to continuous passive motion (CPM). An experimental investigation in the rabbit. Clin Med 1987;10(Suppl):B127. Abstract.

26. Salter RB, Simmonds DF, Malcolm BW, et al. The effects of continuous passive motion on the healing of articular cartilage defects: an experimental investigation in rabbits. J Bone Joint Surg 1975;57A:570. Abstract.

27. Salter RB, Simmonds DF, Malcolm BW, et al. The biological effect of continuous passive motion on the healing of full-thickness defects in articular cartilage. J Bone Joint Surg 1980; 62A:1232–1251.

28. Van Royen BJ, O'Driscoll SW, Wouter JAD, Salter RB. Comparison of the effects of immobilization and continuous passive motion on surgical wound healing in the rabbit. Plast Reconstr Surg 1986;78:360–366.

29. Wall PD, Melzack R. Textbook of pain. Edinburgh: Churchill Livingstone, 1984.

30. Zarnett R, Salter RB. Periosteal neochondrogenesis for biological resurfacing joints: its cellular origin. Can J Surg 1989;32(3):171–174.

31. Zarnett R, Delaney JP, O'Driscoll SW, et al. Cellular origin and evolution of neochondrogenesis in major full-thickness defects of a joint surface treated by free autogenous periosteal grafts and subjected to continuous passive motion in rabbits. Clin Orthop 1987;222:267.

32. Zarnett R, Valasquez R, Salter RB. The effects of continuous passive motion on knee ligament reconstruction with carbon fibre. J Bone Joint Surg 1991;73B:47–52.

Index

Books are properly compared to tools of which the index is a handle
—John Shaw Billings